Transcultural Concepts in Nursing Care

Transcultural Concepts in Nursing Care

Fifth Edition

Margaret M. Andrews, PhD, RN, CTN, FAAN
Director and Professor of Nursing
School of Health Professions and Studies
University of Michigan – Flint
Flint, Michigan

Joyceen S. Boyle, PhD, RN, FAAN, CTN
Associate Dean for Academic Affairs
College of Nursing
University of Arizona
Tucson, Arizona

 Wolters Kluwer | Lippincott Williams & Wilkins
Health
Philadelphia · Baltimore · New York · London
Buenos Aires · Hong Kong · Sydney · Tokyo

Acquisitions Editor: Hilarie Surrena
Managing Editor: Michelle Clarke
Senior Production Editor: Marian A. Bellus
Director of Nursing Production: Helen Ewan
Senior Managing Editor / Production: Erika Kors
Art Director, Design: Joan Wendt
Art Director, Illustration: Brett MacNaughton
Senior Manufacturing Manager: William Alberti
Manufacturing Coordinator: Karin Duffield
Indexer: Greystone Indexing
Compositor: Spearhead

5th Edition

9 8 7 6 5 4 3 2 1

Library of Congress Cataloging-in-Publication Data

Library of Congress Cataloging-in-Publication Data
Andrews, Margaret M.
Transcultural concepts in nursing care / Margaret Andrews, Joyceen Boyle. —5th ed.
     p. ; cm.
  Includes bibliographical references and index.
  ISBN-13: 978-0-7817-9037-6
  ISBN-10: 0-7817-9037-9
  1. Transcultural nursing.   I. Boyle, Joyceen S.   II.   Title.
[DNLM: 1.   Transcultural Nursing. WY 107 A563t 2008]

RT86.54.A53 2008
362.17′3—dc22   2007022190

Care has been taken to confirm the accuracy of the information presented and to describe generally accepted practices. However, the authors, editors, and publisher are not responsible for errors or omissions or for any consequences from application of the information in this book and make no warranty, expressed or implied, with respect to the currency, completeness, or accuracy of the contents of the publication. Application of this information in a particular situation remains the professional responsibility of the practitioner; the clinical treatments described and recommended may not be considered absolute and universal recommendations.

The authors, editors, and publisher have exerted every effort to ensure that drug selection and dosage set forth in this text are in accordance with the current recommendations and practice at the time of publication. However, in view of ongoing research, changes in government regulations, and the constant flow of information relating to drug therapy and drug reactions, the reader is urged to check the package insert for each drug for any change in indications and dosage and for added warnings and precautions. This is particularly important when the recommended agent is a new or infrequently employed drug.

Some drugs and medical devices presented in this publication have Food and Drug Administration (FDA) clearance for limited use in restricted research settings. It is the responsibility of the health care provider to ascertain the FDA status of each drug or device planned for use in their clinical practice.

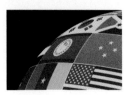

CONTRIBUTORS

Patricia A. Hanson, PhD, RN, APRN, GNP
Professor
College of Nursing & Health
Madonna University
Livonia, Michigan

Paula Herberg, PhD, RN
Professor and Chair
Department of Nursing
California State University, Fullerton
Fullerton, California

Kathryn Hopkins Kavanagh, PhD, RN

Jana Lauderdale, PhD, RN
Assistant Dean for Cultural Diversity
Vanderbilt University
School of Nursing
Nashville, Tennessee

Patti Ludwig-Beymer, PhD, RN, CTN, FAAN
Administrative Director for Nursing Research
and Education
Edward Hospital & Health Services
Naperville, Illinois

Margaret A. McKenna, PhD, MPH, MN
Principal
ConTEXT Sociocultural Research & Consulting;
Program Manager
Northwest Institute for Children and Families
School of Social Work;
Clinical Associate Professor
Department of Health Services
University of Washington
Seattle, Washington

Dula F. Pacquiao, EdD., RN, CTN
Associate Professor
Director
Stanley Bergen Center for Multicultural
Education, Research, and Practice
University of Medicine and Dentistry
of New Jersey
School of Nursing
Newark, New Jersey

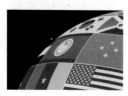

REVIEWERS

Rita Bergevin, MA, RN, BC
Clinical Assistant Professor of Nursing
Decker School of Nursing
Binghamton University, SUNY
Binghamton, New York

Sharon Aneta Bryant, PhD
Associate Professor
Decker School of Nursing
Binghamton University, SUNY
Binghamton, New York

Jo Ann Himaya, RN, PhD
Associate Professor of Nursing
Northwestern State University of Louisiana
Shreveport, Louisiana

Dorothy Hubbard, PhD, RN
Associate Professor
Northwestern State University of Louisiana
Shreveport, Louisiana

Barbara A. Ihrke, RN, PhD
Chair, Division of Nursing
Indiana Wesleyan University
Marion, Indiana

Sherry Knoppers, RN, PhDc
Nursing Faculty
Grand Rapids Community College
Grand Rapids, Michigan

Malgosia E. Krasuska, RN, MSN, PhD
Associate Professor
Decker School of Nursing
Binghamton University, SUNY
Binghamton, New York

Eloise T. Lewis, RN, MSN
Associate Professor
Ivy Tech Community College of Indiana
Columbus, Indiana

Joan Such Lockhart, PhD, RN, CORLN, AOCN, CNE, FAAN
Professor & Associate Dean for Academic Affairs
Duquesne University School of Nursing
Pittsburgh, Pennsylvania

Ruby S. Morrison, DSN, RN, CMAC
Associate Professor
Capstone College of Nursing, The University of Alabama
Tuscaloosa, Alabama

Sandra J. Mixer, MSN, RN
Assistant Professor of Nursing
Middle Tennessee State University
Murfreesboro, Tennessee

Jenny Radsma, PhD, RN
Associate Professor of Nursing
University of Maine at Fort Kent
Fort Kent, Maine

Amelia Siatkowski, RN, MSN
Instructor
School of Nursing
Southern Illinois University at Edwardsville
Edwardsville, Illinois

Gale A. Spencer, PhD, RN
Professor and Decker Chair in Community Health
Binghamton University, SUNY
Binghamton, New York

Kathryn Sridaromont
Associate Professor
School of Nursing
Texas Tech University Health Sciences Center
Lubbock, Texas

Mary Welhaven, PhD, RN
Professor
Winona State University Rochester Center
Rochester, Minnesota

Judy Darlene Welsh, RN, MSN
Lecturer
University of Kentucky
Lexington, Kentucky

Rick Zoucha, APRN, BC, DNSc, CTN
Associate Professor
Duquesne University School of Nursing
Pittsburgh, Pennsylvania

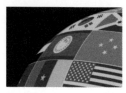

FOREWORD

The 21st century has found nurses and other health professionals eager to learn about different cultures of the world and to provide effective culturally based health care. Fortunately, this was anticipated in the early 1950s when I foresaw that nurses and other health professionals needed to become educated and competent to function with people of diverse cultures. Today, transcultural nursing has been soundly established, and with the major purpose to provide culturally competent health care for immigrants, refugees, and people of many different cultural backgrounds.

This Fifth Edition of *Transcultural Concepts in Nursing Care*, by Drs. Andrews and Boyle is an important and major contribution to transcultural nursing. The book is updated to help nurses functioning in different clinical contexts to become knowledgeable and competent to practice transcultural nursing. Nothing is more rewarding and encouraging than to see former students become dynamic leaders to advance knowledge in their areas of expertise and to transmit such insights to future generations of students. Drs. Andrews and Boyle have been these active and dynamic leaders, teachers, and researchers who have played a major role in shaping the world of transcultural nursing over the past several decades. They are committed leaders who want to make transcultural nursing a meaningful and useful reality for nurses. Their leadership has been demonstrated in community nursing, consultation, education, research, and administration. Their accomplishments are well known and reflected in this new edition.

This Fifth Edition reflects the authors' creative work to refine, explicate, and expand transcultural nursing knowledge and practices throughout the life cycle and in different clinical and community-based contexts. Several chapters have been revised and updated to integrate transcultural nursing concepts and principles into all areas of nursing. Much of the new content is evidence-based practice based on transcultural assessments and the use of transcultural concepts and principles. International health with a transcultural nursing perspective is a new addition to this book and is most welcome with global care essential today. Most encouraging and rewarding has been the use of the theory of Culture Care Diversity and Universality as the philosophical, theoretical, and practice guide to help nurses discover ways to provide competent, safe, and meaningful care to clients of similar and diverse cultures. The Sunrise Enabler, along with Leininger's other enablers and the three creative new modes of arriving at transcultural care decision or action are valued and demonstrated in this book.

Most importantly, this edition reflects the authors' scholarly ability to draw upon past historical developments in transcultural nursing but especially to draw upon important concepts, principles, and new research findings to promote and maintain culturally competent care. This book reveals the cumulative growth and use of transcultural nursing knowledge over the past five decades. This is most encouraging to witness since my first book, *Nursing and Anthropology*, was published in 1970, and followed by the definitive transcultural nursing publications in 1978, 1995, 2000, and 2006. These scholarly developments are reflected in this new edition and are hallmarks of genuine transcultural nursing authors as they build upon and advance transcultural nursing knowledge in significant ways. A highly valuable and special feature of this book is that the authors have incorporated comparative cultural care practices in community and clinical settings using ethical values and research findings. A unique feature is that different cultural contexts are emphasized to increase nurses' knowledge of the importance of context. I contend that the readers will find this Fifth Edition extremely helpful as they teach and mentor undergraduate students in transcultural nursing courses and clinical settings. This book is a valuable stepping stone for students to pursue graduate study in transcultural nursing because it provides a sound and broad foundation for transcultural nursing. This book will complement the new and comprehensive Leininger-McFarland transcultural nursing book as students pursue further theoretical, clinical, and research graduate education in transcultural

nursing. Drs. Andrews and Boyle are to be highly commended for their diligent and creative work in updating and expanding transcultural nursing knowledge and practices with this most recent edition. It is a very important publication to advance transcultural nursing and to guide students in providing culturally competent, safe, and meaningful care to people of diverse cultures.

Madeleine M. Leininger, PhD, LHD, DS, RN, CTN, FAAN, FRCNA

Founder and Leader of Transcultural Nursing and Human Care Theory and Research

Professor Emeritus of Nursing, Wayne State University (Detroit) and

Professor, University of Nebraska (Omaha)

Transcultural Global Nursing Consultant and Lecturer residing in Omaha, Nebraska

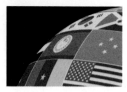

PREFACE

In the mid 1950s, the nurse-anthropologist Dr. Madeleine M. Leininger envisioned *transcultural nursing* as a formal area of study and practice for nurses. Since that time, there has been a major cultural care movement, as there is now a keen interest by many health care professionals in culturally competent care. The influence of transcultural nursing has spread to many countries in the world. In addition, transcultural nursing has influenced other health-related disciplines, including medicine, pharmacy, physical therapy, occupational therapy, social work, and many other fields. *Culturally competent care* is now an expected standard of care for individuals, families, groups, and communities and many state and national accrediting bodies include criteria related to the cultural needs of patients.

Our major contribution to transcultural nursing in all five editions of *Transcultural Concepts in Nursing Care* has been a synthesis of transcultural theories, models, and research studies compiled into a comprehensive text. Our primary goal has been to advance the use of transcultural knowledge in nursing practice and to develop *cultural competence* in the care of individuals and groups. While we hope that every reader will draw his or her own conclusions, we believe that we have made a significant contribution to incorporating cultural knowledge in nursing care and providing a state-of-the-art text in this exciting area of nursing called *transcultural nursing*.

Initially published in 1989, *Transcultural Concepts in Nursing Care* began as a collegial effort among faculty and doctoral students at the University of Utah College of Nursing to help us expand and clarify our view of transcultural nursing. Many of the chapter authors were teaching

undergraduate students, and we were looking for articles and textbooks to help us in both classroom and clinical practice settings. We had strong clinical backgrounds and an interest in solving practice problems, so we wanted a textbook that would apply transcultural nursing concepts to clinical practice. In particular, we wanted a text that undergraduate students would find interesting, challenging and, above all, helpful in providing culturally competent nursing care for patients from diverse backgrounds. We have a strong commitment to theory developing in nursing that helped us develop an evidence-based theoretical framework for transcultural nursing practice. In this fifth edition, we have many of the same contributors, but have been pleased to have other transcultural nursing experts join us.

Many contributors teach in baccalaureate, masters, and/or doctoral programs. Over the years we have explored ways to creatively and effectively teach our students how to apply transcultural concepts to practice, with the goal of developing their knowledge and skill in providing culturally competent and culturally congruent nursing care. The Commission on Collegiate Nursing Education, the National League for Nursing, most state boards of nursing, and other accrediting and certification bodies require or strongly encourage the inclusion of cultural aspects of care in nursing curricula. This underscores the importance of the purpose, goal, and objectives for *Transcultural Concepts in Nursing Care, Fifth Edition*.

Purpose: To contribute to the development of theoretically based transcultural nursing knowledge and the advancement of transcultural nursing practice.

Goal: To increase the delivery of culturally competent care to individuals, families, groups, communities and institutions.

Objectives:

1. To apply a transcultural nursing framework to guide nursing practice in diverse health care settings across the lifespan.
2. To analyze major concerns and issues encountered by nurses in providing transcultural nursing care to individuals, families, groups, communities, and institutions.
3. To expand the theoretical bases for using concepts from the natural and behavioral sciences and from the humanities to provide culturally congruent nursing care.

We believe that cultural assessment skills, combined with the nurse's critical thinking abilities, will provide the necessary knowledge on which to base transcultural nursing care. Using this approach, nurses will be able to provide culturally competent and contextually meaningful care for clients—individuals, families, groups, communities, and institutions.

Given that nurses are likely to encounter people from literally hundreds of different cultures, we believe this approach is more effective than simply memorizing the esoteric health beliefs and practices of a litany of different groups. Thus, we believe that nurses must acquire the knowledge and skills needed to assess and care for clients from virtually any and all cultural groups that they might encounter in their professional careers.

We would like to comment on the extensive progress that has been made in nursing education, practice, and research in terms of cultural awareness, sensitivity, and competence during the past decade. Although there remains much work to be done, we are pleased that many clinicians, educators, researchers, administrators, and consultants have, with increasing frequency, integrated transcultural nursing concepts into their respective areas of expertise. Similarly, the authors of nursing and health care textbooks and other publications often integrate transcultural nursing into their work or invite certified trans-cultural nurses to do so. While we are pleased with this trend, we also recognize that there remains a need for a comprehensive text that provides nurses with the theoretical foundations for transcultural nursing, develops competence in cultural assessment, and systematically applies transcultural concepts across the lifespan. We also believe that there are contemporary health care issues, problems, and challenges that warrant critical analysis, thus making a text such as *Transcultural Concepts in Nursing Care, Fifth edition,* a useful adjunct to general and specialty nursing texts.

In light of the development of this book through four editions, it is not surprising to discover that the fifth edition of Transcultural Concepts in Nursing Care strongly reflects the current challenges faced by nurses who are practicing in a changing clinical environment. Overall, the authors and contributors share a commitment to:

- Foster the development and maintenance of a disciplinary knowledge base and expertise in culturally congruent care.
- Synthesize existing theoretical and research knowledge regarding nursing care of different ethnic/minority, marginalized, and disenfranchised populations.
- Identify evidence-based practice and best practices in the care of diverse individuals, groups, and communities.
- Create an interdisciplinary knowledge base that reflects heterogeneous health care practices within various cultural groups.
- Identify, describe, and examine methods, theories, and frameworks appropriate for development knowledge that will improve health and nursing care to minority, underrepresented, disenfranchised and marginalized populations.

Recognizing Individual Differences and Acculturation

When considering transcultural nursing issues, nurses and other health care professionals are, with increasing frequency, referring to the federally defined population categories (i.e., White, Black, Hispanic Asian/Pacific Islander, and American Indian/Alaska Native). The creation of these defined population categories by the United States government has had a tremendous impact on our conceptualization of the various groups that constitute our society. The unique characteristics and individual differences of the five cultural groups have often been ignored, along with the impact acculturation has had on these groups. The outcomes are reminiscent of the melting pot metaphor, only now we have five or six pots instead of one. While the most recent census enabled citizens to self-identify with more than one group, the data remain far from perfect in describing the multicultural, multiethnic, and multiracial composition of contemporary society in the United States. Canada, Australia, the United Kingdom, and many other nations, both Eastern and Western, continue to struggle with the challenges of diversity in society.

We believe it is tremendously important to recognize the myriad of health-related beliefs and practices that exist within the population categories. For example, the differences are rarely recognized among people who identify themselves as Hispanic/Latino: this group includes people from along the U.S.-Mexico border, Puerto Rico, Mexico, Spain, Guatemala, or "Little Havana" in Miami, who may have some similarities but who also may have distinct cultural differences.

We would like to comment briefly on the terms minority and ethnic minorities. These terms are perceived to be offensive by some because they connote inferiority and marginalization. Although we have used these terms occasionally, we prefer to make reference to a specific subculture or culture whenever possible. We refer to categorizations according to race, ethnicity, religion, or a combination, such as ethnoreligion (e.g., Amish), but we make every effort to avoid using any label in a pejorative way. We do believe, however, that the concepts or terms minority or ethnicity are limiting, not only for those to whom the label may be applied, but also for nursing theory and practice.

Critical Thinking Linked to Delivering Culturally Competent Care

We believe that cultural assessment skills, combined with the nurse's critical thinking ability, will provide the necessary knowledge on which to base transcultural nursing care. Using this approach, we are convinced that nurses will be able to provide culturally competent and contextually meaningful care for clients from a wide variety of cultural backgrounds, rather than simply memorizing the esoteric health beliefs and practices of any specific cultural group. We believe that nurses must acquire the skills needed to assess clients from virtually any and all groups that they encounter throughout their professional life.

New to the Fifth Edition

All content in this edition has been reviewed and updated to capture the nature of the changing health care delivery system and to explain how nurses and other health care providers can use culturally competent skills to improve the care of clients, families, groups, and communities.

New Chapter

We welcome back a former contributor to the text, Dr. Paula Herberg, who currently is Associate Professor and Chair of the Department of Nursing at the California State University, Fullerton, CA. Dr. Herberg was a contributor to the first three editions of Transcultural Concepts in Nursing Care. She has practiced internationally for many years and is eminently qualified to write a new chapter on International Nursing.

We have maintained the same conceptual framework for the text, focusing on the life span first and then on specialty areas within transcultural nursing. We have updated all chapters, reorganized and revised to make the content current, and more readable and succinct. In doing so, we recognized that the major contributions of many of the nurse-anthropologists who laid the foun-

dations for transcultural nursing along with
Leininger have ceased publishing in retirement.
We especially acknowledge our dear colleague
Agnes Aamodt, PhD, RN, FAAN, a retired nurse-
anthropologist who died in 2006. We have relied
on her original work for many years.

Chapter Pedagogy

Learning Activities

All of the chapters include review questions as
well as learning activities to promote critical
thinking. In addition, each chapter includes
chapter objectives and key terms to help readers
understand the purpose and intent of the content they will be reading. Many of the chapters
include up-to-date and challenging case studies.

Evidence-Based Practice

Current research studies related to the content of
the chapter are presented as Evidence-Based
Practice boxes. We have included a section in
each box describing appropriate clinical applications derived from the research.

Case Studies Based on Actual Clinical
or Research Experiences

Case Studies based on the authors' actual clinical
experiences and research findings are presented
to make conceptual linkages and to illustrate
how concepts are applied in health care settings.

Text Organization

Part One: Historical and Theoretical
Foundations of Transcultural Nursing

The first section focuses on the historical and
theoretical aspects of transcultural nursing. The
development of transcultural nursing frameworks that include concepts from the natural
and behavioral sciences are described as they
apply to nursing practice. Because nursing perspectives are used to organize the content in
Transcultural Concepts in Nursing Care, the
reader will not find a chapter purporting to
describe the nursing care of a specific cultural

group. Instead, the nursing needs of culturally
diverse groups are used to illustrate cultural concepts used in nursing practice. Chapter 1 provides an overview of the historical and theoretical
foundations of transcultural nursing and Chapter 2 introduces key concepts associated with cultural competence. In Chapter 3, we discuss the
domains of cultural knowledge that are important in cultural assessment and describe how this
cultural information can be incorporated into all
aspects of nursing care. Chapter 4 provides a
summary of the major cultural belief systems
embraced by people of the world with special
emphasis on their health-related and culturally
based values, attitudes, beliefs and practices.

Part Two: A Developmental Approach
to Transcultural Nursing

Chapters 5 through 8 use a developmental
framework to discuss transcultural concepts
across the lifespan. The care of childbearing
women and their families, children, adolescents,
middle-aged adults, and the elderly is examined,
and information about various cultural groups is
used to illustrate common transcultural nursing
issues, trends and concerns.

Part Three: Nursing in Multicultural
Health Care Settings

In the third section of the text, we explore the
components of cultural competence in mental
health and in family and community health care
settings. We also examine cultural competence in
health care organizations and cultural diversity
in the health care workforce. The clinical application of concepts throughout this section uses situations commonly encountered by nurses and
describes how transcultural nursing principles
can be applied in diverse settings. The chapters in
this section are intended to illustrate the application of transcultural nursing knowledge to nursing practice.

Part Four: Contemporary Challenges
in Transcultural Nursing

In the fourth section of the text, Chapters 13 to
16, we look at selected contemporary issues and

challenges that face nursing and health care. In Chapter 13, we critically examine the fourth vital sign—pain—from a transcultural perspective, building on and synthesizing the extensive body of research on transcultural aspects of pain. In Chapter 14, we review major religious traditions of North America and the interrelationships among religion, culture, and nursing. Recognizing the numerous moral and ethical challenges in contemporary health care as well as within transcultural nursing, Chapter 15 discusses cultural competence in ethical and moral dilemmas from a transcultural perspective. Chapter 16, a new chapter, provides an overview of International Nursing and provides a global perspective of what is done in the international arena to promote human development and health. This chapter highlights the field of international nursing and the ways in which nurses from the United States can contribute to the global efforts to improve the health status of the world's peoples.

Margaret M. Andrews, PhD, RN, FAAN CTN
Joyceen S. Boyle, PhD, RN, FAAN, CTN

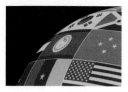

ACKNOWLEDGMENTS

We are so pleased to acknowledge the assistance and support of our families, friends, and colleagues in making this book possible. We also appreciate the help of the many nursing faculty members, practitioners, and students who have offered helpful comments and suggestions. We have found it helpful to call upon many of our colleagues for advice in this new edition. Particular appreciation is extended to Teresa and Neil Cooper who provided another memorable photograph for us.

We would like to acknowledge Betsy Gentzler, Associate Development Editor, Lippincott Williams & Wilkins. Betsy worked with us during the first part of the preparation for the 5th edition. Michelle L. Clarke, Managing Editor, Lippincott, Williams & Wilkins, stepped in during the second half of the project. She supported and encouraged us through the process of reviews and revisions, as well as helped with editorial concerns along the way. A special word of thanks to Margaret Zuccarini, Senior Acquisitions Editor who, although she did not directly work with us on this edition, has provided encouragement each time we have seen her at national meetings.

We are grateful for the support of our friends, too numerous to list by name, who often stopped by our office, emailed, or phoned to express their interest. Each year at the Annual Transcultural Nursing Conference, numerous colleagues have purchased our book as well as provided positive feedback and encouragement. We have been most appreciative of their interest and support.

Last, once again we would like to thank each other for what is a professional lifetime of friendship that has withstood the test of time and now five editions of this book. We started this course in 1983 with sharpened pencils and yellow legal pads with our first edition and have progressed to emails, computers, and fax machines. Through it all, we have found our professional endeavors in transcultural nursing and the friends we have made to be both satisfying and rewarding.

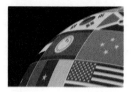

CONTENTS

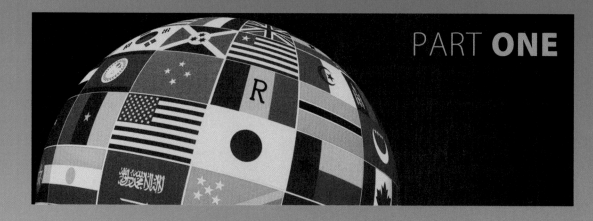

PART **ONE**

HISTORICAL AND THEORETICAL FOUNDATIONS OF TRANSCULTURAL NURSING

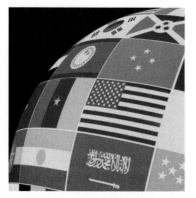

CHAPTER 1

Theoretical Foundations of Transcultural Nursing

Margaret M. Andrews

KEY TERMS

Anthropology
Culture-specific nursing care
Culture-universal nursing
  care
Cultural competence

Cultural congruence
Culturally congruent care
Diversity
Ethnocentric
Leininger's Sunrise Model

Leininger's Theory of Culture
  Care Diversity and
  Universality
Panethnic minority groups
Transcultural nursing

LEARNING OBJECTIVES

1. Examine the historical origins of transcultural nursing with special emphasis on its roots in anthropology.
2. Critically analyze the need for transcultural nursing in contemporary society.
3. Critically analyze prevailing nursing paradigms and nursing theories from a transcultural nursing perspective.
4. Identify resources available in transcultural nursing and health care.

During the past 6 decades, transcultural nursing's foundress Dr. Madeleine M. Leininger and thousands of other nurses from around the world have worked diligently to establish **transcultural nursing** as a formal area of academic study and practice. Since its initial conception in the 1950s to its formal creation as a specialty and new discipline within the profession in the 1960s and 1970s, a substantial and important body of transcultural theoretical, research-, and evidence-based knowledge has been generated by nurse scholars on every continent. In a historical and interpretive narrative highlighting the major features of the evolution of transcultural nursing as a specialty and discipline, Dr. Leininger describes her philosophical thoughts as she contemplated developing a new field of knowledge in nursing and health care: "It is amazing what some women and men dare to do with their ideas over time and in many places in the world. Creative thinking and actions are often needed. Indeed, the nursing world needed transcultural nursing as essential to meet a changing world and changing health needs. . . . it is new ideas, education and practices that are essential to transform old practices and ideas into new ones" (Leininger, in press).

The term *transcultural nursing* is sometimes used interchangeably with *cross-cultural, intercultural,* or *multicultural* nursing. In analyzing the Latin derivations of the prefixes associated with these terms, you will notice that *trans* means *across, inter* means *between,* and *multi* means *many.* Given these derivations, it is understandable that various words have been used with similar connotative meaning (Andrews, 1992, 1995). Some

3

people have used the term *ethnic nursing care* (Orque, Bloch, & Monrroy, 1983) or have referred to *caring for people of color* (Branch & Paxton, 1976).

Approximately 30 years ago, nurse–anthropologists debated the conceptual differences between transcultural and cross-cultural nursing, and debate has continued. We have chosen to use transcultural nursing in this book in recognition of the historical and theoretical contributions of Dr. Madeleine M. Leininger, a nurse–anthropologist who, in the mid-1950s, envisioned transcultural nursing as a formal area of study and practice for nurses and coined the term *transcultural nursing* (Andrews & Boyle, 1997; Leininger, 1995, 1999; Leininger & McFarland, 2002; Leininger & McFarland, 2006). In her classic work, *Nursing and Anthropology: Two Worlds to Blend*, Dr. Leininger notes that "the fields of anthropology and nursing must be interdigitated so that each field will profit from the contribution of the other…. It is apparent that if these two fields were sharing their special knowledge and experiences, both would undoubtedly see new pathways in thinking and research" (Leininger, 1970).

As the name implies, transcultural nursing goes across cultural boundaries in a search for the essence of nursing. Transcultural nursing is the blending of anthropology and nursing in both theory and practice (Daugherty & Tripp-Reimer, 1985; Lipson & Bauwens, 1988; McKenna, 1984; Osborne, 1969). **Anthropology** refers to the study of humans and humankind, including their origins, behavior, social relationships, physical and mental characteristics, customs, and development through time and in all places in the world. Recognizing that nursing is an art and a science, transcultural nursing enables us to view our profession from a cultural perspective. Transcultural nursing is not just for immigrants, people of color, or members of the federally defined **panethnic minority groups**, i.e., Blacks, Hispanics, Asians/Pacific Islanders, and American Indians/Alaska Natives. Everyone has a cultural heritage, including nurses, patients, and other members of the health care team; the latter groups might be referred to as being members of occupational or professional cultures (Andrews & Boyle, 1997; Andrews & Boyle, 2002). There also are many other examples of *nonethnic cultures,* such as the culture of poverty or affluence, culture of the deaf or hearing impaired and the blind or visually impaired, and the gay, lesbian, and transgender cultures.

Transcultural nursing is a specialty within nursing focused on the comparative study and analysis of different cultures and subcultures. These groups are examined with respect to their caring behavior, nursing care, and health–illness values, beliefs, and patterns of behavior. The goal of transcultural nursing is to develop a scientific and humanistic body of knowledge in order to provide **culture-specific** and **culture-universal nursing care** practices to individuals, families, groups, and communities from diverse backgrounds. *Culture-specific* refers to particular values, beliefs, and patterns of behavior that tend to be special or unique to a group and that do not tend to be shared with members of other cultures. *Culture-universal* refers to the commonly shared values, norms of behavior, and life patterns that are similarly held among cultures about human behavior and lifestyles (Leininger, 1978, 1991, 1995; Leininger & McFarland, 2002).

Transcultural nursing requires sophisticated assessment and analytic skills and the ability to plan, design, implement, and evaluate nursing care for individuals, families, groups, and communities representing various cultures. You must also be able to apply knowledge related to the culture of organizations, institutions, and agencies, especially those concerned with health and nursing.

The Importance of Transcultural Nursing

Leininger (1995) cites eight factors that influenced her to establish transcultural nursing:

1. There was a marked increase in the migration of people within and between countries worldwide. Transcultural nursing is

needed because of the growing diversity that characterizes our national and global populations. In its broadest sense, **diversity** refers to differences in race, ethnicity, national origin, religion, age, gender, sexual orientation, ability or disability, social and economic status or class, education, and related attributes of groups of people in society.

2. There has been a rise in multicultural identities, with people expecting their cultural beliefs, values, and lifeways to be understood and respected by nurses and other health care providers.
3. The increased use of health care technology sometimes conflicts with cultural values of clients, such as Amish prohibitions against using certain apnea monitors, IV pumps, and other such health care technologic devices in the home.
4. Worldwide, there are cultural conflicts, clashes, and violence that have an impact health care as more cultures interact with one another.
5. There was an increase in the number of people traveling and working in many different parts of the world.
6. There was an increase in legal suits resulting from cultural conflict, negligence, ignorance, and imposition of health care practices.
7. There has been a rise in feminism and gender issues, with new demands on health care systems to meet the needs of women and children.
8. There has been an increased demand for community and culturally based health care services in diverse environmental contexts.

Let's examine a few clinical examples of ways in which transcultural nursing can be used in the care of people with diverse backgrounds. Transcultural nursing enables nurses to communicate more effectively with clients from diverse cultural and linguistic backgrounds and to assist those with mental health problems. Transcultural nursing enables nurses to more accurately assess the cultural expression of pain and to provide culturally appropriate interventions to prevent or alleviate discomfort. Last, incidents have been reported in which parents have been arrested for child abuse because culturally based child-rearing practices were poorly understood. Transcultural nursing is a vehicle for assessing the parent–child relationship and for encouraging forms of parental discipline that promote the health and well-being of children and prevent physical or emotional harm (Andrews, 1992, 1995; Flaskerud, 2000; Leininger, 1997; Leininger & McFarland, 2002, 2006; Mahoney & Engebretson, 2000).

Throughout this book, we shall examine various ways in which transcultural nursing facilitates nurses' knowledge and skill in caring for people from diverse backgrounds. Although much of the emphasis will be on diversity, we shall also explore the universal attributes that we have in common with other members of the human race, such as the need for food, sleep, shelter, safety, and human interaction. Let us now examine some key developments in transcultural nursing from a historical perspective.

History of Transcultural Nursing

In the 1950s, Dr. Madeleine M. Leininger noted cultural differences between patients and nurses while working with emotionally disturbed children. This clinical experience led her in 1954 to study cultural differences in the perceptions of care, and in 1965 she earned a doctorate in cultural anthropology from the University of Washington (Leininger, 1995; Leininger & McFarland, 2002, 2006; Reynolds & Leininger, 1993). Leininger recognized that one of anthropology's most important contributions to nursing was the realization that health and illness states are strongly influenced by culture. Table 1-1 gives a summary of Dr. Leininger's contributions to the development of transcultural nursing.

To help develop, test, and organize the emerging body of knowledge in transcultural nursing,

TABLE 1–1 *Contributions of Madeleine Leininger to the Development of Transcultural Nursing*

Date	Achievement and Contribution
1954	Dr. Madeleine Leininger noticed and studied the cultural differences in the perception of care
1965	Leininger earned a doctorate in cultural anthropology (U. of Washington)
1965–1969	Leininger offered first courses and telelectures offered in transcultural nursing (U. of Colorado School of Nursing)
	Established first PhD nurse-scientist program combining anthropology and nursing (U. of Colorado School of Nursing)
1973	First academic department in transcultural nursing established (U. of Washington School of Nursing)
1974	Transcultural Nursing Society established as the official organization of transcultural nursing
1975	First national transcultural nursing conference, *Care of Infants and Children*, held at Snowbird, Utah; thereafter annual conferences held at various locations in the U.S., Canada, the Netherlands, Finland, Australia, Spain, and United Kingdom
1978	First advanced degree programs (master's and doctoral) established (U. of Utah School of Nursing)
1988	Transcultural Nursing Society initiated certification examinations: Certified Transcultural Nurse (CTN)
1989	Journal of Transcultural Nursing (JTN) first published as official publication of the Transcultural Nursing Society with Dr. Madeleine Leininger as founding editor. Goal of the JTN: to disseminate transcultural ideas, theories, research findings, and/or practice experiences
1991	Dr. Leininger published *Culture Care Diversity and Universality: A Theory of Nursing*, in which she outlined her theory (Culture Care Diversity and Universality and the Sunrise Model) and its research applications
1995	Dr. Leininger published *Transcultural Nursing: Concepts Theories, Research and Practices* (2nd edition)
2000	As part of a longstanding history of collaboration with Madonna University (Livonia, Michigan), Dr. Leininger negotiated to build the Transcultural Nursing Society's World Headquarters as part of a new wing of the building that houses the College of Nursing and Health
2002	Dr. Leininger (with co-author Dr. Marilyn McFarland) published *Transcultural Nursing: Concepts, Theories, Research, and Practices* (3rd edition)
2004	Installation of the Founder and Presidential Photos in the Global Transcultural Nursing Headquarters and induction as a charter member of the Transcultural Nursing Scholars (TNS)
2006	Dr. Leininger (with co-author Dr. Marilyn McFarland) published *Culture Care Diversity and Universality: A Worldwide Theory for Nursing*
2006	Dr. Leininger released a series of three DVDs: *The Life Career of Leininger, The Theory of Culture Care,* and *Conversation with a Legend*
2007 to present	A member of the Transcultural Nursing Society's Board of Directors and Professor Emerita at Wayne State University and the University of Nebraska, Dr. Leininger continues to be active as a transcultural nurse consultant, scholar, researcher, speaker, and leader in the field of transcultural nursing

Table based, in part, on Transcultural Nursing Society. (2007). Transcultural Nursing Society: Historical moments. Transcultural Nursing Society Newsletter, 16(1), 9.

it is necessary to have a specific conceptual framework from which various theoretical statements can emerge. **Leininger's Sunrise Model** (Figure 1–1) is based on the concept of cultural care and shows three major nursing modalities that guide nursing judgments and activities to provide **culturally congruent care**—that is, care that is beneficial and meaningful to the people

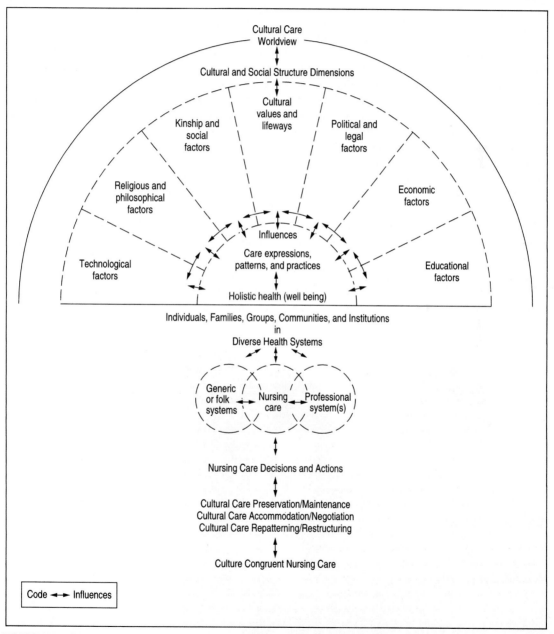

FIGURE 1-1. Leininger's Sunrise enabler to depict the Theory of Cultural Care Diversity and Universality. (Reprinted by permission from Leininger, M. M., & McFarland, M. R. [2006]. Culture care diversity and universality: A worldwide theory for nursing [2nd ed., p. 25]. Sudbury, MA: Jones & Bartlett, Publishers.)

being served (Leininger, 1991, 1995; Leininger & McFarland, 2002).

Leininger's Theory of Culture Care Diversity and Universality focuses on describing, explaining, and predicting nursing similarities and differences focused primarily on human care and caring in human cultures. Leininger uses worldview, social structure, language, ethnohistory, environmental context, and the generic (folk) and professional systems to provide a comprehensive and holistic view of influences in culture care. Culturally based care factors are recognized as major influences on human expressions and experiences related to health, illness, and well-being or on facing disabilities or death. The three modes of nursing decisions and actions—culture care preservation and/or maintenance, culture care accommodation and/or negotiation, and culture care repatterning and/or restructuring—are presented to demonstrate ways to provide culturally congruent nursing care (Leininger, 1991, 1995; Leininger & McFarland, 2002). Among the strengths of Leininger's theory is its flexibility for use with individuals, families, groups, communities, and

institutions in diverse health systems. Leininger's Sunrise Model depicts components of the Theory of Cultural Care Diversity and Universality, and it provides a visual schematic representation of the key components of the theory and the interrelationships among its parts. As the world of nursing and health care has become increasingly multicultural, the theory's relevance has increased as well. For further information about Dr. Leininger and her Theory of Culture Care Diversity and Universality, visit either Dr. Leininger's Web site (www.madeleine-leininger.com) or the Transcultural Nursing Society's Web site (www.tcns.org).

Critical Analysis of Transcultural Nursing

Transcultural nursing has been criticized for its definitional, theoretical, and practical limitations. You are encouraged to think critically as you examine some of the major criticisms of transcultural nursing. Recognizing that all nursing theories have limitations, you are urged to

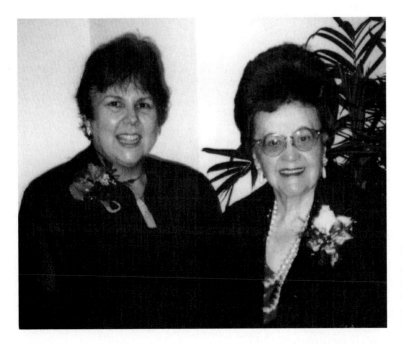

FIGURE 1-2. Author Dr. Margaret Andrews (*left*) and Transcultural Nursing Foundress, and Dr. Madeleine Leininger (*right*), at a meeting of The American Academy of Nursing.

critically reflect on ways in which the limitations can be addressed or overcome.

Major Criticisms

Let us begin by examining the criticism that transcultural nursing contains ambiguous terminology and lacks clarity in describing key concepts (Habayeb, 1995; Mulholland, 1995). For example, nurses have struggled to achieve clarity in concepts such as cultural awareness, cultural sensitivity, **cultural competence**, and **cultural congruence**. Color, religion, and geographic location are most often used to narrowly define culture and highlight cultural diversity, which is often portrayed as a minority/majority issue. Discrepancies in definition arise when one fails to recognize that every person has a cultural heritage. Talabere (1996) suggests that cultural diversity is itself an **ethnocentric** term because it focuses on "how different the other person is from me" rather than "how different I am from the other." In using the term *cultural diversity*, the White panethnic group is frequently viewed as the norm against which the differences in everyone else (ethnocentrically referred to as non-Whites) are measured or compared.

Another criticism of transcultural nursing models is their failure to recognize the relationship between knowledge and power and their inattention to the complexities associated with prejudice, discrimination, and racism (cf. Gustafson, 1999; Price & Cortis, 2000). Although Leininger and other transcultural nurses address the need to consider the political, economic, and social dimensions in their theoretical formulations, transcultural nursing has been criticized for doing too little to encourage nurses to be actively involved in setting political, economic, and social policy agendas.

Culley (1996) criticizes transcultural nursing for failing to recognize the power relations that exist between groups. When clients from traditionally underrepresented groups fail to behave as a nurse expects, the behavior is sometimes referred to as *noncompliant,* a term with a negative connotation that is sometimes used synonymously with *different, deviant, abnormal,* or *pathologic.* Problems are thought to be generated by customs or traditions deemed by the nurse to be "inappropriate," a judgment that may be the result of personal bias, lack of knowledge concerning the cultural context in which these customs are practiced, the nurse's inexperience, or other factors. As a result, complex sociocultural phenomena are often reduced to overgeneralized stereotypes. For example, some North American nurses are critical of the role of women in traditional African and Middle Eastern cultures. In concentrating on culturally determined gender issues, you might ignore or minimize the significance of power, inequality, and racism as embedded in structures or institutions (Gustafson, 1999; Price & Cortis, 2000), factors that fundamentally affect the health of cultural groups and their members' access to quality health care. The same criticism might be applied to nursing's failure to address other forms of bias, prejudice, discrimination, and social injustice.

Juntunen (2007) has criticized Leininger for generalizing her research by creating lists of the culture care values, meanings, and action modes of each of the cultures that she and her disciples have studied. These generalizations foster stereotyping and fail to consider the variations within cultures that influence the ways in which people express their cultural orientation. Lastly, every belief and practice has both cultural and individual or familial determinants.

Finally, transcultural nursing has been criticized for embracing models based on the assumption that understanding one's own culture and the culture of others creates tolerance and respect for people from diverse backgrounds. It has become apparent that the mere awareness of one's own culture and that of others is insufficient for the alleviation and potential eradication of prejudice, bigotry, racial, ethnic, or cultural conflicts, discrimination, or ethnic violence. Rather, nursing students, nurses, and other health care providers must have positive experiences with members of other cultures and learn to genuinely value the contributions all cultures make to our multicultural society.

Response to Criticisms

In the remainder of this book, we, the authors, will attempt to address these criticisms of transcultural nursing through our approach to topics. It should be noted, however, that many of the issues raised by critics have deeply rooted historical, socioeconomic, religious, cultural, and political origins. Because the nursing profession is a microcosm of society, it mirrors the biases and prejudices found in the larger social order. It is unrealistic to expect that transcultural nursing can reverse all the inequalities cited by the critics. It is realistic, however, to expect more definitional, conceptual, and theoretical clarity. It also is realistic to expect nurses to become increasingly active in setting political, economic, and social policy agendas at the local, state/provincial, national, and international levels.

For example, you can empower yourself and your profession by running for elected offices; supporting candidates with health-related agendas congruent with your own; voting for candidates from diverse cultural backgrounds; using print, broadcast, and Web-based media to influence public opinion; and joining professional organizations or unions that employ professional lobbyists to represent them. You have the power to confront prejudice and discrimination by refusing to tolerate ethnic jokes and other expressions of prejudice in health care or educational settings. You can use peer pressure to change culturally insensitive or offensive behavior by others. You can also work with others to ensure that medical and surgical procedures, health-related appointments, and schedules are congruent with the religious and cultural calendars of clients, staff, and students.

Nurse educators can examine admission and recruitment policies, curricula, pedagogy, academic calendars, and teaching strategies from a transcultural nursing perspective. Nurse researchers need to ensure that diversity is represented in the population studied, that appropriate translation and interpretation have been used for non–English-speaking informants or subjects, and that research instruments are appropriate for use with diverse populations. Finally, nurses in key administrative positions can critically assess the organizational climate and culture for its encouragement of diversity, examine the organization's administrative hierarchy for the presence of diversity in leadership positions, evaluate its commitment to culturally sensitive and appropriate personnel policies, and foster an openness to different perspectives on leadership and management. The examples cited are intended to be illustrative, not exhaustive.

A variety of organizations, professional publications, and electronic resources support the development of transcultural nursing and health. With the proliferation of electronic resources available to search for subjects related to transcultural nursing and health, it is important for you to keep abreast of computer-based tools that enable you to obtain the information you need on a wide variety of transcultural subjects. Andrews, Burr, & Janetos (2004) provide suggestions for narrowing and focusing your search using important research databases such as Medline, Cumulative Index to Nursing and Allied Health Literature (CINAHL), Educational Resources Information Center (ERIC), and Psychological Abstracts (PsycINFO). Selected Web sites for U.S. government agencies, organizations, and commercial groups that concern transcultural nursing and health care are also described in brief annotations. Table 1–2 provides some basic information on selected resources.

Standards for Transcultural Nursing

Under the leadership of the Minnesota Chapter of the Transcultural Nursing Society, standards for transcultural nursing have been developed based on Leininger's Theory of Culture Care Diversity and Universality (Leininger, 1991, 1995, 1998; Leininger & McFarland, 2002) and Campinha-Bacote's Model of Cultural Competence (Campinha-Bacote, 2002). The Standards for Transcultural Nursing were developed to foster excellence in transcultural nursing practice, provide criteria for the evaluation of transcultural nursing, create a tool for teaching and learning,

TABLE 1–2 *Selected Resources for Transcultural Nursing*

Professional Resources	Description	Description and Purpose
Professional Organizations	Council on Nursing and Anthropology Association (CONAA) (1968)	Organization for nurse–anthropologists, transcultural nurses, and anthropologists Purpose: promotes interdisciplinary research exchange
	Transcultural Nursing Society (TNS) (1974)	Organization of transcultural nurses Purpose: to promote transcultural nursing knowledge and competencies globally through education, research, consultation, and clinical services
	Council on Cultural Diversity of the American Nurses' Association (ANA, 1978)	ANA Council of transcultural nurses Purpose: to focus on diversity issues in clinical practice
	International Association of Human Caring (1987)	Organization of qualitative researchers, some of whom are nurses Purpose: to explore the cultural similarities and differences in expressions of human care
	Committee on Cultural Diversity	Committee established by the American Academy of Nursing Purpose: to develop guidelines for culturally competent nursing
Refereed Printed Materials on Transcultural Nursing and Health	*Journal of Transcultural Nursing*	Only publication focused on transcultural nursing theory, research methods, consultation, teaching, and clinical community practices
	Journal of Multicultural Nursing and Health (JMCNH)	Interdisciplinary; addresses multiculturalism in nursing education and/or health
	Journal of Cultural Diversity	Focuses on cultural diversity theory and principles from a variety of perspectives
	Association of Black Nursing Faculty (ABNF) *Journal*	Documents the distinct nature and health care needs of the Black patient
	International Nursing Review	Both published by the International Council of Nurses
	International Journal of Nursing Studies	
Nonrefereed Print Materials	*Minority Nurse Newsletter*	Examines minority issues affecting patient care and nursing education
	Closing the Gap (newsletter)	Published by the Federal Office of Minority Health; focuses on federal interventions aimed at improving the health of panethnic groups
	IHS Primary Care Provider (newsletter)	Published by the Federal Indian Health Service; free to nursing and medical students and health care providers

(Continued on following page)

Professional Resources	Description	Description and Purpose
TABLE 1–2 *Selected Resources for Transcultural Nursing (continued)*		
Electronic Resources	www.tcns.org	Official Web site for the Transcultural Nursing Society, provides information about membership in the organization, conferences, regional workshops, transcultural nursing certification, and the *Journal of Transcultural Nursing;* useful links to other Web sites of relevance to transcultural nursing

increase the public's confidence in the nursing profession, and advance the field of transcultural nursing. The general membership of the Transcultural Nursing Society subsequently reviewed and approved the standards, which, effective fall 2008, will form the foundation for the Transcultural Nursing Certification Exam. Each of the eight transcultural nursing standards is accompanied by rationale, process criteria, and outcome criteria. The eight standards are (1) Theoretical Foundations of Transcultural Nursing, (2) Cultural Information Gathering, (3) Caring and Healing Systems, (4) Cultural Health Patterns and Caring Practices, (5) Health Care Planning, (6) Evaluation, (7) Research, and (8) Professional Development. These eight standards were developed to assist nurses in providing culturally competent and culturally congruent care, a topic that will be discussed in more depth in Chapter 2. Standards provide clarity in direction for nursing practice, reflect values and priorities in professional practice, define accountability to the public, and provide a clear framework for evaluation of transcultural nursing practice (Leuning, Swig-gum, Wieger, & McCullough-Zander, 2002; Transcultural Nursing Certification Committee, 2007).

Summary

In this introductory chapter, we have examined the historical origins of transcultural nursing as a blending of two fields: anthropology and nursing. Founded by nurse–anthropologist Dr. Madeleine M. Leininger, transcultural nursing has provided a theoretical foundation to guide nurses in the provision of culturally congruent and competent care for individual clients and patients of all ages, families, groups, and communities. Transcultural nursing also enables nurses to examine the cultural dimensions of health and nursing organizations, institutions, and agencies. Leininger's Theory of Culture Care Diversity and Universality and her Sunrise Model were introduced. Finally, selected resources in transcultural nursing and health care were identified.

REVIEW QUESTIONS

1. Conceived in the early 1950s by nurse-anthropologist Dr. Madeleine M. Leininger, the term *transcultural nursing* was coined in 1970 with her seminal work *Nursing and Anthropology: Two Worlds to Blend.* Define transcultural nursing in your own words.

2. Summarize the historical development of transcultural nursing since its founding by Dr. Madeleine Leininger.

3. Review the limitations of transcultural nursing cited by critics. What can be done to address the criticisms?

4. Identify electronic and print resources in transcultural nursing and health.

CRITICAL THINKING ACTIVITIES

1. Visit the Transcultural Nursing Society's official Web site (www.tcns.org).
   a. Briefly summarize the information you found at the Web site.
   b. Critically evaluate the strengths and limitations of this information source and the data available.
   c. What clinical relevance does the electronic information on transcultural nursing have for you as a nurse?
   d. Visit links to other related Web sites on transcultural nursing.

2. Using CINAHL, enter the words *transcultural nursing* and search for references cited during the past year. How many references are identified? What are the subcategories under which you can narrow your search? If you want information about a specific cultural, ethnic, or minority group, what keywords will help you to narrow the search? Consult a reference librarian for assistance if you need help.

REFERENCES

Andrews, M. M. (1992). Cultural perspectives on nursing in the 21st century. *Journal of Professional Nursing, 8*(1), 1–9.

Andrews, M. M. (1995). Transcultural nursing: Transforming the curriculum. *Journal of Transcultural Nursing, 6*(2), 4–9.

Andrews, M. M., & Boyle, J. S. (1997). Competence in transcultural nursing care. *American Journal of Nursing, 97*(8), 16AAA–16DDD.

Andrews, M. M., & Boyle, J. S. (2002). Transcultural concepts in nursing care. *Journal of Transcultural Nursing, 13*(3), 178–180.

Andrews, M. M., Burr, J., & Janetos, D. H. (2004). Searching electronically for information on transcultural nursing and health subjects. *Journal of Transcultural Nursing, 15*(3), 242–247.

Branch, M. F., & Paxton, P. P. (Eds.). (1976). *Providing safe nursing care for ethnic people of color.* New York: Appleton-Century-Crofts.

Campinha-Bacote J. (2002). The Process of Cultural Competence in the Delivery of Healthcare Services: a model of care. *Journal of Transcultural Nursing, 13*(3), 181–184.

Culley, L. (1996). A critique of multiculturalism in health care: The challenge for nursing education. *Journal of Advanced Nursing, 23,* 564–570.

Dougherty, M. C., & Tripp-Reimer, T. (1985). The interface of nursing and anthropology. *Annual Review of Anthropology, 14,* 219–241.

Flaskerud, J. H. (2000). Ethnicity, culture and neuropsychiatry. *Issues in Mental Health Nursing, 21*(5), 5–29.

Gustafson, D. L. (1999). Toward inclusionary practices in the education of nurses: A critique of transcultural nursing theory. *The Alberta Journal of Educational Research, 45*(4), 468–470.

Habayeb, G. L. (1995). Cultural diversity: A nursing concept not yet reliably defined. *Nursing Outlook, 43*(5), 224–227.

Juntunen, A. (2007). Professional and lay care in the Tanzanian village of Ilembula (Doctoral dissertation, University of Oulu). Retrieved March 18, 2007, from http://herkules.oulu.fi/isbn9514264312/isbn9514264312.pdf

Leininger, M. M. (1970). *Nursing and anthropology: Two worlds to blend.* New York: John Wiley & Sons.

Leininger, M. M. (1978). *Transcultural nursing: Concepts, theories and practices.* New York: John Wiley & Sons.

Leininger, M. M. (1991). *Culture care diversity and universality: A theory of nursing.* New York: National League for Nursing.

Leininger, M. M. (1995). *Transcultural nursing: Concepts, theories, research and practices.* New York: McGraw-Hill.

Leininger, M. M. (1997). Future directions in transcultural nursing in the 21st century. *International Nursing Review, 44*(1), 19–23.

Leininger, M. M. (1998). Twenty five years of knowledge and practice development transcultural nursing society annual research conferences. *Journal of Transcultural Nursing, 9*(2), 72–74.

Leininger, M. M. (1999). What is transcultural nursing and culturally competent care? *Journal of Transcultural Nursing, 10*(1), 9.

Leininger (in press). The evolution of transcultural nursing with breakthroughs to discipline status. *Journal of Transcultural Nursing.*

Leininger, M. M., & McFarland, M. R. (2002). *Transcultural nursing: Concepts, theories and practices.* New York: McGraw-Hill.

Leininger, M. M., & McFarland, M. R. (2006). *Culture care diversity and universality: A worldwide theory for nursing* (2nd ed.). Sudbury, MA: Jones & Bartlett, Publishers.

Leuning, C. J., Swiggum, P. D., Wieger, H. M. B., & McCullough-Zander, K. (2002). Proposed standards for transcultural nursing. *Journal of Transcultural Nursing, 13*(1), 40–46.

Lipson, J., & Bauwens, E. (1988). Uses of anthropology in nursing. *Practicing Anthropology, 10,* 4–5.

Lipson, J. G. (1999). Cross-cultural nursing: The cultural perspective. *Journal of Transcultural Nursing, 10*(1), 7.

Mahon, P. Y. (1997). Transcultural nursing: A source guide. *Journal of Nursing Staff Development, 13*(4), 218–222.

Mahoney, J. S., & Engebretson, J. (2000). The interface of anthropology and nursing guiding culturally competent care in psychiatric nursing. *Archives of Psychiatric Nursing, 14*(4), 183–190.

McKenna, M. (1984). Anthropology and nursing: The interaction between two fields of inquiry. *Western Journal of Nursing Research, 6*(4), 423–431.

Mulholland, J. (1995). Nursing humanism and transcultural theory: The "bracketing out" of reality. *Journal of Advanced Nursing, 22,* 442–449.

Orque, M. S., Bloch, B., & Monrroy, L. S. (1983). *Ethnic nursing care.* St. Louis: C.V. Mosby.

Osborne, O. (1969). Anthropology and nursing: Some common traditions and interests. *Nursing Research, 18*(3), 251–255.

Price, K. M., & Cortis, J. D. (2000). The way forward for transcultural nursing. *Nurse Education Today, 20*(3), 233–243.

Reynolds, C. L., & Leininger, M. M. (1993). *Madeleine Leininger: Cultural care diversity and universality theory.* Newbury Park, NJ: Sage.

Talabere, L. R. (1996). Meeting the challenge of culture care in nursing: Diversity, sensitivity, and congruence. *Journal of Cultural Diversity, 3*(2), 53–61.

Transcultural Nursing Certification Committee. (2007, March 23–25). *Transcultural Nursing Certification revision.* Conducted at Transcultural Nursing Certification Committee Meeting, Fenton, Michigan.

Transcultural Nursing Society. (2007). Transcultural Nursing Society: Historical moments. *Transcultural Nursing Society Newsletter, 16*(1), 9.

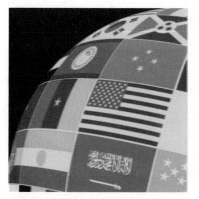

CHAPTER 2

Culturally Competent Nursing Care

Margaret M. Andrews

KEY TERMS

Collateral relationships
Cross-cultural communication
Cultural code
Cultural competence
Culturally congruent care
Cultural self-assessment

Distance
Environmental context
Eye contact
Individual cultural
  competence
Linguistic competence

Nonverbal communication
Proxemics
Sick role behavior
Silence
Space
Touch

LEARNING OBJECTIVES

1. Analyze the complex integration of knowledge, attitudes, and skills needed for cultural competence.
2. Explore cross-cultural communication as the foundation for the provision of culturally competent nursing care.
3. Identify strategies for promoting effective cross-cultural communication in multicultural health care settings.

When the author recently conducted an Internet search for **cultural competence**, using the popular search engine Google, more than 27,700,000 "hits" resulted. These fell into two major categories: (1) *organizational cultural competence* and (2) *individual cultural competence*, usually in reference to nurses, physicians, social workers, or others in health care, education, or social services professionals.

According to the National Center for Cultural Competence (Georgetown University Center for Child and Human Development, n.d.), cultural competence requires that *organizations* have the following characteristics:

- A defined set of values and principles and demonstration of behaviors, attitudes, poli-

cies, and structures that enable them to work effectively cross-culturally.
- The capacity to (1) value diversity, (2) conduct self-assessment, (3) manage the dynamics of difference, (4) acquire and institutionalize cultural knowledge, and (5) adapt to diversity and the cultural contexts of the communities they serve.
- Incorporation of the previously mentioned items in all aspects of policy making, administration, practice, and service delivery, and systematic involvement of consumers, key stakeholders, and communities.

Individual cultural competence refers to a complex integration of knowledge, attitudes, beliefs, skills, and encounters with those from

15

cultures different from one's own that enhances cross-cultural communication and appropriate and effective interactions with others (American Academy of Nursing, 1992, 1993; Campinha-Bacote, 2000, 2003; Geron, 2002). Cultural competence has been defined as a process, as opposed to an end point, in which the nurse continuously strives to work effectively within the cultural context of an individual, family, or community from a diverse cultural background (Andrews & Boyle, 1997; Campinha-Bacote, 2000, 2003; Campinha-Bacote & Munoz, 2001; Wells, 2000; Smith, 1998). Campinha-Bacote (2003) defines cultural competence as "the ongoing process in which the healthcare professional continuously strives to seek the ability and availability to work effectively within the cultural context of the client (individual, family, community). This process involves the integration of cultural desire, cultural awareness, cultural knowledge, cultural skill and cultural encounters" (Campinha-Bacote, 2003, p. 14).

In addition to cultural competence, some experts have noted the considerable impact that **linguistic competence** by health care providers has on clients' access and response to health care services. Cultural and linguistic competence refers to an ability by health care providers and health care organizations to understand and effectively respond to the cultural and linguistic needs brought by clients to the health care encounter. Summarized in Box 2–1 are the 14 recommended standards for culturally and linguistically appropriate health care services proposed by the U.S. Department of Health and Human Services, Office of Minority Health (2000). These standards identify the 14 standards and include a definition of culturally competent care, as well as standards concerning language access, required organizational supports, implementation guidelines, the relationship between the standards and existing laws, diverse and culturally competent staff, data collection, and information dissemination.

Instead of using the term *cultural competence*, Leininger (1991, 1995, 1999; Leininger & McFarland, 2005) prefers *culturally congruent care*, which she defines as the provision of care that is meaningful and fits with cultural beliefs and lifeways. Leininger's definition of culturally congruent care is holistic and focuses on the complex interrelationship of lifeways, religion, kinship, politics, law, education, technology, language, **environmental context**, and worldview—all factors that contribute to culturally congruent care.

Because you may encounter clients from literally hundreds of cultures in your professional career and clients of mixed cultural heritage, it is virtually impossible to know about the culturally based, health-related beliefs and practices of them all. It is, however, possible to master the knowledge and skills associated with cultural assessment and learn about some of the cultural dimensions of care for clients representing the groups most frequently encountered. In-depth knowledge of several cultures is often a reasonable goal if you live in a large urban center characterized by a high degree of diversity.

Cultural Self-Assessment

Before you can provide culturally competent care for people from diverse backgrounds, it's important to engage in a **cultural self-assessment**. When interacting with clients from various cultural backgrounds, you must be aware of your own cultural values, attitudes, beliefs, and practices. To gain insight into the way that you relate to various groups of people in society, describe your level of response to the groups identified in Box 2–2.

Through self-assessment, it is possible to gain insights into the health-related values, attitudes, beliefs, and practices that have been transmitted to you by your own family. These insights also enable you to overcome ethnocentric tendencies and cultural stereotypes, which are vehicles for perpetuating prejudice and discrimination against members of certain groups.

After you have engaged in a cultural self-assessment, it is possible to conduct a cultural assessment of others.

BOX 2-1

Office of Minority Health Standards for Culturally and Linguistically Appropriate Health Care by Health Care Organizations

- Promote and support attitudes, behaviors, knowledge, and skills necessary for staff to work respectfully and effectively with patients and each other in a culturally diverse work environment
- Have a comprehensive management strategy, including strategic goals, plans, policies, procedures, and designated staff responsible for implementation
- Utilize formal mechanisms of community and consumer involvement in the development and execution of service delivery
- Develop and implement a strategy to recruit, retain, and promote qualified diverse and culturally competent administrative, clinical, and support staff who are trained to address the needs of racial and ethnic communities
- Require and arrange for ongoing education and training for administrative, clinical, and support staff in culturally and linguistically competent delivery of service
- Provide all clients having limited English proficiency with access to bilingual interpretation services
- Provide oral and written notices, including translated signage at key points of entry, to clients in their primary language, informing them of their right to receive interpreter services
- Translate and make available signage and commonly used written patient educational materials in the predominant language(s) in the service area

- Ensure that interpreters and bilingual staff can demonstrate bilingual proficiency and receive training that includes the skills and ethics of interpreting
- Ensure that the clients' primary spoken language and self-identified race/ethnicity are included in the health care organization's information system
- Use a variety of methods to collect and utilize accurate demographic, cultural, epidemiological, and clinical outcome data for racial and ethnic groups and become informed about the ethnic/cultural needs, resources, and assets of the surrounding community
- Undertake ongoing organizational self-assessments of cultural and linguistic competence and measure for access, satisfaction, quality, and outcome using internal audits and performance improvement programs
- Develop structures and procedures to address cross-cultural ethical and legal issues in health care delivery and complaints or grievances by patients and staff about unfair, culturally insensitive, or discriminatory treatment, or difficulty in accessing services, or denial of services
- Prepare an annual progress report documenting progress in implementing these standards, including information on programs, staffing, and resources

Source: Office of Minority Health (2000). National standards on culturally linguistically appropriate services (CLAS). *Federal Register* 65(247), 80865–80879. Department of Health and Human Services, U.S. Public Health Service. Washington, D.C. *www.omhre.gov/clas/ds.htm*

Cultural Assessment

The author believes that cultural assessment is the foundation for culturally competent and culturally congruent nursing care. Appendix A contains the Andrews/Boyle Transcultural Nursing Assessment Guide for Individuals and Families, an instrument that is intended to help you to ask key questions during your assessment interview. Please refer to Chapter 3, Cultural Competence in the Health History and Physical Examination, for a complete discussion of cultural assessment.

Skills Needed for Cultural Competence

The term *cultural competence* implies that you have developed certain psychomotor or behavioral skills. Box 2–3 contains selected examples of these skills, and others will be presented throughout the text. It should be noted that mastery of some skills, such as the assessment of

BOX 2-2

How Do You Relate to Various Groups of People in the Society?

Described below are different levels of response you might have toward a person.

Levels of Response

1. *Greet*: I feel I can *greet* this person warmly and welcome him or her sincerely.
2. *Accept*: I feel I can honestly *accept* this person as he or she is and be comfortable enough to listen to his or her problems.
3. *Help*: I feel I would genuinely try to *help* this person with his or her problems as they might relate to or arise from the label-stereotype given to him or her.
4. *Background*: I feel I have the *background* of knowledge and/or experience to be able to help this person.
5. *Advocate*: I feel I could honestly be an *advocate* for this person.

The following is a list of individuals. Read down the list and place a checkmark next to anyone you would *not* "greet" or would hesitate to "greet." Then move to response level 2, "accept," and follow the same procedure. Try to respond honestly, not as you think might be socially or professionally desirable. Your answers are only for your personal use in clarifying your initial reactions to different people.

Level of Response

Individual	1 Greet	2 Accept	3 Help	4 Background	5 Advocate
1. Haitian	☐	☐	☐	☐	☐
2. Child abuser	☐	☐	☐	☐	☐
3. Jew	☐	☐	☐	☐	☐
4. Person with hemophilia	☐	☐	☐	☐	☐
5. Neo-Nazi	☐	☐	☐	☐	☐
6. Mexican American	☐	☐	☐	☐	☐
7. IV drug user	☐	☐	☐	☐	☐
8. Catholic	☐	☐	☐	☐	☐
9. Senile, elderly person	☐	☐	☐	☐	☐
10. Teamster Union member	☐	☐	☐	☐	☐
11. Native American	☐	☐	☐	☐	☐
12. Prostitute	☐	☐	☐	☐	☐
13. Jehovah's Witness	☐	☐	☐	☐	☐
14. Cerebral palsied person	☐	☐	☐	☐	☐
15. ERA proponent	☐	☐	☐	☐	☐
16. Vietnamese American	☐	☐	☐	☐	☐
17. Gay/lesbian	☐	☐	☐	☐	☐
18. Atheist	☐	☐	☐	☐	☐
19. Person with AIDS	☐	☐	☐	☐	☐

(Continued on following page)

BOX 2-2 (continued)

How Do You Relate to Various Groups of People in the Society?

Level of Response

Individual	1 Greet	2 Accept	3 Help	4 Background	5 Advocate
20. Communist	☐	☐	☐	☐	☐
21. Black American	☐	☐	☐	☐	☐
22. Unmarried expectant teenager	☐	☐	☐	☐	☐
23. Protestant	☐	☐	☐	☐	☐
24. Amputee	☐	☐	☐	☐	☐
25. Ku Klux Klansman	☐	☐	☐	☐	☐
26. White Anglo-Saxon	☐	☐	☐	☐	☐
27. Alcoholic	☐	☐	☐	☐	☐
28. Amish person	☐	☐	☐	☐	☐
29. Person with cancer	☐	☐	☐	☐	☐
30. Nuclear armament proponent	☐	☐	☐	☐	☐

Scoring Guide: The previous activity may help you anticipate difficulty in working with some clients at various levels. The 30 types of individuals can be grouped into 5 categories: ethnic/racial, social issues/problems, religious, physically/mentally handicapped, and political. Transfer your checkmarks to the following form. If you have a concentration of checks within a specific category of individuals or at specific levels, this may indicate a conflict that could hinder you from rendering effective professional help.

Level of Response

Individual	1 Greet	2 Accept	3 Help	4 Background	5 Advocate
Ethnic/racial					
1. Haitian American	☐	☐	☐	☐	☐
6. Mexican American	☐	☐	☐	☐	☐
11. Native American	☐	☐	☐	☐	☐
16. Vietnamese American	☐	☐	☐	☐	☐
21. Black American	☐	☐	☐	☐	☐
26. White Anglo-Saxon	☐	☐	☐	☐	☐
Social issues/problems					
2. Child abuser	☐	☐	☐	☐	☐
7. IV drug user	☐	☐	☐	☐	☐
12. Prostitute	☐	☐	☐	☐	☐
17. Gay/lesbian	☐	☐	☐	☐	☐
22. Unmarried expectant teenager	☐	☐	☐	☐	☐
27. Alcoholic	☐	☐	☐	☐	☐
Religious					
3. Jew	☐	☐	☐	☐	☐
8. Catholic	☐	☐	☐	☐	☐
13. Jehovah's Witness	☐	☐	☐	☐	☐
18. Atheist	☐	☐	☐	☐	☐
23. Protestant	☐	☐	☐	☐	☐
28. Amish person	☐	☐	☐	☐	☐

(Continued on following page)

BOX 2-2 (continued)

How Do You Relate to Various Groups of People in the Society?

	Level of Response				
	1	2	3	4	5
Individual	Greet	Accept	Help	Background	Advocate
Physically/mentally handicapped					
4. Person with hemophilia	☐	☐	☐	☐	☐
9. Senile elderly person	☐	☐	☐	☐	☐
14. Cerebral palsied person	☐	☐	☐	☐	☐
19. Person with AIDS	☐	☐	☐	☐	☐
24. Amputee	☐	☐	☐	☐	☐
29. Person with cancer	☐	☐	☐	☐	☐
Political					
5. Neo-Nazi	☐	☐	☐	☐	☐
10. Teamster Union member	☐	☐	☐	☐	☐
15. ERA proponent	☐	☐	☐	☐	☐
20. Communist	☐	☐	☐	☐	☐
25. Ku Klux Klansman	☐	☐	☐	☐	☐
30. Nuclear armament proponent	☐	☐	☐	☐	☐

Reproduced with permission of the Association for the Care of Children's Health, 7910 Woodmont Avenue, Suite 300, Bethesda, MD 20814, from E. Randall-David (1989). *Strategies for Working with Culturally Diverse Communities and Clients*, pp. 7–9.

cyanosis in people with darkly pigmented skin, might be critical for a patient's survival. Other skills may be helpful in promoting hygiene or comfort, but they do not have such dire consequences. Because communication is a skill foundational to all nursing interactions, the remainder of this chapter will focus on this important topic.

Cross-Cultural Communication

Communication is an organized, patterned system of behavior that regulates and makes possible all nurse-client interactions. It is the exchange of messages and the creation of meaning. Because communication and culture are acquired simultaneously, they are integrally linked. In effective communication there is mutual understanding of the meaning attached to the messages. Barriers to communication include differences in language, worldview, and values. It is estimated that up to 90% of all difficulties in nurse-client interactions have resulted from miscommunication.

To begin the discussion on **cross-cultural communication**, it is necessary to examine the ways in which people from various cultural backgrounds communicate with one another. In addition to oral and written communication, messages are conveyed nonverbally through gestures, body movements, posture, tone of voice, and facial expressions (Figure 2–1).

Frequently overlooked is the context in which communication occurs. The environmental context imparts its own message and is influenced by the setting, the purposes of the communication, and the perceptions of the nurse and client concerning time, space, distance, touch, modesty, and other factors. For example, let us imagine you know that a Mexican-American patient is extremely anxious about having a mammogram.

BOX 2-3

Selected Examples of Psychomotor Skills Useful in Transcultural Nursing

Assessment

- Techniques for assessing biocultural variations in health and illness, e.g., assessing cyanosis, jaundice, anemia, and related clinical manifestations of disease in darkly pigmented clients; differentiating between mongolian spots and ecchymoses (bruises)
- Measurement of head circumference and fontanelles in infants using techniques not in violation of taboos for selected cultural groups
- Growth and development monitoring for children of Asian heritage, using culturally appropriate growth grids
- Cultural modification of the Denver II and other developmental tests used for children
- Conducting culturally appropriate obstetric and gynecologic examinations of women from various cultural backgrounds

Communication

- Speaking and writing the language(s) used by clients
- Using alternative methods of communicating with non–English-speaking clients and families when no interpreter is available (e.g., pantomime)

Hygiene

- Skin care for clients of various racial/ethnic backgrounds
- Hair care for clients of various ethnic/racial backgrounds, e.g., care of African-American clients' hair

Activities of Daily Living

- Assisting Chinese-American clients to regain use of chopsticks as part of rehabilitation regimen after a stroke
- Assisting paralyzed Amish client with dressing when buttons and pins are used
- Assisting West African client who uses "chewing stick" with oral hygiene

Religion

- Emergency baptism and anointing of the sick for Catholics
- Care before and after ritual circumcision by *mohel* (performed 8 days after the birth of a male Jewish infant)

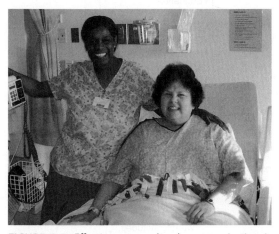

FIGURE 2-1. Effective cross-cultural communication is vital to the establishment of a strong nurse-patient relationship. It is important to understand both verbal and nonverbal cues when communicating with people from various cultural backgrounds. (© Copyright M. Andrews)

After the procedure, you intend to send an empathetic, caring message by remarking, "It's all over, Señora Garcia." Señora Garcia bursts into tears because she believes she has been diagnosed with terminal breast cancer. Needless to say, even communication between individuals having the same cultural background may be fraught with pitfalls. When you communicate with others from cultural backgrounds unlike your own and with those for whom English is a second language, the probability of miscommunication increases significantly. In promoting effective cross-cultural communication, you should avoid technical jargon, slang, colloquial expressions, abbreviations, and excessive use of medical terminology.

Lipson and Steiger (1996) suggest affective, cognitive, and behavioral strategies for effective cross-cultural communication. In the affective domain, they suggest respect for, appreciation of, and comfort with cultural differences; enjoyment of learning through cultural exchange; ability to observe behavior without judging; awareness of one's own cultural values and biases; and belief in cultural relativity: that there are many acceptable cultural ways. In the cognitive domain, they emphasize knowledge about different cultures, ability to recognize when there is a cultural explanation for an interpersonal problem, understanding that meanings can differ for others, and understanding the sociopolitical system with respect to its treatment of minorities. In the behavioral domain (communication skills), they advocate flexibility in verbal and nonverbal communication styles; ability to speak slowly and clearly without excessive slang; ability to encourage others to express themselves; ability to communicate sincere interest, empathy, and patience; and ability to observe and intervene when misunderstanding occurs.

Important factors to consider for cross-cultural communication include communication with family members and significant others; space, distance, and intimacy; nonverbal communication; language; and sick role behaviors (Figure 2–2).

Communication with Family Members and Significant Others

Knowledge of a client's family and kinship structure helps you to ascertain the values, decision-making patterns, and overall communication

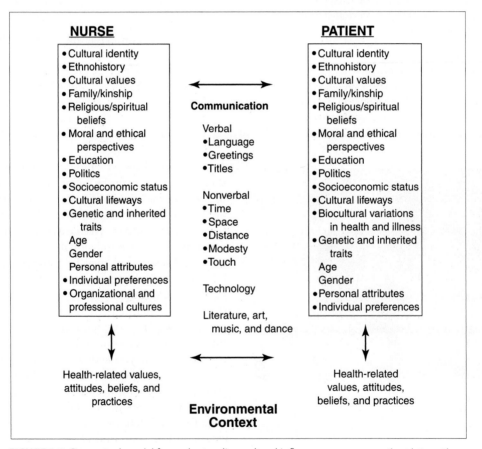

FIGURE 2-2. Conceptual model for understanding cultural influences on nurse-patient interactions.

within the household. It is necessary to identify the significant others whom clients perceive to be important in their care and who may be responsible for decision making that affects their health care. For example, for many clients, familism—which emphasizes interdependence over independence, affiliation over confrontation, and cooperation over competition—may dictate that important decisions affecting the client be made by the family, not the individual alone. When you work with clients from cultural groups that value cohesion, interdependence, and collectivism, you may perceive the family as being overly involved and usurping the autonomy of the client. Clients are likely to perceive the involvement with family as a source of mutual support, security, and fulfillment.

The family is the basic social unit in which children are raised and learn culturally based values, beliefs, and practices about health and illnesses. The essence of family consists of living together as a unit. Relationships that may seem obvious sometimes warrant further exploration when the nurse interacts with clients from culturally diverse backgrounds. For example, most European Americans define siblings as two persons with either the same mother, the same father, the same mother and father, or the same adoptive parents. In some Asian cultures, a sibling relationship is defined as any infants breastfed by the same woman. In other cultures, certain kinship patterns, such as maternal first cousins, are defined as sibling relationships. In some African cultures, anyone from the same village may be called brother or sister.

Members of some ethnoreligious groups (e.g., Roman Catholics of Italian, Polish, Spanish, or Mexican descent) recognize relationships such as godmother or godfather, in which an individual who is not the biologic parent promises to assist with the moral or spiritual development of an infant and agrees to care for the child in the event of parental death. The godparent makes these promises during the religious ceremony of baptism.

In communicating with the parent or parent surrogate of infants and children, it is important to identify the primary provider of care and the key decision maker who acts on behalf of the child. In some instances, this person may not be the biologic parent. Among some Hispanic groups, for example, female members of the nuclear or extended family such as sisters and aunts are primary providers of care for infants and children. In some African-American families, the grandmother may be the decision maker and primary caretaker of children. To provide culturally congruent care, you must be certain that you are effectively communicating with the appropriate decision maker(s).

When making health-related decisions, some members of culturally diverse backgrounds in which lineal relationships predominate may seek assistance from other members of the family. It is sometimes culturally expected that a relative (e.g., parent, grandparent, eldest son, or eldest brother) will make decisions about important health-related matters. For example, in many Asian cultures, it is the obligation and duty of the eldest son to assume primary responsibility for his aging parents and to make health care decisions for them. If **collateral relationships** are valued, decisions about the client may be interrelated with the impact of illness on the entire family or group. For example, among the Amish, the entire community is affected by the illness of a member because the community pays for health care from a common fund, members join together to meet the needs of both the sick person and his or her family throughout the illness, and the roles of dozens of people in the community are likely to be affected by the illness of a single member. The individual values orientation concerning relationships is predominant among the dominant cultural majority in North America. Although members of the nuclear family may participate to varying degrees, decision making about health and illness is often an individual matter.

Cultural Perspectives on Intimacy

Interactions between you and your client are influenced by the degree of intimacy desired, which may range from very formal interactions to close personal relationships. For example, some clients of Asian origin expect you and other health care providers to be authoritarian, directive, and detached. In seeking health care, some clients of Chinese descent may expect you to know intuitively what is wrong with them, and you may actually lose some credibility by asking a fairly standard interview question such as, "What brings you here?" The Asian-American patient may be thinking, "Don't you know why I'm here? You're supposed to be the one with all the answers." The reserved interpersonal behavior characteristics of many Asian Americans may leave you with the impression that the client agrees with or understands your explanation. Nodding or smiling by Asians may simply reflect their cultural value for interpersonal harmony, not agreement with what you have said. The emphasis on social harmony among Asian-North American clients may prevent their full expression of concerns or feelings.

In Thai culture, a high value is placed on *kreengcaj*, or awareness and anticipation of the feelings of others by kindness and the avoidance of interpersonal conflict. By obtaining validation of assumptions, you may distinguish between genuine concurrent and socially compliant client responses aimed at maintaining harmony. This may be accomplished by inviting the client to respond frankly to suggestions or by giving the client "permission" to disagree.

By contrast, Appalachian clients often have close family interaction patterns that lead them to expect close personal relationships with health care providers. The Appalachian client may evaluate your effectiveness on the basis of interpersonal skills rather than professional competencies. Some Appalachian clients may be uncomfortable with the impersonal orientation of most health care institutions.

Among some Hispanic groups, such as Mexican Americans and Cuban Americans, *simpatia* and *personalismo* should be considered. *Simpatia* refers to the need for smooth or harmonious interpersonal relationships, characterized by courtesy, respect, and the absence of critical or confrontational behavior. The concept of *personalismo* emphasizes intimate personal relationships. Persons of Latin American or Mediterranean origins often expect a high degree of intimacy and may attempt to involve you in their family system by expecting you to participate in personal activities and social functions. These individuals may come to expect personal favors that extend beyond the scope of what you believe to be professional practice, and they may feel it is their privilege to contact you at home during any time of the day or night for care. If your cultural value system emphasizes a high level of personal privacy, you may choose to give clients the agency's phone number and address rather than disclose information about your personal residence.

Because initial impressions are so important in all human relationships, cross-cultural considerations concerning introductions warrant a few brief remarks. To ensure that a mutually respectful relationship is established, you should introduce yourself and indicate to the client how you prefer to be called: by first name, last name, and/or title. You should elicit the same information from the client because this enables you to address the person in a manner that is culturally appropriate.

Nonverbal Communication

Because **nonverbal communication** patterns vary widely across cultures, nurses must be alert for cues that convey cultural differences in the use of silence, eye contact, touch, space, distance, and facial expressions. Cultural influences on appropriate communication between individuals of different genders also need to be considered.

Silence

Wide cultural variation exists in the interpretation of **silence**. Some individuals find silence extremely uncomfortable and make every effort to fill conversational lags with words. By contrast, many Native North Americans consider silence essential to understanding and respecting the other person. A pause following your question signifies that what has been asked is important enough to be given thoughtful consideration. In traditional Chinese and Japanese cultures, silence may mean that the speaker wishes the listener to consider the content of what has been said before continuing. Other cultural meanings of silence may be found. English persons and Arabs may use silence out of respect for another's privacy, whereas French, Spanish, and Russian persons may interpret it as a sign of agreement. Asian cultures often use silence to demonstrate respect for elders. Among some African Americans, silence is used in response to a question perceived as inappropriate.

Eye Contact

The use of **eye contact** is among the most culturally variable nonverbal behaviors that clients will use to communicate with you. Although most nurses have been taught to maintain eye contact when speaking with clients, individuals from culturally diverse backgrounds may attribute other culturally based meanings to this behavior. Asian, Native North American, Indochinese, Arab, and Appalachian clients may consider direct eye contact impolite or aggressive, and they may avert their own eyes when talking with you. Native North Americans often stare at the floor during conversations—a culturally appropriate behavior indicating that the listener is paying close attention to the speaker. Some African Americans use oculistics (eye rolling) in response to what is perceived to be an inappropriate question. Among Hispanic clients, respect dictates appropriate deferential behavior in the form of downcast eyes toward others on the basis of age, sex, social position, economic status, and position of authority. Elders expect respect from younger individuals, adults from children, men from women, teachers from students, and employers from employees. In the nurse-client relationship with Hispanic clients, eye contact is

expected of you but will not necessarily be reciprocated by the client.

In some cultures, including Arab, Latino, and African-American groups, modesty for both women and men is interrelated with eye contact. Muslim-Arab women achieve modesty, in part, by avoiding eye contact with males (except for one's husband) and keeping the eyes downcast when encountering members of the opposite sex in public situations. In many cultures, the only woman who smiles and establishes eye contact with men in public is a prostitute. Hasidic Jewish males also have culturally based norms concerning eye contact with females; you may observe a Hasidic Jewish man avoiding direct eye contact and turning his head in the opposite direction when walking past or speaking to a woman. The preceding examples are intended to be illustrative, not exhaustive.

Touch

You are urged to give careful consideration to issues concerning **touch**. While we recognize the often-reported benefits in establishing rapport with clients through touch, including the promotion of healing through therapeutic touch, physical contact with clients conveys various meanings cross-culturally. In many Arab and Hispanic cultures, male health care providers may be prohibited from touching or examining part or all of the female body. Adolescent girls may prefer female health care providers or may refuse to be examined by a male. You should be aware that the client's significant others also may exert pressure by enforcing these culturally meaningful norms in the health care setting.

In some cultures, there are strict norms related to touching children. Many Asians believe that touching the head is a sign of disrespect because it is thought to be the source of a person's strength. You need to be aware that patting a child on the head or examining the fontanelles of a Southeast Asian infant should be avoided or done only with parental permission. Whenever possible, you should explore alternative ways to express affection or to obtain information necessary for assessment of the client's condition. For example, you might ask the mother to hold the child on her lap while you observe for other manifestations of increased intracranial pressure or signs of premature fontanelle closure. You might also try placing your hand over the mother's while asking for a description of what she feels.

Space and Distance

The concepts of **space** and **distance** are significant in cross-cultural communication. The perception of appropriate distance zones varies widely among cultural groups. Although there are individual variations in spatial requirements, people of the same culture tend to act in similar ways. For example, if you are of European North American heritage, you may find yourself backing away from clients of Hispanic, East Indian, or Middle Eastern origins who frequently seem to invade your personal space. Such behavior by these clients is probably an attempt to bring you closer into the space that is comfortable to them. Although you may be uncomfortable with close physical proximity to these clients, they are perplexed by your distancing behavior and may perceive you as aloof and unfriendly.

Because individuals are usually notconsciously aware of their personal space requirements, they frequently have difficulty understanding a different cultural pattern. For example, sitting in close proximity to another person may be perceived by one client as an expression of warmth and friendliness but by another as a threatening invasion of personal space. According to Watson (1980), Americans, Canadians, and British require the most personal space, whereas Latin Americans, Japanese, and Arabs need the least.

In the early 1960s, Edward T. Hall pioneered the study of **proxemics**, which focuses on how people in various cultures relate to their physical space. Although there are intercultural variations, the intimate distance in interpersonal interactions ranges from 0 to 18 inches. At this distance, people experience visual detail and each other's odor, heat, and touch. Personal distance varies from 1.5 to 4 feet, the usual space within which communication between friends and acquaintances occurs. Nurses frequently interact with clients in the intimate or personal distance zones. Social distance refers to 4 to 12 feet, whereas anything greater than 12 is considered public distance (Hall, 1963).

Sex and Gender

Nonverbal behaviors are culturally significant, and failure to adhere to the **cultural code** (set of rules or norms of behavior used by a cultural group to guide behavior and to interpret situations) is viewed as a serious transgression. Violating norms related to appropriate male-female relationships among various cultures might jeopardize your therapeutic relationship with clients and their families. Among Arab Americans, you may find that adult males avoid being alone with members of the opposite sex (except for their wives) and are generally accompanied by one or more male companions when interacting with females. The presence of the companion(s) conveys that the purpose of the interaction is honorable and that no sexual impropriety will occur. Some women of Middle Eastern origin do not shake hands with men, nor do men and women touch each other outside the marital relationship. Given that clients who have recently immigrated are in various stages of assimilation, traditional customs such as these may or may not be practiced. If in doubt, you should ask the client or observe the client's behaviors, preferably at the time of admission.

A brief comment about same-sex relationships is warranted. In some cultures, it is considered an acceptable expression of friendship and affection to openly and publicly hold hands with or embrace members of the same sex without any sexual connotation being associated with the behavior. For example, you may note that although a Nigerian-American woman may not demonstrate overt affection for her husband or other male family members, she will hold hands with female relatives and friends while walking or talking with them. You may find that clients display similar behaviors toward you, and you should feel free to discuss cultural differences and similarities openly with the client. The discussion should include how each person feels about the cultural practice and exploration of mutually acceptable—and unacceptable—avenues for communicating.

Language

In the United States, nearly 45 million people, age 5 five years or older, speak a language other than English at home (U.S. Census Bureau, 2000). Summarized in Table 2–1 are the numbers of Americans who speak other languages and who report that they have difficulty speaking English well.

According to the U.S. Census Bureau (U.S. Department of Commerce [DOC], U.S. Census Bureau, 2003), nearly 1 in 5 people, or 47 million U.S. residents age 5 and older, speak a language other than English at home. Fifty-five percent of the people who spoke a language other than English at home reported they spoke English "very well."

Other than English, Spanish is the major language spoken in the United States, and it is spoken by 31 million U.S. citizens age 5 and older; eleven million of those individuals indicated that they speak *only* Spanish. The Western states are home to more than one-third (37%) of all those who spoke a language other than English at home, the highest proportion of any region. California led the states (39%), followed by New Mexico (37%) and Texas (31%) (U.S. DOC, U.S. Census Bureau, 2003).

After English (215.4 million speakers) and Spanish (31 million), Chinese (2 million) was the language most commonly spoken at home, eclipsing French, German, and Italian during the decade of the '90s. Of the 20 non-English languages spoken most widely at home, the largest proportional increase since the last census in 1990 has been Russian. Speakers of this language nearly tripled, from 242,000 to 706,000. The second-largest increase was among French Creole speakers (including Haitian Creoles), whose numbers more than doubled, from 188,000 to 453,000 (U.S. DOC, U.S. Census Bureau, 2003).

TABLE 2-1 *Summary of Languages Spoken at Home*

Language Spoken at Home	Estimate
Population 5 Years Old and Older	268,110,961
English only	216,176,111
Language other than English	51,934,850
Speak English less than "very well"	23,142,029
Spanish or Spanish Creole	32,184,293
Speak English less than "very well"	15,396,674
Other Indo-European languages	9,929,004
Speak English less than "very well"	3,302,077
Asian and Pacific Islander languages	7,769,500
Speak English less than "very well"	3,828,819
Other languages	2,052,053
Speak English less than "very well"	614,459

Adapted from: U.S. Census Bureau (2005). *2005 American Community Survey.* Retrieved from www.factfinder.census.gov.

USE OF INTERPRETERS

One of the greatest challenges in cross-cultural communication occurs when you and your client speak different languages. After assessing the language skills of non–English-speaking clients, you may find yourself in one of two situations: either struggling to communicate effectively through an interpreter or communicating effectively when there is no interpreter. See Box 2-4.

NON–ENGLISH-SPEAKING PATIENTS AND INTERPRETERS

Interviewing the non–English-speaking person requires a bilingual interpreter for full communication. Even a person from another culture or country who has a basic command of English (someone for whom English is a second language) may need an interpreter when faced with the anxiety-provoking situation of entering a hospital, encountering a strange symptom, or discussing a sensitive topic such as birth control or gynecologic or urologic concerns. Ideally, a trained medical interpreter should be used. This person knows interpreting techniques, has a health care background, and understands patients' rights. The trained interpreter is also knowledgeable about cultural beliefs and health practices. This person can help you to bridge the cultural gap and can give advice concerning the cultural appropriateness of your recommendations.

Although you will be in charge of the focus and flow of the interview, the interpreter should be viewed as an important member of the health care team. It is tempting to ask a relative, a friend, or even another client to interpret because this person is readily available and likely is anxious to help. However, this violates confidentiality for the client, who may not want personal information shared. Furthermore, the friend or relative, though fluent in ordinary language usage, is likely to be unfamiliar with medical terminology, hospital or clinic procedures, and health care ethics.

Whenever possible, work with a bilingual member of the health care team. In ideal circumstances, you should ask the interpreter to meet the client beforehand to establish rapport and to obtain basic descriptive information about the client such as age, occupation, educational level, and attitude toward health care. This eases the interpreter into the relationship and allows the client to talk about aspects of his or her life that are relatively nonthreatening.

When using an interpreter, you should expect that the interaction with the client will require more time than is needed in the care of English-speaking clients. It will be necessary to organize nursing care so that the most important interactions or procedures are accomplished first before any of the parties (including yourself) becomes fatigued.

Both you and the client should speak only a sentence or two and then allow the interpreter time to translate. You should use simple language, not medical jargon that the interpreter must simplify before it can be translated. Summary translation—allowing a person to speak in his or her native language and then having an interpreter summarize what was said—goes faster and is useful for teaching relatively simple health techniques with which the interpreter is already familiar. Be alert for nonverbal cues as the client talks; he or she can give valuable data. A skilled interpreter also will note nonverbal messages and pass them on to you (Nailon, 2004, 2006). Evidence-based Practice Box 2-1 examines nurses' concerns and practices using interpreters in the care of Latino patients in the emergency department.

The Joint Commission on Accreditation of Healthcare Organizations and the American Hospital Association both require that accommodations be made for patients who lack proficiency in English, and some states have passed laws requiring health care organizations to provide interpreters for their non–English-speaking patients. Box 2-5 provides a summary of suggestions for the selection and use of an interpreter and for overcoming language barriers when an interpreter is unavailable. Although the use of an interpreter is ideal, you will need a strategy for promoting effective communication when none is present.

BOX 2-4

Overcoming Language Barriers

Use of an Interpreter

- Before locating an interpreter, be sure that the language the client speaks at home is known, considering it may be different from the language spoken publicly (e.g., French is sometimes spoken by well-educated and upper-class members of certain Asian or Middle Eastern cultures).
- Avoid interpreters from a rival tribe, state, region, or nation (e.g., a Palestinian who knows Hebrew may not be the best interpreter for a Jewish client).
- Be aware of gender differences between interpreter and client. In general, same gender is preferred.
- Be aware of age differences between interpreter and client. In general, an older, more mature interpreter is preferred to a younger, less experienced one.
- Be aware of socioeconomic differences between interpreter and client.
- Ask the interpreter to translate as closely to verbatim as possible.
- Expect an interpreter who is not a relative to seek compensation for services rendered.

Recommendations for Institutions

- Maintain a computerized list of interpreters who may be contacted as needed.
- Network with area hospitals, colleges, universities, and other organizations that may serve as resources.
- Utilize the translation services provided by telephone companies (e.g., American Telephone and Telegraph Company).

What to Do When There Is No Interpreter

- Be polite and formal.
- Greet the person using the last or complete name. Gesture to yourself and say your name. Offer a handshake or nod. Smile.
- Proceed in an unhurried manner. Pay attention to any effort by the patient or family to communicate.

- Speak in a low, moderate voice. Avoid talking loudly. Remember that there is a tendency to raise the volume and pitch of your voice when the listener appears not to understand. The listener may perceive that the nurse is shouting and/or angry.
- Use any words known in the patient's language. This indicates that the nurse is aware of and respects the client's culture.
- Use simple words, such as *pain* instead of *discomfort*. Avoid medical jargon, idioms, and slang. Avoid using contractions. Use nouns repeatedly instead of pronouns. Example: Do *not* say, "He has been taking his medicine, hasn't he?" Do say, "Does Juan take medicine?"
- Pantomime words and simple actions while verbalizing them.
- Give instructions in the proper sequence. Example: Do *not* say, "Before you rinse the bottle, sterilize it." Do say, "First, wash the bottle. Second, rinse the bottle."
- Discuss one topic at a time. Avoid using conjunctions. Example: Do *not* say, "Are you cold and in pain?" Do say, "Are you cold [while pantomiming]?" Are you in pain?"
- Validate whether the client understands by having him or her repeat instructions, demonstrate the procedure, or act out the meaning.
- Write out several short sentences in English, and determine the person's ability to read them.
- Try a third language. Many Indochinese speak French. Europeans often know three or four languages. Try Latin words or phrases, if the nurse is familiar with that language.
- Ask who among the client's family and friends could serve as an interpreter.
- Obtain phrase books from a library or bookstore, make or purchase flash cards, contact hospitals for a list of interpreters, and use both formal and informal networking to locate a suitable interpreter.

Adapted from M. Andrews (2004). Transcultural considerations in health assessment. In C. Jarvis, *Physical Examination and Health Assessment* (p. 69). Philadelphia: W.B. Saunders. Reprinted by permission.

Evidence-Based Practice 2–1:

Use of Interpreters in the Care of Latino Patients in the Emergency Department

Nearly one-fourth of Latinos residing in the United States live in *linguistically isolated* households, which means that all household members age 14 and older have at least some difficulty speaking and understanding English. When these individuals visit the emergency department, they may fail to receive care in a timely and culturally appropriate manner because a medically trained interpreter is unavailable. Nurses are cognizant of the need for accurate communication in meeting the nursing care needs of their Spanish-speaking patients/clients and sometimes turn to family members or untrained interpreters due to the urgency of the patient's medical situation.

This phenomenological study focuses on the nursing care of Latinos in the emergency department and the manner in which nurses from four hospitals in the Northwest approached the cultural and language needs of their Latino patients. Using unstructured interviews and participant observation, the researcher studied 22 nurse-patient encounters, 16 of which involved the use of an interpreter. The majority of the 15 nurses who participated in the study had minimal to limited Spanish-speaking ability and required the assistance of an interpreter.

Clinical Applications

The findings from the study include the following clinical implications:

- Lack of interpreter availability impedes nurses' involvement with non–English-speaking patients and reduces the amount of time nurses spend with them.
- Nurses' skills relative to work with interpreters, interpreter availability, engagement, and accuracy enhance or impede effective care.
- Nurses and interpreters should receive training to prepare them to work effectively with each other so that meaningful, accurate, and culturally appropriate communication results with non–English-speaking Latino patients and their families.
- Linguistic differences challenge effective care provision by nurses, including the tendency to defer valuable and expensive time involving an interpreter to the physician.
- Nurses tend to take shortcuts when assessing non–English-speaking Latino patients in the emergency department by relying too much on vital signs and observation of patients rather than gathering firsthand information from the patient.
- If interpreters are used, nurses tend to involve them for discharge teaching but not always during the assessment or provision of care.
- Culturally competent care requires accurate communication.
- Strong administrative support is necessary for cultural competence, including funding to train interpreters and nurses to facilitate effective nurse-patient communication for non–English-speaking patients.

Nailon, R. E. (2006). Nurses' concerns and practices with using interpreters in the care of Latino patients in the emergency department. *Journal of Transcultural Nursing, 17*(2), 119–128.

BOX 2-5

National Council for Interpreters in Health Care

The National Council on Interpreting in Health Care (2006) has developed the first set of national standards for medical interpreting professionals in the United States. The 32 national standards provide guidelines on the following nine issues:

- Accuracy: To enable other parties to know precisely what each speaker has said.
- Confidentiality: To honor the private and personal nature of the health care interaction and maintain trust among all parties.
- Impartiality: To eliminate the effect of interpreter bias or preference.
- Respect: To acknowledge the inherent dignity of all parties in the interpreted encounter.
- Cultural Awareness: To facilitate communication across cultural differences.
- Role Boundaries: To clarify the scope and limits of the interpreting role to avoid conflicts of interest.
- Professionalism: To uphold the public's trust in the interpreting profession.
- Professional Development: To attain the highest possible level of competence and service.
- Advocacy: To prevent harm to parties whom the interpreter serves.

Sick Role Behaviors

If you find yourself feeling uncomfortable because a client is asking too many questions, assuming a defensive posture, or otherwise showing discomfort, it might be appropriate to pause for a moment to examine the source of the conflict from a transcultural perspective. During ill-ness, culturally acceptable **sick role behavior** may range from aggressive, demanding behavior to silent passivity. Researchers have found that complaining, demanding behavior during illness is often rewarded with attention among Jewish and Italian groups. Because Asian and Native North American patients are likely to be quiet and compliant during illness, they may not receive the attention they need. Children are socialized into culturally acceptable sick role behaviors at an early age.

Clients of Asian heritage may provide you with the answers that they think are expected. This behavior is consistent with the dominant cultural value for harmonious relationships with others. Thus, you should attempt to phrase questions or statements in a neutral manner that avoids foreshadowing an expected response.

Summary

In this chapter we have explored culturally competent and culturally congruent nursing care as well as the importance of linguistic competence. We have discussed cultural self-assessment and encouraged you to gain insights into your own attitudes and beliefs about different ethnic, religious, and social groups.

Most of the chapter has focused on the complex, multifaceted topic of cross-cultural communication, including aspects of verbal and nonverbal communication that enable nurses to provide culturally competent and culturally congruent nursing care.

REVIEW QUESTIONS

1. Summarize the key standards for culturally and linguistically competent health care recommended by the Office of Minority Health, U.S. Department of Health and Human Services.
2. Critically examine the strategies for promoting effective cross-cultural communi-cation between nurses and clients. Identify actions that you can take to overcome communication barriers when caring for non–English-speaking clients.
3. What are the major languages spoken in households in the United States and Canada?

CRITICAL THINKING ACTIVITIES

1. After critically analyzing the definitions of cultural competence presented in the chapter, craft a definition of the term in your own words.

2. To provide culturally competent nursing care, you should engage in a cultural self-assessment. Answer the questions in Box 2–2, How Do You Relate to Various Groups of People in the Society?, and score your answers using the guide provided. What did you learn about yourself? How would you learn more about the background of those groups mentioned, including information about their health-related beliefs and practices? What resources might you use in your search for information?

3. At the request of the Bureau of Primary Health Care, Health Resources and Services Administration, in the U.S. Department of Health and Human Services, staff at the National Center for Cultural Competence (NCCC) developed the *Cultural Competence Health Practitioner Assessment* which is available online. Visit the Web site at http://www11.Georgetown.edu/research/gucchd/nccc/features/CCHPA.html and complete this assessment.

4. After identifying someone for whom English is a second language, ask the person what he or she believes (a) promotes effective communication and (b) sets up barriers to effective communication. What has the person found to be most challenging in communicating health-related needs to physicians, nurses, and other health care providers?

5. Interview a nurse with experience in caring for clients whose primary language is not English. What challenges does the nurse report in communicating with these clients? What strategies does the nurse use to promote effective cross-cultural communication? How effective does the nurse believe these strategies have been in the care of these clients?

REFERENCES

American Academy of Nursing. (1992). AAN expert panel report: Culturally competent health care. *Nursing Outlook, 40,* 277–283.

American Academy of Nursing. (1993). *Promoting cultural competence in and through nursing education.* New York: Subpanel on Cultural Competence in Nursing Education, American Academy of Nursing.

Andrews, M. M., & Boyle, J. S. (1997). Competence in transcultural nursing care. *American Journal of Nursing, 98*(8), 16AAA–16DDD.

Campinha-Bacote, J. (2000). A model of practice to address cultural competent health care in the home. *Home Care Provider, 5*(6), 213–219.

Campinha-Bacote, J. (2002). The process of cultural competence in the delivery of healthcare services: A Model. *Journal of Transcultural Nursing, 13,* 181–184.

Campinha-Bacote, J. (2003). *The process of cultural competence in the delivery of healthcare services* (4th ed.). Cincinnati, OH: Transcultural C.A.R.E. Associates.

Campinha-Bacote, J., & Munoz, C. (2001). A guiding framework for delivering culturally competent services in case management. *The Case Manager, 12*(2), 48–52.

Georgetown University Center for Child and Human Development, National Center for Cultural Competence (NCCC). (n.d.). *Foundations of cultural and linguistic competence.* Retrieved August 19, 2006, from www.gucchd.georgetown.edu/nccc

Georgetown University Center for Child and Human Development, NCCC. (1999). *Cultural Competence Health Practitioner Assessment.* Available at http://www11.Georgetown.edu/research/gucchd/nccc/features/CCHPA.html

Geron, S. M. (2002). Cultural competency: How is it measured? Does it make a difference? *Generations, 26*(3), 39–45.

Hall, E. (1963). Proxemics: The study of man's spatial relationships. In I. Gladstone (Ed.). *Man's image in medicine and anthropology* (pp. 109–120). New York: International University Press.

Leininger, M. M. (1991). *Culture care diversity and universality: A theory of nursing.* New York: National League for Nursing Press.

Leininger, M. M. (1995). *Transcultural nursing: Concepts, theories, research and practices*. New York: McGraw-Hill.

Leininger, M. M. (1999). What is transcultural nursing and culturally competent care? *Journal of Transcultural Nursing, 10*(1), 9.

Leininger, M. M., & McFarland, M. R. (2002). *Transcultural nursing: Concepts, theories, research and practices*. New York: McGraw-Hill.

Lipson, J. G., & Steiger, N. J. (1996). *Self-care nursing in a multicultural context*. Thousand Oaks, CA: Sage.

Nailon, R. E. (2004). Expertise in the care of Latinos: An interpretive study of culturally congruent nursing practices in the emergency department. *Dissertation Abstracts International, 65,* 12B. (UMI No. 3158546)

Nailon, R. E. (2006). Nurses' concerns and practices with using interpreters in the care of Latino patients in the emergency department. *Journal of Transcultural Nursing, 17*(2), 119–128.

National Council on Interpreting in Health Care. (2002). *Models for the provision of health care interpreter training*. Retrieved August 19, 2006, from www.ncih.org

Smith, L. S. (1998). Concept analysis: Cultural competence. *Journal of Cultural Diversity, 5*(1), 4–10.

U.S. Census Bureau. (2000). *2000 census of population and housing*. Washington, DC: U.S. Government Printing Office. www.census.gov. Retrieved April 12, 2007.

U.S. Department of Commerce, U.S. Census Bureau. (2003, October 8). Nearly 1-in-5 speak a foreign language at home. Press release retrieved on August 19, 2006, from www.census.gov/Press-Release/www/releases.language3.pdf

U.S. Department of Health and Human Services, Office of Minority Health. (2000). National standards on culturally and linguistically appropriate services (CLAS), *Federal Register, 65*(247), 80865–80879. Retrieved from www.omhrc.gov/clas/ds.htm

Watson, O. M. (1980). *Proxemic behavior: A cross-cultural study*. The Hague, Netherlands: Mouton Press.

Wells, M. I. (2000). Beyond cultural competence: A model for individual and institutional cultural development. *Journal of Community Health Nursing, 17*(4), 189–199.

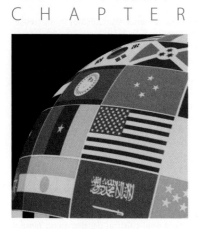

CHAPTER 3

Cultural Competence in the Health History and Physical Examination

Margaret M. Andrews

Cultural assessment, or *culturologic nursing assessment,* refers to a systematic, comprehensive examination of individuals, families, groups, and communities regarding their health-related cultural beliefs, values, and practices. The goal of cultural assessment is to determine the explicit nursing and health care needs of people and to intervene in ways that are culturally congruent and meaningful (cf. Leininger, 1995; Leininger & McFarland, 2002). Because they deal with cultural values, belief systems, and lifeways, cultural assessments tend to be broad and comprehen-

sive, although it is possible to focus on a smaller segment. Cultural assessment consists of both *process* and *content. Process* refers to your approach to the client, consideration of verbal and nonverbal communication, and the sequence and order in which data are gathered. The *content* of the cultural assessment consists of the actual data categories in which information about clients is gathered.

This chapter will be divided into two major sections: (1) transcultural perspectives on the health history and (2) transcultural perspectives on the physical examination. Ideally, the cultural assessment should be integrated into the overall assessment of the client, family, group, and/or community. It is usually impractical to expect that nurses will have the time to conduct a separate cultural assessment, so questions aimed at gathering cultural data should be integrated into the overall assessment.

In Appendix A you will find the Andrews and Boyle **Transcultural Nursing Assessment Guide for Individuals and Families**. The major categories in this guide include cultural affiliations, values orientation, communication, health-related beliefs and practices, nutrition, socioeconomic considerations, organizations providing cultural support, education, religion, cultural aspects of disease incidence, biocultural variations, and developmental considerations across the life span.

Transcultural Perspectives on the Health History

The purpose of the health history is to gather *subjective data*—a term that refers to things that people say about themselves. The health history provides a comprehensive overview of a client's past and present health, and it examines the manner in which the person interacts with the environment. The health history enables the nurse to assess health strengths, including cultural beliefs and practices that might influence the nurse's ability to provide culturally competent nursing care. The history is combined with the *objective data* from the physical examination and the laboratory results to form a diagnosis about the health status of a person (Jarvis, 2004).

For the well client, the history is used to assess lifestyle, which includes activity, exercise, diet, and related personal choices that enable you to identify potential risk factors for disease. For the ill client, the health history includes a chronologic record of the health problem(s). For both well and ill clients, the health history is a screening tool for abnormal symptoms, health problems, and concerns. The health history also

provides you with valuable information about the coping strategies used previously by clients (Jarvis, 2004).

In many health care settings, the client is expected to fill out a printed history form or checklist. From a transcultural perspective, this approach has both positive and negative aspects. On the positive side, this approach provides the client with ample time to recall details such as relevant family history and the dates of health-related events such as surgical procedures and illnesses. It is expedient for nurses because it takes less time to review a form than to elicit the information in a face-to-face or telephone interview.

However, this approach has limitations. First, the form is likely to be in English. Those whose primary language is not English might find the form difficult or impossible to complete accurately. Although some health care facilities provide forms translated into Spanish, French, or other languages known to be spoken by relatively large numbers of people who use the facility, it is costly to translate forms into multiple languages. In some instances, the literal translation of medical terms isn't possible. In other instances, the symptom or disease is not recognized in the culture with which the client identifies. For example, in asking about symptoms of depression, there might be many cultural factors that influence the client's interpretation of the question. In Chinese languages, there is no literal translation for the word *depression*. In Chinese culture it is more acceptable to somaticize emotional pain with expressions of physical discomfort such as chest pain or "heaviness of the heart." If health care providers fail to understand the cultural meaning of the symptom "heaviness of the heart," unnecessary, invasive, and costly tests might be performed to rule out cardiovascular disease. In some instances, clients might be unable to read or write in any language; thus, an assessment of the client's literacy level should precede the use of printed history forms or checklists.

Although there is wide variation in health history formats, most contain the following categories: *biographic data, reason for seeking care, present health or history of present illness, past history, family and social history,* and *review of systems.* This chapter will not cover a comprehensive overview of all data categories in a health history; it will present only those relative to the provision of culturally congruent and culturally competent nursing care.

Biographic Data and Source of History

In addition to the standard descriptive information about clients (name, address, phone, age, gender, and so forth), it is necessary to record who has furnished the data. Whereas this is usually the client, the source might be a relative or friend. Note whether an interpreter is used and indicate his or her relationship to the client. Be sure to document the *specific language* spoken by the client, e.g., Mandarin Chinese (compared with Cantonese Chinese or other dialects).

Although the biographic information might seem straightforward, several cultural variations in recording age are important to note. In some Asian cultures, an infant is considered to be one year old at birth. Among some South Vietnamese immigrants who migrated to the United States during the Vietnam War, there might be inaccuracies in the reported age. These inaccuracies occurred in response to U. S. immigration laws in the 1960s and 1970s, which attempted to limit the numbers of Southeast Asians entering the United States.

One of the first areas that you should assess is the client's cultural affiliation. With what cultural group(s) does the client report affiliation? Where was the client born? What is the **ethnohistory** of the client? Knowledge of the client's ethnohistory is important in determining his or her risk factors for genetic and acquired diseases and in understanding the client's cultural heritage. How many years have the client and his or her family lived in this country? If the client is a recent immigrant, ask him or her to describe what the migration experience was like.

Reason for Seeking Care

The *reason for seeking care* refers to a brief statement describing in clients' own words why they are visiting a health care provider. In the past, this statement has been called the *chief complaint,* a term that is now avoided because it focuses on illness rather than wellness and tends to label the person as a complainer. All symptoms are believed to have cultural meanings, and the nurse should realize that they are usually more than manifestations of a biologic reality.

Symptoms are defined as phenomena experienced by individuals that signify a departure from normal function, sensation, or appearance and that might include physical aberrations. By comparison, *signs* are objective abnormalities that the examiner can detect on physical examination or through laboratory testing. As individuals experience symptoms, they interpret them and react in ways that are congruent with their cultural norms. Symptoms cannot be attributed to another person; rather, individuals experience symptoms from their knowledge of bodily function and sociocultural interactions. Symptoms are perceived, recognized, labeled, reacted to, ritualized, and articulated in ways that make sense within the cultural worldview of the person experiencing them (Good & Good, 1980; Wenger, 1993).

Symptoms are defined according to the client's perception of the meaning attributed to the event. This perception must be considered in relation to other sociocultural factors and biologic knowledge. People develop culturally based explanatory models to explain how their illnesses work and what their symptoms mean. The search for cultural meaning in understanding symptoms involves a translation process that includes both the nurse's worldview and the client's. You need to assess the symptoms within the client's sociocultural and ethnohistorical context. It is important to use the same terms for symptoms that clients use. For example, if the client refers to "swelling" of the leg, refrain from medicalizing that to "edema." Knowledge of the cultural expression of symptoms will influence the decisions you make and will facilitate your ability to provide culturally congruent or culturally competent nursing care (Wenger, 1993).

Present and Past Illnesses

Table 3–1 provides an alphabetic listing of selected diseases and their increased or decreased prevalence among members of certain cultural groups. Accurate assessment and evaluation of the present and past illnesses requires knowledge of the biocultural aspects of acute and chronic diseases. The distribution of selected genetic traits and disorders prevalent among children from selected cultural groups is presented in Chapter 6, Transcultural Perspectives in the Nursing Care of Children.

Culture-Bound Syndromes

Although all illness might be culturally defined, the term **culture-bound syndromes** refers to disorders restricted to a particular culture or group of cultures because of certain psychosocial characteristics of those cultures. Culture-bound syndromes are often referred to as folk illnesses in which alterations of behavior and experience are prominent features. More than 200 culture-bound syndromes have been identified. For example, anorexia nervosa is believed to be a Western culture-bound syndrome because the condition is largely confined to Western cultures or to non-Western cultures undergoing the process of westernization, such as Japan. Culture-bound syndromes are thought to be illnesses created by personal, social, and cultural reactions to malfunctioning biologic or psychologic processes and can be understood only within defined contexts of meaning and social relationships (Kleinman, 1980). When you encounter clients with culture-bound syndromes, it is important to find out what they and other concerned individuals believe is happening. What prior efforts for help or cure have been tried? What were the results? It is impossible to produce a definitive list of all culture-bound syndromes, but Table 3–2 summarizes selected examples that are found in specific cultural groups. For a more comprehensive list of culture-

bound syndromes and descriptions of them, visit http://experts.about.com/c/c/cu/Culture-bound_syndrdome.htm.

Current Medications

In the health history you should note the name, dose, route of administration, schedule, frequency, purpose, and length of time of each medicine that has been taken. It is also important to note all prescription and over-the-counter medications, including herbs that clients might purchase or grow in home gardens. Because of cultural differences in people's perception of what substances are considered medicines, it is important to ask about specific items by name. For example, you should inquire about vitamins, birth control pills, aspirin, antacids, herbs, teas, inhalants, poultices, vaginal and rectal suppositories, ointments, and any other items taken by the client for therapeutic purposes.

PLANT-DERIVED DRUGS

In particular, it is important to be aware of the widespread use of **plant-derived medications** among various cultures (Table 3–3). Since prehistoric times, people have attempted to identify plants, marine organisms, arthropods, animals, and minerals with healing properties. According the World Health Organization, 80% of people residing in less developed countries use traditional medicine, including medicinal plants, for their major primary health care needs. Although the exact number of plants being used medicinally worldwide is unknown, approximately 5% of the 250,000 known species of plants have ever been studied for bioactive compounds that might have healing effects. (It is estimated that approximately 75% of the plant-derived drugs currently used in the United States and Canada were discovered as a result of chemical studies designed to isolate the active ingredients responsible for the use of the plants in traditional medicine. These drugs are derived from approximately 90 of the 250,000 known species of plants on this planet.) The global market for plant-derived drugs is worth an estimated $18 billion and is projected to grow to $26 billion by 2011.

TABLE 3-1 *Biocultural Aspects of Disease*

Disease	Remarks
Alcoholism	Indians have double the rate of Whites; lower tolerance to alcohol among Chinese and Japanese North Americans
Anemia	High incidence among Vietnamese because of the presence of infestations among immigrants and low iron diets; low hemoglobin and malnutrition found among 18.2% of Native North Americans, 32.7% of Blacks, 14.6% of Hispanics, and 10.4% of White children under 5 years of age
Arthritis	Increased incidence among Native North Americans Blackfoot 1.4% Pima 1.8% Chippewa 6.8%
Asthma	Six times greater for Native North American infants <1 year; same as general population for Native North Americans aged 1–44 years
Bronchitis	Six times greater for Native North American infants <1 year; same as general population for Native North Americans aged 1–44 years. Main cause of death for Aboriginal Canadian infants in the postnatal period
Cancer	Nasopharyngeal: high among Chinese North Americans and Native Americans Breast: Black women 1 1/2 times more likely than White Colorectal: Blacks 40% higher than Whites Esophageal: No. 2 cause of death for Black men aged 35–54 years *Incidence:* White men 3.5/100,000 Black men 13.3/100,000 Liver: Highest among all ethnic groups are Filipino Hawaiians Latinos have twice the rate of Whites Stomach: Black men twice as likely as White men; low among Filipinos Cervical: 120% higher in Black women than in White women Mexican American and Puerto Rican women 2–3 times higher than Whites Uterine: 53% lower in Black women than White women Prostate: Black men have highest incidence of all groups Most prevalent cancer among Native North Americans: biliary, nasopharyngeal, testicular, cervical, renal, and thyroid (females) cancer Lung cancer among Navajo uranium miners 85 times higher than among White miners Most prevalent cancer among Japanese North Americans: esophageal, stomach, liver, and biliary cancer Among Chinese North Americans, there is a higher incidence of nasopharyngeal and liver cancer than among the general population
Cholecystitis	*Incidence:* Whites 0.3% Puerto Ricans 2.1% Native Americans 2.2% Chinese 2.6%
Colitis	High incidence among Japanese North Americans
Diabetes mellitus	Three times as prevalent among Filipino North Americans as Whites; higher among Hispanics than Blacks or Whites

(Continued on following page)

TABLE 3-1 *Biocultural Aspects of Disease* (continued)

Disease	Remarks
	Death rate is 3–4 times as high among Native North Americans aged 25–34 years, especially those in the West such as Utes, Pimas, and Papagos
	Complications
	Amputations: Twice as high among Native North Americans vs. general U.S. population
	Renal failure: 20 times as high as general U.S. population, with tribal variation, e.g., Utes have 43 times higher incidence
G-6-PD deficiency	Present among 30% of Black males
Influenza	Increased death rate among Native Americans aged 45+
Ischemic heart disease	Responsible for 32% of heart-related causes of death among Native Americans; Blacks have higher mortality rates than all other groups
Lactose intolerance	Present among 66% of Hispanic women; increased incidence among Blacks and Chinese
Myocardial infarction	Leading cause of heart disease in Native Americans, accounting for 43% of death resulting from heart disease; low incidence among Japanese Americans
Otitis media	7.9% incidence among school-aged Navajo children versus 0.5% in Whites
	Up to 1/3 of Eskimo children <2 years have chronic otitis media
	Increased incidence among bottle-fed Native Americans and Eskimo infants
Pneumonia	Increased death rate among Native North Americans aged 45+
Psoriasis	Affects 2–5% of Whites but <1% of Blacks; high among Japanese Americans
Renal disease	Lower incidence among Japanese North Americans
Sickle cell anemia	Increased incidence among Blacks
Trachoma	Increased incidence among Native North Americans and Eskimo children (3 to 8 times greater than general population)
Tuberculosis	Highest among Asian Americans & Pacific Islanders;
	Increased incidence among Native North Americans
	Apache 2.0%
	Sioux 3.2%
	Navajo 4.6%
	Aboriginals living on Canadian reserves are 10 times more likely to have TB than non-Aboriginal Canadians
	Non-Whites 5.2 times more than Whites
Ulcers	Decreased incidence among Japanese North Americans

Table based on data accessed on January 1, 2007, at American Cancer Society (www.cancer.org); American Diabetes Association (www.diabetes.org); American Heart Association (www. americanheart.org); Health Canada (http://www.hc-sc.gc.ca/fnih-spni/pubs/gen/stats_profil_e.html); Office of Minority Health (http://www.omhrc.gov/omh/whatsnew/2pgwhatsnew/special128a.htm); National Center for Health Statistics (http://www.cdc.gov/nchs); National Center on Minority Health & Health Disparities, National Institutes of Health (ncmhd.nihgov); Spotlight on Minority Health (http://www.cdc.gov/omh/populations/populations.htm)

TABLE 3-2 *Selected Culture-Bound Syndromes*

Group	Disorder	Remarks
Blacks, Haitians	Blackout	Collapse, dizziness, inability to move
	Low blood	Not enough blood or weakness of the blood that is often treated with diet
	High blood	Blood that is too rich in certain things because of the ingestion of too much red meat or rich foods
	Thin blood	Occurs in women, children, and old people; renders the individual more susceptible to illness in general
	Diseases of hex, withchcraft, or conjuring	Sense of being doomed by spell; gastrointestinal symptoms, e.g., vomiting; hallucinations; part of voodoo beliefs
Chinese/Southeast Asians	*Koro*	Intense anxiety that penis is retracting into body
Greeks	Hysteria	Bizarre complaints and behavior because the uterus leaves the pelvis for another part of the body
Hispanics	*Empacho*	Food forms into a ball and clings to the stomach or intestines, causing pain and cramping
	Fatigue	Asthma-like symptoms
	Mal ojo, "evil eye"	Fitful sleep, crying, diarrhea in children caused by a stranger's attention; sudden onset
	Pasmo	Paralysis-like symptoms of face or limbs; prevented or relieved by massage
	Susto	Anxiety, trembling, phobias from sudden fright
Japanese	*Wagamama*	Apathetic childish behavior with emotional outbursts
Korean	*Hwa-byung*	Multiple somatic and psychologic symptoms; "pushing up" sensation of chest; palpitations, flushing, headache, "epigastric mass," dysphoria, anxiety, irritability, and difficulty concentrating; mostly afflicts married women
Native Americans	Ghost	Terror, hallucinations, sense of danger
North India Indians	Ghost	Death from fever and illness in children; convulsions, delirious speech (or incessant crying in infants); choking, difficulty breathing; based on Hindu religious beliefs and curing practices
Whites	Anorexia nervosa	Excessive preoccupation with thinness; self-imposed starvation
	Bulimia	Gross overeating and then vomiting or fasting

Currently respiratory problems such as asthma represent the largest medical application of plant-derived drugs, accounting for 24% of total sales of plant-derived medicines. In the future, cancer treatment is expected to become the largest application of plant-derived drugs, cap-turing 24% of the market by 2011 (BCC Research, 2006; Ma et al., 2005) (Figure 3–1).

Many of the active ingredients in plant-derived drugs or herbs are unknown and remain largely unregulated by government agencies, except for customs officials who make efforts to

TABLE 3-3 *Herbal Remedies*	

Aloe Vera

Aloe Vera

Source	Leaf of *Aloe barbadensis* Mill. (family Liliaceae)
Action	Topical analgesic, anti-inflammatory, antibacterial, and antifungal agent
Traditional Uses	Applied topically for treatment of inflammation, minor burns, sunburn, cuts, bruises, and abrasions Orally, aloe juice was used for gastrointestinal upset, arthritis, diabetes mellitus, and gastric ulcers
Current Uses	Promotes wound healing in soft tissue injuries Prevents wound pain by inhibiting the action of the pain-producing agent bradykinin May prevent progression of skin damage from electrical burns and frostbite Prevention of wound infection because of its antibacterial and antifungal properties Used in a wide variety of ointments, creams, lotions, and shampoos
Dosage	Apply topically as needed
Warnings	Rarely, skin rash follows topical application May cause burning if applied after removal of acne scars To avoid deterioration of active ingredients, use the fresh gel and avoid diluted extracts When taken internally as aloe latex, it causes intestinal cramping and may lead to ulcers and bowel irritation

Dong-Quai (Chinese Angelica)

Angelica sinensis

Source	Dried root of a member of the parsley family
Action	Smooth muscle relaxant; antispasmodic
Traditional Uses	A highly regarded herb in Chinese medicine, dong-quai means "proper order"; used to suppress menstruation, cleanse the blood, and promote harmony in the body In the West, used to regulate menstrual periods, symptoms of menopause, and premenstrual syndrome (PMS)
Current Uses	Relaxes uterine muscle and improves circulation to the uterus. Improves circulation and lowers blood pressure; reduces inflammation, pains, and spasm; increases number of red blood cells and platelets. Protects liver from toxins
Dosage	5–12 g (1 to 3 teaspoons) daily
Warnings	Contraindicated for pregnant and breast-feeding women and persons with abdominal distention or diarrhea Large doses may cause contact dermatitis and photodermatitis

(Continued on following page)

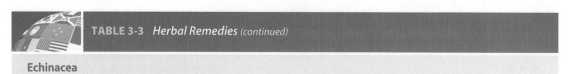

TABLE 3-3   *Herbal Remedies* (continued)

Echinacea

Echinacea angustifolia, E. pallida, E. pururea

Source	Member of the daisy family; also known as purple coneflower
Action	Reduces cold symptoms
Traditional Uses	Used by Native Americans in poultices, mouthwashes, and teas for colds, cancer, and other disorders Some herbalists consider it a blood purifier and an aid to fighting infections
Current Uses	Enhances the immune system by stimulating the production of white blood cells needed to fight infection or cancer
Dosage	Follow directions on label; needed at onset of symptoms; usually taken for no longer than 2 weeks
Warnings	Contraindicated for pregnant or breast-feeding women, children, and those who are allergic to ragweed. Not recommended for people with severely compromised immune systems such as those with HIV/AIDS, tuberculosis, or multiple sclerosis Look for reputable suppliers, because a high percentage of the root currently marketed is adulterated with less expensive inactive substitutes

Evening Primrose Oil

Oenothera biennis

Source	Seeds of the wildflower evening primrose
Action	Antihypertensive, immunostimulant, weight reduction
Traditional Uses	Used by Native Americans for food; in eastern North America, used to treat obesity and hemorrhoids; new settlers to North America used the plant for gastrointestinal upsets and sore throats
Current Uses	Used as a dietary supplement for essential fatty acids; believed to help asthma, migraine headaches, inflammations, PMS, diabetes mellitus, and arthritis; also believed to lower blood pressure and lower cholesterol, slow the progression of multiple sclerosis, promote weight loss without dieting, alleviate hangovers, and moisturize dry eyes, brittle hair, and fingernails
Dosage	Follow directions on label; will take at least 1 month to experience benefits
Warnings	Side effects include occasional reports of headache, nausea, and abdominal discomfort; not recommended for children Some capsules may be altered with other types of oil such as soy or safflower

Ginger

Current Uses	Effective in reducing morning sickness and postoperative nausea for some people; used in China to treat first- and second-degree burns
Dosage	Boil 1 oz dried ginger root in 1 cup water for 15 to 20 minutes Follow label directions on ginger supplements

(Continued on following page)

TABLE 3-3   *Herbal Remedies* (continued)

Warning	Large doses may cause central nervous system depression and cardiac arrhythmias
	Side effects include heartburn
	Contraindicated in the presence of gallbladder disease

Ginkgo

Ginkgo biloba

Source	Extract from leaves of the ginkgo tree, a living fossil, believed to be more than 200 million years old
Action	Antioxidant; improves blood circulation
Traditional Uses	Used in China since the 15th century for cough, asthma, diarrhea, skin lesions, and removal of freckles
Current Uses	Promotes vasodilation and improves circulation of blood; may be an effective free radical scavenger or antioxidant; improves short-term memory, attention span, and mood in early stages of Alzheimer's disease by improving oxygen metabolism in the brain
Dosage	Range: 120–160 mg TID
	May take 6–8 weeks before results are evident
Warnings	Large doses may cause irritability, restlessness, diarrhea, nausea, and vomiting
	Some people (who are also sensitive to poison ivy) are unable to tolerate even low doses
	Contraindicated for women who are pregnant or breast-feeding
	Contraindicated for persons with clotting disorders
	Not recommended for children

Ginseng (American and Asian)

Panax quinquefolius (American)

Panax ginseng (Asian)

Source	Dried root of several species of the genus *Panax* of the family Aralaceae
Action	Tonic
Traditional Uses	Treatment of anemia, atherosclerosis, edema, ulcers, hypertension, influenza, colds, inflammation, and disorders of the immune system (American)
	In traditional China, used for treatment of shock, diaphoresis, dyspnea, fever, thirst, irritability, diarrhea, vomiting, abdominal distention, anorexia, and impotence; considered a "heat-raising" tonic for the blood and circulatory system (Asian)
Current Uses	Used to enhance sexual experience and treat impotence, though there is no current research to support this claim (American)
	In Germany may be labeled as a tonic to treat fatigue, reduced work capacity. In some parts of Asia, used for lack of concentration and for convalescence (Asian)
	Improved sense of well-being (Asian)

(Continued on following page)

TABLE 3-3 *Herbal Remedies* (continued)

Dosage	American: Follow directions on label Asian: 100 mg BID
Warnings	American: May cause headaches, insomnia, anxiety, breast tenderness, rashes, asthma attacks, hypertension, cardiac arrhythmias, and postmenopausal uterine hemorrhage Should be used with caution for the following conditions: pregnancy, insomnia, hay fever, fibrocystic breasts, asthma, emphysema, hypertension, clotting disorders, and diabetes mellitus Asian: Same as American

Gotu Kola

Centella asiatica

Source	Dried and powdered leaves of a member of the parsley family
Action	Improves memory
Traditional Uses	In ancient India, considered a rejuvenating herb that increases intelligence, longevity, and memory while slowing the aging process In China, used as a tea for colds and for lung and urinary tract infections, and topically for snakebite, wounds, and shingles Recommended for treatment of mental disorders, hypertension, abscesses, rheumatism, fever, ulcers, skin lesions, and jaundice
Current Uses	Acceleration of wound healing, diuretic, treatment of phlebitis
Dosage	Follow directions on label; lower dose needed for children and older adults
Warnings	Sides effects include headaches and skin rash Contraindicated for pregnant or breast-feeding women and children younger than 2 years Contraindicated when using tranquilizers or sedatives

Saint John's Wort

Hypericum perforatum

Source	Tea made from the leaves and flowering tops of the perennial *Hypericum perforatum*, which is particularly abundant on June 24th, the feast of St. John the Baptist
Action	Antidepressant
Traditional Uses	Used in 1st-century Greece for wound healing and menstrual disorders, and as a diuretic In 19th-century North America, used for its astringent, wound healing, diuretic, and mild sedative effects
Current Uses	Treatment of mild to moderate depression; effects are linked to various substances that act as monoamine oxidase (MAO) inhibitors
Dosage	300 mg daily

(Continued on following page)

TABLE 3-3 *Herbal Remedies* (continued)

Warnings	Fair-skinned people may experience urticaria or vesicular skin lesions upon exposure to sunlight
	Reduces effectiveness of some anticancer agents
	Clinical manifestations of depression should be considered seriously
	Encourage client to see a mental health care provider
Valerian	
Valeriana officinalis	
Source	Dried rhizome and roots of the tall perennial *Valeriana officinalis*
Action	Mild tranquilizer and sedative
Traditional Uses	Used by the ancient Greeks for the treatment of epilepsy and menstrual disorders, and as a diuretic
	Used by 17th- and 18th-century Europeans as an antispasmodic and sedative
	Listed as an official remedy in the *United States Pharmacopoeia* from 1820 to 1936
Current Uses	Used as a mild tranquilizer and sedative; relieves muscle spasms
	Especially effective for insomniac persons and older adults
Dosage	300–400 mg daily; take 1 hour before bedtime as a sleeping aid
Warnings	Reported side effects include headache, gastrointestinal upset, and excitability
	Signs of overdose include severe headache, restlessness, nausea, morning grogginess, or blurred vision
	Must not be taken in combination with other tranquilizers or sedatives
	Client should be cautioned against operating a motor vehicle after ingesting

Table based on data accessed on January 1, 2007, at The Alternative Medicine Home Page (http://www.pitt.edu/~cbw/herb.html); MedlinePlus Herbal Medicine (www.nlm.nih.gov/medlineplus/herbalmedicine.html); National Center for Complementary and Alternative Medicine (http://www.nccam.gov); Sloan-Kettering: About Herbs, Botanicals and Other Products (http://www.mskcc.org/mskcc/html/11570.cfm).

control the flow of illegal drugs. Fresh or dried herbs are usually brewed into a tea, with the dosage adjusted according to the chronicity or acuteness of the illness, age, and size of the patient. Traditional Chinese medicine usually is used only as long as symptoms persist. Some patients extend the same logic to Western biomedicine. For example, they might stop taking an antibiotic as soon as the symptoms subside instead of completing the course of treatment for the prescribed length of time. Be sure to consider the potential interaction of herbs with Western biomedicines. The root of the shrub *ginseng*, for example, is widely used for the treatment of arthritis, back and leg pains, and sores. Because ginseng is known to potentiate the action of some antihypertensive drugs, you must ask the patient whether he or she is experiencing side effects or toxicity, and monitor blood pressure frequently. It might be necessary to withhold doses of the prescribed antihypertensive medicine if the blood pressure is low or to ask the client to discontinue or reduce the strength of the ginseng. When assessing the patient's use of traditional Chinese medicine, you should be aware that some Chinese North Americans who use herbs topically do not consider them to be drugs. For further information about herbs, the nurse should ask the patient and family, consult with an herbalist, search for reputable sources on

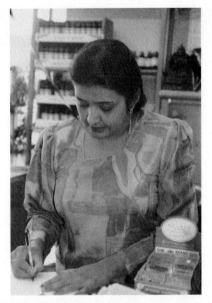

FIGURE 3-1. Shopkeeper of Indian ancestry sells herbal remedies used in Ayurvedic healing in a neighborhood store that attracts recent immigrants from India. People from diverse backgrounds who embrace Ayurvedic medicine also patronize the store, which sells prepackaged herbal remedies and dried herbs used to brew teas.

the Internet; or check reference books on herbal remedies.

Dosage Modifications

As indicated in Table 3–4, there is growing evidence-based data indicating that modifications in dosages of some drugs should be made for members of selected racial and ethnic groups. It might be difficult to develop ethnic-specific norms for drug dosages because of intermarriage, individual differences (e.g., weight and body fat index), and related factors. It is possible, however, to alert nurses to the variations that occur in side effects, adverse reactions, and toxicity so that clients from diverse cultural backgrounds can be monitored for possible untoward clinical manifestations.

MEDICATION ADMINISTRATION

If the medication prescribed, its route of administration, or the substances given with it conflict

with clients' adherence to the yin/yang, hot/cold, or other belief system, it is unlikely that they will follow your advice concerning the medication. The nurse should be aware that some clients of Latino, Middle Eastern, and Asian heritage believe that it is important to take medicine with certain beverages or foods to provide the necessary balance for health. If clients give cues that they are uncomfortable with the beverage or food being used in the health care setting, discuss alternatives. For example, in most health care facilities, medications are given with cold water, but they could be given with hot water, tea, coffee, or a similar beverage if the client believes that such a beverage would promote healing. Some Mexican Americans believe that grapefruit juice has healing properties, so you might contact the dietary department to ensure that this juice is available when medications are administered. If the cultural healing beliefs and practices of the client are incorporated into medication administration, there is a higher probability that the client will believe in the healing properties of the drugs and will continue to take them as prescribed after discharge.

Family and Social History

In addition to diagramming a family tree to identify familial relationships and the presence of disease conditions among those related to the client, you should assess the broader socioeconomic factors influencing the client. The health history should include in-depth data pertaining to the client's family and/or close social friends, including identification of *key decision makers*. Although personal financial information is often a sensitive topic, it is important to determine the overall economic factors that influence a client. For example, regardless of race or ethnicity, people from lower socioeconomic categories have poorer health and shorter lives. Unfortunately, there is a disproportionately high level of poverty among Blacks, Latinos/Latinas, First Nation People of Canada, and North American Indians/Alaska Natives. Economic factors have

TABLE 3-4 *Cultural Differences in Response to Drugs*

Drug Category	Remarks
Arab Americans	
Antiarrhythmics	Some may need lower dosage
Antihypertensives	Some may need lower dosage
Neuroleptics	Some may need lower dosage
Opioids	Some may require higher dosage because of diminished ability to metabolize codeine to morphine
Psychotropics	Some may need lower dosage
Asian/Pacific Islanders	
Be aware that drugs are part of the yin/yang belief system embraced by some Asian Americans and that herbal remedies may be used in addition to prescription drugs Be sure to consider lower body weight and mass when calculating doses	
Narcotic analgesics	Chinese may be less sensitive to the respiratory depressant and hypotensive effects of morphine but more likely to experience nausea; Chinese have a significantly higher clearance of morphine
Antihypertensives	Respond best to calcium antagonists
Neuroleptics	Require lower dose
Psychotropics	Require lower dose, sometimes as little as half the normal dose for tricyclic antidepressants (TCAs) and lithium
Fat-soluble drugs	On average, Asian Americans have a lower percentage of body fat, so dosage adjustments must be made for fat-soluble vitamins and other drugs, e.g., vitamin K used to reverse the anticoagulant effect of Coumadin (warfarin); consider dietary intake of vitamins when calculating doses
Blacks	
Analgesics	Despite decreased sensitivity to pain-relieving therapeutic action of drugs, there are increased gastrointestinal side effects, especially with acetaminophen
Antihypertensives	Respond best to treatment with a single drug (versus combined antihypertensive therapy) Research suggests favorable response to diuretics, calcium antagonists, and alpha-blockers Less responsive to beta-blockers (e.g., propranolol) and angiotensin-converting enzyme (ACE) inhibitors (e.g., enalapril, imidapril) Increased side effects such as mood response (e.g., depression) to thiazides (e.g., hydrochlorothiazide), which may explain reluctance to take drug as prescribed There is little justification to use racial profiling to avoid drug classes. Current research is focusing on differences in the causes of hypertension in Blacks to explain differences in drug responses
Mydriatics	Less dilation occurs with dark-colored eyes
Psychotropics	Increased extrapyramidal side effects with TCAs such as haloperidol

(Continued on following page)

TABLE 3-4   *Cultural Differences in Response to Drugs* (continued)

Drug Category	Remarks
Steroids	When methylprednisolone is used for immunosuppression in renal transplant patients, there is increased toxicity such as steroid-associated diabetes; although Blacks are four times as likely to develop end-stage renal disease as Whites, they have the poorest long-term graft survival of any ethnic group
Tranquilizers	15–20% are poor metabolizers of Valium (diazepam)

Hispanics

Drug Category	Remarks
Psychotropics	May require lower dosage and experience higher incidence of side effects with TCAs

Greeks, Italians, and others of Mediterranean Descent with G-6-PD Deficiency

Drug Category	Remarks
Oxidating drugs	The following drugs may precipitate a hemolytic crisis: primaquine, quinidine, thiazolsulfone, furazolidone, haloperidol, nitrofural, naphthalene, toluidine blue, phenylhydrazine, chloramphenicol, aspirin

Jewish North Americans (Ashkenazi)

Drug Category	Remarks
Psychotropics	Agranulocytosis develops in 20% when clozapine is used to treat schizophrenia; thus, the granulocyte count should be checked before the drug is administered

Native North Americans

Drug Category	Remarks
Muscle relaxants	Alaskan Eskimos may experience prolonged muscle paralysis and an inability to breathe without mechanical ventilation for several hours postoperatively when succinylcholine has been administered in surgery

Table based partially on data from
Bloche, M. G. (2006). Race, money, and medicines. *The Journal of Law, Medicine, & Ethics, 34*(3), 555–558.
Davies, S. (2006). Pharmacogenetics, pharmacogenomics and personalized medicine: Are we there yet? *Hematology,* 2006, 111–117.
Harty, L., Johnson, K., & Power, A. (2006). Race and ethnicity in the era of emerging pharmacogenomics. *Journal of Clinical Pharmacology, 46,* 405–407.
Lin, K., Anderson, D., & Poland, R. (1995). Ethnicity and psychopharmacology: Bridging the gap. *Psychiatric Clinics of North America, 18*(3), 635–647.
Ma, J. K., Chikwamba, R., Sparrow, P., Fischer, R., Mahoney, R., & Twyman, R. M. (2005). Plant-derived pharmaceuticals—the road forward. *Trends in Plant Science, 10*(12), 580–585.
Mathis, A. S., & Knipp, G. T. (2002). Do sex and ethnicity influence drug pharmacokinetics in solid organ transplantation? *Graft, 5*(50), 294–302.
Overfield, T. (1995). *Biologic variation in health and illness.* New York: CRC Press.
Schultz, J. (2003). FDA guidelines on race and ethnicity: Obstacle or remedy? *Journal of the National Cancer Institute, 95*(6), 425–426.
Zhou, H. H., Sheller, J. R., Nu, H., Wood, M., & Wood, A. J. J. (1993). Ethnic differences in response to morphine. *Clinical Pharmacology and Therapeutics, 54*(3), 507–513.

been identified as causes of less favorable outcomes among clients with cancer. Research suggests that this is caused by a lack of health insurance and/or diminished access to health care services, both of which contribute to a situation in which less affluent clients receive diagnosis and treatment later in the course of the disease. See Appendix A for suggested interview questions aimed at eliciting information about family and social history.

Review of Systems

The purposes of the review of systems are to evaluate the past and present health state of each body system, to provide an opportunity for the client to report symptoms not previously stated, and to evaluate health promotion practices. Knowledge of current research on diseases prevalent in specific ethnic and racial groups might be useful in asking appropriate questions in the review of systems. For example, if the nurse is gathering review of systems information from a middle-aged African-American man, it is useful to know that there is a statistically higher incidence of hypertension, sickle cell anemia, and diabetes in this group than in counterparts from other racial and ethnic groups. This will assist in customizing the review of systems questions and ensuring that symptoms of disease specific to the client's ethnic or racial heritage are included.

Transcultural Perspectives on the Physical Examination

The purpose of this discussion is to identify selected **biocultural variations** that nurses sometimes encounter when conducting the physical examination of clients from different cultural backgrounds. Accurate assessment and

evaluation of clients require knowledge of normal biocultural variations among healthy members of selected populations. You must also possess assessment skills that will enable you to recognize variations that occur in illness. The following remarks are intended to be illustrative, not exhaustive. As more research on biocultural variations is conducted, undoubtedly there will be additions and perhaps some modifications. The author would like to note that the data in the following section is evidence-based and reflects the findings of classic studies that have been conducted over a period of years. The work of Dr. Theresa Overfield, a renowned nurse–anthropologist who has published extensively on biological variations in health and illness, has been cited frequently in the discussion of biocultural variations that follows.

Biocultural Variations in Measurements

Height

Summarized in Table 3–5 are average heights for men and women from selected cultural groups that have been studied. In all groups, *height* increases up to 1.5 inches as socioeconomic status improves. First-generation immigrants might be up to 1.5 inches taller than their counterparts in the country of origin because of (1) better nutrition and (2) decreased interference with growth by infectious diseases. During the past decade, the overall height of men from the

TABLE 3-5 *Biocultural Variations in Height for Selected Groups*

Height (in inches) for all groups

All groups of men	White American	African American	Mexican American	Asian
69.1	69.1	69.2	67.2	65.7
All groups of women				
63.7	63.8	63.8	61.8	60.3

Table developed using data from Overfield, T. (1995). *Biologic variation in health and illness.* New York: CRC Press.

United States increased by 0.7 inches, whereas women from the United States grew an average of 0.5 inches taller (Overfield, 1995).

Body Proportions

Biocultural variations are found in the *body proportions* of individuals, largely because of differences in bone length. In examining sitting/standing height ratios, you will notice that Blacks of both genders have longer legs and shorter trunks than Whites. Because proportionately most of the weight is in the trunk, White men appear more obese than their Black counterparts. The reverse is true of women. Clients of Asian heritage are markedly shorter, weigh less, and have smaller body frames than their White counterparts and/or the overall population (Overfield, 1995).

Weight

Biocultural differences exist in the amount of body fat and the distribution of fat throughout the body. As a general rule, people from the lower socioeconomic class are more obese than those from the middle class, who are more obese than members of the upper class. On average, Black men weigh less than their White counterparts throughout adulthood (166.1 pounds versus 170.6 pounds). The opposite is true of women. Black women are consistently heavier than White women at every age (149.6 pounds versus 137 pounds). Between the ages of 35 to 64 years, Black women weigh on average 20 pounds more than White women. Mexican Americans weigh more in relation to height than non-Hispanic Whites because of differences in truncal fat patterns. Most differences in the amount of body fat are related to socioeconomic factors, which in turn influence nutrition and exposure to communicable diseases. Around the world, people in cold climates tend to have more body fat, whereas those residing in warmer areas have less. Blacks have smaller skinfold thicknesses on their trunks and arms than do their White counterparts. Bottle-fed infants are heavier on average than those who are breast-fed, although their lengths are similar (Overfield, 1995).

Biocultural Variations in Vital Signs

Although the average pulse rate is comparable across cultures, there are racial and gender differences in *blood pressure*. Black men have lower systolic blood pressures than their White counterparts from ages 18 to 34, but between the ages of 35 and 64 it reverses: Blacks have an average systolic blood pressure of 5 mm Hg higher. After age 65 there is no difference between the two races. Black women have a higher average systolic blood pressure than their White counterparts at every age. After age 45, the average blood pressure of Black women might be as much as 16 mm Hg higher than that of White women in the same age group (Overfield, 1995).

Biocultural Variations in General Appearance

In assessing general appearance, you should survey the person's entire body. You will want to note the general health state and any obvious physical characteristics and readily apparent biologic features unique to the individual. In assessing the client's general appearance, you should consider four areas: physical appearance, body structure, mobility, and behavior. *Physical appearance* includes age, gender, level of consciousness, facial features, and skin color (evenness of color tone, pigmentation, intactness, presence of lesions or other abnormalities). *Body structure* includes stature, nutrition, symmetry, posture, position, and overall body build or contour. *Mobility* includes gait and range of motion. *Behavior* includes facial expression, mood and affect, fluency of speech, ability to communicate ideas, appropriateness of word choice, grooming, and attire or dress (Jarvis, 2004).

In assessing a client's hygiene, it is useful to ask about typical bathing habits and customary use of various hygiene-related products. People in most cultures in the United States and Canada make a great effort to disguise their natural body odors by bathing frequently, using douches, or applying antiperspirants, colognes, and/or perfumes with scents that are deemed to be desirable. Ironically, some colognes and perfumes such as those with musk oil are marketed in the United States and Canada because of their more "natural" odor, which is alleged to give the wearer more sex appeal. Recent immigrants from some arid nations where water is scarce might bathe less frequently than those from countries where water is more abundant.

Biocultural Variations in Skin

An accurate and comprehensive examination of the skin of clients from culturally diverse backgrounds requires that you possess knowledge of biocultural variations and skill in recognizing color changes, some of which might be subtle. Awareness of normal biocultural differences and the ability to recognize the unique clinical manifestations of disease are developed over time as you gain experience with clients having various skin colors.

The assessment of a client's skin is subjective and is highly dependent on your observational skill, ability to recognize subtle color changes, and repeated exposure to individuals having various gradations of skin color. *Melanin* is responsible for the various colors and tones of skin observed in different people. Melanin protects the skin against harmful ultraviolet rays—a genetic advantage accounting for the lower incidence of skin cancer among darkly pigmented Black and Native North American clients.

Normal skin color ranges widely. Some health care practitioners have made attempts to describe the variations by labeling their observations with some of the following adjectives: *copper, olive, tan,* and various shades of *brown (light, medium, and dark)*. In observing pallor in clients, the term *ashen* is sometimes used. Of most clinical significance, particularly for clients whose health condition might be linked to changes in skin color, is your ability to establish a reliable description of a baseline color and subsequently to recognize when variations occur in the same individual.

Mongolian Spots

Mongolian spots are irregular areas of deep blue pigmentation, are usually located in the sacral and gluteal areas but sometimes occur on the abdomen, thighs, shoulders, or arms. During embryonic development, the melanocytes originate near the embryonic nervous system in the neural crest. They then migrate into the fetal epidermis. Mongolian spots consist of embryonic pigment that has been left behind in the epidermal layer during fetal development. The result looks like a bluish discoloration of the skin.

Mongolian spots are a normal variation in children of African, Asian, or Latin descent. By adulthood, these spots become lighter but usually remain visible. Mongolian spots are present in 90% of Blacks, 80% of Asians and Native North Americans, and 9% of Whites (Overfield, 1995). If you are unfamiliar with Mongolian spots, it is important to exercise caution so as not to confuse them with bruises. Recognition of this normal variation is particularly important when you are dealing with children who might be erroneously identified as victims of child abuse, causing much anguish to the parents or guardians.

Vitiligo

Vitiligo, a condition in which the melanocytes become nonfunctional in some areas of the skin, is characterized by unpigmented skin patches. Vitiligo affects an estimated 2–4 million Americans, primarily dark-skinned individuals. Clients with vitiligo also have a statistically higher-than-normal risk for pernicious anemia, diabetes mellitus, and hyperthyroidism. These factors are believed to reflect an underlying genetic abnormality. There are numerous online sites with information about vitiligo including Vitiligo Support International (www.vitilgosupport.org) and the National Vitiligo Foundation (www.nvfi.org).

Hyperpigmentation

Other areas of the skin affected by hormones and, in some cases, differing for people from certain ethnic backgrounds are the sexual skin areas, such as the nipples, areola, scrotum, and labia majora. In general, these areas are darker than other parts of the skin in both adults and children, especially among African-American and Asian clients. When assessing these skin surfaces on dark-skinned clients, you must observe carefully for erythema, rashes, and other abnormalities because the darker color might mask their presence.

Cyanosis

Cyanosis is the most difficult clinical sign to observe in darkly pigmented persons. Because peripheral vasoconstriction can prevent cyanosis, you need to be attentive to environmental conditions such as air conditioning, mist tents, and other factors that might lower the room temperature and thus cause vasoconstriction. For the client to manifest clinical evidence of cyanosis, the blood must contain 5 g of reduced hemoglobin in 1.5 g of methemoglobin per 100 mL of blood (Overfield, 1995).

Given that most conditions causing cyanosis also cause decreased oxygenation of the brain, other clinical symptoms, such as changes in the level of consciousness, will be evident. Cyanosis usually is accompanied by increased respiratory rate, use of accessory muscles of respiration, nasal flaring, and other manifestations of respiratory distress. You must exercise caution when assessing persons of Mediterranean descent for cyanosis because their circumoral region is normally dark blue.

Jaundice

In both light- and dark-skinned clients, **jaundice** is best observed in the sclera. When examining culturally diverse individuals, exercise caution to avoid confusing other forms of pigmentation with jaundice. Many darkly pigmented people, e.g., African Americans, Filipinos, and others, have heavy deposits of subconjunctival fat that contains high levels of carotene in sufficient quantities to mimic jaundice. The fatty deposits become denser as the distance from the cornea increases. The portion of the sclera that is revealed naturally by the palpebral fissure is the best place to accurately assess color. If the palate does not have heavy melanin pigmentation, jaundice can be detected there in the early stages (i.e., when the serum bilirubin level is 2 to 4 mg/100 mL). The absence of a yellowish tint of the palate when the sclerae are yellow indicates carotene pigmentation of the sclerae rather than jaundice. Light- or clay-colored stools and dark golden urine often accompany jaundice in both light- and dark-skinned clients. If you are to distinguish between carotenemia and jaundice, it will be necessary to inspect the posterior portion of the hard palate using bright daylight or good artificial lighting (Overfield, 1995).

Pallor

When assessing for **pallor** in darkly pigmented clients, you might experience difficulty because the underlying red tones are absent. This is significant because these red tones are responsible for giving brown or black skin its luster. The brown-skinned individual will manifest pallor with a more yellowish brown color, and the black-skinned person will appear ashen or gray. Generalized pallor can be observed in the mucous membranes, lips, and nail beds. The palpebrae, conjunctivae, and nail beds are preferred sites for assessing the pallor of anemia. When inspecting the conjunctiva, you should lower the lid sufficiently so you can see the conjunctiva near the inner and outer canthi. The coloration is often lighter near the inner canthus.

In addition to changes seen on skin assessment, the pallor of impending shock is accompanied by other clinical manifestations, such as increasing pulse rate, oliguria, apprehension, and restlessness. Anemia, particularly chronic iron-deficiency anemia, might be manifested by the characteristic "spoon" nails, which have a concave shape. A lemon-yellow tint of the face and slightly yellow sclerae accompany pernicious anemia, which is also manifested by neurologic deficits and a red, painful tongue. Also, fatigue, exertional dyspnea, rapid pulse, dizziness, and impaired mental function accompany the most severe anemia (Overfield, 1995).

Erythema

You might find that it is difficult to assess **erythema** (redness) in darkly pigmented clients. Erythema is frequently associated with localized inflammation and is characterized by increased skin temperature. The degree of redness is determined by the quantity of blood in the subpapillary plexus, whereas the warmth of the skin is related to the rate of blood flow through the blood vessels. In the assessment of inflammation in dark-skinned clients, it is often necessary to palpate the skin for increased warmth, tautness, or tightly pulled surfaces that might indicate edema, and hardening of deep tissues or blood vessels. You will find that the dorsal surfaces of your fingers will be the most sensitive to temperature sensations. The erythema associated with rashes is not always accompanied by noticeable increases in skin temperature. Macular, papular, and vesicular skin lesions are identified by a combination of palpation and inspection. In addition, it is important that you listen to the client's description of symptoms. For example, persons with macular rashes usually will complain of itching, and evidence of scratching will be apparent. When the skin is only moderately pigmented, a macular rash might become recognizable if the skin were gently stretched. Stretching the skin decreases the normal red tone, thus providing more contrast and making the macules appear brighter. In some skin disorders with a generalized rash, you will observe that the rash is most readily visible on the hard and soft palates (Overfield, 1995).

The increased redness that accompanies carbon monoxide poisoning and the blood disorders collectively known as *polycythemia* can be observed on the lips of dark-skinned clients. Because lipstick masks the actual color of the lips, you should ask the client to remove it prior to inspection.

Petechiae

In dark-skinned clients, **petechiae** are best visualized in the areas of lighter melanization, such as the abdomen, buttocks, and volar surface of the forearm. When the skin is black or very dark brown, petechiae cannot be seen in the skin. Most of the diseases that cause bleeding and the formation of microscopic emboli, such as thrombocytopenia, subacute bacterial endocarditis, and other septicemias, are characterized by petechiae in the mucous membranes and skin. Petechiae are most easily seen in the mouth, particularly the buccal mucosa, and in the conjunctiva of the eye (Overfield, 1995).

Ecchymoses

In assessing **ecchymotic lesions** caused by systemic disorders, you will find them in the same locations as petechiae, although their larger size makes them more apparent on dark-skinned individuals. When you are differentiating petechiae and ecchymoses from erythema in the mucous membrane, pressure on the tissue will momentarily blanch erythema but not petechiae or ecchymoses.

Normal Age-Related Skin Changes

Although aging is accompanied by the growing presence of wrinkles in all cultures, Blacks, Asian Americans, American Indians, and Eskimos wrinkle later in life than their Anglo American counterparts. Light skin shows the effects of sun damage more than dark skin, regardless of race or ethnicity. The area of the skin that is exposed to the sun shows the effects of aging more than protected skin, such as those parts covered by clothing. Regardless of climate, dry skin is inevitable in individuals older than 70 years of age. In part, dry skin is caused by transepidermal water loss, which decreases in older adults. African Americans have a significantly higher transepidermal water loss than Whites, which correlates with the water content of the stratum corneum layer of the skin. Because the number of *moles* increases with age, they are thought to be the result of long-term exposure to the sun. People with lighter skin have more moles than those with darkly pigmented skin. Whites have more moles than Asian North Americans or African Americans (Overfield, 1995).

Nurses and other health care providers often overestimate or underestimate age when dealing with clients whose cultural heritage is different from their own. Whites tend to underestimate the age of Africans, Asians, and North American Indians, whereas African Americans, Asians, and North American Indians tend to overestimate the age of White clients (Overfield, 1995).

Biocultural Variations in Body Secretions

The *apocrine* and *eccrine sweat glands* are important for fluid balance and for thermoregulation. Approximately 2 to 3 million glands open onto the skin surface through pores and are responsible for the presence of sweat. When they are contaminated by normal skin flora, odor results. Most Asians and Native North Americans have a mild to absent body odor, whereas Whites and African Americans tend to have strong body odor.

Eskimos have made an environmental adaptation whereby they sweat less than Whites on their trunks and extremities but more on their faces. This adaptation allows for temperature regulation without causing perspiration and dampness of their clothes, which would decrease their ability to insulate against severe weather and would pose a serious threat to their survival.

The amount of chloride excreted by sweat glands varies widely, and African Americans have lower salt concentrations in their sweat than do Whites. A study of Ashkenazi Jews (of European descent) and Sephardic Jews (of North African and Middle Eastern descent) revealed that those of European origin had a lower percentage of sweat chlorides (Levin, 1966). This variation might be significant in the care of clients with renal or cardiac conditions or of children with cystic fibrosis (Overfield, 1995).

Biocultural Variation in the Head, Eyes, Ears, and Mouth

Hair

Perhaps one of the most obvious and widely variable cultural differences occurs with assessment of the hair. African Americans' hair varies widely in texture. It is very fragile and ranges from long and straight to short, spiraled, thick, and kinky. The hair and scalp have a natural tendency to be dry and to require daily combing, gentle brushing, and the application of oil. By comparison, clients of Asian backgrounds generally have straight, silky hair.

Obtaining a baseline hair assessment is significant in the diagnosis and treatment of certain disease states. For example, hair texture is known to become dry, brittle, and lusterless with inadequate nutrition. The hair of Black children with severe malnutrition, as in the case of marasmus, frequently changes not only in texture but also in color. The child's hair often becomes straighter and turns a reddish copper color. Certain endocrine disorders are also known to affect the texture of hair.

Although gray hair correlates with age for both men and women, there are cultural differences in the rate of hair graying. Whites gray significantly faster than any other group. The hair of 66% of fair-haired individuals, but only 37% of dark-haired persons, is fully white by age 60 (Overfield, 1995). Among Asian Americans, graying might be delayed significantly, with some in their eighth or ninth decade of life showing little or no graying.

Eyes

Biocultural differences in both the structure and the color of the eyes are readily apparent among clients from various cultural backgrounds. Racial differences are evident in the palpebral fissures. Persons of Asian background are often identified by their characteristic epicanthal eye folds, whereas the presence of narrowed palpebral fissures in non-Asian individuals might be diagnostic of a serious congenital anomaly known as *Down syndrome or trisomy 21.*

There is culturally based variability in the color of the iris and in retinal pigmentation: Darker irises are correlated with darker retinas. Clients with light retinas generally have better night vision but can experience pain in an environment that is too light. The majority of African Americans and Asians have brown eyes, whereas many individuals of Scandinavian descent have blue eyes (Overfield, 1995).

It is clinically relevant that differences in visual acuity occur among people from different cultures. Blacks have poorer corrected visual acuity than Whites. The visual acuity of Hispanic Americans is between that of Blacks and Whites. American Indians are comparable to Whites in visual acuity, whereas Japanese and Chinese Americans have the poorest corrected visual acuity because of a high incidence of myopia (Overfield, 1995).

Ears

It does not take long to notice that ears come in a variety of sizes and shapes. Earlobes can be free-standing or attached to the face. Ceruminous glands are located in the external ear canal and are functional at birth. Cerumen is genetically determined and comes in two major types: (1) dry cerumen, which is gray and flaky and frequently forms a thin mass in the ear canal, and (2) wet cerumen, which is dark brown and moist. Asians and Native North Americans (including Eskimos) have an 84% frequency of dry cerumen, whereas African Americans have a 99% frequency and Whites have a 97% frequency of wet cerumen (Overfield, 1995). The clinical significance of this occurs when you are examining or irrigating the ears. You should be aware that the presence and composition of cerumen are not related to poor hygiene, and caution should be exercised to avoid mistaking flaky, dry cerumen for the dry lesions of eczema.

Hearing gradually declines with age, especially in the high frequencies. After age 40, men have poorer hearing than women. Blacks have better hearing at high and low frequencies, whereas Whites have better hearing at middle frequencies. Blacks are less susceptible to noise-induced hearing loss (Overfield, 1995).

Mouth

Oral hyperpigmentation also shows variation by race. Usually absent at birth, hyperpigmentation increases with age. By age 50 years, 10% of Whites and 50 to 90% of African Americans will show oral hyperpigmentation, a condition believed to be caused by a lifetime of accumulation of postinflammatory oral changes (Overfield, 1995).

Cleft uvula, a condition in which the uvula is split either completely or partially, occurs in 18% of some Native North American groups and 10% of Asians. The occurrence in Whites and Blacks is rare. *Cleft lip* and *cleft palate* are most common in Asians and Native North Americans and least common in African Americans (Overfield, 1995).

Leukoedema, a grayish white benign lesion occurring on the buccal mucosa, is present in 68% to 90% of Blacks but only 43% of Whites. Care should be taken to avoid mistaking leukoedema for oral thrush or related infections that require treatment with medication (Overfield, 1995).

Teeth

Because teeth are often used as indicators of developmental, hygienic, and nutritional adequacy, you should be aware of biocultural differences. Although it is rare for a White baby to be born with teeth (1 in 3,000), the incidence rises to 1 in 11 among Tlingit Indian infants and to 1 or 2 in 100 among Canadian Eskimo infants. Although congenital teeth are usually not problematic, extraction is necessary for some breast-fed infants (Overfield, 1995).

The size of teeth varies widely, with the teeth of Whites being the smallest, followed by Blacks and then Asians and Native North Americans. The largest teeth are found among Eskimos and Australian Aborigines. Larger teeth cause some groups to have prognathic (protruding) jaws, a condition that is seen more frequently in African and Asian North Americans. The condition is normal and does not reflect a serious orthodontic problem.

Agenesis (absence of teeth) varies by race, with missing third molars occurring in 18% to 35% of Asians, 9% to 25% of Whites, and 1% to 11% of Blacks. Throughout life, Whites have more tooth decay than Blacks, which might be related to a combination of socioeconomic factors and biocultural variation. Complete tooth loss occurs more often in Whites than in African Americans despite the higher incidence of periodontal disease in Blacks. Approximately one third of

Whites 45 years or older have lost all their teeth, compared with 25% of Blacks in the same age group (Overfield, 1995).

The differences in tooth decay between African Americans and Whites can be explained by the fact that African Americans have harder and denser tooth enamel, which makes their teeth less susceptible to the organisms that cause caries. The increase in periodontal disease among African Americans is believed to be caused by poor oral hygiene. When obvious signs of periodontal disease are present, such as bleeding and edematous gums, a dental referral should be initiated (Overfield, 1995).

Biocultural Variations in the Mammary Venous Plexus

Regardless of gender, the superficial veins of the chest form a network over the entire chest that flows in either a transverse or a longitudinal pattern. In the transverse pattern, the veins radiate laterally and toward the axillae. In the longitudinal pattern, the veins radiate downward and laterally like a fan. These two patterns occur with different frequencies in the two populations that have been studied. The recessive longitudinal pattern occurs in 6% to 10% of White women and in 30% of Navajos. The only known alteration of either pattern is produced by breast tumor. Although this variation has no clinical significance, it is mentioned so that if nurses note its presence during physical assessment, they will recognize it as a nonsignificant finding (Overfield, 1995).

Biocultural Variation in the Musculoskeletal System

Many normal biocultural variations are found in clients' musculoskeletal systems. The long bones of Blacks are significantly longer, narrower, and denser than those of Whites. Bone density measured by race and gender shows that Black males have the densest bones, thus accounting for the relatively low incidence of osteoporosis in this population. Bone density in Chinese, Japanese,

and Eskimos is below that of Whites (Overfield, 1995).

Curvature of the body's long bones varies widely among culturally diverse groups. Native North Americans and First Nation People have anteriorly convex femurs, whereas Blacks have markedly straight femurs, and Whites have intermediate femurs. This characteristic is related to both genetics and body weight. The femurs of thin Blacks and Whites have less curvature than average, whereas those of obese Blacks and Whites display increased curvatures. It is possible that the heavier density of the bones of Blacks helps to protect them from increased curvature caused by obesity (Overfield, 1995). Table 3–6 summarizes biocultural variations occurring in the musculoskeletal system that have been identified through observation and study of people from various cultures and subcultures.

Biocultural Variations in Illness

Researchers have abundant evidence that there is a relationship between ethnicity and the incidence of certain diseases across the life span, from infancy to old age. The distribution of selected genetic traits and disorders prevalent among infants and children from selected cultural groups is shown in Chapter 6. Table 3–7 provides an alphabetical listing of selected diseases and their increased or decreased prevalence among members of certain cultural groups. A knowledge of normal biocultural variations and those occurring during illness helps nurses to conduct more accurate, comprehensive, and thorough physical examinations of clients from diverse cultures.

Laboratory Tests

You should be aware that biocultural variations occur with some laboratory test results, such as measurement of *hemoglobin, hematocrit, cholesterol, serum transferrin,* and *blood glucose.* You also will want to consider cultural differences in the

TABLE 3-6 *Biocultural Variations in the Musculoskeletal System*

Component	Remarks		
Bone			
Frontal	Thicker in Black males than in White males		
Parietal occiput	Thicker in White males than in Black males		
Palate	Tori (protuberances) along the suture line of the hard palate		
	Problematic for denture wearers		
	Incidence:		
	Blacks	20%	
	Whites	24%	
	Asians	Up to 50%	
	Native Americans	Up to 50%	
Mandible	Tori (protuberances) on the lingual surface of the mandible near the canine and premolar teeth		
	Problematic for denture wearers		
	Most common in Asians and Native Americans; exceeds 50% in some Eskimo groups		
Humerus	Torsion or rotation of proximal end with muscle pull		
	Whites > Blacks		
	Torsion in Blacks is symmetric; torsion in Whites tends to be greater on right side than left side		
Radius	Length at the wrist variable		
Ulna	Ulna or radius may be longer		
	Equal length		
	Swedes	61%	
	Chinese	16%	
	Ulna longer than radius		
	Swedes	16%	
	Chinese	48%	
	Radius longer than ulna		
	Swedes	23%	
	Chinese	10%	
Vertebrae	Twenty-four vertebrae are found in 85% to 93% of all people; racial and sex differences reveal 23 or 25 vertebrae in select groups		
	Vertebrae	Population	
	23	11% of Black females	
	25	12% of Eskimo and Native American males	
	Related to lower back pain and lordosis		
Pelvis	Hip width is 1.6 cm (0.6 in) smaller in Black women than in White women; Asian women have significantly smaller pelvises		
Femur	Convex anterior	Native American	
	Straight	Black	
	Intermediate	White	

(Continued on following page)

TABLE 3-6 *Guide for Using the Culturally Competent Model* (continued)

Component	Remarks	
Second tarsal	Second toe longer than the great toe	
	Incidence:	
	Whites	8–34%
	Blacks	8–12%
	Vietnamese	31%
	Melanesians	21–57%
	Clinical significance for joggers and athletes	
Height	White males are 1.27 cm (0.5 in.) taller than Black males and 7.6 cm (2.9 in.) taller than Asian males	
	White females = Black females	
	Asian females are 4.14 cm (1.6 in.) shorter than White or Black females	
Composition of long bones	Longer, narrower, and denser in Blacks than in Whites; bone density in Whites > Chinese, Japanese, and Eskimos	
	Osteoporosis lowest in Black males; highest in White females	
Muscle		
Peroneus tertius	Responsible for dorsiflexion of foot	
	Muscle absent:	
	Asians, Native Americans, and Whites	3–10%
	Blacks	10–15%
	Berbers (Sahara desert)	24%
	No clinical significance because the tibialis anterior also dorsiflexes the foot	
Palmaris longus	Responsible for wrist flexion	
	Muscle absent:	
	Whites	12–20%
	Native Americans	2–12%
	Blacks	5%
	Asians	3%
	No clinical significance because three other muscles are also responsible for flexion	

Based on data reported by T. Overfield. (1995). *Biologic variation in health and illness: Race, age, and sex differences.* New York: CRC Press.

results of tests conducted during pregnancy. The *multiple-marker screening* test and two tests of *amniotic fluid constituents* are used to screen pregnant women for potential fetal problems. Although the reasons for these differences are unknown, genetic, environmental, dietary, socioeconomic, cultural, and lifestyle factors are being studied to determine the extent to which they contribute to the differences in test results. Table 3-8 identifies biocultural variations and their clinical significance for selected laboratory tests.

Clinical Decision Making and Nursing Actions

After you have completed a comprehensive cultural assessment, you are ready to analyze your subjective and objective data, set mutual goals

TABLE 3-7 *Distribution of Selected Genetic Traits and Disorders by Population or Ethnic Group*

Ethnic or Population Group	Genetic or Multifactorial Disorder Present in Relatively High Frequency
Aland Islanders	Ocular albinism (Forsius-Eriksson type)
Amish	Limb girdle muscular dystrophy (IN—Adams, Allen counties)
	Ellis–van Creveld syndrome (PA—Lancaster county)
	Pyruvate kinase deficiency (OH—Mifflin county)
	Hemophilia B (PA—Holmes county)
Armenians	Familial Mediterranean fever
	Familial paroxysmal polyserositis
Blacks (African)	Sickle cell disease
	Hemoglobin C disease
	Hereditary persistence of hemoglobin F
	G-6-PD deficiency, African type
	Lactase deficiency, adult
	β-thalassemia
Burmese	Hemoglobin E disease
Chinese	α-thalassemia
	G-6-PD deficiency, Chinese type
	Lactase deficiency, adult
Costa Ricans	Malignant osteopetrosis
Druze	Alkaptonuria
English	Cystic fibrosis
	Hereditary amyloidosis, type III
Eskimos	Congenital adrenal hyperplasia
	Pseudocholinesterase deficiency
	Methemoglobinemia
French Canadians (Quebec)	Tyrosinemia
	Morquio syndrome
Finns	Congenital nephrosis
	Generalized amyloidosis syndrome, V
	Polycystic liver disease
	Retinoschisis
	Aspartylglycolsaminuria
	Diastrophic dwarfism
Gypsies (Czech)	Congenital glaucoma
Hopi Indians	Tyrosinase-positive albinism
Icelanders	Phenylketonuria
Irish	Phenylketonuria
	Neural tube defects
Japanese	Acatalasemia
	Cleft lip/palate
	Oguchi disease

(Continued on following page)

TABLE 3-7 *Distribution of Selected Genetic Traits and Disorders by Population or Ethnic Group* (continued)

Ethnic or Population Group	Genetic or Multifactorial Disorder Present in Relatively High Frequency
Jews	
Ashkenazi	Tay-Sachs disease (infantile)
	Niemann-Pick disease (infantile)
	Gaucher disease (adult type)
	Familial dysautonomia (Riley-Day syndrome)
	Bloom syndrome
	Torsion dystonia
Sephardi	Factor XI (PTA) deficiency
	Familial Mediterranean fever
	Ataxia-telangiectasia (Morocco)
	Cystinuria (Libya)
	Glycogen storage disease III (Morocco)
Orientals	Dubin-Johnson syndrome (Iran)
	Ichthyosis vulgaris (Iraq, India)
	Werdnig-Hoffman disease (Karaite Jews)
	G-6-PD deficiency, Mediterranean type
	Phenylketonuria (Yemen)
	Metachromatic leukodystrophy (Habbanite Jews, Saudi Arabia)
Lapps	Congenital dislocation of hip
Lebanese	Dyggve-Melchoir-Clausen syndrome
Mediterranean people (Italians, Greeks)	G-6-PD deficiency, Mediterranean type
	β-thalassemia
	Familial Mediterranean fever
Navajo Indians	Ear anomalies
	Joseph disease
Polynesians	Clubfoot
Poles	Phenylketonuria
Portuguese	Joseph disease
Nova Scotia Acadians	Niemann-Pick disease, type D
Scandinavians (Norwegians, Swedes, Danes)	Cholestasis-lymphedema syndrome (Norwegians)
	Sjögren-Larsson syndrome (Swedes)
	Krabbe disease
Scots	Phenylketonuria
	Phenylketonuria
	Cystic fibrosis
	Hereditary amyloidosis, type III
Thoi	Lactase deficiency, adult
	Hemoglobin E disease
Zuni Indians	Tyrosinase-positive albinism

From Cohen, F. L. (1984). *Clinical Genetics in Nursing Practice* (pp. 23–24). Philadelphia: J.B. Lippincott. Reprinted by permission.

TABLE 3-8 *Biocultural Variations and Clinical Significance for Selected Laboratory Tests*

Test	Remarks
Hemoglobin/hematocrit	1 g lower for Blacks than other groups; Blacks < counterparts in other groups
Serum transferrin	Biocultural variation in children aged 1–3 1/2 years Mean for Blacks 22 mg/100 mL > Whites *Note:* May be due to lowered hemoglobin and hematocrit levels found in Blacks *Clinical significance:* Transferrin levels increase in the presence of anemia, thus influencing the diagnosis, treatment, and nursing care of children with anemia
Serum cholesterol	Biocultural variation across the life span Birth — Blacks = Whites Childhood — Blacks 5 mg/100 mL > Whites; Pima Indians 20–30 mg/100 mL > Whites Adulthood — Blacks < Whites; Pima Indians 50–60 ml/100 mL < Whites *Clinical significance:* Prevention, treatment, and nursing care of clients with cardiovascular disease
High-density lipoproteins (HDLs)	Biocultural variation in adults Blacks > Whites Asians ≥ Whites Mexican North Americans < Whites
Ratio of HDL to total cholesterol	Blacks < Whites
Low-density lipoproteins (LDLs)	Biocultural variation in adults Blacks < Whites *Clinical significance:* Prevention, treatment, and nursing care of clients with cardiovascular disease
Blood glucose	Biocultural variation in adults North American Indians, Hispanics, Japanese > Whites Blacks = Whites (for equivalent socioeconomic groups) *Clinical significance:* Diagnosis, treatment, and nursing care of adults with hypoglycemia and diabetes mellitus
Multiple-marker screening	Biocultural variations in blood levels for protein and hormones in pregnant women Alphafetoprotein (AFP), hCG, and estriol levels in Black and Asian women > Whites *Clinical significance:* High AFP levels signal that the woman is at increased risk for being delivered of an infant with spina bifida and neural tube defects, whereas low levels may signal Down syndrome; Down syndrome also is associated with low levels of estriol and high levels of hCG

(Continued on following page)

TABLE 3-8 *Biocultural Variations and Clinical Significance for Selected Laboratory Tests (countinued)*

Test	Remarks
	Black and Asian American women have higher average levels of AFP, hCG, and estriol than White counterparts Using a single median for women of all cultures: ■ Causes Black and Asian women to be *falsely* identified as being *at risk* for having infants with spina bifida and neural tube defects; by being classified as *high risk*, women are more likely to be subjected to invasive and expensive procedures such as amniocentesis; some may elect to abort the pregnancy based on screening test results ■ *Inappropriately lowers* the identified Down syndrome risk for Black and Asian women
Lecithin/sphingomyelin ratio	Biocultural variations in amniotic fluid measures of fetal pulmonary maturity Blacks have higher ratios than Whites from 23 to 42 weeks gestation *Clinical significance:* The ratio is used to calculate the risk of respiratory distress in premature infants: lung maturity in Blacks is reached 1 week earlier than in Whites (34 versus 35 weeks); racial differences should be considered in making decisions about inducing labor or delivering by cesarean section

Table based on data from
Allanson, A., Michie, S., & Matreau, T. M. (1997). Presentation of screen negative results on serum screening for Down's Syndrome. *Journal of Medical Screening, 4*(1), 21–22.
Chapman, S. J., Brumfield, C. G., Wenstrom, K. D., & DuBard, M. B. (1997). Pregnancy outcomes following false-positive multiple marker screening test. *American Journal of Perinatology, 14*(8), 475–478.
O'Brien, J. E., Dvorin, E., Drugan, A., Johnson, M. P., Yaron, Y., & Evans, M. I. (1997). Race-ethnicity-specific variation in multiple-marker biochemical screening: Alpha-fetoprotein, hCG, and estriol. *Obstetrics and Gynecology, 89*(3), 355–358.
Overfield, T. (1995). *Biologic variation in health and illness: Race, age, and sex differences.* New York: CRC Press.

with the client, develop a plan of care, make referrals as needed, and implement a plan of care, either alone or with others. Before **clinical decision making** or **nursing actions** can occur, you should identify the client's strengths and limitations, including his or her social support network: family, friends, clergy, and other visitors from the client's place of worship, ethnic or cultural organizations, or other sources that can be mobilized to assist the client. Next, you will want to determine whether there are client goals or needs for which professional nursing care is required.

Modes to Guide Nursing Judgments, Decisions, and Actions

Leininger (1991; Leininger & McFarland, 2002) suggests three major modalities to guide nursing judgments, decisions, and actions for the purpose of providing culturally congruent care that is beneficial, satisfying, and meaningful to the people served by nurses. The three modes are *cultural preservation or maintenance, cultural care accommodation or negotiation,* and *cultural care repatterning or restructuring.* Let us briefly examine each of these modes.

Cultural preservation or maintenance refers to "those professional actions and decisions that help people of a particular culture to retain and/or preserve relevant care values so that they can maintain their well-being, recover from illness, or face handicaps and/or death" (Leininger, 1991; Leininger & McFarland, 2002).

Cultural care accommodation or negotiation refers to professional actions and decisions that help people of a designated culture to adapt to or to negotiate with others for beneficial or satisfying health outcomes with professional care providers (Leininger, 1991; Leininger & McFarland, 2002). Cultural negotiation is sometimes referred to as *culture brokering.*

Cultural care repatterning or restructuring refers to professional actions and decisions that help clients reorder, change, or greatly modify their lifeways for new, different, and beneficial health care patterns while respecting the clients' cultural values and beliefs and still providing more beneficial or healthier lifeways than before the changes were coestablished with the clients (Leininger, 1991; Leininger & McFarland, 2002).

These modes are care-centered and based on use of the client's care knowledge. Negotiation increases understanding between the client and the nurse and promotes culturally congruent nursing care.

Evaluation

Evaluation of the effectiveness of clinical decisions and nursing actions should occur in collaboration with the client and his or her significant others—which may include members of the extended family, traditional healers, those with culturally determined nonfamilial relationships, and friends. A careful evaluation of each component of the transcultural nursing interaction should be undertaken in collaboration with the client. It may be necessary to gather further data, reinterpret existing findings, redefine mutual

nurse-client goals, or renegotiate the roles and responsibilities of nurses, clients, and members of their support system.

The previous discussion has focused to a large extent on the individual during the period of hospitalization or while being cared for by nurses in the home or community environment. Next, we will look at the issue of evaluation after discharge. In the current managed care environment, there is growing emphasis on client *outcomes* and reported satisfaction with the care provided by nurses and other health care providers. You will need to participate in the establishment of *quality assurance, total quality management,* and/or *continuous quality improvement* initiatives aimed at gathering information from clients about their overall satisfaction with care. You also need to ensure that the process and instruments are culturally appropriate. For example, how are the needs of linguistically diverse clients met? Is translation or interpretation available? Are the questions asked in a culturally appropriate manner? It is imperative that nurses be included in all aspects of the evaluation and that they use feedback to improve their nursing care in the future.

Summary

In this chapter we have examined transcultural perspectives on the health history and physical examination, key components of the cultural assessment. In the first section we have provided an overview of the major data categories that nurses should consider if they are to demonstrate cultural competence in conducting the health history. In the second section we have identified biocultural variations in the physical examination in health and illness. In the final section we have examined cultural factors that influence clinical decision making, nursing actions, and evaluation.

1. In your own words, describe the key components of cultural assessment.
2. Analyze the difference in body proportions, height, and weight among clients from diverse cultural backgrounds, and indicate the reasons for differences among the groups.
3. Compare and contrast your approach to the assessment of light- and dark-skinned clients for cyanosis, jaundice, pallor, erythema, and petechiae.
4. Review the biocultural variations in laboratory tests for hemoglobin, hematocrit, serum cholesterol, serum transferrin, multiple-marker screening, and amniotic fluid constituents.
5. Critically analyze the reasons for the current interest in ethnopharmacology by nurses, physicians, pharmacists, and other health care providers. How does knowledge of ethnopharmacology and cultural differences in response to medications facilitate your ability to provide culturally competent and congruent nursing care?

CRITICAL THINKING ACTIVITIES

1. Critically analyze the instrument, tool, or form used by nurses when conducting an initial patient or resident *admission assessment* at a hospital, extended care facility, or other health care agency in terms of its relevance to the health and nursing needs of persons from diverse cultures. From a transcultural nursing perspective, identify the *strengths* and *limitations* of the admission assessment instrument. What suggestions would you make to enhance the effectiveness of the instrument in assessing the cultural needs of newly admitted patients or residents? Be sure to consider the *practical* constraints that nurses face in the current managed care environment, such as time limitations, external forces that require us to care for increasingly large numbers of patients, and other constraints, before you suggest modifications.

2. Using the Andrews and Boyle Transcultural Nursing Assessment Guide for Individuals and Families (Appendix A), answer the questions in each data category as they apply to *yourself*. As you write your responses to the questions, critically reflect on your own health-related cultural values, attitudes, beliefs, and practices.

3. Using the Andrews and Boyle Transcultural Nursing Assessment Guide for Individuals and Families (Appendix A), interview someone from a cultural background different from your own to assess his or her health-related cultural values, attitudes, beliefs, and practices. After you have completed the interview, compare and contrast those responses with your own responses in Question 2. Identify the ways in which you are *alike*. Critically analyze the *differences* as potential sources of cross-cultural conflict, and explore ways in which they might influence the nurse-client interaction.

4. Conduct a head-to-toe physical examination of a person from a racial background different from your own. Summarize your findings in writing. In a constructively self-critical manner, reflect on what aspects of the exam were (a) easiest and (b) most difficult for you. Try to determine the reason(s) why some aspects were relatively easy or difficult for you. What further information or skill development would assist you in gaining confidence in your ability to conduct physical examinations on people from diverse racial backgrounds?

REFERENCES

BCC Research. (2006). *Plant-derived drugs: Products, technology, applications* [Report]. Retrieved from www.the-infoshop. com/study/bc41846-plant-derived-drugs.html; retrieved April 12, 2007.

Bloche, M. G. (2006). Race, money, and medicines. *The Journal of Law, Medicine, & Ethics, 34*(3), 555–558.

Davies, S. (2006). Pharmacogenetics, pharmacogenomics and personalized medicine: Are we there yet? *Hematology*, 2006, 111–117.

Good, B. J., & Good, M. J. (1980). The meaning of symptoms: A cultural hermeneutic model for clinical practice. In L. Eisenberg & A. Kleinman (Eds.). *The relevance of social science for medicine.* Boston: D. Reidel.

Harty, L., Johnson, K., & Power, A. (2006). Race and ethnicity in the era of emerging pharmacogenomics. *Journal of Clinical Pharmacology, 46,* 405–407.

Jarvis, C. (2004). *Physical examination and health assessment.* Philadelphia: W.B. Saunders.

Kleinman, A. (1980). *Patients and healers in the context of culture.* Berkeley, CA: University of California Press.

Kleinman, A., Eisenberg, L., & Good, B. (1978). Culture, illness and care: Clinical lessons from anthropologic and cross-cultural research. *Annals of Internal Medicine, 88,* 251–258.

Leininger, M. M. (1991). *Culture care diversity and universality: A Theory of Nursing.* New York: NLN Press.

Leininger, M. M. (1995). *Transcultural nursing: Concepts, theories, research and practices.* New York: McGraw-Hill.

Leininger, M. M., & McFarland, M. R. (2002). *Transcultural nursing: Concepts, theories, research and practices.* New York: McGraw-Hill.

Levin, S. (1966). Effect of age, ethnic background and disease on sweat chloride. *Israeli Journal of Medical Science, 2*(3), 333–337.

Ma, J. K., Chikwamba, R., Sparrow, P., Fischer, R., Mahoney, R., & Twyman, R. M. (2005). Plant-derived pharmaceuticals—the road forward. *Trends in Plant Science, 10*(12), 580–585.

Mathis, A. S., & Knipp, G. T. (2002). Do sex and ethnicity influence drug pharmacokinetics in solid organ transplantation? *Graft, 5*(50), 294–302.

Overfield, T. (1995). *Biologic variation in health and illness: Race, age and sex differences.* New York: CRC Press.

Schultz, J. (2003). FDA Guidelines on Race and Ethnicity: Obstacle or remedy? *Journal of the National Cancer Institute, 95*(6), 425–426.

Wenger, A. F. (1993). Cultural meaning of symptoms. *Holistic Nursing Practice, 7*(2), 22–35.

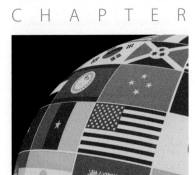

CHAPTER 4

The Influence of Cultural and Health Belief Systems on Health Care Practices

Margaret M. Andrews

In this chapter we shall examine the major cultural belief systems embraced by people from diverse cultures and explore the characteristics of three of the most prevalent worldviews, or paradigms, related to health-illness beliefs: the magico-religious, the scientific/biomedical, and the holistic health paradigms. We shall explore self-treatment, professional care systems, and folk (indigenous, traditional, generic) care systems and their respective healers. After analyzing the influence of culture on symptoms and sick role and illness behaviors, we shall examine selected complementary and alternative thera-pies used to treat physical and psychological diseases and illnesses.

Cultural Belief Systems

Cultural meanings and **cultural belief systems** develop from the shared experiences of a group in society and are expressed symbolically. The use of symbols to define, describe, and relate to the world around us is one of the basic characteristics of being human. One of the most common expressions of symbolism is the **metaphor**. In metaphor, one aspect of life is connected to another through a shared symbol. For example, the phrases "what a tangled web we weave" and "all the world's a stage" express metaphorically the relationship between two normally disparate concepts (such as human deception and a spider's web). People often use metaphors as a way of thinking about and explaining life's events.

Every group of people has found it necessary to explain the phenomena of nature. From the explanations developed emerges a common belief system. The explanations usually involve metaphoric imagery of magical, religious, natural/holistic, or biological form. The range of explanations is limited only by the human imagination.

The set of metaphoric explanations used by a group of people to explain life's events and to offer solutions to life's mysteries can be viewed as the group's **worldview**. A worldview can also be defined as a major paradigm. A **paradigm**, like any general perspective, is a way of viewing the world and the phenomena in it. A paradigm includes the assumptions, premises, and glue that hold together a prevailing interpretation of reality. Paradigms are slow to change and do so only if and when their explanatory power has been exhausted.

The worldview developed reflects the group's total configuration of beliefs and practices and permeates every aspect of life within the culture of that group. Members of a culture share a worldview without necessarily recognizing it. Thinking itself is patterned on this worldview because the culture imparts a particular set of symbols to be used in thinking. Because these symbols are taken for granted, people do not normally question the cultural bias of their very thoughts. The use in the United States of the term *American* reflects such an unconscious cultural bias. This term is understood by citizens of the United States to refer only to themselves collectively; although in reality, it is a generic term referring to anyone in this hemisphere, including Canadians, Mexicans, Colombians, and so on.

Another example of symbolism and worldview can be seen in the way nurses use terms such as *nursing care, health promotion,* and *illness and disease.* Nurses often take for granted that all their clients define and relate to these concepts in the same way they do. This reflects an unconscious belief that the same cultural symbols are shared by all and therefore do not require reinterpretation in any given nurse–client context. Such an assumption accounts for many of the problems nurses face when they try to communicate with others who are not members of the health profession culture.

Health Belief Systems

Generally, theories of health and disease or illness causation are based on the prevailing worldview held by a group. These worldviews include a group's health-related attitudes, beliefs, and practices and frequently are referred to as health belief systems. People embrace three major **health belief systems** or worldviews: magico-religious, scientific, and holistic, each with its own corresponding system of health beliefs. In two of these worldviews, disease is thought of as an entity separate from self, caused by an agent that is external to the body but capable of "getting in" and causing damage. This causative agent has been attributed to a variety of natural and supernatural phenomena.

Magico-Religious Health Paradigm

In the **magico-religious paradigm**, the world is an arena in which supernatural forces dominate. The fate of the world and those in it, including humans, depends on the actions of God, or the gods, or other supernatural forces for good or evil. In some cases, the human individual is at the mercy of such forces regardless of behavior. In other cases, the gods punish humans for their transgressions. Many Latino, African American, and Middle Eastern cultures are grounded in the magico-religious paradigm. Magic involves the calling forth and control of supernatural forces for and against others. Some African and Caribbean cultures, e.g., voodoo, have aspects of magic in their belief systems. In Western cultures there are examples of this paradigm in which metaphysical reality interrelates with human society. For instance, Christian Scientists believe that physical healing can be effected through prayer alone.

Ackerknecht (1971) states that "magic or religion seems to satisfy better than any other device a certain eternal psychic or 'metaphysical' need of mankind, sick and healthy, for integration and harmony." Magic and religion are logical in their own way, but not on the basis of empiric premises; that is, they defy the demands of the physical world and the use of one's senses, particularly observation. In the magico-religious paradigm, disease is viewed as the action and result of supernatural forces that cause the intrusion of a disease-producing foreign body or the entrance of a health-damaging spirit.

Widespread throughout the world are five categories of events that are believed to be responsible for illness in the magico-religious paradigm. These categories, derived from the work of Clements (1932), are sorcery, breach of taboo, intrusion of a disease object, intrusion of a disease-causing spirit, and loss of soul. One of these belief categories, or any combination of them, may be offered to explain the origin of disease. Eskimos, for example, refer to soul loss and breach of taboo (breaking a social norm, such as committing adultery). West Indians and some Africans and African Americans believe that the malevolence of sorcerers is the cause of many conditions. *Mal ojo,* or the evil eye, common in Latino and other cultures, can be viewed as the intrusion of a disease-causing spirit.

In the magico-religious paradigm, illness is initiated by a supernatural agent with or without justification, or by another person who practices sorcery or engages the services of sorcerers. The cause-and-effect relationship is not an organic one; rather, the cause of health or illness is mystical. Health is seen as a gift or reward given as a sign of God's blessing and goodwill. Illness may be seen as a sign of God's special favor insofar as it gives the affected person the opportunity to become resigned to God's will, or it may be seen

as a sign of God's possession or as a punishment. For example, in many Christian religions, the faithful gather communally to pray to God to heal the ill or to practice healing rituals such as laying on of hands or anointing the sick with oil.

In addition, in this paradigm, health and illness are viewed as belonging first to the community and then to the individual. Therefore, one person's actions may directly or indirectly influence the health or illness of another person. This sense of community is virtually absent from the other paradigms.

Scientific or Biomedical Health Paradigm

The **scientific paradigm** is the newest and most removed from the interpersonal human arena of life. According to this worldview, life is controlled by a series of physical and biochemical processes that can be studied and manipulated by humans. Several specific forms of symbolic thought processes characterize the scientific paradigm. The first is determinism, which states that a cause-and-effect relationship exists for all natural phenomena. The second, mechanism, relates life to the structure and function of machines; according to mechanism, it is possible to control life processes through mechanical, genetic, and other engineered interventions. The third form is reductionism, according to which all life can be reduced or divided into smaller parts; study of the unique characteristics of these isolated parts is thought to reveal aspects or properties of the whole. One idea of reductionism is Cartesian dualism: the idea that the mind and the body can be separated into two distinct entities. The final thought process is objective materialism: What is real can be observed and measured. There is a further distinction between subjective and objective realities in this paradigm.

In general, the scientific paradigm disavows the metaphysical, though in recent years, there has been growing recognition that the positive and negative effects on health brought about by religious and holistic practices can be measured scientifically. When beneficial effects are identified, some who embrace the scientific paradigm include these practices in what is sometimes referred to as *integrative medicine*. The scientific paradigm usually ignores the holistic forces of the universe as well, unless explanations for such forces fit into the symbolic forms discussed previously. Members of most Western cultures, including the dominant cultural groups in the United States and Canada, espouse this paradigm. When the scientific paradigm is applied to matters of health, it is often referred to as the *biomedical model*.

Biomedical beliefs and concepts dominate medical thought in Western societies and must be understood to appreciate the practice of modern health care. In the biomedical model, all aspects of human health can be understood in physical and chemical terms. This fosters the belief that psychological processes can be reduced to the study of biochemical exchanges. Only the organic is real and worthy of study. Effective treatment consists of physical and chemical interventions, regardless of human relationships.

In this model, disease is viewed metaphorically as the breakdown of the human machine as a result of wear and tear (stress), external trauma (injury, accident), external invasion (pathogens), or internal damages (fluid and chemical imbalances or structural changes). Disease is held to cause illness, to have a more or less specific cause, and to have a predictable time course and set of treatment requirements. This paradigm is similar to the magico-religious belief in external agents, having replaced supernatural forces with infectious agents.

Using the metaphor of the machine, Western medicine uses specialists to take care of the "parts"; "fixing" a part enables the machine to function. The computer is the analogy for the brain; engineering is a task for biomedical practitioners. The discovery of DNA and human genome research have led to the field of genetic engineering, an eloquent biomedical metaphor. The symbols used to discuss health and disease reflect the North American cultural values of aggression and mastery: Microorganisms attack the body, war is raged against these invaders,

money is donated for the campaign against cancer, and illness is a struggle in which the patient must put up a good defense. The biomedical model defines health as the absence of disease or the signs and symptoms of disease. To be healthy, one must be free of all disease.

Holistic Health Paradigm

In the **holistic paradigm**, the forces of nature itself must be kept in natural balance or *harmony*. Human life is only one aspect of nature and a part of the general order of the cosmos. Everything in the universe has a place and a role to perform according to natural laws that maintain order. Disturbing these laws creates imbalance, chaos, and disease. The holistic paradigm has existed for centuries in many parts of the world, particularly in North American Indian cultures and Asian cultures. It is gaining increasing acceptance in the United States and Canada because it complements a growing awareness that the biomedical view fails to account fully for most diseases as they naturally occur.

The holistic paradigm seeks to maintain a sense of balance or harmony between humans and the larger universe. Explanations for health and disease are based not so much on external agents as on imbalance or disharmony among the human, geophysical, and metaphysical forces of the universe. For example, in the biomedical model, the cause of tuberculosis is clearly defined as the invasion of mycobacterium. In the holistic paradigm, whereby disease is the result of multiple environment–host interactions, tuberculosis is caused by the interrelationship of poverty, malnutrition, overcrowding, and mycobacterium.

The term *holistic*, coined in 1926 by Jan Christian Smuts, defines an attitude or mode of perception in which the whole person is viewed in the context of the total environment. Its Indo-European root word, *kailo*, means "whole, intact, or uninjured." From this root have come the words *hale, hail, hallow, holy, whole, heal,* and *health*. The essence of health and healing is the quality of wholeness we associate with healthy functioning and well-being.

In this paradigm, health is viewed as a positive process that encompasses more than the absence of signs and symptoms of disease. It is not restricted to biologic or somatic wellness but rather involves broader environmental, sociocultural, and behavioral determinants. In this model, diseases of civilization, such as unemployment, racial discrimination, ghettos, and suicide, are just as much illnesses as are biomedical diseases.

Metaphors used in this paradigm, such as *healing power of nature, health foods,* and *Mother Earth,* reflect the connection of humans to the cosmos and nature. Voltaire's statement that an efficient physician is one who successfully bemuses the patient so that nature can affect a cure stems from this belief. The belief system of Florence Nightingale, who emphasized nursing's control of the environment so that patients could heal naturally, was also holistic.

A strong metaphor in the holistic paradigm is exemplified by the Chinese concept of **yin and yang,** in which the forces of nature are balanced to produce harmony. The *yin* force in the universe represents the female aspect of nature. It is characterized as the negative pole, encompassing darkness, cold, and emptiness. The *yang,* or male force, is characterized by fullness, light, and warmth. It represents the positive pole. An imbalance of forces creates illness.

Illness is the outward expression of disharmony. This disharmony may result from seasonal changes, emotional imbalances, or any other pattern of events. Illness is not perceived as an intruding agent but as a natural part of life's rhythmic course. Going in and out of balance is seen as a natural process that happens constantly throughout the life cycle. No sharp line is drawn between health and illness; both are seen as natural and as being part of a continuum. They are aspects of the same process, in which the individual organism changes continually in relation to the changing environment.

In the holistic health paradigm, because illness is inevitable, perfect health is not the goal. Rather, achieving the best possible adaptation to the environment by living according to society's rules and caring appropriately for one's body is the ultimate aim. This places a greater emphasis on preventive and maintenance measures than does Western biomedicine.

Another common metaphor for health and illness in the holistic paradigm is the **hot/cold theory of disease.** This is founded on the ancient Greek concept of the four body humors: yellow bile, black bile, phlegm, and blood. These humors are balanced in the healthy individual. The treatment of disease becomes the process of restoring the body's humoral balance through the addition or subtraction of substances that affect each of these humors. Foods, beverages, herbs, and other drugs are all classified as hot or cold depending on their effect, not their actual physical state. Disease conditions are also classified as either hot or cold. Imbalance or disharmony is thought to result in internal damage and altered physiologic functions. Medicine is directed at correcting the imbalance as well as restoring body functioning. Each cultural group defines what it believes to be hot and cold entities, and little agreement exists across cultures, although the concept of hot and cold is itself widespread, being found in Asian, Latino, Black, Arab, Muslim, and Caribbean societies.

Health and Illness Behaviors

The series of behaviors typifying the health-seeking process have been labeled *health and illness behaviors.* These behaviors are expressed in the roles people assume after identifying a symptom. Related to these behaviors are the roles individuals assign to others and the status given to the role players. People assume various types of behaviors once they have recognized a symptom. **Health behavior** is any activity undertaken by a person who believes himself or herself to be healthy for the purpose of preventing disease or detecting disease in an asymptomatic stage. **Illness behavior** is any activity undertaken by a person who feels ill for the purpose of defining the state of his health and of discovering a suitable remedy. **Sick role behavior** is any activity undertaken by a person who considers himself ill for the purpose of getting well.

Three sets of factors influence the course of behaviors and practices carried out to maintain health and prevent disease: (1) one's beliefs about health and illness; (2) personal factors such as age, education, knowledge, or experience with a given disease condition; and (3) cues to action, such as advertisements in the media, the illness of a relative, or the advice of friends.

A useful model of illness behavior has been proposed by Mechanic (1978), who outlines 10 determinants of illness behavior that are important in the help-seeking process (Table 4–1). Knowledge of these factors can help the nurse appreciate the client's behaviors and decisions about seeking and complying with health care. Awareness of these motivational factors can help nurses offer the appropriate assistance to clients as they work through the illness process.

Types of Healing Systems

The term *healing system* refers to the accumulated sciences, arts, and techniques of restoring and preserving health that are used by any cultural group. In complex societies in which several cultural traditions flourish, healers tend to compete with one another and/or to view their scopes of practice as separate from one another. In some instances, however, practitioners may make referrals to different healing systems. For example, a nurse may contact a rabbi to assist a Jewish patient with spiritual needs, or a *curandero* may advise a Mexican-American patient to visit a physician or nurse practitioner for an antibiotic when traditional practices fail to heal a wound.

Self-Care

For common minor illnesses, an estimated 70% to 90% of all people initially try **self-care** with over-the-counter medicines, megavitamins, herbs, exercise, and/or foods that they believe have healing powers. Many self-care practices

have been handed down from generation to generation, frequently by oral tradition. When self-treatment is ineffective, people are likely to turn to *professional* and/or *folk* (indigenous, generic, traditional) healing systems. Or perhaps it might be more accurate to say that professional health care procedures include those that supplement or substitute for self-care practices. Self-care is the largest component of the North American health care system and accounts for billions of dollars in revenue annually (Vallerand, Fouladabakhsh, & Templin, 2004).

Professional Care Systems

According to Leininger (1991, 1997; Leininger & McFarland, 2002), **professional care systems** are formally taught, learned, and transmitted professional care, health, illness, wellness, and related knowledge and practice skills that prevail in professional institutions, usually with multidisciplinary personnel to serve consumers. Professional care is characterized by specialized education and knowledge, responsibility for care, and expectation of remuneration for services rendered. Nurses, physicians, physical therapists, and other licensed health care providers are examples of professionals who constitute professional care systems in North America and other parts of the world.

Folk Healing System

A **folk healing system** is a set of beliefs that has a shared social dimension and reflects what people actually do when they are ill versus what society says they ought to do according to a set of social standards (Wing, 1998). According to Leininger (1991; Leininger & McFarland, 2002), all cultures of the world have had a lay health care system, which is sometimes referred to as indigenous or generic. Although the terms *complementary, alternative,* and *naturalistic healing* are sometimes used interchangeably with folk healing systems, the key consideration that defines folk systems is their history of tradition. Many

TABLE 4-1 *Mechanic's Determinants of Illness Behavior*

Determinant	Description
Quality of symptom	The more frightening or visible the symptom, the greater is the likelihood that the individual will intervene.
Seriousness of symptom	The perceived threat of the symptom must be serious for action to be taken. Often others will step in if the person's behavior is considered dangerous (e.g., suicidal behavior) but will be unaware of potential problems if the person's behavior seems natural ("he always acts that way").
Disruption of daily activities	Behaviors that are very disruptive in work or other social situations are likely to be labeled as illness much sooner than the same behaviors in a family setting. An individual whose activities are disrupted by a symptom is likely to take that symptom seriously even if on another occasion he would consider the same symptom trivial (e.g., acne just before a date).
Rate and persistence of symptom	The frequency of a symptom is directly related to its importance; a symptom that persists is also likely to be taken seriously.
Tolerance of symptom	The extent to which others, especially family, tolerate the symptom before reacting varies; individuals also have different tolerance thresholds.
Sociocognitive status	A person's information about the symptom, knowledge base, and cultural values all influence that person's perception of illness.
Denial of symptom	Often, the individual or family members need to deny a symptom for personal or social reasons. The amount of fear and anxiety present can interfere with perception of a symptom.
Motivation	Competing needs may motivate a person to delay or enhance symptoms. A person who has no time or money to be sick will often not acknowledge the seriousness of symptoms.
Assigning of meaning	Once perceived, the symptom must be interpreted. Often people explain symptoms within normal parameters ("I'm just tired").
Treatment accessibility	The greater the barriers to treatment—whether psychologic, economic, physical, or social—the greater the likelihood that the symptom will not be interpreted as serious or that the person will seek an alternative form of care.

From Mechanic, D. (1978). *Medical sociology,* 2nd ed. New York: The Free Press, a Division of Macmillan, Inc. Copyright © 1978 by David Mechanic. By permission.

folk healing systems have endured over time and rely on oral tradition for the transmission of beliefs and practices from one generation to the next. A folk healing system is a mixture of non-professional systems and uses healing practices that are learned informally. The folk healing system is often divided into secular and sacred components.

Most cultures have **folk healers** (sometimes referred to as traditional, indigenous, or generic healers), most of whom speak the native tongue of the client, sometimes make house calls, and usually charge significantly less than healers practicing in the biomedical or scientific health care system (Leininger, 1997; Leininger & McFarland, 2002). In addition, many cultures have lay midwives (e.g., *parteras* for Hispanic women), *doulas* (support women for new mothers and babies), or other health care providers available for meeting the needs of clients. Table 4–2 identifies indigenous or folk healers for selected groups.

If clients use folk healers, these healers should be an integral part of the health care team and should be included in as many aspects of the client's care as possible. For example, you might

TABLE 4-2 *Healers and Their Scope of Practice*

Culture/Folk Practitioner	Preparation	Scope of Practice
Hispanic		
Family member	Possesses knowledge of folk medicine	Common illnesses of a mild nature that may or may not be recognized by modern medicine
Curandero	May receive training in an apprenticeship; may receive a "gift from God" that enables him or her to cure; knowledgeable in use of herbs, diet, massage, and rituals	Treats almost all of the traditional illnesses; some may not treat illness caused by witchcraft for fear of being accused of possessing evil powers; usually admired by members of the community
Espiritualista or spiritualist	Born with the special gifts of being able to analyze dreams and foretell future events; may serve apprenticeship with an older practitioner	Emphasis on prevention of illness or bewitchment through use of medals, prayers, amulets; may also be sought for cure of existing illness
Yerbero	No formal training Knowledgeable in growing and prescribing herbs	Consulted for preventive and curative use of herbs for both traditional and Western illnesses
Sabador	Knowledgeable in massage and manipulation of bones and muscles	Treats many traditional illnesses, particularly those affecting the musculoskeletal system; may also treat nontraditional illnesses
Black		
"Old lady"	Usually an older woman who has successfully raised her own family; knowledgeable in child care and folk remedies	Consulted about common ailments and for advice on child care; found in rural and urban communities
Spiritualist	Called by God to help others; no formal training; usually associated with a fundamentalist Christian church	Assists with problems that are financial, personal, spiritual, or physical; predominantly found in urban communities
Voodoo priest and priestess or *Houngan* and *Mambo*	May be trained by other priests(esses). In the U.S. the eldest son of a priest becomes a priest; the daughter of a priest(ess) becomes a priestess if she is born with a veil (amniotic sac) over her face	Knowledgeable about properties of herbs; interpretation of signs and omens; able to cure illness caused by voodoo; uses communication techniques to establish a therapeutic milieu like a psychiatrist; treats Blacks, Mexican Americans, and Native Americans
Chinese		
Herbalist	Knowledgeable in diagnosis of illness and herbal remedies	Both diagnostic and therapeutic; diagnostic techniques include interviewing, inspection, auscultation, and assessment of pulses
Acupuncturist	3 1/2 to 4 1/2 years (1,500 to 1,800 hours) of courses on acupuncture, Western anatomy & physiology, Chinese herbs; usually requires a period of apprenticeship, learning from someone else who is licensed or certified	Diagnosis and treatment of yin/yang disorders by inserting needles into *meridians,* pathways through which life energy flows; when heat is applied to the acupuncture needle, the term *moxibustion* is used

(Continued on following page)

TABLE 4-2 *Healers and Their Scope of Practice (continued)*

Culture/Folk Practitioner	Preparation	Scope of Practice
	Licensure required in North America	May combine acupuncture with herbal remedies and/or dietary recommendations Acupuncture is sometimes used as a surgical anesthetic
Amish		
Braucher or baruch-doktor	Apprenticeship	Men or women who use a combination of modalities including physical manipulation, massage, herbs, teas, reflexology, and *brauche*, folk-healing art with origins in 18th and 19th century Europe; especially effective in the treatment of bedwetting, nervousness, and women's health problems; may be generalist or specialist in practice; some set up treatment rooms; some see non-Amish as well as Amish patients
Lay midwives	Apprenticeship	Care for women before, during, and after delivery
Greek		
Magissa "magician"	Apprenticeship	Woman who cures *matiasma* or evil eye May be referred to as doctor
Bonesetters	Apprenticeship	Specialize in treating uncomplicated fractures
Priest (Orthodox)	Ordained clergy Formal theological study	May be called on for advice, blessings, exorcisms, or direct healing
Native Americans		
Shaman	Spiritually chosen Apprenticeship	Uses incantations, prayers, and herbs to cure a wide range of physical, psychologic, and spiritual illnesses
Crystal gazer, hand trembler (Navajo)	Spiritually chosen Apprenticeship	Diviner diagnostician who can identify the cause of a problem, either by using crystals or placing hand over the sick person; does not implement treatment

Adapted with permission from Hautman, M. A. (1979). Folk health and illness beliefs. *Nurse Practitioner, 4*(4), 23, 26–27, 31.

include the folk healer in obtaining a health history and in determining what treatments already have been used in an effort to bring about healing. In discussing traditional remedies, it is important to be respectful and to listen attentively to healers who effectively combine spiritual and herbal remedies for a wide variety of illnesses, both physical and psychological in origin. Chapter 14 provides detailed information about the religious beliefs and spiritual healers in major religious groups.

Complementary and Alternative Medicine

Complementary and Alternative Medicine (CAM) is an umbrella term for hundreds of therapies based on health care systems of people from around the world. Some CAM therapies have ancient origins in Egyptian, Chinese, Greek, and Native North American cultures. Others, such as osteopathy and magnet therapy, have evolved in more recent times. *Western biomedicine*, or **allopathic medicine**, is the reference point, with all other therapies being considered complementary (in addition to) or alternative (instead of) to it. Coined by homeopathic physician Samuel Hahnemann in the 19th century, *allopathic medicine* is used most often to refer to conventional medical practice, which emphasizes killing bacteria and suppressing symptoms. Conventional medicine (or more accurately health care) is practiced by those who have earned either MD (medical doctor) or DO (doctor of osteopathy) degrees and by other related health professionals such as registered nurses, physical therapists, and psychologists. Some dietary supplements have been incorporated into conventional medicine. For example, research has demonstrated that folic acid prevents certain birth defects and that a regimen of vitamins and zinc can slow the progression of age-related macular degeneration (National Eye Institute, 2001).

The National Center for Complementary and Alternative Medicine (NCCAM), the U.S. Federal Government's lead agency for scientific research on CAM, has defined CAM as a group of diverse medical and health care systems, practices, and products that are not currently considered to be part of conventional or allopathic medicine. NCCAM's mission is to examine complementary and alternative healing practices in the context of rigorous science, train CAM researchers, and disseminate authoritative information to the public and professionals. While some scientific evidence exists to support the safety and efficacy of selected CAM therapies, there needs to be a great deal more research on most of these therapies before their safety and efficacy can be documented for treating the diseases or medical conditions for which they are used (Ernst, et al., 2001; Fontaine, 2001; Keegan, 2001; National Center for Complementary and Alternative Medicine, 2007). The list of what is considered to be CAM changes continually as those therapies that are proven to be safe and effective become adopted into conventional health care and as new approaches to health care emerge (Balneaves, 2006; Burke, et al., 2005; Burrowes & Brommage, 2006; Chong, 2006; Foster, 1996; Fouladabakhsh, et al. (2005); Grzywacz, 2006;

Hsiao et al., 2006; Jagtenberg, 2006; Kuhn & Winston (2000); Lenacher, et al. (2006); Magin, 2006; Menzies, 2006; National Center for Complementary and Alternative Medicine, 2007; Taylor, 2006). NCCAM classifies CAM therapies into five categories:

1. *Alternative medical systems* are built upon complete systems of theory and practice. Often these systems have evolved apart from and earlier than the conventional medical approach used in the United States or Canada. Examples of alternative medical systems that have developed in Western cultures include homeopathic medicine and naturopathic medicine. Examples of systems that have developed in non-Western cultures include traditional Chinese medicine and Ayurveda, which originated in India.
2. *Mind–body medicine* uses a variety of techniques designed to enhance the mind's capacity to affect bodily functions and symptoms. Some techniques that were considered CAM in the past have become mainstream (e.g., patient support groups and cognitive-behavioral therapy). Other mind–body techniques are still considered CAM, including meditation, prayer, mental healing, and therapies that use creative outlets such as art, music, or dance.
3. *Biologically based therapies* in CAM use substances found in nature, such as herbs, foods, and vitamins. Some examples include dietary supplements, herbal products, and the use of other so-called "natural" but as yet scientifically unproven therapies (e.g., using shark cartilage to treat cancer).
4. *Manipulative and body-based methods* in CAM are based on manipulation and/or movement of one or more parts of the body. Some examples include chiropractic or osteopathic manipulation, and massage.
5. *Energy therapies* involve the use of energy fields in two ways:
   a. *Biofield therapies* are intended to affect energy fields that purportedly surround

and penetrate the human body. The existence of such fields has not yet been scientifically proven. Some forms of energy therapy manipulate biofields by applying pressure and/or manipulating the body by placing the hands in, or through, these fields. Examples include qigong, Reiki, and Therapeutic Touch.

b. *Bioelectromagnetic-based therapies* involve the unconventional use of electromagnetic fields, such as pulsed fields, magnetic fields, or alternating-current or direct-current fields.

Box 4–1 identifies selected CAM therapies currently used by people in the United States and Canada to promote health and prevent and treat disease.

Summary

In this chapter we have examined the major cultural belief systems embraced by people of the world, including the top three: magico-religious, scientific, and holistic health paradigms or worldviews. We examined self-treatment, professional care systems, and folk (indigenous, traditional, or generic) care systems and the types of healers who practice in them. After analyzing the influence of culture on symptoms and sick role behavior, we explored complementary and alternative medicine and healing modalities that are frequently used to treat physical and psychological conditions.

BOX 4-1

Selected Complementary and Alternative Therapies

Acupuncture ("AK-yoo-pungk-cher") refers to a family of procedures involving stimulation of anatomical points on the body by a variety of techniques. The acupuncture technique that has been most studied scientifically involves penetrating the skin with thin, solid, metallic needles that are manipulated by the hands or by electrical stimulation. When heat is applied to the needles, it is referred to as moxibustion ("mox-eh-BUST-chun").

Aromatherapy ("ah-roam-uh-THER-ah-py") involves the use of essential oils (extracts or essences) from flowers, herbs, and trees to promote health and well-being.

Ayurveda ("ah-yur-VAY-dah") includes diet and herbal remedies and emphasizes the use of body, mind, and spirit in disease prevention and treatment.

Chiropractic ("kie-roh-PRAC-tic") focuses on the relationship between bodily structure (primarily that of the spine) and function, and how that relationship affects the preservation and restoration of health. Chiropractors use manipulative therapy as an integral treatment tool.

Dietary supplements are products (other than tobacco) taken by mouth that contain a *dietary ingredient* intended to supplement the diet. *Dietary ingredients* may include vitamins, minerals, herbs or other botanicals, amino acids, and substances such as enzymes, organ tissues, and metabolites. *Dietary supplements* come in many forms, including extracts, concentrates, tablets, capsules, gelcaps, liquids, and powders. In the United States and Canada they have special requirements for labeling and are considered foods, not drugs.

Homeopathic ("home-ee-oh-PATH-ic") **medicine** is a CAM alternative medical system. In homeopathic medicine, there is a belief that "like cures like," meaning that small, highly diluted quantities of medicinal substances are given to cure symptoms, even though the same substances given at higher or more concentrated doses would actually cause those symptoms.

Massage ("muh-SAHJ") therapists manipulate muscle and connective tissue to enhance function of those tissues and promote relaxation and well-being.

(Continued on following page)

BOX 4-1 (continued)

Selected Complementary and Alternative Therapies

Naturopathic ("nay-chur-o-PATH-ic") **medicine**, or naturopathy, is based on the premise that there is a healing power in the body that establishes, maintains, and restores health. Practitioners work with the patient with a goal of supporting this power through treatments such as nutrition and lifestyle counseling, dietary supplements, medicinal plants, exercise, homeopathy, and traditional Chinese medicine.

Osteopathic ("ahs-tee-oh-PATH-ic") **medicine** is a form of conventional medicine that, in part, emphasizes diseases arising in the musculoskeletal system. There is an underlying belief that all of the body's systems work together, and disturbances in one system may affect function elsewhere in the body. Some osteopathic physicians practice osteopathic manipulation, a full-body system of hands-on techniques to alleviate pain, restore function, and promote health and well-being.

Qigong ("chee-GUNG") is a component of traditional Chinese medicine that combines movement, meditation, and regulation of breathing to enhance the flow of qi (pronounced "chee" and meaning *vital energy*) in the body, improve blood circulation, and enhance immune function.

Reiki ("RAY-kee") is a Japanese word representing *Universal Life Energy*. Reiki is based on the belief that when spiritual energy is channeled through a Reiki practitioner, the patient's spirit is healed, which in turn heals the physical body.

Therapeutic Touch is based on the premise that it is the healing force of the therapist that affects the patient's recovery; healing is promoted when the body's energies are in balance, and by passing their hands over the patient, healers can identify energy imbalances.

Traditional Chinese medicine (TCM) is the current name for an ancient system of health care from China. TCM is based on a concept of balanced qi or *vital energy*, which is believed to flow throughout the body. Qi regulates a person's spiritual, emotional, mental, and physical balance and is influenced by the opposing forces of yin (negative energy) and yang (positive energy). Disease is proposed to result from the flow of qi being disrupted and yin and yang becoming imbalanced. Among the components of TCM are herbal and nutritional therapy, restorative physical exercises, meditation, acupuncture, and remedial massage.

National Center for Complementary and Alternative Medicine. (2007). *What is complementary and alternative medicine?* (NCCAM Publication No. D347). Retrieved January 28, 2007, from http://nccam.nih.gov/health/whatiscam/

REVIEW QUESTIONS

1. In your own words, describe what is meant by the following terms: (a) cultural belief system, (b) worldview, and (c) paradigm.
2. What are the primary characteristics of the three major health belief systems: magicoreligious, scientific, and holistic paradigms?
3. What are the differences between professional and folk care systems?

4. What is allopathic medicine?
5. What is the primary mission of the National Center for Complementary and Alternative Medicine (NCCAM)?
6. Identify the seven major categories of complementary and alternative medicine as defined by the National Center for Complementary and Alternative Medicine.

CRITICAL THINKING ACTIVITIES

1. Select a complementary or alternative practice that you would like to know more about, e.g., acupuncture, chiropractic, or homeopathy. Search the Internet for information about this practice, and go to a library to conduct background research. After you have learned more about the practice, contact a healer who uses the type of practice that interests you and ask the following questions:
   a. How did you prepare to be a practitioner of _____?
   b. What do you believe are the major benefits of _____ to patients?
   c. What health-related conditions do you believe respond best to _____?
   d. Are there any risks to clients resulting from the use of _____?

2. According to the World Health Organization, 80% of the people in the world use complementary and alternative medicine for the treatment of common illnesses. Select a common illness, such as upper respiratory infection, arthritis, or a similar condition, and identify the various complementary and alternative approaches to allopathic medicine that clients might use. What is the efficacy of each intervention that you have identified? How effective do you think the complementary and alternative practices are compared with allopathic medicine?

3. The herb echinacea is frequently used for the prevention and treatment of the common cold. If a patient asked your opinion about the use of echinacea, how would you reply? Would you recommend that the patient use this herb for treatment of a cold? Explain why or why not.

4. Visit three of the following Web sites for further information about specific types of alternative and complementary medicine.
   Acupressure and Massage
   Acupressure Institute
   http://www.acupressure.com
   American Massage Therapy Association
   http://www.amtamassage.org/
   International Massage Association
   http://www.imagroup.com
   Rolf Institute of Structural Integration
   http://www.rolf.org
   Acupuncture and Chinese Medicine
   American Association of Oriental Medicine (provides referrals to acupuncturists in local areas)
   http://www.aaom.org
   National Acupuncture and Oriental Medicine Alliance
   http://www.acuall.org/
   Aromatherapy
   American Alliance of Aromatherapy
   http://www.healthy.net/aromatherapy
   National Association for Holistic Aromatherapy
   http://www.naha.org/

Ayurvedic Medicine

Ayurvedic Institute

http://www.ayurveda.com

Biofeedback

Association for Applied Psychophysiology and Biofeedback

http://www.aapb.org

Chiropractic

American Chiropractic Association

http://www.amerchiro.org

International Chiropractors Association

http://www.chiropractic.org

Dietary Supplements

Office of Dietary Supplements, National Institutes of Health (NIH)

http://ods.od.nih.gov

International Bibliographic Information on Dietary Supplements (IBIDS) database

http://ods.od.nih.gov/Health_Information/IBIDS.aspx

U.S. Food and Drug Administration (FDA) Center for Food Safety and Applied
  Nutrition

http://www.cfsan.fda.gov/

Toll-free U.S. phone no.: 1-888-723-3366

Information includes *Tips for the Savvy Supplement User: Making Informed Decisions
  and Evaluating Information* (U.S. Food and Drug Administration, Center for Food
  Safety and Applied Nutrition, 2002) and updated safety information on
  supplements (www.cfsan.fda.gov/~dms/ds-warn.html). Adverse effects from
  a supplement can be reported to the FDA's MedWatch program, which collects
  and monitors such information (1-800-FDA-1088 or www.fda.gov/medwatch).

Environmental Medicine

American Academy of Environmental Medicine

http://www.aaem.com/

Guided Imagery

Academy for Guided Imagery

http://www.academyforguidedimagery.com/

Herbal Medicine

American Botanical Council

http://www.herbalgram.org

American Herbalist Guild

http://www.americanherbalistsguild.com/

Herb Research Foundation

http://www.herbs.org

Hypnosis

American Board of Hypnotherapy

http://www.abh-abnlp.com/

Mind/Body Medicine

Benson-Henry Institute for Mind Body Medicine

http://mindbody.harvard.edu/home/

Center for Mind/Body Medicine
http://www.cmbm.org/

Music Therapy

American Music Therapy Association
http://www.musictherapy.org

Naturopathic Medicine

American Association of Naturopathic Physicians
http://www.naturopathic.org

Qigong

The Qigong Institute
http://www.qigonginstitute.org/main_page/main_page.php

REFERENCES

Ackernecht, E. (1971). Natural diseases and rational treatment in primitive medicine. *Bulletin of the History of Medicine, 19,* 467–497.

Andrews, M. M., Herberg, P., and Rigdon, I. (1983). *A comparison of three health–illness paradigms.* Unpublished manuscript.

Balneaves, L. G. (2006). Levels of commitment: Exploring complementary therapy use by women with breast cancer. *Journal of Alternative and Complementary Medicine, 12*(5), 459–466.

Burke, A., Upchurch, D. M., Dye, C., & Chyu, L. (2005). Acupuncture use in the United States: Findings from the National Health Interview Survey. *Journal of Alternative and Complementary Medicine, 12*(7), 639–648.

Burrowes, J. D., & Brommage, D. (2006). Issues in renal nutrition: Focus on nutritional care for nephrology patients. Herbs and dietary supplement use with stage 5 chronic kidney disease. *Nephrology Journal, 33*(1), 85–88.

Chong, O. (2006). An integrative approach to addressing clinical issues in complementary and alternative medicine in an outpatient oncology center. *Clinical Journal of Oncology Nursing, 10*(1), 83–92.

Clements, F. E. (1932). Primitive concepts of disease. *University of California Publications in Archeology and Ethnology, 32*(2), 185–252.

Ernst, E., Pittler, M. H., Stevinson, C., & White, A. (2001). *The desktop guide to complementary and alternative medicine: An evidence-based approach.* New York: Mosby.

Fontaine, K. L. (2000). *Healing practices: Alternative therapies for nursing.* Upper Saddle River, NJ: Prentice Hall.

Foster, S. (1996). *Herbs for your health.* Loveland, CO: Interweave Press.

Fouladabakhsh, J. M., Stommel, M., Given, B., & Given, C. (2005). Predictors of use of complementary and alternative therapies by cancer patients. *Oncology Nursing Forum, 32*(6), 115–123.

Grzywacz, J. G., (2006). Older adults' use of complementary and alternative medicine for mental health: Findings from the 2002 National Health Interview Survey. *Journal of Alternative and Complementary Medicine, 12*(5), 467–473.

Hsiao, A., Wong, M. D., Goldstein, M. S., Yu, H. J., Andersen, R. M., & Brown, E. R., et al. (2006). Variation in complementary and alternative medicine (CAM) use across racial/ethnic groups and the development of ethnic-specific measures of CAM use. *Journal of Alternative and Complementary Medicine, 12*(3), 281–290.

Jagtenberg, T. (2006). Evidence-based medicine and naturopathy. *Journal of Alternative and Complementary Medicine, 12*(3), 323–328.

Keegan, L. (2001). *Healing with complementary and alternative therapies.* Albany, NY: Delmar.

Kuhn, M. A., & Winston, D. (2000). *Herbal therapy and supplements: A scientific and traditional approach.* Philadelphia: Lippincott Williams & Wilkins.

Leininger, M. M. (1991). *Culture care diversity and universality: A theory of nursing.* New York: National League for Nursing Press.

Leininger, M. M. (1997). Founder's focus alternative to what? Generic vs. professional caring, treatments and healing modes. *Journal of Transcultural Nursing, 91*(1), 37.

Leininger, M. M., & McFarland, M. R. (2002). *Transcultural nursing: Concepts, theories, research and practices.* New York: McGraw-Hill.

Lengacher, C. A., Bennett, M. P., Kip, K. E., Gonzalez, L., Jacobsen, P., & Cox, C. E. (2006). Relief of symptoms, side effects, and psychological distress through complementary and alternative medicine for women with breast cancer. *Oncology Nursing Forum, 33*(1), 97–104.

Magin, P. J. (2006). Complementary and alternative therapies in acne, psoriasis, and atopic dermatitis. *Journal of Alternative and Complementary Medicine, 12*(5), 451–457.

Mechanic, D. (1978). *Medical sociology* (2nd ed.). New York: Free Press.

Menzies, V. (2006). Effects of guided imagery on outcomes of pain, functional status, and self-efficacy in persons diagnosed with fibromyalgia. *Journal of Alternative and Complementary Medicine, 12*(1), 23–30.

Monte, T. (1997). *The complete guide to natural healing.* New York: Berkeley Publishing Group.

National Center for Complementary and Alternative Medicine. (2007). *What is complementary and alternative medicine?* (NCCAM Publication No. D347). Retrieved January 28, 2007, from http://nccam.nih.gov/health/whatiscam/

National Eye Institute. (2001). *Antioxidant vitamins and zinc reduce risk of vision loss from age-related macular degeneration* [Press release]. Retrieved January 28, 2007, from http://nccam.nih.gov/health

Taylor, D. N. (2006). Health care industry shaping chiropractic's future. *Journal of the American Chiropractic Association, 43*(6), 19–23.

U.S. Food and Drug Administration, Center for Food Safety and Applied Nutrition. (2002). *Tips for the savvy supplement user: Making informed decisions and evaluating information.* Retrieved from http://www.cfsan.fda.gov/~dms/ds-savvy.html

Vallerand, A. H., Fouladbakhsh, J. M., & Templin, T. (2004). Use of complementary and alternative therapies in urban, suburban, and rural communities. *American Journal of Public Health, 93*(6), 923–925.

Wing, D. M. (1998). A comparison of traditional folk healing concepts with contemporary healing concepts. *Journal of Community Health Nursing, 15*(3), 143–154.

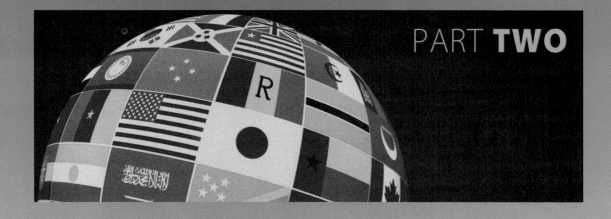

PART TWO

TRANSCULTURAL NURSING: ACROSS THE LIFESPAN

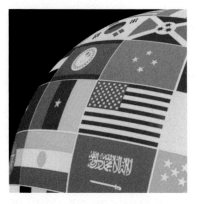

CHAPTER 5

Transcultural Perspectives in Childbearing

Jana Lauderdale

This chapter will explore how **culture** influences the experience of **childbearing**. The experience of the woman and that of her significant other during pregnancy, birth, and the postpartum period are discussed. Recommendations for practice are outlined in each section for nurses caring for childbearing women and their families. Also presented are discussions related to culturally specific circumstances and behaviors of the childbearing woman and her family for consideration.

Overview of Cultural Belief Systems and Practices Related to Childbearing

Childbearing is a time of transition and social celebration of central importance in any society, signaling a realignment of existing cultural roles and responsibilities, psychologic and biologic states, and social relationships. The different ways in which a particular society views this transitional period and manages childbirth are dependent on the culture's consensus about health, medical care, reproduction, and the role and status of women (Dickason, Silverman, & Schult, 1994).

Pregnancy and childbirth practices in contemporary Western society have seen dramatic changes over the past 2 decades. An increase in the number of women in the work force, advances in reproductive technology, self-care, alternative therapies, the explosion of health information available to consumers on the Internet, and the influx of immigrants and refugees are but a few of the trends that require nurses to examine and rethink how we can better care for our clients (Tiedje, 2000). The dominant medical practices related to pregnancy and childbirth in the United States and Canada include the use of various state-of-the-art technologies such as fetal monitoring devices and sometimes cesarean sections. Medical care focuses on the pregnant woman and fetus; the father and other family members or significant others, if they are included at all, are relegated to observer rather than participant status. The dominant cultural practices or rituals in the United States and Canada include formal prenatal care (including childbirth classes), ultrasonography to view the fetus, and hospital delivery. Monitoring fetal status, inducing labor, providing anesthesia for labor and delivery, and placing the woman in the lithotomy position during the birth are all part of routine hospital care in modern North American health care facilities. A highly specialized group of nurses, obstetricians, perinatologists, and pediatricians actively monitors the mother's physiologic status, delivers the infant, and provides newborn care. However, because there is not total cultural agreement about the value of these practices, some health care providers elect to offer their pregnant clients alternative health care services. These alternatives include in-hospital and freestanding birth centers and care by nurse practitioners and nurse midwives, who promote family-centered care and emphasize pregnancy as a normal process requiring minimal technologic intervention.

Additionally, subcultures within the United States and Canada have very different practices, values, and beliefs about childbirth and the roles of women, men, social support networks, and health care practitioners. They include proponents of the "back to nature" movement, who are often vegetarian, use lay midwives for home deliveries, and practice herbal or naturopathic medicine. Other groups that might have distinct cultural practices include African Americans, American Indians, Hispanics, Middle Eastern groups, Orthodox Jewish groups, and Asians, among others. Additionally, religious background, regional variations, age, urban or rural background, sexual preference, and other individual characteristics all might contribute to cultural differences in the experience of childbirth.

Great variations exist in the social class, ethnic origin, family structure, and social support networks of women, men, and families in the United States and Canada. Despite these differences, many health care providers assume that the changes in status and rites of passage associated with pregnancy and birth are experienced similarly by all people. In addition, many of the traditional cultural beliefs, values, and practices related to childbirth have been viewed by some professional nurses as "old-fashioned" or "old wives' tales." Although some of these customs are changing rapidly, many women and families are attempting to preserve their own valued patterns of experiencing childbirth. In recent years, nurses and other health professionals have attempted to understand the client's lifestyle, value system, and health and illness behaviors so that effective interventions can be implemented to reduce risks in a manner that is culturally congruent with community, group, and individual values.

Fertility Control and Culture

The literature provides limited information regarding cultural beliefs and practices related to the control of fertility. A woman's fertility varies depending on several factors, including the likelihood of sterility as well as the probability of conceiving and of intrauterine mortality. In addition, the duration of a postpartum period, during which a woman is unlikely to ovulate or conceive, also influences fertility. These variables are further modified by cultural and social variables, including marriage and residence patterns, diet, religion, the availability of abortion, the incidence of venereal disease, and the regulation of birth intervals by cultural or artificial means. The focus of this section is on influences affecting reproductive rights and population control.

In 2001, approximately one-half of pregnancies in the United States were unintended (Finer, 2006), and the United States has set a national goal of decreasing unintended pregnancies to 30% by 2010. Unintended pregnancy has been cited as a core concept in understanding the fertility of populations and the unmet need for contraception (Centers for Disease Control and Prevention [CDC])). Santelli et al. (2003) reports unintended pregnancy can have numerous negative effects on the mother and the fetus, including a delay in prenatal care, continued or increased tobacco and alcohol use, and increased physical abuse during pregnancy, any of which can lead to preterm labor or low birth weight infants. Luker (1999) suggests the pattern of *when* unintended pregnancy occurs has changed from the end of the reproductive cycle (when family size is complete) to the start of the cycle (when to start a family). The author believes the result is caused by a change in social mores sanctioning motherhood outside of marriage, contraception availability, earlier sexual activity, and multiple partners. One of the goals of Healthy People 2010 is to decrease unintended pregnancies from 49% to 30% by 2010 (U.S. Department of Health and Human Services, 2000). Programs aimed at reducing or preventing unintended pregnancy must build on the cultural meaning of the problem and focus on the processes women and their partners use to make fertility decisions.

Commonly used methods of contraception in the United States and Canada include hormonal methods, intrauterine devices (IUDs), permanent sterilization, and to a lesser degree, barrier and "natural" methods. Natural methods of family planning are based on the recognition of fertility through signs and symptoms and abstinence during periods of fertility. The religious beliefs of some cultural groups might affect their use of **fertility controls** such as abortion or artificial regulation of conception; for example, Roman Catholics might follow church edicts against artificial control of conception, and Mormon families might follow their church's teaching regarding the spiritual responsibility to have large families and promote church growth (Andrews & Hanson, 2003). The ability to control fertility successfully also requires an understanding of the menstrual cycle and the times and conditions under which pregnancy is more or less likely to occur—in essence, an understanding of bodily functions. When these functions change, the woman might perceive the changes as abnormal or unhealthy. Because the use of artificial methods of fertility control might alter the body's usual cycles, women who use them might become anxious, consider themselves ill, and discontinue the method. American Indian women monitor their monthly bleeding cycles closely and believe in the importance of monthly menstruation for maintaining harmony and physical well-being. Contraceptives such as the IUD are generally better accepted than hormonal methods because of the normal or increased flow associated with the IUD. Because the mechanism of action of an IUD might include the expulsion of a fertilized ovum, some women oppose use of the IUD for religious reasons.

In a study by Yusu, Siedlecky, and Byrnes (1993), 980 Turkish, Lebanese, and Vietnamese immigrant women living in Sydney, Australia, were surveyed regarding family planning. The Lebanese and Turkish women were better informed about the more modern forms of contraception (the pill, condoms, and IUDs) than were Vietnamese women. At the time of the study, the pill and traditional methods (abstinence, prolonged breast-feeding, rhythm, and withdrawal) were the most common forms of birth control, regardless of ethnicity. However, Turkish women continued to rely on abortion as a means of contraception as well. Condom use was low among Lebanese husbands but high among the young Turkish and Vietnamese groups. IUDs were used more often among Turkish women, and sterilization was the contraceptive method of choice for both Lebanese and Turkish women over the age of 40.

In 2006, the CDC reported that there are approximately 10 million refugees and 25 million internally displaced persons worldwide. As a result of fleeing their home countries, women and children (80%) were identified as most vulnerable to poor reproductive illness and outcomes (CDC, Division of Reproductive Health, National Center for Chronic Disease Prevention and Health Promotion, 2006). The CDC has developed a refugee program with a focus on refugee reproductive health. The goals for the program are presented in Box 5-1. Women living in refugee situations encounter many barriers to

---

BOX 5-1

CDC Refugee Reproductive Health Activities Goals

1. Initiate epidemiologic studies to evaluate the reproductive health status of women in refugee and IDP settings to better provide information to improve service, quality, and accessibility.
2. Design, implement, and evaluate reproductive health rapid assessment tools and behavioral and epidemiologic surveillance systems appropriate to refugee settings.
3. Design, recommend, and evaluate interventions and "best practices" identified through epidemiologic research, rapid assessment, and surveillance.
4. Strengthen the capacity of the refugee/IDP community, as well as the agencies providing health services, to collect and use data to improve reproductive health status and services.
5. Translate and communicate study findings and best practices to refugees and supporting agencies.

CDC, Division of Reproductive Health, National Center for Chronic Disease Prevention and Health Promotion, Atlanta, GA. (2006). Retrieved from http://www.cdc.gov

---

contraceptive use (see Evidence-Based Practice 5-1).

Religious beliefs can also influence birth control choices. For example, the Hindu religion teaches that the right hand is clean and the left is dirty. The right hand is for holding religious books and eating utensils, and the left hand is used for dirty things, such as genitals. This belief complicates the use of contraceptives requiring the use of both hands, such as a diaphragm (Bromwich and Parson, 1990). Buddhism values a celibate life and natural things. Modern contraceptives are not considered natural by this group and are therefore unacceptable. Traditional Mayan women in Guatemala believe strongly in privacy; therefore, skirts are kept on during intercourse and childbirth. Some women also believe it is improper to touch or expose their genitals, making traditional birth control methods such as abstinence or the rhythm method much more acceptable (Cosminsky, 1982). In some African cultures, the view of birth spacing has traditionally been to impose a taboo on postpartum sexual activity, with some women leaving their home for as long as 2 years to avoid pregnancy (Miller, 1992). The influence of religious beliefs on birth control choices can vary within and between groups.

In a study by Otoide, Oronsaye, & Okonofua (2001), Nigerian adolescents participated in focus groups to explore their level of understanding regarding contraception. The researchers were aware that in this particular group there is a low level of contraceptive use but a high reliance on abortion. According to the results, the participants perceived that modern contraceptives would have a prolonged, adverse effect on future fertility, whereas abortion was seen as an immediate solution to unplanned pregnancy. This indicates a need to educate Nigerian adolescents regarding contraceptive action and side effects versus the use of unsafe abortion practices. Few cultural groups give unqualified social approval to abortion. In the United States and Canada, religious affiliation is the variable most closely associated with attitudes toward abortion. Women from traditional societies are questioning long-held beliefs related to fertility control (see Evidence-Based Practice 5-2).

Evidence-Based Practice 5–1:

Barriers to Contraceptive Use for Women Living in the Khao Phlu Refugee Camp in Thailand

By use of focus groups, 102 women living in the Khao Phlu refugee camp in Thailand were studied, along with 10 midwives and traditional birth attendants who provided care for the women at the maternal and child health center serving the refugees. Information was gathered regarding the women's knowledge of contraceptives, beliefs, and practices. According to the results, 82% of the women wanted to stop or delay childbearing, but only 12% reported using some sort of contraception. The reasons for lack of contraceptive use included the refugee situation itself (i.e., uncertainty regarding their future), displacement of family or support system, cultural conflicts regarding modern contraceptive use, fear of side effects, lack of information, current illness, and discomfort level for asking about contraception. Additionally, almost 40% of the women had no knowledge of what contraceptive methods were available at the health center that served the camp. Few of the midwives and none of the women or traditional birth attendants were aware of emergency contraception.

Clinical Application

The results suggest that the stress of the refugee situation itself, along with cultural influences and the inaccessibility of contraceptives, had an effect on acceptance and use. Nurses working with refugee women must be aware of the issues to provide culturally competent care in matters regarding contraception practices.

Morrison, V. (2000). Contraceptive need among Cambodian refugees in Khao Phlu camp. *International Family Planning Perspectives, 26*(4), 188–192.

Nurses providing family planning services must take care to be culturally sensitive so that women can be assisted in defining their own attitudes, beliefs, and sense of gynecologic well-being regarding fertility control.

Pregnancy and Culture

All cultures recognize **pregnancy** as a special transition period, and many have particular customs and beliefs that dictate activity and behavior during pregnancy. Recent reports of childbirth customs in the United States and Canada have focused on accounts of differing beliefs and practices relative to pregnancy among various ethnic and cultural groups. This section describes some of the biologic and cultural variations that might influence the provision of nursing care during pregnancy.

Biologic Variations

Knowledge of certain biologic variations resulting from genetic and environmental backgrounds is important for nurses who care for childbearing families. For example, pregnant women who have the sickle cell trait and are heterozygous for the sickle cell gene are at increased risk for asymptomatic bacteriuria and urinary tract infections such as pyelonephritis. Obviously, this places them at greater-than-normal risk for premature labor as well. Although heterozygotes are found most commonly among African Americans (8% to 14%), individuals living in the United States and Canada who are of

Evidence-Based Practice 5–2:

Perceptions of abortion among Hmong women.

Using a qualitative approach, in-depth interviews and participant observation were conducted to explore perceptions of abortion and cultural values related to childbearing in a Hmong community in Melbourne, Australia. The findings were twofold: The majority of the women were knowledgeable about indigenous fertility control practices, including abortion, and secondly, there is a growing discontent among younger Hmong women with the societal norm that dictates abortion rights belong only to women who are older and have many children to ensure the family lineage. The younger women voiced feelings of being pressured by their families to produce many children or fear of causing a "cosmological" imbalance of their society. Many identified a need to feel in control of their fertility, and abortion was viewed as one such control being denied. This has been a source of growing conflict, with more and more women going against traditional teachings.

Clinical Application

Nurses working with this population of women must learn to balance fertility education with cultural expectations. Educating Hmong women of childbearing age on fertility issues will prove challenging as old customs and values are questioned and tested and must be handled in a way that brings young and old into discussions for the purpose of exploring fertility options acceptable to all.

Liamputtong, P. (2003). Abortion—It is for some women only! Hmong women's perceptions of abortion. *Health Care for Women International, 24*(3): 230–241.

Mediterranean ancestry, as well as of Germanic and Native North American descent, might occasionally carry the trait (Overfield, 1985; Perry, 2000). If both parents are heterozygous, there is a one-in-four chance that the infant will be born with sickle cell disease.

Another important biologic variation relative to pregnancy is diabetes mellitus. The incidence of non-insulin-dependent and gestational diabetes is much higher than normal among some Native North American groups—a problem that increases maternal and infant morbidity. Illnesses that are common among European North Americans might manifest themselves differently in Native North American clients. For example, an American Indian woman might have a high blood sugar level but be asymptomatic for diabetes mellitus. It is important to be aware that the mortality rate in pregnant American Indian

women with diabetes is higher than in White European American women. Diabetes during pregnancy, particularly with uncontrolled hyperglycemia, is associated with an increased risk of congenital anomalies, stillbirth, macrosomia, birth injury, cesarean section, neonatal hypoglycemia, and other problems.

Because long-term studies have been conducted among the Pima Indians of Arizona, we know that they have a very high incidence of gestational diabetes. Because some of the children born to Pima mothers after the studies began are now 28 to 30 years old, we can understand how a mother's diabetes can influence a child's health in adulthood. Researchers have found that the children of women with diabetes during pregnancy have a higher risk of becoming obese and getting diabetes earlier in life than those born to mothers who had normal blood sugar. We now

Evidence-Based Practice 5–3:

HIV Knowledge Among Pregnant Korean Women

The findings indicated that Korean women were knowledgeable about HIV infection and AIDS but were less knowledgeable about transmission. A group singled out in the study as being at particular risk of HIV transmission to their unborn fetuses was Korea's upper middle-class pregnant women. Korean women are tolerant of extramarital sex, which is considered a norm within Confucianism. Foreign travel of Korean businessmen, along with their higher socioeconomic status, makes extramarital sex affordable within and outside of Korea. Contact with prostitutes is increased, with subsequent exposure of the wife to sexually transmitted diseases. Koreans' belief that to go outside the family for help when caring for a family member with the HIV virus will bring shame to the family increases the need for health care providers to be culturally sensitive. To prevent rejection and shame, the woman might not reveal her diagnosis, which has obvious implications for prenatal care and subsequent care of the mother and baby.

Clinical Application

Pregnancy is a time when most pregnant women are very aware of the health of their unborn babies. Education focusing on HIV transmission might be especially meaningful to women during this time. Because the family is the mainstay of the support system in this culture, every effort must be made to include selected members in the care of the pregnant woman and her education.

Chang, S. (1996). HIV/AIDS related knowledge, attitudes, and preventive behavior of pregnant Korean women. *Image: Journal of Nursing Scholarship, 28*(4), 321–324.

know there is a nongenetic cause of diabetes, the diabetic intrauterine environment, which poses problems for the child that extend well beyond birth (Chamberlain, n.d.).

Korea is another area in Southeast Asia where cultural mores might put pregnant women at risk. Evidence-Based Practice 5–3 describes how and why pregnant women in Korea's upper middle class might be at increased risk of HIV transmission to their unborn fetuses.

Cultural Variations Influencing Pregnancy Outcomes

Several cultural variations might influence pregnancy outcomes. Those highlighted in this chapter include alternative lifestyle choices, nontraditional support systems, cultural beliefs related to parental activity during pregnancy, and food taboos and cravings. Nurses must be able to differentiate among beliefs and practices that are harmful, benign, and health promoting. Few cultural customs related to pregnancy are dangerous; although they might cause a woman to limit her activity and her exposure to some aspects of life, they are rarely harmful to herself or her fetus.

Alternative Lifestyle Choices

Despite recent cultural changes that have made it more acceptable for women to have careers and pursue alternative lifestyles, the dominant cultural expectation for North American women remains motherhood within the context of the nuclear family. Changing cultural expectations have influenced many middle-class North American women and couples to delay childbearing until their late 20s and early 30s and to have small families. Some women are making choices regarding childbearing that might not involve a marital relationship.

For another group of mothers who choose not to parent, the choices are not as clear. **Infant relinquishment** is in direct conflict with Western ideal cultural values, which suggest that all parents want a child. Nurses must examine their own cultural values when caring for women in this situation, making certain to avoid negatively stereotyping mothers who decide to relinquish their babies for adoption. The decision to relinquish is almost always difficult, and the birth mother does not forget the experience. Not all infant relinquishments result merely from the mother "not wanting the baby." For example, Native North Americans living on reservations have been known to relinquish young and older children in the hope that their children will have "a better life off the reservation." Even with such good intentions, the relinquishment is difficult for all concerned. In a study of the experience of infant relinquishment by Lauderdale and Boyle (1994), the most common reasons given by birth mothers for relinquishment were strictly altruistic: The birth mothers wanted a better life for the baby than they believed they could offer, and they wanted the baby to have both a mother and a father. Box 5–2 lists considerations in the nursing care of relinquishing birth mothers who are making this difficult decision.

Lesbian couple childbearing occurs in another subculture of pregnant women with special needs. This group of women faces psychosocial dilemmas related to their lifestyle and social stigma. The most common fear reported by lesbian mothers is the fear of unsafe and inadequate care from the practitioner once the mother's sexual orientation is revealed (Youngkin, Davis, & Fogel, 1998; Spinks, Andrews, & Boyle, 2000). This situation will require health care providers to examine their own cultural value systems. Keep in mind that lesbian parents are dedicated to bringing a new life safely into the world to love and care for to the best of their abilities—the same hopes all parents have for their newborns. McManus, Hunter, and Renn (2006) further support past studies, indicating four areas in their review of the literature that were significant in

---

BOX 5-2

Considerations in the Care of Relinquishing Birth Mothers

1. During pregnancy, be open to the discussions of single parenting or adoption; be supportive of the woman's decision.
2. Encourage early and appropriate prenatal care.
3. During hospitalization, acknowledge the adoption as a loss; discuss the grief and grieving process with the birth mother.
4. Accept the birth mother as a "real mother," encourage questions, discuss her hospital expectations.
5. Encourage the midwife and/or obstetrician and the pediatrician to provide follow-up care to the birth mother.
6. Include the birth mother in postpartum teaching as appropriate.
7. Assist with the creation of memories in the form of picture taking, saving locks of hair, making footprints, or other acts that have meaning to the birth mother.
8. If desired by the birth mother, allow a formal closure ceremony. Examples of closure could be a quiet "good-bye" between mother and infant or a prayer with family and clergy present. This is important because it facilitates the grief and grieving process.
9. After relinquishment, it might be helpful for the birth mother to link with other mothers who have successfully coped with a similar experience. Support groups can be located in association with hospitals, adoption agencies, and other interested community agencies.
10. Encourage postpartum follow-up so that the birth mother's physical and emotional recovery can be monitored.

---

regards to lesbians considering parenting: (1) sexual orientation disclosure to providers and finding sensitive caregivers, (2) conception options, (3) assurance of partner involvement, and (4) how to legally protect both the parents and the child. Lesbian and heterosexual pregnancies have many similarities, and health care providers should not overlook the parallels. Issues of sexual activity, psychosocial changes related to attaining the traditionally defined maternal tasks of pregnancy

(Rubin, 1984), and birth education all need to be addressed with lesbian couples. Special needs of the lesbian couple requiring assessment include social discrimination, family and social support networks, obstacles in becoming pregnant (i.e., coitus versus artificial insemination), lesbian maternal role development, legal issues of adoption by the partner, and coparenting roles.

Buchholz's qualitative study (2000) examined the childbirth experiences of lesbian couples. The researcher focused on the positive aspects of the experience and the reasons why they were positive for the mother. Preparation of the nursing staff before the couples' arrival in the delivery area was seen by the couples as helpful. This preparation assisted the staff with the execution of the couple's birth plan and helped identify, ahead of time, nurses who would prefer not to work with the couple. The nurses' inclusion of the mother's partner in the labor and delivery process, by acknowledging their approaching parenthood and allowing the partner to assist with newborn care after delivery, was seen as positive. The nursing staff conveyed support by using comforting gestures, checking with the couple frequently, answering questions, and just "being there" for them (Buchholz, 2000).

This study identified two major concerns of lesbian couples. The first centered on legal issues such as power of attorney, visiting restrictions for the partner, and birth certificate information (father identification). The second dealt with the couple's attention to nurses' behavioral cues and questioning whether busyness on the part of the nurses might somehow equate to discomfort with the situation.

To meet lesbian parents' special needs and provide sensitive and appropriate care, nurses must come to understand the lifestyle and culture of the lesbian couple and work with them in addressing both their physical and their psychosocial concerns. Equally important, nurses must understand their own cultural values and norms, being careful not to impose them on couples with special needs. Last, hospital policies and procedures might need to be adapted to reflect the changing times, lifestyles, attitudes, and needs of all our clients.

Maternal Role Attainment Alterations

Maternal role attainment is an attribute many times taken for granted in Western culture. If you give birth and become a mother, the assumption is you automatically become "maternal" and successfully care for and nurture your infant. However, many factors can affect maternal role attainment, including separation of mother and infant in cases such as illness, incarceration, or adoption, to name only a few. An example of successful maternal role attainment superimposed with a chronic illness is described in a phenomenological study that explored factors affecting maternal role attainment in Thai HIV-positive mothers selected for their successful adaptation to the maternal role. The results indicated six internal and external factors used to assist in attainment: (1) setting a purpose of raising their babies; (2) keeping their HIV status secret; (3) maintaining feelings of autonomy and optimism by living as if nothing were wrong, i.e., normalization; (4) belief of quality versus quantity of support from husbands, mothers, or sisters; (5) hope for a cure; and (6) belief that their secret is safe with their health care providers. The study results indicated that while the diagnosis of HIV created challenges in attaining their mothering role, the women's feelings of shame of infection (seen as a disease of prostitutes in Thai culture) were buffered by their will to live, love for, and hope for a future with their children. The researcher notes in Thai society, women are the major agents of socialization in a child's life. As such, the knowledge gained by studying how HIV-positive Thai mothers manage the dual demands of survival and the attainment of the maternal role will help health care providers as they work to care for and provide support to women in these circumstances (Jirapaet, 2001).

Nontraditional Support Systems

A cultural variation that has important implications is a woman's perception of the need for formalized assistance from health care providers during the antepartum period. Western medicine is generally perceived as having a curative rather than a preventive focus. Indeed, many health care providers view pregnancy as a disaster waiting to happen, a physiologic state that at any moment will become pathologic. Because many cultural groups perceive pregnancy as a normal physiologic process, not seeing pregnant women as ill or in need of the curative services of a doctor, women in these diverse groups often delay seeking, or even neglect to seek, prenatal care.

Pregnant women and their partners are placing increased emphasis on the quality of pregnancy and childbirth, and many childbearing women rely on nontraditional support systems. For couples who are married, White, middle class, and infrequent users of their extended family for advice and support in childbirth-related matters, this kind of support might not be crucial. However, for other more traditional cultural groups, including African Americans, Hispanics, Filipinos, Asians, and Native Americans, the family and social network (especially the grandmother or other maternal relatives) may be of primary importance in advising and supporting the pregnant woman.

It is essential that the nurse do a thorough cultural assessment to ascertain how much the pregnant woman uses nontraditional support systems and/or Western health care during her pregnancy. Once this assessment is complete and a trusting relationship has been established, the woman's pregnancy can be managed and consideration given to all the components that both she and the nurse believe are important for a successful outcome. An example of how women's perceptions for the need of antepartum care might vary is described in Evidence-Based Practice 5–4.

Cultural Beliefs Related to Activity During Pregnancy

Cultural variations also involve beliefs about activities during pregnancy. A belief is something held to be actual or true on the basis of a specific rationale or explanatory model. **Prescriptive beliefs,** which are phrased positively, describe expectancies of behavior; the more common restrictive beliefs, which are phrased negatively, limit choices and behaviors. Many people believe that the activities of the mother—and to a lesser extent of the father—influence newborn outcome. Box 5–3 describes some prescriptive and restrictive beliefs and taboos that provide cul-

tural boundaries for parental activity during pregnancy. These beliefs are attempts to increase a sense of control over the outcome of pregnancy.

Positive or prescriptive beliefs might involve wearing special articles of clothing, such as the *muneco* worn by some traditional Hispanic women to ensure a safe delivery and prevent morning sickness. Other beliefs and practices involve ceremonies and recommendations about physical and sexual activity. One event in which a prescriptive belief might cause harm occurs when there is a poor neonatal outcome and the mother blames herself. For example, the mother whose fetus has died as a result of a cord accident, and who believed that hanging laundry caused the cord to encircle the baby's neck or body, might experience severe guilt. The nurse who is sensitive to the mother's anguish might say, "Many people say that if you reach over your head during pregnancy, it will cause the cord to wrap around the baby's neck. Have you heard this belief?" Once the woman responds, the nurse can explore her feelings about the practice. Do others in her family or social support network share her belief? The nurse might share her own views by saying, "I have not read in any medical or nursing books that this practice is related to cord problems, although I know many people share your belief." The discussion can then continue focusing on the feelings and perceptions of the event as it is experienced by the woman and her family.

Negative or **restrictive beliefs** are widespread and numerous. They include activity, work, and sexual, emotional, and environmental prescriptions. **Taboos,** or restrictions with serious supernatural consequences, include the Orthodox Jewish avoidance of baby showers and divulgence of the infant's name before the infant's official naming ceremony (Bash, 1980). A Hispanic taboo involves the traditional belief that an early baby shower will invite bad luck, or *mal ojo,* the evil eye (Spector, 2003).

Food Taboos and Cravings

Among many cultures, a traditional belief was that the mother had little control over the outcome of pregnancy except through the avoidance of foods that are considered taboo. Another tra-

Evidence-Based Practice 5–4:

Amish Women and Perinatal Beliefs

Fifteen Amish women from Ohio described their perinatal beliefs and how they used the available health care system during a total of 76 pregnancies. Before the study, local health care providers commonly believed that Amish women underutilized available prenatal and birth care resources. The Amish women used perinatal care based on their beliefs about pregnancy and childbirth and in relation to cost, transportation, and child care. The women reported initiating prenatal care earlier for first pregnancies and progressively later with increasing parity and with the increasing knowledge that pregnancy was indeed a "nonproblematic" condition. However, all the women reported seeking immediate medical attention if a serious problem arose, e.g., bleeding. During pregnancy, vitamins and herbal teas were commonly used in preparation for childbirth and usually were recommended by Amish family members or a midwife. Usual daily routines were encouraged to continue throughout pregnancy. A normal pregnancy course for an Amish woman consisted of following recommendations on vitamin and herb use from family and friends, going to a physician for prenatal care, and finally being delivered out of the hospital (either at home or at the Amish birthing center) by a midwife. Hospitals were spoken of positively in terms of "safety" and "getting additional rest." Negative statements about the hospital experience involved "lack of privacy" and "high cost." The findings also indicated that Amish women are not opposed to the technologic aspects of childbirth but that they selected modern technology to meet their individual and cultural needs.

Clinical Application

This finding is consistent with other research, which has shown that selective use of modern technology is a critical means of cultural preservation for the Amish community in modern society (Kraybill, 1989). This study emphasized the need to look beyond conformity and homogeneity when providing health care to the culturally different childbearing woman.

In the preceding examples of nontraditional support during pregnancy, it is evident that women use a variety of sources, including family, friends, and traditional healers. It is the nurse's responsibility to accurately assess each woman's situation, experience, and cultural value system so that culturally competent care can be offered.

Campanella, K., Korbin, J., & Acheson, L. (1993). Pregnancy and childbirth among the Amish. *Social Science Medicine* 36(3), 333–342.

---

ditional belief in many cultures is that a pregnant woman must be given the food that she smells to eat, otherwise the fetus will move inside of her and a miscarriage will result (Spector, 2003). Spicy, cold, and sour foods are often the foods to be avoided during pregnancy.

Some pregnant women experience pica: the craving for and ingestion of nonfood substances, such as clay or laundry starch. Some Hispanic women prefer the solid milk of magnesia that can be purchased in Mexico, whereas other women eat the ice or frost that forms inside refrigerator units. The causes of pica are poorly understood, but there are some cultural implications because women from certain ethnic or cultural groups experience this disorder. In the United States, pica is common in African-American women raised in the rural South and in women from

BOX 5-3

Cultural Beliefs Regarding Activity and Pregnancy

Prescriptive Beliefs

- Remain active during pregnancy to aid the baby's circulation (Crow Indian)
- Remain happy to bring the baby joy and good fortune (Pueblo and Navajo Indian, Mexican, Japanese)
- Sleep flat on your back to protect the baby (Mexican)
- Keep active during pregnancy to ensure a small baby and an easy delivery (Mexican and Cambodian Canadian)
- Continue sexual intercourse to lubricate the birth canal and prevent a dry labor (Haitian, Mexican)
- Continue daily baths and frequent shampoos during pregnancy to produce a clean baby (Filipino)

Restrictive Beliefs

- Avoid cold air during pregnancy (Mexican, Haitian, Asian)
- Do not reach over your head or the cord will wrap around the baby's neck (African American, Hispanic, White, Asian)
- Avoid weddings and funerals or you will bring bad fortune to the baby (Vietnamese)
- Do not continue sexual intercourse or harm will come to you and baby (Vietnamese, Filipino, Samoan)
- Do not tie knots or braid or allow the baby's father to

do so because it will cause difficult labor (Navajo Indian)
- Do not sew (Pueblo Indian, Asian)
- Avoid heavy physical work, eat rich and healthy foods, and get frequent rest (Iranian Canadian)

Taboos

- Avoid lunar eclipses and moonlight or the baby might be born with a deformity (Mexican)
- Do not walk on the streets at noon or 5 o'clock because this might make the spirits angry (Vietnamese)
- Do not join in traditional ceremonies like Yei or Squaw dances or spirits will harm the baby (Navajo Indian)
- Do not get involved with persons who cast spells or the baby will be eaten in the womb (Haitian)
- Do not say the baby's name before the naming ceremony or harm might come to the baby (Orthodox Jewish)
- Do not have your picture taken because it might cause stillbirth (African American)
- During the postpartum period, avoid visits from widows, women who have lost children, and people in mourning because they will bring bad fortune to the baby (South Asian Canadian)

From Waxler-Morrison, N., Andrews, J., & Richardson, E. (1990). *Cross-cultural caring: A handbook for health professionals in Western Canada.* Vancouver, BC: University of British Columbia Press.

lower socioeconomic levels. The phenomenon of pica has been described in Kenya, Uganda, and Saudi Arabia (Boyle & Mackey, 1999).

Cultural Issues Impacting Prenatal Care

Morgan's study (1996) of African-American women explored beliefs, practices, and values related to prenatal care. The findings indicated that many of the women in urban areas lacked trust and were apprehensive about their current life circumstances. Establishing a good relationship and providing a safe environment increased attendance at prenatal clinics. Urban African-

American women indicated that they had less support than their contemporaries in the rural South. Nurses should be encouraged to set up peer social and educational groups for women who are similar to those in this study. In addition, the findings indicated that adherence to folk health care beliefs and practices were prevalent among study participants. Nurses must learn more about the practices of their clients and have a nonjudgmental attitude. Acceptance of alternative healers might even be therapeutic and helpful for many clients.

In a study by Berry (1999), Mexican-American women participated in an ethnonursing study focusing on the meanings and experiences attached to generic care (family and extended family pregnancy guidance) and professional care during pregnancy. Significant themes for generic culture care were identified as protection of the mother and fetus by elder Mexican-American women, who were affected by religious and family practices, and the value attached to the family providing care for the mother and being with her. Professional culture care themes included (1) respecting the family roles of caring for the mother in relation to age and gender, (2) expressing concern, knowledge, protection, and explanations and attending to the needs of the mother, (3) using the Spanish language while caring for the mother, and (4) believing that professional prenatal care was valued by the women even though access was in many cases problematic.

Incorporating the value of respect into the culture care of Mexican-American pregnant women can be achieved on many levels and might be demonstrated by the following practices:

1. Supporting the religious or spiritual needs of clients by helping to locate religious advisors and providing time for prayer when indicated
2. Addressing clients by last name and conversing with clients about their families before the initiation of care
3. Acknowledging elder generic guidance during pregnancy and, when appropriate, incorporating these practices into the client's care
4. Respecting the family's beliefs in a male authority as the protector and final decision maker
5. Encouraging a client to include her spouse in prenatal visits when decisions regarding care must be made, or making the information available for the client to take home for approval, especially when consents are required (Berry, 1999).

Both studies (Morgan, 1996; Berry, 1999) reported similar barriers to prenatal care access, including (1) lack of telephones for communicating with health care providers, (2) lack of transportation to the clinics, (3) legal issues surrounding immigration that affected access, (4) bureaucratic paperwork, and (5) inflexible clinic schedules. Nurses need to exercise creativity when solving these problems. For instance, they can explore the possibility that city or county governments will provide free transportation to health care sites for women in need of such assistance. Nurses can support the development of telephone health information systems in appropriate languages to explain access to health care, especially for newly immigrated clients. And last, nurses can rethink and restructure clinic schedules to include weekend and evening appointments as one way of easing the burden of access (Berry, 1999).

Traditional beliefs surrounding care during pregnancy when interfaced with Western medicine has, in some situations, forced an adjustment in the way Mexican-American women engage in pregnancy care behaviors. Mexican-American childbearing women seem to represent a healthy model for preventing low birth weight infants. However, acculturation to U.S. lifestyle may also put them at an increased risk for poor birth outcomes (Martin et al., 2004). An ethnographic study in California examined the influence of acculturation on pregnancy beliefs and practices of Mexican-American childbearing women. Lagana (2003) reported that "selective biculturalism" emerged as a protective approach to stress reduction and health promotion. The women interviewed indicated that regardless of the level of acculturation to U.S. culture, during pregnancy, they returned to traditional Mexican practices. Such practices include a low-fat, high-protein, natural diet (eat right—*come bien*); exercise for well-being (walk—*camina*); and avoidance of worry or stress, which could have a negative effect on the pregnancy outcome (don't worry—*no se preocupe*). They described the family as a major support during pregnancy but also valued the economic and personal freedom available to women in the United States. The resulting conflicts lead to the adoption of a "selective bicultural perspective." This perspective allowed the women to maintain or reject cultural practices as needed. The fact that the women in this study lived in a largely Latino town might have limited their bicultural stress, whereas Mexican pregnant women living in a more heterogeneous environment might experience higher levels of stress related to cultural conflicts. The author suggests, "It is likely that some cultural traits protective of pregnancy are lost through the process of acculturation" (Lagana, 2003, p. 123). This statement indicates that health care providers need to consider not only the support from family and social support networks, but also explore the impact of stress from cultural conflicts on pregnancy outcomes.

Cultural Interpretation of Obstetric Testing

Many women do not understand the emphasis that Western prenatal care places on urinalysis, blood pressure readings, and abdominal measurements. For traditional women from the Middle East, the vaginal examination might be so intrusive and embarrassing that they might avoid prenatal visits or request a female physician or midwife (Lipson, Hosseini, Omidian, & Edmonston, 1995). Common discomforts of pregnancy might be managed with folk, herbal, home, or over-the-counter remedies on the advice of a relative (generally the maternal grandmother) or friends (Spector, 2003). Health care providers can attempt to meet the needs of women from traditional cultures by explaining health regimens so that they have meaning within the cultural belief system. However, such explanations are only an initial step. Nursing visits can be made to the home, or group prenatal visits might be made based on self-care models instituted by nurses in local community centers. Additionally, nurses can incorporate significant others into the plan of care. During prenatal visits, nurses can provide information on normal fetal growth and development, and they can discuss how the health and behavior of the mother and those around her can influence fetal outcome.

Cultural Preparation for Childbirth

Preparation for childbirth can be developed through programs that allow for cultural variations, including classes during and after the usual clinic hours in busy urban settings, teen-only classes, single-mother classes, group classes combined with prenatal checkups at home, classes on rural reservations, and presentations that incorporate the older "wise women" of the community. In addition, nurses can organize classes in languages other than English.

Birth and Culture

Beliefs and customs surrounding the experience of labor and delivery are influenced by the fact that the physiologic processes are basically the same in all cultures. Factors such as cultural attitudes toward the achievement of birth, methods of dealing with the pain of labor, recommended positions during delivery, the preferred location for the birth, the role of the father and the family, and expectations of the health care practitioner might vary according to the degree of acculturation to Western childbirth customs, geographic location, religious beliefs, and individual preference.

Traditionally, cultures have viewed the birth of a child in two very different ways; for example, the birth of the first son may be considered a great achievement worthy of celebration, or the birth may be viewed as a state of defilement or pollution requiring various purification ceremonies. In general North American culture, birth is often viewed as an achievement—unfortunately not for the mother but rather for the medical staff. The obstetrician "manages" the labor and "delivers" the infant; for this active role, the doctor is often profusely thanked even before the mother is praised or congratulated. Gifts and celebrations are centered on the newborn rather than the mother. The recent consumer movement in childbirth and the upsurge of feminism has caused some redefinition of the cultural focus and has encouraged women and their partners to assume active roles in the management of their own health and birth experiences. Unfortunately, some women who have prepared themselves for a totally "natural" childbirth might feel disappointment and a sense of failure if they require analgesia or a cesarean section.

Traditional Home Birth

All cultures have an approach to birth rooted in a tradition in which childbirth occurs at home, within the province of women. For generations, traditions among the poor included the use of "granny" midwives by rural Appalachian Whites and southern African Americans and *parteras* by Mexican Americans. A dependence on self-management, a belief in the normality of labor and birth, and a tradition of delivery at home might influence some women to arrive at the hospital only in advanced labor. The need to travel a long distance to the closest hospital might also be a factor contributing to arrival during late labor or to out-of-hospital delivery for many American Indian women living on rural, isolated reservations. Izugbara and Ukwayi (2004) report that in rural Nigeria, women use traditional birth homes operated by birth assistants, and the impetus for home birth is for reasons of geography (i.e., rural isolation, economic and cultural factors). Such "homes" are used for all manner of women's health care, including births, abortions, family planning, and the treatment of sexually transmitted infections (STIs). These traditional birth homes are critical for the delivery of health care to these women and children. The authors report that there is a need to integrate these "homes" into their mainstream health care delivery system in order to increase responsiveness to local communities.

This raises the question of how many informal systems are operating in the United States among rural/or traditional women with no access to mainstream health care, and how can they be identified and integrated in order to have the best of both worlds? One such example currently in existence involves Latinos in the United States, which are one of the most medically underserved populations (Doty, 2003). Latino women have the highest birthrate among ethnic groups in the United States, but because of unaffordable insurance, program cuts, and limited access to appro-

priate prenatal care, this group of women and their unborn babies are placed in a precarious situation (Martin et al., 2004). It has been recommended to integrate the informal Latino care system with the mainstream in such a way as to ensure a complementary system. Latinos informal care system for pregnant women includes the use of lay midwives (*parteras*), labor and postpartum support persons (*doulas*), and health workers in the community (*promotoras*). McGlade, Somnath, and Dahlstrom (2004) describe how community lay workers can be used for outreach, including sharing information regarding availability of formal care, empowering women with cultural care knowledge to continue to work with pregnant women in order to preserve healthy Latino customs that might otherwise be lost to acculturation, and continuing to provide the social support system that is known to be of such benefit to this group of women. Some U.S. clinics have taken this information to heart and have incorporated these recommendations with great success.

The literature offers yet another example of the impact culture has on perinatal care practices. Walsh (2006) examined the beliefs and practices of an indigenous Guatemalan community's traditional birth attendants (TBAs) by using ethnographic methods, identifying the major themes as sacred calling (being called to service by God or a saint), sacred knowledge (skills learned through dreams or visions via communication with God), and sacred rituals (candles, incense, and other religious artifacts to create a sacred environment, along with prayer). The researcher found that most commonly the birth attendant in Guatemala is the *comadrona,* a woman in the community who is trusted and has a calling for the role of a midwife. The women may or may not have training, and because many lack formal training, they are often blamed for the high mortality rates. Currently, most health care practices in urban and rural areas use Western approaches; however, traditional Guatemalan villages continue to use TBAs. The midwives in the highlands were found to attend monthly meetings in which nurses and physicians offer education on obstetrical problems and emergencies. Walsh (2006) reported the *comadronas* are incorporating the information and skills learned in the monthly training sessions into their practices. These findings would indicate that as health care groups work to design programs to improve health outcomes, integrating cultural beliefs and rituals into health care training might ultimately improve health outcomes. As our immigration numbers continue to grow, hopefully, so too will the number of health care institutions that strive to integrate these informal systems into their models for care.

Support During Childbirth

Despite the traditional emphasis on female support and guidance during labor, the inclusion of spouses and male partners in North American labor and birth rooms has been seen as positive by women of many cultures. Women from diverse cultures report a desire to have husbands or partners present for the birth. Unfortunately, some North American hospitals still maintain rules that limit the support person to the spouse or that prevent a husband from attending the birth unless he has attended a formal childbirth education program with his wife. Fortunately, this situation has changed a great deal in the past few years so that husbands or partners now make important contributions in supporting and helping pregnant women during labor (Figure 5–1).

Another source of conflict is the desire of many women to have the mother or some other female relative or friend present during labor and birth. Because many hospitals have rules limiting the number of persons present, the mother might be forced to make a difficult choice among the persons close to her.

For an Orthodox Jewish woman in labor and for reasons of modesty, a woman of choice from the community may be the labor support person (Lewis, 2003). The spouse may elect to stay in the labor room provided the mother's private parts are covered. Similar findings are reported from women of Islamic, Chinese, and Asian Indian backgrounds. Practices followed by these groups might include strict religious and cultural prohibitions against viewing the woman's body by *either* the husband or any other man, or they might practice separation of the husband and wife once the "bloody show" or cervical dilation has occurred (Meleis & Sorrell, 1981; Callister, Semenic, & Foster, 1999). Other noteworthy considerations when caring for laboring Orthodox Jewish couples include keeping the laboring

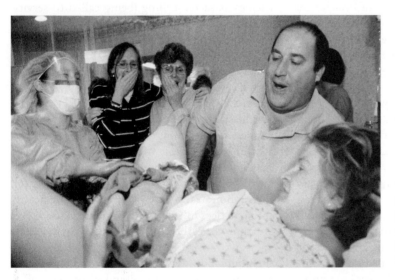

FIGURE 5-1. These family members provide comfort, emotional support, and coaching throughout the entire labor and delivery. (© Copyright B. Proud)

mother's head covered at all times, perhaps by providing her with a surgical cap, and allowing an Orthodox man to pick up his newborn directly from the crib versus having a female nurse or physician hand him the newborn because practicing Orthodox men are not allowed contact with adult women other than their spouses (Lewis, 2003). Nurses must determine how much personal control and involvement are desired by a woman and her family during the birth experience. Due to a wide variation of customs and beliefs, it is always best for the nurse to ask patients directly about the level of observance followed so that hospital practices can be aligned with individual's needs.

For particular groups of women, religion or spirituality is central to their belief system and is the guiding factor in the childbirth experience. A study by Callister et al. (1999) of Orthodox Jewish and Mormon childbearing women investigated the meaning of culture and religion as they relate to childbirth. Evidence-Based Practice 5–5 high-

lights the study's findings and clinical applications.

Cultural Expression of Labor Pain

Although the pain threshold is remarkably similar in all persons regardless of gender, social, ethnic, or cultural differences, these differences play a definite role in a woman's perception of labor pain. Because nurses care for women and families from a variety of cultural backgrounds in labor and birth, they must know and understand how culture mediates pain (Lee & Essoka, 1998; Weber, 1996). In the past it was commonly believed that women from Asian and Native North American cultures were stoic and did not feel pain in labor (Bachman, 2000). Such views are ethnocentric and should be avoided. Many factors interact to influence labor and the perception of pain. They include cultural attitudes toward the normalcy and conduct of birth, expectations of how a woman should act in labor, the

Evidence-Based Practice 5–5:
Culture, Religion, and Childbirth.

This descriptive phenomenological study investigated the spiritual and cultural meanings of childbirth from the perspectives of 30 Canadian Orthodox Jewish childbearing women and 30 American Mormon childbearing women. Five themes were described: (1) the significance of a shared connectedness with others and God, (2) description of birth as a "bittersweet paradox," (3) sense of empowerment, (4) the importance and value placed on childbearing and childrearing, and (5) the spiritual essence of giving birth.

Clinical Application

Listening to women describe significant life events assists nurses as they work with clients to define their health care needs. For these women, spirituality and culture are inextricably woven into the fabric of childbearing practices. Nurses caring for culturally diverse clients must strive to understand the personal meaning and the spiritual essence of birth for each woman and family and respect the expressions of these beliefs by supporting their religious rituals and practices.

Callister, L. C., Semenic, S., & Foster, J. C. (1999). Cultural and spiritual meanings of childbirth. *Journal of Holistic Nursing, 17*(3), 280–295.

role of significant others, and the physiologic processes involved.

Callister and Vega (1998) reported that Guatemalan women in labor tend to vocalize their pain. Coping strategies include moaning or breathing rhythmically and massaging the thighs and abdomen. Japanese, Chinese, Vietnamese, Laotian, and other women of Asian descent maintain that screaming or crying out during labor or birth is shameful; birth is believed to be painful but something to be endured (Lee & Essoka, 1998; Weber, 1996; Bachman, 2000). Although many women from diverse cultures are deemed unprepared by some health professionals because they do not use formal breathing and relaxation techniques, women often use culturally appropriate ways of preparing for labor and delivery. These methods might include assisting with childbirth from the time of adolescence, listening to birth and baby stories told by respected elderly women, or following special dietary and activity prescriptions during the antepartal period.

Birth Positions

Numerous anecdotal reports in the literature describe "typical" birth positions for women of diverse cultures, from the seated position in a birth chair favored by Mexican-American women to the squatting position chosen by Laotian Hmong women. The nurse who cares for laboring women must realize, however, that the choice of positions is influenced by many factors other than culture and that the socialization that occurs when a woman arrives in a labor and delivery unit might prevent her from stating her preference.

Economically disadvantaged women from culturally diverse backgrounds have few birth options; most labor and give birth in large public hospitals. Routine patterns of care and decreased individualization are common in these institutions. These and other problems, such as language barriers, make the provision of culturally competent care during the birth process a challenge. However, any special provisions or attempts to understand the client from her perspective will be received with cooperation and gratitude. Recommendations for intrapartum nursing care of the culturally diverse pregnant woman are presented in Box 5–4.

Cultural Meaning Attached to Infant Gender or Multiple Births

The meaning that parents attach to having a son, a daughter, or multiple births varies from culture to culture. Traditionally, the male gender is highly regarded, which places female infants in a position of "less than favorable." In certain Asian and Islamic cultures, it is believed that a male child is preferable to a female child. Twin births also carry a significance that varies from culture to culture. Twins may be viewed as something very special, while other cultural groups may view multiple births more negatively. In these situa-

---

BOX 5-4

Intrapartum Nursing Care for Culturally Diverse Women

1. If you are unable to speak the woman's language, talk with an English-speaking relative or arrange for an interpreter.
2. If your nursing agency commonly cares for culturally diverse clients, find out whether other nurses have had experiences with similar clients. Share resources and your expertise with staff members.
3. Attempt to gain as much information as possible by completing a cultural assessment.
4. Elicit the mother's expectations about her labor and delivery experience.
5. Ask if she wants a support person with her? If so, have her identify that person.
6. Explore with her any cultural rituals she wants incorporated into her plan of care. If requests are manageable, honor them.
7. Be patient, draw pictures, gesture. Identify key words from family or the interpreter that you will need to be able to express yourself to her, for example, push, blow, pant, stop.

tions, the nurse might find the best course of action is simply to point out all the positive attributes of the newborn.

Culture and the Postpartum Period

Western medicine considers pregnancy and birth the most dangerous and vulnerable time for the childbearing woman. However, other cultures place much more emphasis on the postpartum period. Many cultures have developed practices that balance and cushion this special time of vulnerability for the mother and the infant. Such strategies are thought to mobilize support for the new mother. Interestingly, support that comes from family and friends is usually considered "nontraditional" in approach by Western medicine. These cultural differences, particularly as they relate to restrictive dietary customs, activity levels, and certain taboos and rituals associated with purification and seclusion, might seem unusual to the nurse but have been noted to positively influence the mother's postpartum mental health, thus reducing the incidence of problems such as postpartum depression (Stewart & Jambunathan, 1996). Evidence-Based Practice 5-6 describes postpartum depression among Hmong women.

Posmontier and Horowitz's (2004) review of the literature reports that postpartum depression (PPD) occurs in a wide variety of cultures worldwide. While it is apparent that the majority of PPD research has been conducted with Western cultures (Affonso, De, Horowitz, & Mayberry, 2000), reporting of the phenomenon in non-Western culture may be hindered by culturally unacceptable labeling of the disorder, variance of symptoms from group to group, or differences in diagnostic standards from culture to culture

---

Evidence-Based Practice 5-6:

Hmong Women and Postpartum Depression

Postpartum depression in Western culture has been documented. The literature suggests that one cause of postpartum depression is lack of supportive practices surrounding childbirth. This study explored postpartum depression in Hmong women living in the United States. The results indicated these women perceived themselves to be supported during pregnancy and after delivery. The high levels of support received from spouses and family, combined with the practice of a 30-day rest period, might have made them less vulnerable to depression. The only symptoms of depression reported were related to living in a culture and environment different from their own and having to use a foreign language.

Clinical Application

Be sensitive to the fact that Hmong women have difficulty in learning English because of child care responsibilities and possibly the lack of a formal education. Encourage family involvement in the woman's nursing care plan during and after pregnancy. Provide referrals for opportunities to learn English-speaking skills and employment skills to facilitate the woman's adjustment to North American culture.

Stewart, S., & Jumbunathan, J. (1996). Hmong women and postpartum depression. *Health Care for Women International, 17,* 319–330.

(Yoshida, Yamashita, Ueda, & Tashiro, 2001; Committee on Cultural Psychiatry, 2002; American Psychiatric Association, 2000). Insights provided by the literature suggest nurses should assess all new mothers of diverse backgrounds for culture-specific signs of PPD. Women may express symptoms as somatic in nature, especially in cultures that have no name or definition for PPD, such as the Korean culture (Posmontier & Horowitz, 2004). In order to provide culturally competent nursing care for childbearing women and families from diverse backgrounds, nurses need to incorporate culturally sensitive assessments into their models of care in order to identify significant aspects that can be combined with Western approaches of care.

Routine postpartum nursing care usually includes encouraging a healthy diet, adequate fluid intake, and self-care practices such as good hygiene practices, sitz baths, showering, bathing, ambulation, and exercise. However, these practices, common in North American obstetric care, might seem strange and even dangerous to women of other cultural groups. Nurses must take time not only to teach their clients, but to listen to them, making accommodations and being flexible when possible. In many cultures, the concept of postpartum vulnerability is based on one or more beliefs related to imbalance or "pollution." **Imbalance** is perceived to be the result of disharmony caused by the processes of pregnancy and birth, and **pollution** is seen to be caused by the "unclean" bleeding associated with birth and the postpartum period (Horn, 1981). Restitution of physical balance and purification might occur through many mechanisms, including dietary restrictions, ritual baths, seclusion, restriction of activity, and other ceremonial events.

Hot/Cold Theory

Central to the belief of perceived imbalance in the mother's physical state is adherence to the **hot/cold theories** of disease causation. Pregnancy is considered a "hot" state. Because a great deal of the heat of pregnancy is thought to be lost during the birth process, postpartum practices focus on restoring the balance between the hot/cold beliefs, or yin and yang. Common components of this theory focus on the avoidance of cold, in the form of either air or food. This real fear of the detrimental effects of cold air and water in the postpartum period can cause cultural conflict when the woman and infant are hospitalized. Nurses must assess the woman's beliefs regarding bathing and other self-care practices in a nonjudgmental manner.

Many women will pretend to follow the activities suggested by nurses, to the point of pretending to shower while in reality avoiding the nurses' prescriptions. The common use of perineal ice packs and sitz baths to promote healing can be replaced with the use of heat lamps, heat packs, and anesthetic or astringent topical agents for those who prefer to avoid cold influences. The routine distribution of ice water to all postpartum women is another aspect of care that can be modified to meet women's culturally diverse needs. Offering women a choice of water at room temperature, warm tea or coffee, broth, or another beverage should satisfy most women's needs for warmth, along with the offering of additional bed blankets.

Postpartum Dietary Prescriptions and Activity Levels

Dietary prescriptions are also common in this period. The nurse might note that a woman eats little "hospital" food and relies on family and friends to bring food to her while she is in the hospital. If there are no diet restrictions for health reasons, this practice should be respected. Indeed, the nurse should assess what types of food are being eaten by the woman and documenting them as appropriate.

Regulation of activity in relation to the concept of disharmony or imbalance includes the avoidance of air, cold, and evil spirits. Hispanic women are encouraged to stay indoors and avoid strenuous work. Obviously, if pregnancy and birth cause a "hot" state, the woman should avoid "hot" activities such as ironing. Fruits and vegetables and certainly cold drinks might be avoided because they are considered "cold" foods. Some women from traditional cultural groups view themselves as "sick" during the postpartal lochial flow. They might avoid heavy work, showering, bathing, or washing their hair during this vulnerable time. Cultural prescriptions vary regarding when women can return to full activity after childbirth, but many traditional cultures suggest that a woman can resume normal activities in as little as 2 weeks, and some take up to 4 months.

Postpartum Seclusion

The period of postpartum vulnerability and seclusion in most non-Western cultures varies between 7 and 40 days. Hispanic women, especially primigravidas, might follow a set of dietary and activity rules called *la dieta* (Horn, 1981). The Hispanic midwife or *partera* will stay at the home of the mother for several hours after the delivery and will make a follow-up visit the next day.

Placental burial rituals are also part of the traditional Hmong culture, and with the continued growth in the number of Hmong Americans emigrating from California to different areas of the United States, cultural conflicts are common, especially in the areas of reproductive health (Clemings, 2001). In an effort to assimilate, many Hmong have continued to use animistic ceremonies and herbal remedies in addition to using Western medicine. Helsel and Mochel's study (2002) explored Hmong Americans' attitudes regarding placental disposition, cultural values affecting those attitudes, and perceptions of the willingness of Western providers to accommodate Hmong patients' wishes regarding placental disposal. The Hmong believe the placenta is the baby's "first clothing" and must be buried at the family's home, in a place where the soul can find the afterlife garment once the person is deceased. If the soul is unable to find the placental "jacket," it will not be able to reunite with its ancestors and will spend eternity wandering. Helsel and Mochel's study (2002) suggests that even though the Hmong have made giant leaps in transitioning from their traditional culture to that of

Western culture, traditional Hmong beliefs in placental burial persist. Health care providers need to examine their own beliefs and institutional policy regarding the assumption that the placenta is medical waste and consider beliefs that regard the placenta as a necessary vehicle into the afterlife. This change in attitude and behavior by health care professionals would not only serve to accommodate the needs and wishes of traditional cultures, but it would indicate a commitment to provide culturally competent care.

In some cultures, women are considered to be in a state of impurity or pollution during the postpartum period. Consequently, ritual seclusion and elimination of activity might be practiced to reduce the risk of increasing personal vulnerability to the influence of spirits or of spreading evil and misfortune. In many cultures, this time of seclusion coincides with the period of lochial flow or postpartum bleeding. Common taboos include seclusion and avoidance of contact with others, avoidance of contact with food or objects, and avoidance of sexual relations.

Cultural Influences on Breast-feeding and Weaning Practices

In an effort to increase the practice of breast-feeding, the World Health Organization and UNICEF (2004) recommend children worldwide be breast-fed for a minimum of 2 years, with no defined upper limit on the duration. Physiologically, children can be breast-fed over a period of several years. Only a few women in the United States participate in extended breast-feeding (longer than 3 years) for fear of disapproval; therefore, it is usually concealed from family, friends, and health care providers. Dettwyler's work (2004) in this area reports segments of the country where relatively large groups of women nurse longer than 3 years. These areas include Seattle, WA; Salt Lake City, UT; College Station, TX; and Wilmington, DE. Culturally, breast-feeding and weaning can be affected by a variety of values and beliefs related to societal trends, religious beliefs, the mother's work activities, ethnic cultural beliefs, social support, access to information on breast-feeding, and the health care provider's personal beliefs and experiences regarding breast-feeding and/or weaning practices, to name a few.

For breast-feeding women from traditional backgrounds, it is important for nurses to be aware of factors that have been shown to affect the quality and duration of the breast-feeding experience, along with factors impacting weaning practices. McKee, Zayas, and Jankowski (2004) examined predictors of successful breast-feeding initiation and persistence in a sample of low-income African American and Hispanic women in the urban Northeast. The findings indicated that those women with a strong cultural identification and cultural social support, tended to initiate breast-feeding and continue with breast-feeding longer than those in the groups who did not have strong cultural identification. Adolescent African-American and Latina mothers in Chicago were interviewed to explore the teens' perceptions of breast-feeding and what influenced their infant feeding decisions and practices. Reported influences included perceptions of breast-feeding benefits (bonding, baby's health), perceptions of the problems with breast-feeding (pain, embarrassment, no experience with the act of breast-feeding), and respected, influential people (Hannon, Willis, Bishop-Townsend, Martinez, & Scrimshaw, 2000). In a related study of the influence of grandmothers on breast-feeding, Almroth, Mohale, and Latham (2000) indicated maternal grandmothers to be positively influential in sharing information, advising new mothers, and providing hands-on and how-to suggestions. Conversely, Susin, Giugliani, and Kummer (2005) found that grandmothers in Brazil having daily contact with mothers were negatively impacting the duration of breast-feeding, citing that both maternal and paternal grandmothers encouraged the introduction of teas, water, and "other" milk. The study confirmed the need to include grandmothers in breast-feeding education so that they would exert a more positive influence.

In a qualitative study by Ingalsbe (1999) of U.S.-residing, Japanese- and Mexican-born mothers, several cultural practices were found to be influential in the type of infant feeding practiced. The Japanese mothers indicated a reluctance to ask questions of U.S. health providers (believe questioning to be inappropriate), which impacted the quality of information and direct teaching they received during the prenatal and postnatal periods. Many first-time moms in this study chose bottle-feeding as a result. The Mexican mothers described mixing Maizena, a cornstarch powder, with cow's milk, for use in weaning from breast- or bottle-feeding, citing its benefits as a thickening agent, keeping the stomach fuller for longer periods and thereby increasing times between breast- or bottle-feedings as solid foods were introduced. Cultural beliefs of women in Hong Kong indicate that even "Westernized" women hold fast to the basic teachings of Confucius, i.e., the family's well-being is central, the father is the head of the family, and harmony with others is essential (Chen, 2001). If a Chinese breast-feeding mother is told by her spouse or family to wean in order to maintain harmony, she will usually follow their advice (Fok, 1996).

Researchers have studied ethnicity, cultural beliefs or practices, and social mores as a way to understand the influences on infant feeding practices. However, one group, in particular—the Native American population—has been studied less closely (Dodgson, Duckette, Garwick, & Graham, 2002). Breast-feeding among indigenous populations (e.g., Aboriginal/Alaska Native and American Indian women) declined with the advent of infant formula availability. However, there has been a push from within Native American communities to a return to infant feeding "the natural way." Banks (2003) describes how breast-feeding is being successfully promoted among the Kanesatake, a rural Mohawk community in Quebec, Canada, using culturally competent community-based interventions. The promotion strategies include educating extended family on breast-feeding benefits; teaching the nutritional merits of breast-feeding, particularly to the maternal grandmother; addressing the social, emotional, and spiritual aspects of breast-feeding; using the oral tradition as a way to share information, setting the stage for cooperative and interactive learning; and creating teaching methods which avoid conventional courses, lectures, or written materials on infant feeding practices, as native women are not attracted to or affected by these methods. In the Kanesatake project, a respected elder volunteered to promote breast-feeding in her community. After completing a training session she chose to use subtle teaching encounters at banks, grocery stores, and social gatherings as a way to promote breast-feeding. Support groups or "talking circles" were organized for extended family and grandmothers of pregnant women where breast-feeding issues were discussed openly and freely, lead by the elder. This approach is a good example of how community strengths, incorporation of culturally specific learning styles, and cultural sensitivity can be used as the foundation for successful program development. Evidence-Based Practice 5–7 describes the sociocultural patterns that promote breast-feeding or weaning in select Ojibwe communities in Minnesota.

Prior to becoming industrialized, women always breast-fed, and midwives attended births. They had a variety of names: aunties, medicine women, midwives, doulas, or grandmothers (grannies), but whatever their names, they were women that have and still are providing the support necessary for successful birthing and breast-feeding experiences. As immigrants continue to pour into the United States and American-born women adhering to their traditional cultural heritage attempt to make informed decisions regarding infant feeding practices, it is imperative as nurses to examine specific cultural norms and practices that influence breast-feeding outcomes as we work to develop successful strategies.

Cultural Issues Related to Domestic Violence During Pregnancy

Domestic violence has emerged as one of the most significant health care threats for women and their unborn children. Numerous issues cross all cultural boundaries and influence the prevalence and response to domestic violence. These include a history of family violence, sexual abuse experienced as a child, alcohol and drug abuse by the mother or significant other, shame associated with abuse, fear of retaliation by the abuser, or fear of financial implications if the mother leaves the abuser, to cite a few. Outcomes of abuse shared by these women regardless of culture include stress (physical and emotional), poor lifestyle health practices, delayed prenatal care, and lack of support. It has been known for some time (Bewley & Gibbs, 1994) that physical abuse during pregnancy focuses on attack of the abdomen, breasts, and/or genitals, which puts not only the mother, but also the unborn child at risk. Along with the physical abuse comes the psychological consequences, including possible addiction to drugs and alcohol, stress, and depression. These factors not only affect the mother's health but can have a future effect on the newborn and later as the child develops. Many forms of abuse in the pregnant population warrant attention and discussion. However, this discussion will focus on three culturally different groups of women who experience **domestic violence during pregnancy.** They are Hispanic, African American, and American Indian pregnant women. What links these groups of pregnant women are shared ideologies or characteristics that influence their behavior and have profound effects on their pregnancy outcomes. Ideologies of each group will be examined and recommendations identified for nurses working with these vulnerable pregnant women in these unique circumstances.

Information regarding women in abusive situations is scarce, partly because of underreporting. Important information we do know is that abused women are less likely to seek health care because their abuser limits access to resources and that battering occurs more frequently during pregnancy. This has implications for the pregnant woman and places her in double jeopardy, not only for herself, but also for her unborn baby as battering of pregnant women has long been associated with adverse pregnancy outcomes. In a recent National Violence Against Women study

Evidence-Based Practice 5–7:

Breastfeeding Patterns in an Ojibwe Community

Applying a focused ethnographic approach with an ecological framework, interviews with 52 Ojibwe women were conducted. The women were divided into three groups: health or social service providers, breast-feeding women, and resource people. Data collection sites used three rural northern Minnesota reservation communities and an urban Ojibwe community. Variation was found in the extent to which the women incorporated traditional ways into their lives in the indigenous communities studied. Participants identified the importance of family and elders in their decision regarding infant feeding, weaning, and health-seeking behaviors. Analysis revealed four patterns of influence: (1) mixed messages (conflicting information), (2) life circumstances (impoverished neighborhoods, high crime areas, few resources, unstable households), (3) nurturing and support (families and partners who supported their breast-feeding were viewed as helpful along with providers who understood their culture), and (4) traditions (all expressed a desire to return to traditional ways when breast-feeding was the norm, breast milk was seen as the healthiest food for infants, and breast-feeding was viewed as the "natural" and preferred method).

Clinical Application

In order for findings to be useful to tribal communities it is important to share the information with those who have an interest in putting them to good use, such as tribal health boards community leaders, and community agencies representing these interests. Developing breast-feeding support groups composed of indigenous women whose purpose is to address the needs identified by the participants is also needed and incorporates findings into a participatory action model which will assist in developing culturally appropriate breast-feeding programs.

Dodgson, J. E., Duckett, L., Garwick, A., & Graham, B. (2002). An ecological perspective of breastfeeding in an indigenous community. *Sigma Theta Tau International, 34*(3), 235–241.

sponsored by the National Institute of Justice and the Centers for Disease Control and Prevention, it was estimated that 1.9 million women in the United States are assaulted annually (Tjadin & Thoennes, 1998; Rynerson, 2000). During pregnancy, 25% to 45% of women are beaten, and it is estimated that this percentage may be increasing (Rynerson, 2000).

An abused pregnant woman has a greater risk of being delivered of a low birth weight (LBW) infant. One of the associations between abuse and LBW is delay in obtaining prenatal care. Indeed, recent studies suggest that physical and sexual abuse predicts poor health during preg-

nancy and the postpartum period (Leserman, Stewart, & Dell, 1999). Evidence-Based Practice 5–8 discusses delays in obtaining prenatal care as a result of battering.

The legacy of patriarchy, which is deeply embedded in our culture, undoubtedly contributes to violence against women as do other factors, especially alcohol and drug abuse. Other issues associated with violence against women also influence pregnancy outcomes. These include exposure to physical harm or death, delayed prenatal care because of restricted access by the abuser, restricted support-seeking behavior, and exposure to drugs and alcohol.

Evidence-Based Practice 5–8:

Prenatal Care Delays Related to Battering

This study evaluated patterns of abuse during the pregnancies of 132 African American, 208 Hispanic, and 162 White American women from low-income clinics in large metropolitan cities in the West. The researchers found that the incidence of abuse did not vary significantly among ethnic groups and that the abused women from these groups sought prenatal care 6.5 weeks later than did the nonabused group. In this study, 1 in 4 women reported that they had been physically abused since their current pregnancy began, with African American women experiencing the most severe and most frequent abuse.

Clinical Application

Include questions about abuse in every routine history taken during pregnancy in order to identify abused women. Offer information about abuse and available community resources. Women reporting abuse will need further screening with specific tools. Nurses should be aware of subtle signs of abuse. For example, psychosomatic complaints, injuries inconsistent with the explanation, failure to keep clinic appointments, and overprotective partners might be indications of abuse. Become familiar with community resources for referrals.

Taggart, L., & Mattson, S. (1996). Delay in prenatal care as a result of battering in pregnancy: Crosscultural implications. *Health Care for Women International, 17,* 25–34.

Recommendations for health care providers will follow each discussion and will emphasize the importance of culturally competent care to these at-risk clients.

Hispanic Pregnant Women

Although there are many different Hispanic groups, they do share some important commonalities, e.g., religion, customs, and language. As with any cultural group, differences do exist among the members. The incidence of wife abuse among pregnant Hispanic women is not clear in the literature. However, Richwald and McClusky (1985) believe that although violence during pregnancy is likely to be the most common form of family violence, it is also the least reported. Access to health care for pregnant Hispanic women is problematic. Barriers to prenatal health care include lack of health care insurance and low levels of education, both of which may encourage the use of traditional healers and

remedies and might foster mistrust of health care professionals, leading to noncompliance. Hispanic women tend to be in low-paying jobs whose annual earnings are considerably less than those of non-Hispanic women. They also have less education than White women and large, extended households, often made up of several children and extended family members. The economic status of Hispanics, and therefore their health status, is closely tied to economic levels because economic status often determines access to care (Suarez & Ramirez, 1999). These many factors place them at a distinct disadvantage when it comes to accessing prenatal care. Furthermore, these same factors tend to discourage the pregnant Hispanic woman from disclosing a situation of abuse and violence. Her choices are the same as those of other women in abusive situations: She can try to make the relationship work, or she can leave her abuser. If you are poor, have no friends or family members nearby, and have several little children who depend on you, leaving the family provider will be very difficult.

The Hispanic pregnant woman who chooses to leave her abuser must face the reality of language barriers, a poor economic situation, no insurance, and perhaps leaving her traditional family support network. These same factors inhibit the seeking of information regarding resources available to abused women. Even when faced with death, some abused women find it very difficult to expose their private situation to someone outside their cultural circle. Furthermore, certain groups of Hispanic women, such as migrants, are at higher risk because they are separated from family support systems in addition to confronting barriers related to poverty and language.

Nurses and other health practitioners in prenatal clinics are in an ideal position to facilitate a trusting relationship with an abused woman. Good assessment skills are crucial, because the first sign of abuse might not be an admission of abuse but physical findings of trauma. It is also helpful that the nurse have strong interpersonal skills and a genuine interest in Hispanic culture. In this situation, a Spanish-speaking health care provider might be able to form a trusting relationship more quickly, enabling the woman to share information about domestic violence. Recommendations for assistance of abused pregnant Hispanic women include working with and mobilizing support, using the family and kinship structure, educating the abused woman regarding available resources for abused women, encouraging the woman's inner strength, and assisting in the development of skills necessary to mobilize resources.

African American Pregnant Women

Many cultural values of African Americans emphasize the larger Black society rather than focusing on individuals, making "all" collectively responsible for one another (Hine & Thompson, 1998). Therefore, many African American women exist in a social context supported by social connectedness versus that of autonomy. It is difficult to be specific about an assessment of factors related to domestic violence among African American women because of the lack of information. However, poor economic conditions might be a primary reason why violence occurs in African American families because often domestic violence is related to social and economic resources. The risk of wife abuse is thought to increase when the woman has a higher educational status than her partner or when the man is unemployed or has trouble keeping a job. This is often a familiar social situation in African American male–female relationships (Barnes, 1999).

One of the most difficult barriers confronting African American abused women attempting to get help from police or from the legal system is the stereotypical view that violence among African Americans is normal. This view can lead to an unequal response to African American victims of violence.

Again, the nurse in the prenatal setting is in an ideal position to gather information and initiate a trusting relationship. As has been pointed out, the abused pregnant woman in this culture might not be willing to incriminate her mate because she already sees him as a "victim of society." The nurse might need to rely heavily on her assessment and history-taking skills, being particularly alert to instances of trauma and to problems with past pregnancies. Education must stress that although the women see their men as "victims," women cannot and must not tolerate abuse. The nurse can identify shelter facilities in the woman's neighborhood and in other areas. If the woman feels uncomfortable going outside her neighborhood (many do for fear they will not be understood outside their culture) the nurse can encourage her to go to members of her extended family, which might be more acceptable within this culture. What is most important is that she has a plan of what to do, where to go, and who to call for help the next time she is afraid for her own safety. Last, the nurse must realize that in most instances, African American women believe that it is the responsibility of the woman to maintain the family, regardless of other factors. Therefore, African American women may be more likely to stay in an abusive relationship.

American Indian Pregnant Women

Violence within families has not always been part of American Indian society. Before contact with Europeans, American Indian society was based on harmony and respect for nature and all living things, sharing, and cooperation. Contributions from both sexes were valued, and many activities were shared, including the roles of warrior and hunter. As Indian communities strive to maintain cultural ties, the concepts of spirituality (balance, harmony, oneness), passive forbearance (humility, respect, circularity, connection, honor), and behaviors that promote harmonious living are reinforced in daily living (Nichols, 2004). Traditionally, cruelty to women and children resulted in public humiliation and loss of honor. Cultural disintegration, poverty, isolation, racism, and alcoholism are just a few of the problems that have fostered violence in American Indian cultures. Nevertheless, despite its prevalence, cruelty to women and children continues to be viewed by American Indians as a social disgrace (Green, 1996). In a recent study by Bohn (2002), the complicating factor of lifetime abuse events was shown to be a significant contributor to preterm birth and low birth weight infants (meaning not only current abuse by the spouse or significant other but other types of abuse inflicted over the lifetime of the mother). Since the 1970s, American Indian tribes have made an effort to develop programs to meet the many needs of their communities. However, violence against women has not been addressed adequately because of the male-dominated leadership, other needs of the tribes, and the shame associated with abuse (Bohn, 1993). This trend is changing gradually.

Recommendations for health care providers include identification of the abused person by direct questioning in a private setting, following the establishment of a trusting relationship; assessment of the woman's chart or medical record may provide an opening for discussion of abuse-related questions. A physical exam may identify signs of abuse, e.g., injuries to the abdomen, breasts, or genitals, and a thorough history may identify signs of depression, suicide attempts, eating disorders, miscarriages, and/or a history of complications of pregnancy.

In interviews with American Indian women, a sense of humor is most helpful because they view someone with whom they can laugh as easy to talk to. Open-ended questions are preferable. The nurse should also learn to become comfortable with periods of silence after questions. This does not mean that clients are not listening but rather just the opposite. These women think the question is worthy of thoughtful consideration before answering.

Once abuse has been assessed, the extent of abuse must be ascertained. The nurse or practitioner must then intervene by providing information, discussing alternatives, and supporting the woman in her decision. Options should focus on Native North American resources because they will be culturally sensitive to her needs. If only non-Indian resources are available, the nurse should follow through within these agencies. Variables to be considered in a discussion of options should include the woman's support system, her personal and cultural value system, and her financial status.

Abuse within this culture is traditionally handled within the family first. The abused woman might be reluctant to go outside for help because this might cause both families to ostracize her. It is important to know that an American Indian woman considers it a virtue to stay with her mate no matter what the circumstance, especially if the marriage was performed by a traditional medicine man or woman. A woman who chooses to stay with her abuser might do so out of loyalty because he is Indian rather than because he is a man. It is essential to understand that when a woman attempts to leave an abusive relationship, she must know that her health care provider cares about her. Safety for the woman and her unborn baby is the priority. The woman will need phone numbers of shelters, counselors, and legal advisors as well as information about job training and educational opportunities. It is important to focus on her strengths, her sense of humor, and her skills and resources. She must be able to feel hope that both she and her abuser will heal.

Summary

Culture as it relates to pregnancy and childbirth was discussed from many vantage points. Biologic and cultural variations that can affect childbearing outcomes were identified and analyzed. Women choosing alternative childbearing lifestyles were examined. The importance of nontraditional support systems to pregnant women, along with discussions of cultural beliefs and practices as they relate to pregnancy, birth, and the postpartum period, were presented with suggestions for care.

Vulnerable pregnant populations at risk for abuse were selected for examination, including Hispanic, African American, and American Indian pregnant women. Nursing care recommendations were offered for each.

Cultural beliefs and practices are continuously evolving, making it necessary for the nurse to acknowledge the various cultures and explore the meaning of childbearing with each family with whom she has contact. It is also important to remember that behavior must be evaluated from within each person's cultural context so that the care provided is not only knowledge based but meaningful. It is always important for the culturally competent nurse to demonstrate genuine concern, interest, and respect for clients' differing backgrounds. Only when these aspects are fully realized can we develop and provide culturally appropriate care for childbearing women and their families.

REVIEW QUESTIONS

1. List the biologic variations discussed and the implications for nursing care of the childbearing woman and her family.
2. Identify nursing interventions for women who relinquish infants during the postpartum period. Identify the typical cultural values in North American society about women who relinquish their infants.
3. Describe the special needs of lesbian couples during the childbearing process. What are common pejorative values about lesbian mothers?
4. Compare traditional Western medical support for pregnant women with nontradi-

tional support, and describe why both might be critical for successful pregnancy outcomes in culturally diverse women.
5. Describe the differences between prescriptive and restrictive beliefs of a mother's behavior during pregnancy.
6. Describe two barriers that African American women face as they attempt to get help in abusive situations.
7. Describe the issues for consideration when developing a breast-feeding program for a traditional American Indian community.

CRITICAL THINKING ACTIVITIES

1. Critically analyze the culturally competent nursing interventions for a Hispanic woman after fetal demise from a cord accident.
2. Analyze the responses the culturally competent postpartum nurse should initiate when an African American woman refuses to get out of bed and shower?

3. Discuss and critically analyze how you would respond to your labor patient's request to allow her lesbian partner to participate in the birth of their child. What activities would you include in the plan of care? Why?

4. Describe and analyze how the nurse might offer culturally appropriate support to an Orthodox Jewish husband who has followed his cultural traditions and refuses to accept his newborn from a female nurse.

REFERENCES

Affonso, D., De, A., Horowitz, J., & Mayberry, L. (2000). An international study exploring levels of postpartum depressive symptomatology. *Journal of Psychosomatic Research, 49,* 207–216.

Almroth, S. Mohale, M., Latham, M. C. (2000). Unnecessary water supplementation for babies: Grandmothers blame clinics. *Acta Paediatrican, 89,* 1408–1413.

American Psychiatric Association. (2000). *Diagnostic and statistical manual of mental disorders* (4th ed., text revision). Washington, DC: Author.

Andrews, M. M., & Hanson, P. A. (2003). Religion, culture and nursing. In M. M. Andrews & J. S. Boyle (Eds.), *Transcultural concepts in nursing* (4th ed., pp. 432–502). Philadelphia: Lippincott, Williams & Wilkins.

Bachman, J. A. (2000). Management of discomfort. In D. L. Lowdermilk, S. E. Perry, & I. M. Bobak (Eds.), *Maternity and women's health care* (7th ed., pp. 463–487). St. Louis, MO: Mosby.

Banks, J. W. (2003). Ka'nistenhsera Teiakotihsnie's: A native community rekindles the tradition of breastfeeding. *AWHONN Lifelines, 7*(4), 340–347.

Barnes, S. Y. (1999). Theories of spouse abuse: Relevance to African Americans. *Issues in Mental Health Nursing, 20,* 357–371.

Bash, D. M. (1980). Jewish religious practices related to childbearing. *Journal of Nurse-Midwifery, 25*(5), 39–42.

Berry, A. B. (1999). Mexican American women's expressions of the meaning of culturally congruent prenatal care. *Journal of Transcultural Nursing, 10*(3), 203–212.

Bewley, C., & Gibbs, A. (1994). Coping with domestic violence in pregnancy. *Nursing Standard, 8*(50), 25–28.

Bohn, D. K. (1993). Nursing care of Native American battered women. *AWHONN's Clinical Issues in Perinatal and Women's Health Nursing, 4*(3), 424–436.

Bohn, D. K. (2002). Lifetime and current abuse, pregnancy risks, and outcomes among Native American women. *Journal of Health Care for the Poor and Underserved, 13*(2), 184–198.

Boyle, J. S., & Mackey, M. (1999). Pica: Sorting it Out. *Journal of Transcultural Nursing, 10*(1), 65–68.

Bromwich, P., & Parsons, T. (1990). *Contraception: The facts* (2nd ed.). Oxford: Oxford University Press.

Buchholz, S. (2000). Experiences of lesbian couples during childbirth. *Nursing Outlook, 48*(6), 307–311.

CDC. *Unintended pregnancy prevention, home.* Retrieved January 5, 2007, from http://www.cdc.gov/reproductivehealth/UnintendedPregnancy/index.htm

CDC, Division of Reproductive Health and the National Center for Chronic Disease Prevention and Health Promotion. (2006). Retrieved January 5, 2007, from http://www.cdc.gov

Callister, L. C., Semenic, S., & Foster, J. C. (1999). Cultural and spiritual meanings of childbirth: Orthodox Jewish and Mormon women. *Journal of Holistic Nursing, 17*(3), 280–295.

Callister, L. C., & Vega, R. (1998). Giving birth: Guatemalan women's voices. *Journal of Obstetric, Gynecologic, and Neonatal Nursing, 27,* 289–295.

Chamberlain, J. (n.d.). *The Pima Indians: The vicious cycle.* Retrieved January 3, 2007, from National Institutes of Health, National Institute of Diabetes and Digestive and Kidney Diseases Web site: http://diabetes.niddk.nih.gov/dm/pubs/pima/vicious/vicious.htm

Chen, Y.C. (2001). Chinese values, health and nursing. *Journal of Advanced Nursing. 36,* 270–273.

Clemings, R. (2001). Fresno's Hmong leave for new lives. *Fresno Bee,* pp., A1, A12.

Committee on Cultural Psychiatry. (2002). *Cultural assessment in clinical psychiatry.* Washington DC: American Psychiatric Publishing.

Cosminsky, S. (1982). Childbirth and change: A Guatemalan study. In C. P. MacCormack (Ed.), *Etiology of fertility and birth.* New York: Academic Press.

Dettwyler, K. A. (2004). When to wean: Biological versus cultural perspectives. *Clincial Obstetrics and Gynecology. 47*(3): 712–723.

Dickason, E. J., Silverman, B. L., & Schult, M. O. (1994). *Maternal infant nursing care* (2nd ed.). St. Louis, MO: Mosby.

Dodgson, J. E., Duckett, L., Garwick, A., & Graham, B. (2002). An ecological perspective of breastfeeding in an indigenous community. *Journal of Nursing Scholarship, 34*(3), 235–241.

Doty, M. M. (2003). *Hispanic patients' double burden: Lack of health insurance and limited English.* New York, NY: Commonweath Fund.

Finer, L. B. (2006). Disparities in rates of unintended pregnancy in the United States, 1994 and 2001. *Perspectives on Sexual Reproductive Health, 38,* 90–96.

Fok, D. (1996). Cross cultural practice and its influence on breastfeeding—the Chinese culture. *Breastfeeding Review, 4*(1), 13–18.

Green, K. (1996). *Family violence in aboriginal communities: An aboriginal perspective.* Ottawa, ON: National Clearing House on Family Violence.

Hannon, P. R.,Willis, S. K., Bishop-Townsend, V., Martinez, I. M., Scrimshaw, S. C. (2000). African-American and Latina adolescent mothers' infant feeding decisions and breastfeeding practices: A qualitative study. *Journal of Adolescent Health, 26*(6), 399–407.

Helsel, D., & Mochel, M. (2002). Afterbirths in the afterlife: Cultural meaning of placental disposal in a Hmong American community. *Journal of Transcultural Nursing, 13*(4), 282–286.

Hine, D. C., & Thompson, K. (1998). *A shining thread of hope.* New York: Broadway Books.

Horn, B. M. (1981). Cultural concepts and postpartal care. *Nursing and Health Care, 2*(9), 516–517.

Ingalsbe, K. S. (1999). *Infant feeding practices of Japanese and Mexican mothers who live in the United States.* Unpublished doctoral dissertation, Saint Louis University.

Izugbara, C. O., & Ukwayi, J. K. (2004). An intercept study of persons attending traditional birth homes in rural southeastern Nigeria. *Culture, Health & Sexuality. 6*(2), 101–114.

Jirapaet, V. (2001). Factors affecting maternal role attainment among low-income, Thai, HIV-positive mothers. *Journal of Transcultural Nursing, 12*(1), 25–33.

Lagana, K. (2003). Come bien, camina y no se preocupe—Eat right, walk and do not worry: Selective biculturalism during pregnancy in a Mexican American Community. *Journal of Transcultural Nursing, 14*(2), 117–124.

Lauderdale, J., & Boyle, J. (1994). Infant relinquishment through adoption. *Image Journal of Nursing Scholarship, 26*(3), 213–217.

Lee, M., & Essoka, G. (1998). Continuing education. Patient's perception of pain: Comparison between Korean-American and Euro-American obstetric patients. *Journal of Cultural Diversity, 5*(1), 29–40.

Leserman, J., Stewart, J., & Dell, D. (1999). Sexual and physical abuse predicts poor health in pregnancy and postpartum. *Psychosomatic Medicine, 61*, 92.

Lewis, J. A. (2003). Jewish perspectives on pregnancy and childbearing. *The American Journal of Maternal/Child Nursing, 28*(5), 306–312.

Lipson, J. G., Hosseini, M. A., Omidian, P. A., & Edmonston, F. (1995). Health issues among Afghan in California. *Health Care for Women International, 16*(4), 279–286.

Luker, K. C. (1999). A reminder that human behavior frequently refuses to conform to models created by researchers. *Family Planning Perspectives, 31*(5), 248–249.

Martin, J. A., Hamilton, B. E., Sutton, P. D., Ventura, S. J., Menacker, F., & Munson, M. L. (2004). Births: Final data for 2002 [Data file]. *National Vital Statistics Reports, 52*(10). Available from CDC Web site, http://www.cdc.gov

McManus, A. J., Hunter, L. P., & Renn, H. (2006). Lesbian experiences and needs during childbirth: Guidance for health care providers. *Journal of Obstetric, Gynecologic & Neonatal Nursing, 35*(1), 13–23.

McGlade, M. S., Somnath, S., & Dahlstrom, M. (2004). The Latina paradox: An opportunity for restructuring prenatal care delivery. *The American Journal of Public Health, 94*(12), 2062–2065.

McKee, M. D., Zayas, L. H., & Jankowski, K. R. B. (2004). Breastfeeding intention and practice in an urban minority population: Relationship to maternal depressive symptoms and mother-infant closeness. *Journal of Reproductive and Infant Psychology, 22*(3), 167–181.

Meleis, A. I., & Sorrell, L. (1981). Bridging cultures: Arab American women and their birth experiences. *Maternal Child Nursing, 6*, 171–176.

Miller, M. A. (1992). Contraception outside North America: Options and popular choices. *NAACOG's Clinical Issues in Perinatal and Women's Health Nursing, 3*(2), 253–265.

Morgan, M. (1996). Prenatal care of African American women in selected USA urban and rural cultural contexts. *Journal of Transcultural Nursing, 7*(2), 3–9.

Nichols, L. A. (2004). The infant caring process among Cherokee mothers. *Journal of Holistic Nursing, 22*(3), 1–28.

Otoide, V. O., Oronsaye, F., & Okonfua, F. E. (2001). Why Nigerian adolescents seek abortion rather than contraception: Evidence from focus-group discussions. *International Family Planning Perspectives, 27*(2), 77–81.

Overfield, T. (1985). *Biologic variation in health and illness.* Menlo Park, CA: Addison-Wesley.

Perry, S. E. (2000). Medical-surgical problems in pregnancy. In D. L. Lowdermilk, S. E. Perry, & I. M. Bobak (Eds.), *Maternity and women's health care* (7th ed., pp. 887–911). St. Louis, MO: Mosby.

Posmontier, B., & Horowitz, J. (2004). Postpartum practices and depression prevalences: Technocentric and ethnokinship cultural perspectives. *Journal of Transcultural Nursing, 15*(1), 34–43.

Richwald, G. A., & McClusky, T. E. (1985). Family violence during pregnancy. In D. B. Jeliffe & E. F. T. Jeliffe (Eds.), *Advances in international maternal and child health* (pp. 87–96). New York: Oxford University Press.

Rubin, R. (1984). *Maternal identity and the maternal experience.* New York: Springer.

Rynerson, B. C. (2000). Violence against women. In D. L. Lowdermilk, S. E. Perry, & I. M. Bobak (Eds.), *Maternity and women's health care* (7th ed., pp. 225–246). St. Louis, MO: Mosby.

Santelli, J., Rochat, R., Hatfield-Timajchy, K., Gilbert, B., Curtis, K., Cabral, R., et al. (2003). The measurement and meaning of unintended pregnancy. *Perspectives on Sexual and Reproductive Health, 35*(2), 94–101.

Spector, R. (2003). *Cultural diversity in health and illness* (6th ed.). Upper Saddle River, NJ: Prentice Hall Health.

Spinks, V. S., Andrews, J., & Boyle, J. S. (2000). Providing health care for lesbian clients. *Journal of Transcultural Nursing, 11*, 137–143.

Stewart, S., & Jambunathan, J. (1996). Hmong women and postpartum depression. *Health Care for Women International, 17*, 319–330.

Suarez, L., & Ramirez, A. G. (1999). Hispanic/Latino health and disease. In R. M. Huff & M. V. Kline (Eds.), *Promoting health in multicultural populations* (pp.115–136). Thousand Oaks, CA: Sage.

Susin, L. R., Giugliani, E., & Kummer, S. (2005). Influence of grandmothers on breastfeeding practices. *Revista de Saúde Pública / Journal of Public Health, 39*(2), 1–6.

Tiedje, L. B. (2000). Returning to our roots: 25 years of maternal/child nursing in the community. *Maternal/Child Nursing, 25*(6), 315–317.

Tjadin, P., & Thoennes, N. (1998, November). Prevalence, incidence and consequences of violence against women: Findings from the national violence against women survey. *U.S. Department of Justice Research in Brief.* Washington, D.C.: U.S. Department of Justice.

U.S. Department of Health and Human Services. (2000). With understanding and improving health and objectives for improving health. *Healthy People 2010* (2nd ed.). Washington DC: U.S. Government Printing Office.

Walsh, L. (2006). Beliefs and rituals in traditional birth attendant practice in Guatemala. *Journal of Transcultural Nursing, 17*(2), 148–154.

Weber, S. (1996). Cultural aspects of pain in childbearing women. *Journal of Obstetrics, Gynecology, and Neonatal Nursing, 25*(1), 67–72.

World Health Organization and UNICEF. (2004). *Global strategy for infant and young child feeding.* Geneva, Switzerland World Health Organization.

Yoshida, K., Yamashita, H., Ueda, M., & Tashiro, N. (2001). Postnatal depression in Japanese mothers and the reconsideration of "Satogaeri bunben." *Pediatrics International, 43*(2), 189–193.

Youngkin, E. Q., Davis, M. S., & Fogel, C. I. (1998). Health needs of lesbians. In E. Q. Youngkin & M. S. Davis (Eds.), *Women's health: A primary care clinical guide* (2nd ed., pp. 125–135). Stamford, CT: Appleton & Lange.

Yusu, F., Siedlecky, S., & Byrnes, M. (1993). Family planning practices among Lebanese, Turkish and Vietnamese women in Sydney. *Australian New Zealand Journal of Obstetrics and Gynecology, 33*(1), 8–16.

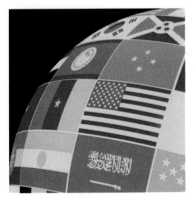

CHAPTER 6

Transcultural Perspectives in the Nursing Care of Children

Margaret M. Andrews

LEARNING OBJECTIVES

1. Examine cultural beliefs and practices related to the health and illness of infants, children, and adolescents.
2. Explore cultural similarities and differences in normal growth and development.
3. Examine biocultural influences on selected acute and chronic conditions affecting infants, children, and adolescents.
4. Apply the transcultural concepts and evidence-based best practices that promote culturally competent care for infants, children, and adolescents.

Society depends on its children for its future and provides its offspring with care, nurturance, and socialization. Cultural survival depends on the transmission of values and customs from one generation to the next, a process that relies on children for its success. In this chapter, the cultural influences on child growth, development, health, and illness will be examined. Figure 6–1 provides a schematic representa-

tion of cultural perspectives on child rearing that include (1) factors that influence parents' child-rearing beliefs and practices, including socioeconomic, educational, political, legal, religious, technological, cultural, and personal characteristics that influence parents; (2) parental beliefs and practices about child rearing and appropriate interpersonal relationships that children have with parents, siblings, extended family members,

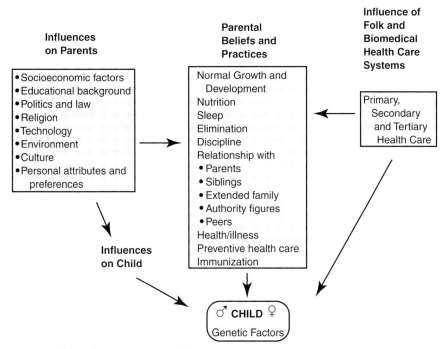

FIGURE 6-1. Cultural perspectives on child rearing.

authority figures, and peers; (3) genetic factors contributing to the child's health and probability of contracting or susceptibility to disease; and (4) influences of folk, traditional or indigenous, and biomedical health care systems on the parents' choices related to primary, secondary, and tertiary health care, including decisions about healers and treatments that are congruent with their cultural beliefs and practices. Figure 6–2 provides a visual representation of the interrelationship among culture, communication, and parental decisions and actions related to child rearing. The clinical relevance of this information for nurses caring for infants, children, and adolescents from diverse cultures will be examined throughout the chapter.

Given that the majority of children are cared for by their natural or adoptive parents, the term *parent* is frequently used in the chapter. However, some children are cared for by grandparents, aunts, uncles, cousins, or those who are unrelated but who function as primary providers of care and/or parent surrogates for varying periods of time. In some cases, the primary provider of care looks after the infant, child, or adolescent for a brief time, perhaps for an hour or two, while the parents are unable to do so. In other cases, this person might function as a long-term or permanent parent substitute even though legal adoption has not occurred. For example, a grandparent might assume responsibility for a child in the event of parental death, illness, disability, or imprisonment. You should be aware that the same factors influencing the parents' cultural perspectives on child rearing also influence others who might care for the child.

Characteristics of the Child Population

Racial and Ethnic Composition

According to Lugaila and Overturf (2004), 72.1 million people under the age of 18 live in the

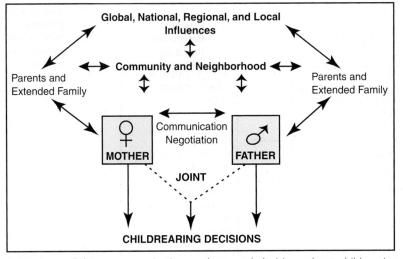

FIGURE 6-2. Culture, communication, and parental decisions about child-rearing practices.

United States; of these, 61% are White, 17% Hispanic (of any race), 15% Black, 3% Asian/Pacific Islander, and 1% Native American/Alaska Native. The number of Hispanic children has increased faster than that of any other group. By 2020, it is projected that more than one in five children in the United States will be of Hispanic origin. It is estimated that by 2020, 40% of school-aged children in the United States will be from federal minority groups. More than 2 million children in the United States are foreign-born, and millions more are the children of recent immigrants. Many of these children constitute the 6.3-million school-age children (14% of the population of the United States, age 5 to 17) who speak a language other than English at home. Approximately two-thirds of these children come from Spanish-speaking homes, and a large percentage of the remainder speaks a variety of Asian languages. Some children of immigrants live in linguistically isolated households: those in which no member age 14 or older speaks English "very well." Nationwide, 4% of children age 5 to 17 live in such households (U.S. Census Bureau, 2000; Lugaila & Overturf, 2004).

Although immigrants and their children are found throughout the United States and Canada, they tend to cluster in certain geographic areas. California, Texas, and New York are homes for almost two-thirds of all foreign-born children. New Mexico, Arizona, New Jersey, and Florida also have relatively high numbers of children whose parents recently immigrated to the United States (U.S. Census Bureau, 2000, 2006; Lugaila & Overturf, 2004). In Canada, most immigrants reside in one of the Canadian Metropolitan Areas (CMAs). Toronto, Vancouver, and Montreal are home for the majority of children of recent immigrants (Statistics Canada, 2004).

Poverty

The impact of poverty on children's health is cumulative throughout the life cycle, with many influences occurring early in life. Halfron & Hochstein (2002) in their Life Course Health Development framework posit that disease in adulthood frequently is the result of early assaults to children's health that become compounded over time. For example, when poverty leads to malnutrition during the so-called "critical period" or the first 2 years of life, the consequences can be catastrophic and irreversible, resulting in damage to the brain, musculoskeletal system, and other parts of the body. If the brain fails to receive sufficient nutrients during the critical period of children's lives, they are likely to experience diminished cognitive development, which leads to poor academic performance in school and later in adulthood to poorer job performance, lower pay, and related outcomes that perpetuate the cycle of poverty and poor health.

Child poverty in the United States continues to grow even though most poor children live in working families. Thirteen million children (one in six) are poor, a number that continues to grow larger each year. A disproportionate number of children from the federal ethnic minority groups live in poverty: one in three African American, American Indian, and Latino children and one in 10 Asian and White, non-Latino children. Children in mother-only family groups are almost five times as likely to be in poverty as those in married-couple families. Research links poverty to numerous risks and disadvantages for children, including increased abuse, neglect, lower reading scores, and overall less success in the classroom, failure, delinquency, malnutrition, and violence (Children's Defense Fund, 2006; Lugaila & Overturf, 2004). To learn more about the characteristics of children and the households they live in, visit www.census.gov/ for the United States and www.statcan.ca/english/census01 for Canada.

Children's Health Status

Indicators of child health status include birth weight, infant mortality, and immunization rates. In general, children from diverse cultural backgrounds have less favorable indicators of health status than their White counterparts. Health status is influenced by many factors, including access to health services. There are numerous barriers to high-quality health care services for minority children such as poverty, geography, lack of cultural competence by health care providers, racism, and other forms of prejudice. Families from diverse cultures might experience difficulties in their interactions with nurses and other health care providers, and these difficulties might have an adverse impact on the delivery of health care. Because ethnic minorities are underrepresented among health care professionals, parents and children often have different cultural backgrounds from their health care providers.

Normal Growth and Development

Although the growth and development of infants and children is similar in all cultures, important racial, ethnic, and gender differences can be identified. From the moment of conception, the developmental processes of the human life cycle take place in the context of culture. Throughout life, culture exerts an all-pervasive influence on the developing infant, child, and adolescent. For example, there is cross-cultural similarity in the sequence and timing of **developmental milestones** in infant development: smiling, separation anxiety, and language acquisition. Developmental researchers who have worked in other cultures have become convinced that human functioning cannot be separated from the cultural and more immediate context in which children develop.

Not all developmental theories formulated on the basis of observations with Western children have cross-cultural generalizability. Investigations of the universality of the stages of development proposed by Piaget, the family role relations emphasized by Freud, and patterns of mother–infant interaction that are taken to indicate security of attachment have resulted in modifications as a result of cross-cultural data.

Growth Patterns

Certain **growth patterns** can be identified across cultural boundaries. For example, regardless of culture, there is a pattern of general-to-specific abilities, from the center of the body to the extremities (proximal-to-distal development) and from the head to the toes (cephalocaudal development). Adult head size is reached by the age of 5 years, whereas the remainder of the body continues to grow through adolescence. Physiologic maturation of organ systems such as the renal, circulatory, and respiratory systems occurs early, whereas maturation of the central nervous system continues beyond childhood.

Other growth patterns seem to be specific to cultural groups. For example, in some cultures, the standard Western developmental pattern of sitting–creeping–crawling–standing–walking–squatting is not followed. The Balinese infant goes from sitting to squatting to standing. Hopi children begin walking about a month and a half later than Anglo-American children, which is paradoxical given the advanced motor development that generally characterizes members of traditional societies. Tooth eruption occurs earlier in Asian and African-American infants than in their White counterparts (Overfield, 1995).

Height and Weight

In the United States, African Americans and Whites differ in mean birth weight, with African Americans being 181 to 240 g lighter. This explains in part why **prematurity**, defined as birth weight less than 2,500 g (5 lb, 8 oz), is twice as common in African Americans as it is in Whites. Chinese, Filipinos, Hawaiians, Japanese, and Puerto Ricans also have lower mean birth weights than Whites in the United States. Significant intertribal variation occurs in the birth weights of Native Americans. For example, the average birth weight among Hopi infant girls is 3,097 g, whereas Cheyenne infant girls weigh, on average, 3,459 g. Native North Americans from British Columbia and Northwestern Ontario have higher mean birth weights than non-Native Canadians. Overall, Native North Americans have a larger number of infants weighing 4,000 g or more at birth—a fact that is believed to be associated with the high incidence of diabetes in Native North Americans (Overfield, 1995).

Although it is difficult to separate nongenetic from genetic influences, some populations are shorter or taller than others during various periods of growth and in adulthood. African-

American infants are approximately three-fourths of an inch shorter at birth than Whites. In general, African-American and White children are tallest, followed by Native Americans; Asian children are shortest. Children of higher socioeconomic status are taller in all cultures. Data on African-American and White children between 1 and 6 years old show that at age 6, African-Americans are taller than Whites. Around age 9 or 10, White boys begin to catch up in height. White girls catch up with their African-American counterparts around 14 or 15 years of age. Around puberty, African-American children begin to slow down in growth, and White children catch up so that the two races achieve similar heights in adulthood. Their sitting/standing height ratios, however, differ. Mexican-American children have sitting/standing height ratios similar to those of White children, indicating similar stature and leg proportions. African-American children have longer legs in proportion to height than other groups (Overfield, 1995).

The growth spurt of adolescence involves the skeletal and muscular systems, leading to significant changes in size and strength in both sexes but particularly in boys. According to Overfield (1995), North American Caucasian youths age 12 to 18 years are 22 to 33 lb heavier and 6 in. taller than Filipino youths the same age. African-American teenagers are somewhat taller and heavier than White teens up to age 15 years old. Japanese adolescents born in the United States or Canada are larger and taller than Japanese who are born and raised in Japan, owing to differences in diet, climate, and social milieu. Adolescence also involves changes in the physiologic functioning of body systems, including the reproductive system.

Infant Attachment

When **infant attachment** is examined, cross-cultural differences become apparent from research on the topic. For example, researchers have discovered that German mothers expect very early autonomy in the child and have few physical interventions as the child plays alone. Among Japanese, there are infrequent mother–

child separations, and the mother has close physical interaction with the child during play. Japanese mothers tend to stay near their infants a great deal, to do many things for them, and to have close physical contact with them. Similarly, Hispanic mothers of Puerto Rican and Dominican ancestry display close mother–child relationships and more verbal and physical expression of parental affection than do European-American parents. Anglo-American mothers tend to have few physical interventions when the child is playing, and they encourage exploration and independence: behaviors that reflect the cultural values of the mothers. Anglo-American mothers tend to give greater emphasis to qualities associated with the mainstream American ideal of individualism such as autonomy, self-control, and activity, whereas Puerto Rican mothers describe children in terms congruent with Puerto Rican cultural emphasis on relatedness, such as affection, dignity, respectfulness, responsiveness to mother and others, and proximity seeking (Zayas & Solari, 1994). Studies suggest that differences in infant attachment are linked to cultural variations in parenting behavior and life experiences. The parents' socialization, values, beliefs, goals, and behaviors are determined in large measure by what their culture defines as good parenting and preferred child behaviors for each gender (Figure 6–3).

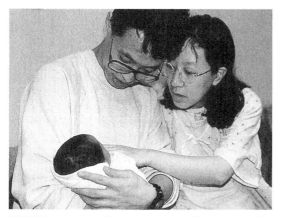

FIGURE 6-3. This Chinese-American family is in the process of developing a strong parent–child bond. (© Copyright Caroline Brown, RNC, MS, DEd)

Crying

Cultural differences exist in mothers' developmental goals for their infants and in the way they perceive, react, and behave in response to their infants' cues, behaviors, and demands. Knowledge of cultural differences in parental responses to crying is relevant for nurses who base their assessment of the severity of an infant's distress according to the parent's interpretation of the crying. You might overestimate or underestimate the seriousness of a problem because of cultural differences in the parent's perception of the infant's distress. You also might misinterpret the degree of parental concern toward an infant if your cultural beliefs and practices differ from those of the parent or other care provider.

Culture-Universal and Culture-Specific Child Rearing

In the following section, some **culture-universal** and **culture-specific child-rearing** values, attitudes, beliefs, and practices will be examined. In reviewing the literature on cultural perspectives on children and adolescents, you will note similarities and differences in the way parents and other primary providers of care relate during various developmental stages. A discussion of culture-universal practices in child rearing will be followed by some remarks about culture-specific practices.

Culture-Universal Child-Rearing Practices

In all cultures, infants and children are valued, treasured, loved, and nurtured because they represent the promise that the human race will continue in future generations. From the moment of birth, differentiation between the sexes is recognized. The early differentiation of gender roles is manifested in gender-specific tasks, play, and dress. Throughout infancy, childhood, and adolescence, girls and boys undergo a process of **socialization** aimed at preparing them to assume adult roles in the larger society into which they have been born or to which they have migrated. Parents and other primary providers of care use various forms of discipline to encourage certain types of behavior and discourage other behaviors in children and adolescents. As children grow and develop, their interaction with others—siblings, extended family members, teachers, religious leaders, peers, and so forth—increases. Children learn communication, language, and other skills needed to interact with people within a cultural context. All parents want to be treated respectfully by their children and want their children to show respect toward selected others in society, the manifestations of which are expressed verbally and nonverbally. When children behave in a manner that is culturally appropriate, they become a source of pride to their parents and bring honor to their family and cultural heritage.

Culture-Specific Child-Rearing Practices

Although there are many universals, most research has focused on culture-specific child-rearing values, attitudes, beliefs, and practices. In other words, there has been a greater interest in cultural differences than in similarities.

A few caveats will be presented before discussing child-rearing practices specific to certain groups. First, child-rearing practices are interrelated with the social, educational, religious, and cultural backgrounds of the parents or other providers of care. Second, it is important to distinguish between cultural practices and those that reflect the economic well-being of the parents and extended family. For example, stereotypes of African Americans suggest that premarital teenage pregnancy is more common and acceptable than among counterparts in other cultures. When socioeconomic factors are considered, however, the myth is shattered. Although African-American adolescents from the lower socioeconomic class have higher rates of teen pregnancy, this is not the case for middle- and upper-class African Americans.

The following discussion will focus on clinically significant child-rearing behaviors among families from diverse cultures. Although it might

be interesting to know, for example, that children are viewed as a gift from God among various ethnic and religious groups, your primary concern is with knowledge that has clinical relevance, such as nutrition, sleep, elimination, parent–child relationships, discipline, and related concepts.

Nutrition: Feeding and Eating Behaviors

In many cultures, breast-feeding is traditionally practiced for varying lengths of time after the birth of an infant: 1 year, 2 years, until the birth of the next child, and so forth. With the growing availability and convenience of bottled formula, manufacturers of these products have launched effective marketing campaigns during recent decades, which have resulted in a decrease in the number of women who breast-feed. You need to be aware that cultural feeding practices might result in threats to the infant's dental health. Studies involving Navajo, Black, Mexican, North American, and other groups demonstrate that caregivers frequently prop a bottle filled with milk, juice, or soda pop with the infant when he or she goes to sleep; this practice is known to cause dental caries. You should teach new mothers about the dangers of propping bottles and encourage them to return to breast-feeding unless it is contraindicated.

In some cultures, mothers might **premasticate**, or chew, the food for infants and young children in the belief that this will facilitate digestion. The practice has been most frequently reported among Black and Hispanic mothers of lower socioeconomic status. From a nutritional perspective, this practice might remove some of the vitamins and minerals from the food before it reaches the infant and make it more acidic. You should warn the mother to refrain from premasticating the food if she has an upper respiratory infection, sore throat, or other condition that could be transmitted to the baby.

Health status is dependent in part on nutritional intake, thus integrally linking the child's nutritional status and health. Although the United States is the world's greatest food-producing nation, nutritional status has not been a priority for many people in this country.

An estimated 1 million children in the United States have malnutrition that is serious enough to interfere with brain development. Many Southeast Asian refugees, for example, were in a prolonged state of malnutrition before emigrating, and undocumented aliens, migrants, poor African Americans in rural and inner-city areas, residents of Appalachia, and others living at the poverty level might be unable to provide their children with an adequate food intake. Likewise, Canadian children living in poverty and those accepted as refugees are more likely to have serious problems associated with malnutrition.

Malnutrition is not found exclusively among children from the lower socioeconomic class. Many middle- and upper-class children, including some obese children, are also malnourished. Obesity frequently begins during infancy, when mothers succumb to cultural pressures to overfeed. For example, among many who identify themselves as Filipino, Vietnamese, and Mexican, to name a few cultures, fat babies generally are considered healthy babies. In most African tribes, fat babies are considered healthy, and mild to moderate obesity is considered a sign of affluence and health later in life.

The popularity of fast-food restaurants and "junk" foods has resulted in a high-calorie, high-fat, high-cholesterol, and high-carbohydrate diet for many children. Parents are frequently involved in numerous activities outside the house and have little time for traditional tasks such as cooking meals. The prevailing attitude among many couples with children is that cooking and housekeeping chores are a choice rather than a necessity. Parents from both affluent and less affluent populations often hold this view toward domestic chores. Because fast foods have intrinsic nutritional value, their benefit needs to be evaluated on the basis of age-specific requirements. For example, the total caloric needs of children of specific ages should be calculated and then compared with total caloric intakes during a typical day (see Evidence-Based Practice 6–1).

The extent to which families retain their cultural practices at mealtime varies widely. Because a hospitalized child's recovery might be enhanced by familiar foods, you need to assess the influence of culture on eating habits. For hospitalized children, you should foster an environment at mealtime that closely simulates the home. Family members can be encouraged to visit during mealtime or to eat with the child if this is appropriate. For example, most Vietnamese parents believe that children should be fed separately from adults and that they should acquire "good table manners" by the age of 5 years. Depending on dietary restrictions necessitated by the child's medical condition, parents should be encouraged to prepare familiar foods at home and bring them to the hospital. The child should be encouraged to eat in the manner that is customary at home. For example, the Asian-American child who eats with chopsticks at home should be encouraged to do so in the hospital.

Sleep

Although the amount of sleep required at various ages is similar across cultures, differences in sleep patterns and bedtime rituals exist. The sleep practices in a family household reflect some of the deepest moral ideals of a cultural community. Nurses working with families of young children in both community and inpatient settings frequently encounter cultural differences in family sleeping behaviors.

Community health, psychiatric, and pediatric nurses who work with young children and their families often assess the family's sleep and rest patterns. On the issue of family cosleeping, nurses traditionally have taken a rigid approach that excludes common cultural practices. Although some degree of **cosleeping**—the practice of parents and children sleeping together for all or part of the night—is common in families with young children, there are marked cultural differences in the proportion who regularly cosleep all night (more than two to three times per week). In a survey of parents of 3- and 4-year-olds of African-American, Hispanic, Vietnamese, Russian, Middle Eastern, and Eastern European descent, Canuso (1996) found that the majority brings their children into bed with them at some

Evidence-Based Practice 6–1:

Best Practices for Preventing Overweight and Obesity in Children from Diverse Cultures

Obesity leads to chronic disease and poor health. Childhood obesity is rising in Canada and other Western industrialized nations at an unprecedented rate. Most experts on obesity agree that the most effective way of curbing the obesity epidemic is through preventive measures. Promoting and protecting the health of children and adolescents in the wake of the growing obesity epidemic requires a comprehensive and carefully constructed plan that draws on past and present research in the area of childhood obesity. The investigator conducted a meta-analysis of research garnered from experts in the areas of child health, immigrant health care, public health, psychology, nutrition, exercise, and health policy on the best ways to prevent and treat obesity in children.

Clinical Applications

- Childhood obesity programs in clinics and schools are helpful in reducing chronic disease risk factor levels (blood fat, blood pressure), reducing body fat, and improving fitness.
- Participating in culturally appropriate physical activities is an important factor in reducing and preventing obesity.
- Involving program participants in the development of programs is important to building acceptance by children, families, and communities.
- Successful programs used multiple strategies such as health education, physical activity, family support, behavior modification, improvement of access to healthy food choices and exercise in schools, and culturally appropriate and meaningful rewards or incentives.

Flynn, M. (2004). Best practices for the prevention of overweight and obesity in children: A focus on immigrants new to industrialized countries. Calgary Health Region. Project No. 6795-15-2002/5440004. Retrieved March 4, 2007, From http://www.hc-sc.gc.ca/sr-sr/finance/hprp-prpms/results-resultats/2004-flynn_e.html.

time. Some parents allow the child into their bed only occasionally, after a nightmare or if the child is upset, whereas others routinely have children crawl in bed with them. A few parents indicated that they sleep with their children all the time.

According to Lozoff, Askew, and Wolf (1996), regular all night cosleeping is most common among African American families (50%), intermediate among Hispanic families (21%), and lowest among White families (<10%). Children might also sleep in the same bed with siblings or members of the extended family. Although the socioeconomic status of the family is known to be a factor, with more cosleeping occurring in families of lower socioeconomic status, some middle- and upper-class families also practice cosleeping. Most White middle-class North Americans believe that infants and children should sleep alone. The values that underlie the custom of having children sleep alone, such as autonomy, privacy, independence, and the primacy of the couple's relationship over the parent–child relationship, are not necessarily shared by parents from diverse cultures who place a higher value on protection of the vulnerable child. Children who cosleep are more likely to wake at night or to have trouble falling asleep alone at bedtime.

To promote rest in the inpatient setting, you need to identify the child's usual pattern by asking the parents about the normal bedtime routine at home. The child might have a favorite toy or story. Depending on the family's religious persuasion, parents might encourage the child to say a prayer at bedtime. You should encourage the child's familiar routine to be continued in the hospital as much as possible.

The type of bed familiar to the child also might vary considerably. In a traditional American Samoan home, infants sleep on a **pandanus mat** covered with a blanket, and sometimes a pillow is used. A **cradleboard** is used by several Native North American nations. Constructed by a family member, a cradleboard is made of cedar, pine, or piñon wood and might be decorated in various ways, depending on the affluence of the family and on tribal customs (Figure 6–4). After completion, the cradleboard is blessed in a traditional manner. The cradleboard helps the infant feel secure and can be moved around with ease

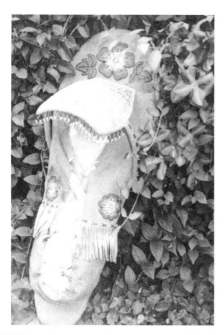

FIGURE 6-4. In most cultures, parents and other care providers use devices that enable the child to sleep while being transported from place to place with relative ease. The use of cradleboards, created many centuries before the infant seat to promote infant mobility and safety, is still prevalent among many Native American nations.

while the family engages in work, travel, or other activities. Although cradleboards have been blamed for exacerbating hip dysplasias in Native infants, diapering counterbalances this by causing a slight abduction of the hips.

In the United States and Canada, the common developmental milestone of sleeping for 8 uninterrupted hours by age 4 to 5 months is regarded as a sign of neurologic maturity. In many other cultures, however, the infant sleeps with the mother and is allowed to breast-feed on demand with minimal disturbance of adult sleep. In such an arrangement, there is less parental motivation to enforce "sleeping through the night," and infants continue to wake up every 4 hours during the night to feed, which is approximately the frequency of feeding during the day. Thus, it appears that this developmental milestone, in addition to its biologic basis, is a function of the context in which it develops.

Elimination

Elimination refers to ridding the body of wastes—a function that is accomplished by the combined work of the gastrointestinal, genitourinary, respiratory, and integumentary systems. Of primary concern to parents is bowel and bladder control, which is the focus of considerable attention by parents of toddlers and preschoolers. Toilet training is a major developmental milestone, perhaps more for the parents than for the child, and is taught through a variety of cultural patterns.

Most children achieve dryness by $2\frac{1}{2}$ to 3 years of age. Bowel training is more easily accomplished than bladder training. Daytime, or diurnal, wetting is less frequent than nighttime, or nocturnal, wetting. Some cultures start toilet training a child before the end of the first year and consider the child a "failure" if dryness is not achieved by 18 months. In other cultures, children are not expected to be dry until 5 years of age. Boys have a more difficult time achieving bladder control than girls.

Constipation in a child is a persistent concern among parents who expect a ritualistic daily pattern. In some cultures, infants are given herbs aimed at purging them when they are a few days, weeks, or months old to remove evil spirits from the body. You should advise the parents against using purgatives in infants because fluid and electrolyte imbalance occurs, and dehydration can ensue rapidly.

The role of the nurse is to acknowledge that toilet training can be taught through a variety of cultural patterns but that physical and psychosocial health are promoted by accepting, flexible approaches. A previously toilet-trained child might become incontinent as a result of the stress of hospitalization but will regain control quickly when returned to his or her familiar home environment. You should reassure parents that regression in hospitalized children is normal and expected.

Menstruation

Ethnicity is the strongest determinant of the duration of menstrual bleeding and of the likelihood that heavy bleeding will occur. In a study of 248 12- to 14-year-old girls of African-American and European descent, Harlow and Campbell (1996) reported that the average duration of bleeding was 5.1 days for African-American girls and 5.6 days for European-American girls. European-American girls were less likely to have an episode of heavy bleeding than were African-American girls. These findings reveal that cultural differences exist in **menstruation** among girls from different groups. The roles of diet, exercise, and stress must also be examined because these factors are known to influence menstruation in women of all ages. Further investigation of potential differences in characteristics of bleeding among various cultural groups might help us understand the reasons for differences in risk of menstrual and uterine abnormalities.

Attitudes toward menstruation are often culturally based, and the adolescent girl might be taught many folk beliefs at the time of puberty. Among Mexican Americans, menstruation is often considered an unpleasant but natural condition requiring circumspect behavior. For example, in traditional Mexican-American families,

menstruating girls and women are not permitted to walk barefooted, wash their hair, or take showers or baths. In encouraging hygienic practices, you should respect cultural directives by encouraging sponge bathing, frequent changing of sanitary pads or tampons, and other interventions that promote cleanliness without violating cultural mandates.

Some Mexican Americans believe that sour or iced foods cause menstrual blood to coagulate, and some Puerto Rican teenagers have been taught that drinking lemon or pineapple juice will increase menstrual cramping. You should be aware of these beliefs and should respect personal preferences concerning beverages. The teenager has probably been taught the folk practices by her mother or by another woman in her family who might be watchful during the girl's menstrual periods. If menstruation coincides with hospitalization, you need to respect the teenager's preferences and might need to reassure the mother or significant other that cultural practices will be respected.

Some Mexican Americans believe that delayed menses are caused by the stoppage of blood flow—a condition treated by the administration of certain herbs. Among other cultural groups, menstrual cramping might be treated with a wide variety of home remedies. You should ask the adolescent girl whether she takes anything special during menstruation or in the absence of menstrual flow. It might be necessary to verify the amount and type of home remedy and to determine its interactive effect with prescription medicines.

Adolescent girls of Islamic religious persuasion, whose heritage might be Palestinian, Lebanese, Jordanian, or Saudi Arabian or from other Near or Middle Eastern nations or some African nations, have cultural and/or religious prohibitions and duties during and after menstruation. In Islamic law, blood is considered unclean. The blood of menstruation, as well as blood lost during childbirth, is believed to render the female impure or potentially polluting.

Because one must be in a pure state to pray, menstruating girls and women are forbidden to perform certain acts of worship such as touching the Qur'an (Koran), entering a mosque, praying, and participating in the feast of Ramadan. During the menstrual period, sexual intercourse is forbidden for both men and women. When the menstrual flow stops, the girl or woman performs a special washing to purify herself.

In Islam, sexual pollution applies equally to men and women. For men, sexual intercourse and the discharge of semen is an act that renders a man impure. A *junub* is a man or woman who has become "impure" because of sexual intercourse and must then perform a ritual washing before being able to perform the prayer (Luna, 1989).

Parent–Child Relationships and Discipline

In some cultures, both parents assume responsibility for the care of children, whereas in other cultures, the relationship with the mother is primary and the father remains somewhat distant (Figure 6–5). With the approach of adolescence, the gender-related aspects of the **parent–child relationship** might be modified to conform with cultural expectations.

Some cultures encourage children to participate in family decision making and to discuss or even argue points with their parents. Some African American families, for example, encourage children to express opinions verbally and to take an active role in all family activities. Many Asian parents value respectful, deferential behavior toward adults, who are considered experienced and wise. Many Asian children are discouraged from making decisions independently. The witty, fast reply that is viewed in some European cultures as a sign of intelligence and cleverness might be punished in some non-Western circles as a sign of rudeness and disrespect.

Physical punishment of Native North American children is rare. Instead of using loud scoldings and reprimands, Native North American

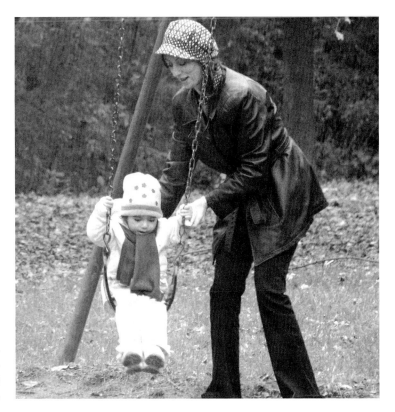

FIGURE 6-5. Culture influences parent–child relationships and age-appropriate activities that promote active, healthy lifestyles for children.

parents generally discipline with a quiet voice, telling the child what is expected. During breastfeeding and toilet training, Native North American children are typically permitted to set their own pace. Parents tend to be permissive and nondemanding.

With the approach of adolescence, parental relationships and discipline generally change. Teens are usually given increasing amounts of freedom and are encouraged to try out adult roles but in a supervised way that enables parents to retain considerable control. In many cultures, adolescent boys are permitted more freedom than girls of the same age.

Child Abuse vs. Folk Healing

Child abuse and neglect have been documented throughout human history and are known across cultures. In the early 1960s, child maltreatment in the United States and Canada became prominent as pediatricians documented radiologic evidence and other symptoms of abuse and neglect in well-publicized reports. International attention to child maltreatment emerged in the late 1970s, and the International Society for the Prevention of Child Abuse and Neglect (ISPCAN) has held international congresses and regional meetings to explore physical abuse and neglect, sexual molestation, child prostitution, nutritional deprivation, emotional maltreatment, and institutional abuse from a cross-national perspective.

Cross-cultural variability in child-rearing beliefs and practices has created a dilemma that makes the establishment of a universal standard for optimal child care, as well as definitions of child abuse and neglect, extremely difficult. Korbin (1991) has identified three levels in formulating culturally appropriate definitions of child maltreatment: (1) cultural differences in child-rearing practices and beliefs, (2) idiosyncratic departure from one's cultural continuum of acceptable behavior, and (3) societal harm to children.

The first level encompasses practices that are viewed as acceptable in the culture in which they occur but are considered abusive or neglectful by outsiders. For example, in Turkey and many Mid-

dle Eastern cultures, despite warm temperatures, infants are covered with multiple layers of clothing and might be observed to sweat profusely because parents believe that young children become chilled easily and die of exposure to the cold. Many African nations continue to practice rites of initiation for boys and girls, usually at the time of puberty. In some cases, ritual circumcision—of both boys and girls—is performed without anesthesia, and the ability to endure the associated pain is considered to be a manifestation of the maturity expected of an adult. In the United States and Canada, the African-American family's focus on physical forms of discipline might present controversial and ethical issues for the nurse.

The second level, idiosyncratic abuse or neglect, signals a departure from the continuum of culturally acceptable behavior. Some societies (Turkish, Mexican, and others), for example, permit fondling of the genitals of infants and young children to soothe them or encourage sleep. However, such fondling of older children or for the sexual gratification of adults would fall outside of the acceptable cultural continuum (Korbin, 1991).

At the third level, societal conditions such as poverty, inadequate housing, poor maternal and child health care, and lack of nutritional resources either contribute powerfully to child maltreatment or are considered maltreatment in and of themselves. African-American children are three times as likely as White children to die of child abuse, but considerable disagreement exists about whether race differences exist in the prevalence of child abuse independently of socioeconomic factors such as income and employment status. You need to become knowledgeable about folk beliefs, child-rearing practices, and cultural variability in defining child maltreatment. Four Southeast Asian folk healing practices that produce physical marks on the child's body are summarized in Table 6-1.

Gender Differences

In all known human societies, adult men differ from adult women in both primary and secondary sex characteristics. On average, men have

TABLE 6-1 *Southeast Asian Folk Healing Practices*

Coining *(Cao gio)*

Appearance	Superficial ecchymotic, nonpainful areas with petechiae, usually appearing between the rib bones on the front and back of the body and resembling strap marks. Coining may also be done along the trachea or on either side of the trachea, vertically along the inner aspect of both upper arms, or along both sides of the spine.
Conditions treated	Pain, colds, heat exhaustion, vomiting, headache.
Procedure	A special menthol oil or ointment is applied to the painful or symptomatic area. Then the edge of a coin is rubbed over the area with firm downward strokes. The procedure is mildly uncomfortable.
Belief	The "coining" exudes the "bad wind." Appearance of a deep reddish-purple skin color is confirmation that the person indeed had "bad wind" in the body and that coining was the appropriate treatment. If only redness appears, the client must consult a healer or doctor for another treatment.
Age of patient	Infants a few months old through seniors.
Practiced by	Mien, Vietnamese, Cambodian (rare), Lao (rare), ethnic Chinese.
Who applies the treatment	Any adult.

Burning *(Poua)*

Appearance	Asymmetric, superficial, painful burns 1/4 inch in diameter, appearing either as a single burn in the center of the forehead or as two nearly symmetrical vertical rows down the front or back of the body, often including the neck.
Conditions treated	Any kind of pain—including pain from a cough or diarrhea—as well as serious conditions such as failure to thrive.
Procedure	A tall, weedlike grass is peeled and allowed to dry. The end is dipped in heated, melted pork lard, and the tip is then ignited and applied to the skin in the area requiring treatment (e.g., joints are burned for failure to thrive). The treatment is painful and always the *treatment of last resort.*
Belief	The burning exudes the noxious element causing the pain or illness.
Age of patient	Infants a few months old through seniors.
Practiced by	Mien, Cambodian (rare).
Who applies the treatment	In Mien culture, the treatment is performed only by a skilled healer. In Cambodian culture, any experienced adult may do it.

Cupping *(Ventouse)*

Appearance	Circular, nonraised, ecchymotic, painful burn marks 2 inches in diameter, usually appearing in symmetric, vertical rows of two to four cups on the left and right sides of the chest, abdomen, and back, or singly as one cup on the forehead. Cupping is rarely practiced in the United States.
Conditions treated	Pain, body ache, headache.

(Continued on following page)

	TABLE 6-1 *Southeast Asian Folk Healing Practices* (continued)
Procedure	Though borrowed from the French, the specific procedure in southeast Asia varies among ethnic groups. The principle is to create a vacuum inside a special cup by igniting alcohol-soaked cotton inside the cup. When the flame extinguishes, the cup is immediately applied to the skin of the painful site. Suction is created, and the skin is pulled up inside the mouth of the cup. The cup remains in place 15 to 20 minutes or until the suction can be easily released. The procedure is painful.
Belief	The suction exudes the noxious element. The greater the "bruise," the greater the seriousness of the illness.
Age of patient	Adults, occasionally teens.
Practiced by	H'mong, Mien, Lao (rare), Cambodian (rare), Vietnamese, ethnic Chinese.
Who applies the treatment	Any adult, except in Vietnamese culture, in which only a skilled nurse or healer may do it.
Pinching (*Bat gio*)	
Appearance	Intensely ecchymotic, isolated, nonsymmetric areas. May be present anywhere on the body, including on the forehead between the eyes, vertically along the trachea, in a "necklace" pattern around the base of the neck, on both sides of the upper chest, on the upper arms (left and right), along the spine, or on either side of the spine.
Conditions treated	Localized pain and a variety of minor and more serious conditions, including lack of appetite, heat exhaustion, dizziness, fainting, blurred vision, any minor illness, cough, fever. Pinching is a *very common* practice.
Procedure	Index and middle finger of one hand are flexed and firmly applied to the skin in a quick, pinching motion. Tiger Balm, a penetrating, mentholated ointment, may be massaged into the area before pinching. The H'mong may pinch first and then prick the area with a sharp needle to draw blood, thus "drawing out" the noxious elements.
Belief	Pinching exudes the bad wind or noxious element.
Age of patient	Children over 10 years old in most cultures; adults only in H'mong culture.
Practiced by	H'mong, Mien, Laotian, Vietnamese, and Cambodian.
Who applies the treatment	Any adult.

From Schreiner, D., Multnomah County Health Services Division. (1981). *S.E. Asian folk healing practices/child abuse?* Paper presented at Indochinese Health Care Conference, Eugene, Oregon. September 18, 1981, pp. 2–5. Reprinted by permission.

a higher oxygen-carrying capacity in the blood, a higher muscle-to-fat ratio, more body hair, a larger skeleton, and greater height. Behaviorally, there are also differences between the two sexes, especially in the division of labor.

For children, gender differences can be identified cross-culturally in six classes of behavior: nurturance, responsibility, obedience, self-reliance, achievement, and independence (Barry, Bacon, & Child, 1967). Differences between boys and girls appear early in life and form the basis for adult roles within a culture. Newborn boys are larger and more vigorously active and have more muscle development, a higher basal metabolic rate, and a higher pain threshold than new-born girls. Newborn girls react more positively to comforting than do newborn boys. By 14 weeks of age, girls might be conditioned through the use of auditory reinforcers, and boys might be conditioned through the use of visual rein-forcers, but not vice versa. By the age of 4 months, girls focus longer than boys on facelike masks, indicating that girls are more interested in faces or facelike configurations (Overfield, 1995).

Variability in sex-role behavior is common. Most people in a society adopt most of the behav-ior defined as appropriate to their biologic sex, but there are many exceptions. Sex roles are themselves highly variable—by age and by social class, among other ways. The stringency of expec-tations also varies, so girls and women in the United States and Canada can violate sex-role norms with fewer explicit sanctions than can boys and men. Across cultures, even the number of sex roles is subject to variations.

Health and Health Promotion

The concept of health varies widely across cul-tures. Regardless of culture, most parents desire health for their children and engage in activities that they believe to be health promoting. Because health-related beliefs and practices are such an integral part of culture, parents might persist with culturally based beliefs and practices even when scientific evidence refutes them, or they might modify them to be more congruent with contemporary knowledge of health and illness.

Illness

The family is the primary health care provider for infants, children, and adolescents. It is the family that determines when a child is ill and decides to seek help in managing an illness. The family determines the acceptability of illness and sick-role behaviors for children and adolescents. Soci-etal trends in illness orientation and economic stress both influence the cultural beliefs that are passed from generation to generation. Health, illness, and treatment (cure/healing) are part of every child's cultural heritage. Every society has an organized response to defined health prob-lems. Certain people are designated as being responsible for deciding who is sick, what kind of sickness the person has, and what kind of treatment is required to restore the person to health.

Research has consistently demonstrated that African-American and Hispanic children are less likely to have seen a physician than are Whites. They also have a lower average number of ambu-latory visits than their White counterparts. Even when children are hospitalized, minorities receive fewer services than do Whites (Federal Interagency Forum on Child and Family Statis-tics, 2006).

Health Belief Systems and Culture-Bound Syndromes

Among many cultural groups, traditional health beliefs coexist with Western medical beliefs. Members of a cultural group choose the compo-nents of traditional or folk beliefs that seem appropriate to them. A Mexican- American fam-ily, for example, might take a child to a physician and either a *curandero* (male) or *curandera* (female)—a traditional healer. After visiting the physician and the *curandero* or *curandera,* the mother might consult with her own mother and then give her sick child the antibiotics prescribed by the physician and the herbal tea prescribed by the traditional healer. If the problem is viral in origin, the child will recover because of innate immunologic defenses, independently of either treatment. Thus, both the herbal tea of the *curan-dero* or *curandera* and the penicillin prescribed by the physician might be viewed as folk remedies; neither intervention is responsible for the child's recovery.

Belief systems about specific symptoms are culturally unique. These are referred to as **culture-bound syndromes**. In Hispanic culture, *susto* is caused by a frightening experience and is recognized by nervousness, loss of appetite, and loss of sleep. Mexican-American babies must be protected from various illnesses. *Pujos* (grunting) is an illness manifested by grunting sounds and protrusion of the umbilicus. It is believed to be caused by contact with a woman who is menstruating or by the infant's own mother if she menstruated sooner than 60 days after delivery.

The evil eye, *mal ojo*, is an affliction feared throughout much of the world. The condition is said to be caused by an individual who voluntarily or involuntarily injures a child by looking at or admiring him or her. The individual has a desire to hold the child, but the wish is frustrated, either by the parent of the infant or by the reserve of the individual. Several hours later, the child might cry and experience fever, vomiting, diarrhea, and loss of appetite. The child's eyes might roll back in the head, and he or she will become listless.

Because the most serious threat to the infant with *mal ojo* is dehydration, the nurse encountering this problem in the community health setting needs to assess the severity of the dehydration and initiate a plan for fluid and electrolyte replacement. You should emphasize the potential seriousness of dehydration to the parents and teach them the warning signs that will alert them to impending danger in the future. A simple explanation of the causes and treatment of dehydration is warranted. If the parents adhere strongly to traditional beliefs, you should respect their desire for the *curandera* to participate in the care. Parents or grandparents might wish to place an amulet, talisman, or religious object such as a crucifix or rosary on the child or near the bed.

Caida de la mollera, or **fallen fontanel**, has a variety of causes for the Mexican American, such as failure of the midwife to press preventively on the palate after delivery. Falling on the head, abruptly removing the nipple from the infant's mouth, and failing to place a cap on the infant's head have also been identified as causes of *caida de la mollera*. The signs of this condition include crying, fever, vomiting, and diarrhea. Given that health care providers frequently note the correspondence of these symptoms with those of dehydration, many parents see *deshidratacion*

(dehydration) or *carencia de agua* (lack of water) as synonymous with *caida de la mollera*. Although regional differences exist, treatment usually is directed at raising the fontanel.

Empacho, a digestive condition recognized by Mexicans, is caused by the adherence of undigested food to some part of the gastrointestinal tract. This condition causes an internal fever, which cannot be observed but which betrays its presence by excessive thirst and abdominal swelling caused by drinking water to quench the thirst. Children who are prone to swallowing chewing gum are most likely to have *empacho*, but it can affect persons of any age.

Among some Hindus from northern India, there is a strong belief in **ghost illness** and **ghost possession**—culture-bound syndromes or folk illnesses based on the belief that a ghost enters its victim and tries to seize his or her soul. If the ghost is successful, it causes death. Illness and the supernatural world are linked by the concepts of fever and the ghost, a supernatural being discussed in the Mahabharata and the Puranas, the Hindu's sacred scriptures.

One sign of ghost illness is a voice speaking through a delirious victim; this may occur in children and adults. Other signs are convulsions and body movements, indicating pain and discomfort, and choking or difficulty breathing. In the case of an infant, incessant crying is a sign. The psychological state of the parents is often involved in the diagnosis, and some believe that ghosts might be cultural scapegoats for the illness and death of children. When an infant or small child becomes ill and dies, a mother or father might be relieved of psychic tension from feelings of personal guilt by transferring the blame for the death to a ghost.

Biocultural Influences on Childhood Disorders

Children are born with a genetic constitution inherited from their parents, who in turn have inherited their own genetic compositions. The child's genetic makeup affects his or her likelihood of both contracting and inheriting specific conditions.

In both children and adults, genetic composition has been demonstrated to affect the individual's susceptibility to specific diseases and disorders. It is often difficult to separate genetic influences from socioeconomic factors such as poverty, lack of proper nutrition, poor hygiene, and such environmental conditions as lack of ventilation, inadequate sanitary facilities, lack of heating during cold weather, and clothing that is insufficient to provide protection during winter months. Other factors responsible for differing susceptibilities to specific conditions are variations in natural and acquired immunity, intermarriage, geographic and climatic conditions, ethnic background, race, and religious practices. Some studies have attempted to explain differences in susceptibility solely on the basis of cultural heritage, but they have not succeeded in doing so. This section examines some common conditions in which genetic constitution seems to be a factor; it is based on research reported by Overfield (1981, 1985).

Immunity

Perhaps one of the most frequently cited examples of the connection between immunity and race is that of malaria and the sickle cell trait in Africans. Black Africans possessing the sickle cell trait are known to have increased immunity to malaria, a serious endemic disease of the tropics. Thus, Blacks with the sickle cell trait survived malarial attacks and reproduced offspring who also possessed the sickle cell trait. As dictated by Mendelian probability, the sickle cell anemia disease eventually developed.

Intermarriage

Intermarriage among certain cultural groups has led to a wide variety of childhood disorders. For example, there is an increased incidence of ventricular septal defects among the Amish and of mental retardation in several other groups. In the extreme, intermarriage among groups having few members can lead to total extinction; the number of Samaritans in Israel, for example, has dwindled to a handful of surviving, aging members.

Geography and Climate

Geographic and climatic factors can be illustrated by the classic example of a common communicable disease of childhood, rubeola (measles). Owing either to mutation of the rubeola virus or to increased individual resistance to the virus, measles became a virtually universal benign childhood disease in many parts of the world during the 19th century. Although the majority of children experienced few ill effects from measles, certain populations, such as children in the Hawaiian Islands, were severely or even mortally affected when explorers and missionaries brought the virus to their lands.

Ethnicity

Although the role of socioeconomic factors in tuberculosis—such as overcrowding and poor nutrition—cannot be disregarded, ethnicity also appears to be a factor in this disease. Groups with a relatively high incidence of tuberculosis are Native North Americans living in the Southwest United States and in northern and prairie regions of Canada, Vietnamese refugees, and Mexican Americans. Ethnicity is also linked to several noncommunicable conditions. For example, Tay-Sachs disease, a neurologic condition affecting Ashkenazic (but not Sephardic) Jews of northeastern European descent, and phenylketonuria (PKU), a metabolic disorder primarily affecting Scandinavians, are congenital abnormalities known to be most prevalent among specific ethnic groups (Overfield, 1981, 1985).

Race

Race has been linked to the incidence of a variety of disorders of childhood. For example, the endocrine disorder cystic fibrosis primarily affects White children, whereas sickle cell anemia has its primary influence among Blacks and those of Mediterranean descent. Black children are known to be at risk for inherited blood disorders, such as thalassemia, G-6-PD deficiency, and hemoglobin C disease. An estimated 70% to 90% of Black children have an enzyme deficiency that results in difficulty with the digestion and metabolism of milk.

Hereditary Predisposition to Disease

The predisposition to certain diseases also has been linked to cultural influences. For example, the incidences of pneumonia and diabetes are especially high among Blacks, and those of dysentery, alcoholism, and suicide are high among Native North American children and adolescents. Mexican-American children are known to succumb to pneumonia more frequently than Anglo North American children of similar socioeconomic status.

Chronic Illness and Disability in Children

Chronic illnesses and **disabilities** have become the dominant health care problem in North America and are the leading causes of morbidity and mortality.

Beliefs Regarding the Cause of Chronic Illnesses and Disabilities

Illness is viewed by many cultures as a form of punishment. The child and/or family with a chronic illness or disability might be perceived to be cursed by a supreme being, to have sinned, or to have violated a taboo. In some cultural groups, the affected child is seen as tangible evidence of divine displeasure, and its arrival is accompanied throughout the community by prolonged private and public discussions about what wrongs the family might have committed.

Inherited disorders and illnesses are frequently envisioned as being caused by a family curse that is passed along from one generation to the next through blood. Within such families, the nurse's desire to determine who is the carrier for a particular gene might be interpreted as an attempt to discover who is at fault and might be met with family resistance.

Folk beliefs mingled with eugenics, particularly throughout western and southern Europe, have resulted in the idea that many chronic conditions, particularly mental retardation, are the products of intermarriage among close relatives. The belief that a chronically ill or disabled child might be the product of an incestuous relation can further complicate attempts to encourage parents to seek assistance.

Among those who believe that chronic illness and disability are caused by an imbalance of hot and cold or yin and yang, the burden of responsibility lies with the affected individual. For many individuals from Latino or Southeast Asian cultures, the cause and potential cure lie within the individual. He or she must try to reestablish equilibrium through regaining balance. Unfortunately for those with permanent disabilities who cannot be fully healed within this conceptual system, society might perceive them as living in a continually impure or diseased state.

Traditional beliefs are tenacious and tend to remain even after genetic inheritance or physiologic patterns of chronic disease progression are explained to the family. Often new information is quickly integrated into the traditional system of folk beliefs, as is evidenced by the addition of currently prescribed medications to the hot/cold classification system embraced by many Hispanic families. An explanation of the genetic transmission of disease might be given to a family, but this does not guarantee that the older belief in a curse or "bad blood" will disappear.

When disability is seen as a divine punishment, an inherited evil, or the result of a personal state of impurity, the very presence of a child or adult with a disability might be something about which the family is deeply ashamed or with which they are unable to cope. In addition to suffering from public disgrace, some parents or families, especially immigrant groups from Eastern Europe and Southeast Asia, might fear that disabled children will be taken away and institutionalized against their will.

Finally, it must be emphasized that some cultural explanations of the cause of chronic disease or disability are quite positive. For example, some Mexican-American parents of chronically ill children believed that a certain number of ill and disabled children would always be born into the world. Many Mexican-American parents who embrace Roman Catholicism believe that God has singled them out for the role because of their past kindnesses to a relative or neighbor who was disabled. They often stated that they welcome the birth of the disabled infant as God's will.

Special Considerations for Adolescents

Culture and Adolescent Development

Adolescence is a developmental passage to adulthood marked by major physical, emotional, and social changes. In many ways, adolescents from different cultural backgrounds grow and develop in similar ways and experience common physical, emotional, and social changes. It is believed that all adolescents show concerns over changes occurring during puberty, such as identity, self-image, increased autonomy, relationships with peers of the opposite sex, and career aspirations. Cultural forces, however, influence the manner in which adolescents respond to these developmental changes.

Havighurst's classic work on adolescent development (1974) identifies eight subtasks that adolescents must complete before entering adulthood: (1) develop new and more relationships with peers, (2) accept a sex role, (3) accept one's physical appearance, (4) become emotionally independent from parents, (5) prepare for marriage and family life, (6) prepare for economic independence, (7) acquire an ideology and value system, and (8) achieve and accept socially responsible behavior. Each task is believed to be important in accomplishing the central task of adolescence: achieving an identity.

Havighurst indicates that the tasks are both historically and culturally relative and acknowledges that variations exist in the type and timing of the tasks faced by adolescents raised in different cultural or subcultural settings. In a cultural–ecologic model, Ogbu (1981) theorizes that development occurs along multiple pathways and suggests that successful development is defined by the culture's "implicit theory of success." This theory is important because it defines for members of the culture the range of available cultural tasks or social positions, their relative value or importance, the competencies essential

for attainment or performance, the strategies for attaining the positions or obtaining the tasks, and the expected penalties and rewards for failures and successes. To achieve culturally defined success, individuals must demonstrate competency at the series of tasks that confront them across the life course. Because the demands and opportunities differ in various cultures or subcultures, however, the competencies required for mastery of cultural tasks also might differ.

From a cultural and developmental task perspective, competent development occurs with successful completion of the tasks that confront the individual at different points in the life course and concomitant development of the social and cognitive skills required by the task and permitted by the culture. Adolescents from a wide range of cultural backgrounds are believed to face different tasks at different points in their lives.

As children grow older they are likely to encounter more people from other cultures and therefore to become increasingly influenced by factors external to their family. By making comparisons between themselves and members of other cultures, adolescents develop a better awareness of their own culture and might begin to select values, behaviors, or attitudes from cultural groups outside the family (Figure 6–6) . The increased sensitivity to cultural differences experienced by adolescents is largely the result of three factors: (1) increased mobility and independence, which permits greater exposure to the world outside the home; (2) growing cognitive ability, which permits greater awareness and understanding of cultural issues; and (3) widening social networks in which diversity manifests itself.

Adolescents who identify with traditionally underrepresented or minority groups are frequently faced with choices about maintaining separateness or going through the process of assimilation or acculturation to the majority group. In assimilation, adolescents take on the values, beliefs, and behaviors of the majority culture and abandon their original ethnic traditions. In acculturation, they accept both their

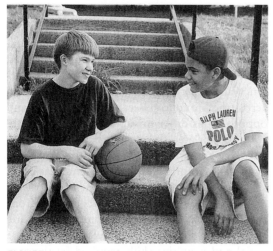

FIGURE 6-6. Adolescents have a need to interact with peers to learn more about themselves and others. (Photo by Melissa Olsen)

own culture and other cultures, adapting elements of each. Acculturated teenagers demonstrate flexibility in adapting their behavior to multiple cultures and are sometimes referred to as having **bicultural** or multicultural competence.

Special Health Care Needs of Adolescents

There are approximately 22 million adolescents in the United States and Canada. Teenagers are in a process of evolving from childhood to adulthood, and they belong not only to the cultural groups that have formed the basis for their values, attitudes, and beliefs, but also to the subculture of adolescents. This subculture links the adolescent with other adolescents through a system of socially transmitted behaviors and belongings, such as clothing, music, and status symbols, including motorcycles, automobiles, videocassettes, compact discs, and stereos. The adolescent subculture has its own set of values, beliefs, and practices that might or might not be in harmony with those of the cultural group that previously guided the teenagers' behaviors.

The society of adolescents is a subculture that is vaguely structured and lacks formal written laws or codes, in which conformity with the peer group is emphasized. One of the most outstanding characteristics of the adolescent subculture is preoccupation with clothing, hairstyles, and grooming. Clothing mirrors the personal feelings of the adolescent and facilitates identity with the peer group.

In the hospital setting, gowns might stifle the individual's sense of identity, so the adolescent should be permitted to wear familiar clothing whenever the style does not interfere with safety, comfort, or hygiene. There is no harm in allowing a small amount of makeup, jewelry, or other items of apparel that might be important to the adolescent.

Whether or not you personally approve of the adolescent's taste in apparel, you should ask the following questions:

- Is the preferred clothing or accessory consistent with the teenager's cleanliness and hygiene? You have the right and responsibility to prohibit the wearing of soiled clothing or to request that clothing be laundered before it is worn.
- Does the clothing or accessory item permit adequate blood circulation? If the clothing is tight or constricting, it might interfere with healing or safety.

To gain the cooperation of the adolescent, you should explain the rationale underlying any concerns about clothing. The adolescent's need to conform to peer norms is important. Rejection by members of the peer reference group might be seen as a fate worse than the illness for which the adolescent is hospitalized.

You might notice that some female refugees or recent immigrants prefer to dress in traditional clothing. Some boys also might elect to wear traditional clothing, but Western-style attire is likely to be more acceptable for men and boys than for women and girls. It is important for the nurse to determine what the adolescent finds most comfortable to wear during hospitalization.

Because of the relationship between some diseases and socioeconomic status, many low-income adolescents from African-American,

Puerto Rican, Mexican-American, and Native American/Canadian subgroups have a higher-than-normal incidence of infectious diseases, orthopedic and visual impairments, mental illness, and untreated dental caries. This group of teenagers from low-income, culturally diverse backgrounds is more vulnerable than normal to illness and is more likely to live in an area in which health care is inadequate or absent. Consequently, low-income teenagers have a wide range of diagnosed and undiagnosed diseases. As these adolescents change from dependent children into independent adults, these disorders might interfere with their development of a positive body image, sexual and personal identity, and value system; with their preparation for citizenship; and with their independence from their parents.

Culturally Competent Nursing Care for Children and Adolescents

A few principles of care for specific cultural groups have been provided to illustrate the practical ways in which culturally competent nursing care should be provided. The examples are intended to be illustrative, not exhaustive.

Nursing Assessment of the Family

Cultural Background

Culture, like language, is acquired early in life, and cultural understanding is typically established by age 5. Every interaction, sound, touch, odor, and experience has a cultural component that is absorbed by the child even when it is not taught directly. Lessons learned at such early ages become an integral part of thinking and behavior. Table manners, the proper behavior when interacting with adults, sick role behaviors, and the rules of acceptable emotional response are anchored in culture. Many beliefs and behaviors learned at an early age persist into adulthood.

Over time, culture has influenced family functioning in many ways, including marriage forms, choice of mates, postmarital residence, family kinship system, rules governing inheritance, household and family structure, family obligations, family–community dynamics, and alternative family formations. These traditions have given families a sense of stability and support from which members draw comfort, guidance, and a means of coping with the problems of life, including physical and mental illness, handicaps, disabilities, dying, and death.

Each family modifies the culture of the larger group in ways that are uniquely its own. Some beliefs, practices, and customs are maintained, whereas others are altered or abandoned. Although it is helpful for you to have a basic knowledge of children's cultural backgrounds, it is also necessary to view each family on an individual basis. Assumptions or biased expectations cannot be allowed to replace accurate assessment. It is essential for you to remember that not all members of a cultural group behave in a stereotypical fashion. For example, although many Chinese North American children behave in the manner congruent with the stereotype—showing respect for authority, polite social behavior, and a moderate-to-soft voice—some are disrespectful, impolite, and boisterous. Individual differences, changing norms over time, the degree of acculturation, the length of time the family has lived in a country, and other factors account for variations from the stereotype.

Family Belief Systems

The behavior of children and adolescents is influenced by child-rearing practices, parental beliefs about involvement with children, and the type and frequency of disciplinary measures. Although both parents exert an influence on the child's orientation to health, research indicates that a wide cultural variability exists, with the mother being the most influential parent in most cultural groups. Thus, identifying the attitudes, values, and beliefs about health and illness held by the parents and other providers of child care is an important part of the cultural assessment of the family.

Mothers' attitudes toward health and illnesses are related to their educational level. Mothers with little formal education tend to be more fatalistic about illness and less concerned with detecting clinical manifestations of disease in their children than are well-educated mothers. The former are also less likely to follow up on precautionary measures suggested by health care providers. A mother who believes that people have no control over whether they become sick is unlikely to have an approach to health in which there is anticipatory guidance or accident prevention and might not comply with recommended immunization schedules. Nursing interventions with a mother who believes that there is much a person can do to keep from becoming ill will be different with regard to the nature of health education and counseling you provide.

With knowledge of the belief system(s) of the family, you have data from which to choose approaches and priorities. For a mother who is not oriented to prevention of illness or maintenance of health, focusing energies on teaching might not be productive; it might be more useful to spend time designing family follow-up care or establishing an interpersonal relationship that invites the parent to follow recommended immunization schedules, well-child care, and other aspects of health promotion. You also should be prepared to understand why the mother who is less educated and embraces a fatalistic philosophy might fail to show up for scheduled well-child appointments but will arrive for an appointment when she believes her child is sick. You might attempt to improve the attendance at well-child care appointments by offering to send reminders (by mail, phone, computer); encouraging mothers to bring grandparents, cousins, friends, or others in a manner that mobilizes the culturally appropriate social support system; and ensuring that the waiting period is reasonable and pleasant (e.g., providing magazines and toys that are culturally appropriate).

Extended Family

Early in the nurse–parent relationship, it is necessary to identify members of the **extended family** who play a significant role in the care of the child. Among families worldwide, the **nuclear family** is a rarity. In only 6% of the world's societies are families as isolated and nuclear as in the United States and Canada. The extended family is far more universally the norm. Kin residence sharing, for example, has long been acknowledged as characteristic of many African-American, Mexican-American, Amish, and other groups.

In societies where the extended family is the norm, parents—particularly those who married at a young age—might be considered too inexperienced to make major decisions on behalf of their child. In these groups, key decisions are frequently made in consultation with more mature relatives such as grandparents, uncles, aunts, cousins, or other kin. Sometimes non-kin are considered to be part of the extended family. In many religions, the members of one's church, synagogue, temple, or mosque are viewed as extended family members who might be relied on for various types of support, including child care. Not coincidentally, members of some congregations refer to one another as brothers and sisters. The Amish family pattern is referred to as *friendscraft*, or three-generational family structure. Amish parents know that they can rely on the support of their entire church community. For example, a young Amish couple might turn to that community for assistance with decision making, finances, and emotional and spiritual support when a child is ill. You should ask the parents if anyone else will be participating in the decision making that affects their child. Once that information is known, you should include the person(s) identified by the parents in the child's plan of care.

The influence of the extended family or the social support network on the child's development becomes particularly important when the number of **single-parent families** in some culturally diverse groups is considered. According to Lugaila and Overturf (2004), 27% of all children in the United States live with only one parent, and 5% live in a household with neither parent present. Although Blacks represent 15% of all children, they account for 32% of all grandchildren, 35% of foster children, and 29% of relatives of the householder other than their sons, daughters, and grandchildren. Seventeen percent of children are of Hispanic heritage and tend to live in households with extended families. Seventy-seven percent of White non-Hispanic children live with two parents. Children born to single mothers are likely to have greater health risks because the social, emotional, and financial resources available to the family are more limited.

The nuclear family is the unit for which most health care programs are designed. Consider the implicit message about the family when you note the number of chairs for visitors typically placed in hospital rooms, physician or nurse practitioner offices, and other health care settings. Although a handful of rural hospitals make special accommodations for the extended and church family of Amish patients to hitch their horses and buggies adjacent to the facility, seldom are the needs of the extended family network accommodated by the majority of health care facilities.

Nursing Interventions

Hair Care

Despite its importance, hair care is sometimes omitted for Black children because White, Hispanic, Asian, and Native American nurses might be unfamiliar with proper care. The hair of Black children varies widely in texture and is usually fragile. Hair might be long and straight or short, thick, and kinky. The hair and scalp have a natural tendency to be dry and to require daily combing, gentle brushing, and application to the scalp of a light oil such as Vaseline or mineral oil. For girls and women (and some adolescent boys), the hair might be rolled on curlers, braided, or left loose according to personal preference. Bobby pins or combs might be used to keep the hair in place. If an individual has cornrowed braids, the scalp might be massaged, oiled, and shampooed without unbraiding the hair.

Some Blacks prefer straightened hair, which might be obtained chemically or thermally. Hair that has been straightened with a pressing comb will return to its naturally kinky state when exposed to moisture or humidity or when hair

---

BOX 6-1

Shampooing the Hair of Black Children and Adolescents

1. Select a mild shampoo. Dandruff is best controlled by shampoos containing zinc pyrithione.
2. Wet hair and apply shampoo directly to scalp. Lather and rinse with warm water.
3. If additional luster and body are desired, add protein conditioner. Allow conditioner to remain in contact with skin for at least 1 full minute, or as directed.
4. Rinse with warm water.
5. Remove excess water with towel, using squeezing motion.
6. Apply small amount of light oil to scalp, using fingertips. Vaseline or mineral oil may be used unless client has a preference for a commercial formula.*

*Note: Chemical relaxers should be applied only by licensed beauticians.

---

growth occurs. Box 6-1 provides a regimen for shampooing the hair of Black children and adolescents.

Children of Asian descent tend to have straight hair that does not require the same amount of care as the hair of most African Americans or Whites. Principles related to personal hygiene apply to children of all racial and ethnic backgrounds, but the specific manner in which care is given might vary widely. When in doubt, you should ask the child's parent or extended family member how hair care is carried out at home. Children might feel more secure if a parent or close family member actually provides the care. If you determine that the child would benefit from care by a familiar caregiver from home, the rationale for requesting family intervention should be explained. Comments that the nursing staff is too busy or uninterested in providing hair care should be avoided; rather, the benefit to the child's security and sense of well-being should be emphasized.

Facial Hair Care

Textural variations are found in the facial hair of culturally diverse boys and men during adolescence and adulthood. Many Asian teenage boys have light facial hair and require infrequent shaving, whereas African-American boys and men tend to have a heavy growth of facial hair requiring regular attention. Some Black teenage boys have tightly curled facial hair, which when shaved curls back on itself and penetrates the skin. This may result in a local foreign-body reaction on the face that can lead to the formation of papules, pustules, and multiple small keloids. Some African-American teens and men might prefer to grow beards rather than shave, particularly when they are ill.

Before shaving a client, you should determine the client's usual method of facial grooming and should attempt to shave or apply depilatories (agents that remove hair) in a similar manner. When using depilatories, you should protect the skin from irritation by keeping the chemical from contacting the client's nose, mouth, eyes, and ears. Straight and safety razors are contraindicated when depilatories are used because they can cause local irritation to the skin.

Skin Care

When bathing a client, you should remember that the washcloth removes some parts of the outermost skin layer. Such sloughed skin, which will be evident on the washcloth and in the bathwater, will vary in color depending on the ethnic group of the person being bathed. The sloughed skin of a darkly pigmented child, for example, will be a brownish black color. This does not mean that the child was dirty; the normal sloughing of skin is simply more evident in darkly pigmented people when compared to lightly pigmented groups. The more melanin that is present, the darker the skin color will be. Because dryness is more evident on darkly pigmented skin, Vaseline, baby oil, lanolin cream, and lotions can be applied after the bath to give the skin a shiny, healthy appearance.

Evaluation of the Nursing Care Plan

To evaluate the effectiveness of the nursing care plan in providing culturally competent care, first you should ask a few probing questions to determine whether the plan was successful in achieving the desired outcomes, including the mutual goals established with the child's parents. Second, if the goals were not met, you should ask a few probing questions to determine the reasons for failure. Were the child's parents included in the planning and implementation of the nursing care? Were extended family members included in the plan? Did the true decision maker in the family participate in the care plan? For example, it might be that the grandmother, grandfather, uncle, aunt, or other extended family member—not the biologic mother or father—is the family decision maker. Third, if the goals were met, the reasons for their success should be evaluated and communicated to other nurses for future reference. Other members of the health care team should be involved in the evaluation, including traditional healers or folk practitioners.

Application of Cultural Concepts to Nursing Care

Case Study 6-1 is presented to demonstrate the application of transcultural nursing concepts, theories, and research findings to clinical nursing practice. The use of the Amish in this case is illustrative of many cultural groups characterized by an extended family network and by cultural beliefs and practices that differ from those of the health care providers of the dominant health care delivery system. The case example warrants attention for the many issues it raises. The cultural concepts relevant to nursing practice in this situation are illustrated in Box 6-2. As shown, the nursing problem is complex and multifaceted. The interconnectedness of the various components of the child's situation with the larger system is often minimized or disregarded. The values and beliefs of both the nurses within the health care delivery system and the Amish extended social network must be considered. For the purpose of analysis, some fundamental conflicts in values and beliefs have been identified.

BOX 6-2

Nursing Plan of Care: Hospitalization of an Amish Child

Goal: Child's recovery and ultimate discharge from the hospital (return to parents) in an optimal state of health. This is a mutual goal of the Amish child's parents and of the health care providers within the health care system. In order to plan care for this child, the nurse needs to examine the underlying attitudes, values, and beliefs of the two groups that are in conflict. Points on which there is agreement must be identified as well.

Amish	**Health Care Providers**
Family	
Large families, agricultural lifestyle, extended sociocultural-religious network of Amish community members who can be counted on to assist the natural parents.	Small family units, urban lifestyle, nuclear family.
Cooperation and support among extended family, especially in stressful "crisis" times such as hospitalization of a child.	Individual responsibility by nuclear family; mother and father primarily responsible.
Amish community members show interest and concern by visiting.	Visiting by grandparents and siblings accepted only under specified conditions (i.e., at times and places convenient for the nurses).
Concept of family includes "nonblood relatives."	Concept of family includes only biologically related persons.
Parental obligations	
Children are a part of a larger cultural group; adult members of the larger community have various relationships and obligations to the children and parents even though they are not biologically related.	Mother and father are responsible for children; *one* adult may stay with patient overnight, preferably natural mother or father. Hospital facilities do not allow for a larger number of visitors, who clutter rooms, violate fire safety rules, and hinder work. A request for information from every visitor is time consuming and perceived as an interruption to the nurse's work.
Economic considerations	
Communal sharing of resources; hospital bill is paid from a common fund; entire bill is paid in cash upon discharge.	Rely on health insurance, using large pools of money derived from insurance premiums for claim payment. Sense of anonymity and impersonal. Government regulation of health care.
Traditional and religious values	
Religious values permeate all aspects of daily living; time set aside daily for prayer and reading of scripture.	Religion is important, in some families often in proportion to the degree of illness; usually worship is limited to a single day of the week, such as Saturday or Sunday.
Illness afflicts both the just and the less righteous and is to be endured with patience and faith.	Illness is part of a cause–effect relationship; science and technology will one day conquer illness.
Protestant work ethic (in an agricultural, rural sense).	Protestant work ethic (in an urban sense).
Dress is according to 19th-century traditions; specific colors and styles indicate marital status.	Fashions occur in trends; wide range of "acceptable" dress.
Married men wear beards; single men are clean-shaven.	Whether a man shaves is a matter of personal preference.
Simple, rural lifestyle; family-oriented living. For religious reasons, avoid "modern" conveniences such as electricity; use candles/kerosene lights, outdoor sanitary facilities.	Use electricity/nuclear energy; indoor plumbing is the norm; view flush toilets as "ordinary."

Similarities and differences also have been indicated in the nursing plan of care.

CASE STUDY 6-1

Maria Gonzalez, an enthusiastic new graduate, argues heatedly with her nursing supervisor, certain that her persuasive, rational approach will win her case, if not the pure "rightness" of her cause. Located approximately 50 miles from a sophisticated urban university medical center is a rural Amish community. With frequent intermarriages have come some serious, but surgically correctable, cardiac defects among the offspring of the Amish. Members of the Amish community have become a familiar nursing "problem" for the staff of this large children's hospital. Arriving in "unreasonably large groups," several adults, adolescent girls, and younger children often come to visit Jeremiah, a 6-month-old with a ventricular septal defect. The problem of overnight accommodation for the extended family, which includes members of the biologic family as well as of the extended Amish community, has become a topic of lively debate among the nursing staff. Sensitive to the cultural practices and beliefs of the Amish child and his family, the new graduate begins her argument on behalf of the family's right to adhere to Amish cultural practices.

The supervisor listens impatiently as Maria argues her case for cultural sensitivity and quickly interrupts Maria with her decision. "These people are such a nuisance. They don't even know how to flush the toilets when they visit the hospital. This isn't a hotel. They can just go back to their horses and buggies, outhouses, and old-fashioned ways. The answer is *NO!* The natural, biologic mother or father may spend the night. Everyone else is to go home. And that's final."

After conducting a cultural assessment, identified mutual goals, and compared underlying attitudes, values, and beliefs among the Amish parents and the health care providers, you are ready to engage in activities that will promote health or identify nursing care problems (sometimes referred to as nursing diagnoses). Having done this, you examine potential nursing interventions from a transcultural perspective. When

nursing care decisions or actions are made, Leininger's (1991, Leininger and McFarland, 2002) cultural care preservation/maintenance, cultural care accommodation/negotiation, and cultural care repatterning/restructuring will be useful in the provision of culture-congruent care. Finally, the nurse, in collaboration with the parents and significant others who might be members of the extended family, should evaluate the effectiveness of the nursing care from a transcultural nursing perspective.

The key to successful nursing care is conducting a comprehensive cultural assessment during which appropriate and relevant cultural information is gathered. In addition, you need to compare these data with what you know about the health care system within your institution or agency. How does change occur? What parts of the system need to be manipulated to bring about the desired change? Who are the key persons to involve in effecting change? In the case involving the Amish child, the nurse is clearly pushing for a policy change, for which she has no support from her immediate nursing supervisor. Is a compromise possible? How legitimate are the arguments against having the extended family room in with the child? Are there legal implications? What ramifications does the proposed change have for the welfare of other patients? Can fire safety regulations be met without necessitating expensive changes in the hospital building? What are the adverse effects on the child if the extended family cannot spend the night? Are the natural parents able to understand the rules of the hospital and to adapt to the situation?

There are no definitive solutions or answers to these questions. This case study is intended to demonstrate the complexity of the problem and to emphasize the necessity for thoughtful analysis of various facets of the problem. The ability to apply knowledge from the liberal arts—psychology, anthropology, religion and theology, history, economics, sociology, and others—to the nursing care of children from culturally diverse backgrounds is invaluable.

If nurses want to provide excellent transcultural nursing care, cultural assessment is the foundation on which it is based. With practice and repeated experiences with assessing children and adolescents from various cultural backgrounds, you will gain the knowledge and skill needed to conduct comprehensive, meaningful cultural assessments. In reflecting on the practical aspects of conducting cultural assessments, some nurses comment on the busy and rapid pace of a typical pediatric unit and argue that there is insufficient time to conduct cultural assessments of their patients. The few minutes needed to take a cursory admission history might be the only time a professional nurse spends in assessing the aspects of the child and family that have cultural significance. Cultural assessment should be an integral part of the admission routine for all children and adolescents, not an additional data category that is perceived to be optional. Other members of the health team frequently overlook cultural information that the nurse fails to obtain during the cultural assessment as well. The missing cultural data might result in an unnecessarily prolonged period of recovery or in care that is culturally inappropriate.

Summary

Culture exerts an all-pervasive influence on infants, children, and adolescents and determines the nursing care appropriate for the individual child, parents, and extended family members. Knowledge of the cultural background of the child and family is necessary for the provision of excellent transcultural nursing care. Your **cross-cultural communication** must convey genuine interest and allow for expression of expectations, concerns, and questions.

Culture influences the child's physical and psychosocial growth and development. Basic physiologic needs such as nutrition, sleep, and elimination have aspects that are culturally determined. Parent–child relationships vary significantly among families of different cultures, and individual differences among those with the same background add to the complexity. Cultural beliefs and values related to health and illness influence health-seeking behaviors by parents and determine the nature of caring and curing expected.

There is a dearth of specific information about adolescents from different cultures. Therefore, health professionals need to learn about, study, and document findings about teenagers. Regardless of the cultural background of an adolescent, the transition has to be made from childhood to adulthood. This can be complicated when the adolescent's values, beliefs, and practices conflict with traditional cultural values or with those of the dominant culture of the United States or Canada in which the teenager lives. The blending of an old culture with a new culture by an adolescent presents problems for the family as well as for the individual.

REVIEW QUESTIONS

1. Analyze the cultural factors that influence parents' child-rearing beliefs and practices. From a transcultural perspective, explore the ways in which parental beliefs influence children's growth and development.
2. Critically examine the framework for socialization of children in the racial and ethnic minorities presented in this chapter. Identify the strengths and limitations of the framework. What challenges do adolescents who are the offspring of mixed marriages face in the process of cultural identification?
3. Compare and contrast the child-rearing practices of at least three cultural groups. Explore the role of extended family members in raising children for each of the three groups. How does the nurse identify key decision makers in the child's family? Critically examine the ways in which extended family members can assist parents during a child's illness.

4. Critically examine the culturally perceived causes of chronic illness and disability in children from diverse cultures. How are the parents' philosophic and religious beliefs interconnected with their explanations for the causes of chronic illness and disability?

5. Compare and contrast the following Hispanic culture-bound syndromes affecting children:

a. *Pujos* (grunting)
b. *Mal ojo* (evil eye)
c. *Caida de la mollera* (fallen fontanel)
d. *Empacho* (a digestive disorder)

6. Critically explore the cultural influences on teen pregnancy. Compare and contrast cultural beliefs about contraceptives for adolescents from different cultures.

CRITICAL THINKING ACTIVITIES

1. To determine your own values and practices that promote an environment conducive to cultural diversity and cultural competency, complete the self-assessment checklist on the Georgetown University's Center for Child and Human Development Web site at www.nasponline.org/resources/culturalcompetence/checklist.aspx. This checklist is designed to heighten your awareness and sensitivity to the importance of cultural diversity and competency in the following categories when caring for children from diverse backgrounds: (1) physical environment, materials, and resources; (2) communication styles; and (3) values and attitudes.

2. Arrange for an observational experience in a classroom at a school known to have children from various cultures. Compare and contrast the behaviors observed. Does the student–teacher interaction vary according to cultural background? What culturally based attitudes, values, and beliefs are reflected in the children's behaviors? If possible, ask the students how they believe they should relate to teachers, nurses, and other adults. Ask the teacher(s) to discuss cultural similarities and differences in the classroom.

3. When caring for a child from a cultural background different from your own, spend time talking with the child's parents or primary provider of care about child-rearing beliefs and practices (e.g., discipline, toilet training, diet, and related topics). Who is the primary provider of care and how do other family members contribute to child rearing? Compare and contrast the parental responses with your own beliefs and practices.

4. When assigned to the pediatric unit, observe the number and relationship of visitors for children from various cultures. Who visits the child? If nonrelative visitors come, what is their relationship to the child? How do various visitors interact with the child? With the parent(s)?

5. When caring for a child from a cultural background different from your own, ask the parent(s) or primary provider(s) of care to tell you what they believe causes the child to be healthy and unhealthy. To what cause(s) do they attribute the current illness or hospitalization? What interventions do they believe will help the child to recover? Are there any healers outside of the professional health care system (e.g., folk, indigenous, or traditional healers) whom they believe could help the child return to health?

6. If your hospital has a playroom, observe the types of toys and books available. For which group(s) is the majority of these items intended? Do books and toys represent various cultures? What is the role of nurses in determining culturally appropriate books and toys? Are there any items you believe should be added to (or removed from) the playroom to better meet the cultural needs of hospitalized children?

REFERENCES

Barry, H., Bacon, M. K., & Child, I. L. (1967). Definitions, ratings, and bibliographic sources of child-training practices of 110 cultures. In C. S. Ford (Ed.), *Cross-cultural approaches* (pp. 293–331). New Haven: HRAF Press.

Canuso, R. (1996). Co-family sleeping: Strange bedfellows or culturally acceptable behavior? *Journal of Cultural Diversity, 3*(4), 109–111.

Children's Defense Fund. (2006). *Improving children's health: Understanding children's health disparities and promising approaches to address them.* Retrieved February 11, 2007, from http://www.childrensdefense.org/site/DocServer/CDF_Improving_Children_s_Health_FINAL.pdf?docID=1781

Federal Interagency Forum on Child and Family Statistics. (2006). *America's children in brief: Key national indicators of well-being, 2006.* Retrieved March 5, 2007, from http://www.childstats.gov/americaschildren

Halfron, N., & Hochstein, M. (2002). Life course health development: An integrated framework for developing health policy and research. *Milbank Quarterly, 80*(3), 433–479.

Havighurst, R. J. (1974). *Developmental tasks and education.* NY: David McKay.

Harlow, S.D., & Campbell, B. (1996). Ethnic differences in the duration and amount of menstrual bleeding during the post menarcheal period. *American Journal of Epidemiology, 144*(10), 988–998.

Korbin, J. E. (1991). Cross-cultural perspectives and research directions for the 21st century. *Child Abuse and Neglect, 15*(Suppl. 1), 67–77.

Leininger, M. M. (1991). *Culture care diversity and universality: A theory of nursing.* NY: National League for Nursing Press.

Leininger, M. M., & McFarland, M. R. (2002). *Transcultural nursing: Concepts, theories, research and practices.* NY: McGraw-Hill.

Lozoff, B., Askew, G. L., and Wolf, A. W. (1996). Cosleeping and early childhood sleep problems: Effects of ethnicity and socioeconomic status. *Developmental and Behavioral Pediatrics, 17*(1), 9–15.

Lugaila, T., & Overturf, J. (2004). *Children and the households they live in: 2000* (CENSR-14). Washington, DC: U.S. Department of Commerce, Economics and Statistics Administration, U.S. Census Bureau. Retrieved February 11, 2007, from http://www.census.gov/prod/2004pubs/censr-14.pdf

Luna, L. J. (1989). *Care and cultural context of Lebanese Muslims in an urban U.S. community: An ethnographic and ethnonursing study conceptualized within Leininger's theory.* Unpublished doctoral dissertation, Wayne State University, Detroit, Michigan.

Ogbu, J. (1981). Origins of human competence: A cultural-ecological perspective. *Child Development, 52,* 413–429.

Overfield, T. (1981). Biological variation: Concepts from physical anthropology. In G. Henderson and M. Primeaux (Eds.), *Transcultural health care.* Menlo Park, CA: Addison-Wesley.

Overfield, T. (1985). *Biologic variation in health and illness: Race, age and sex differences.* Menlo Park, CA: Addison-Wesley.

Overfield, T. (1995). *Biologic variation in health and illness: Race, age and sex differences* (2nd ed.). New York: CRC.

Statistics Canada. (2004). *2001 Census ethnic origin user guide.* Ottawa, ON: Author. Available from http://www.statscan.ca/

U.S. Census Bureau. (2000). *Population estimates and projections: 2000 Census.* Washington, DC: U.S. Government Printing Office.

U.S. Census Bureau. (2006). *Nation's population one-third minority* (CB06-72) [Press release]. Washington, DC: U.S. Department of Commerce. Retrieved February 11, 2007, from www.census.gov/Press-Release/www/releases/archives/population/006808.html

Zayas, L. H., & Solari, F. (1994). Early childhood socialization in Hispanic families: Context, culture, and practice implications. *Professional Psychology: Research and Practice, 25*(3), 2100–2206.

7

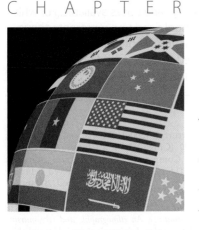

Transcultural Perspectives in the Nursing Care of Adults

Joyceen S. Boyle

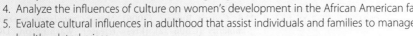

KEY TERMS

Adulthood	Middle adult	Social age
Caregiving	Midlife crisis	Social roles
Developmental crises	"Nerves" ("bad nerves")	Stable adulthood
Developmental tasks	Physiologic development	Stroke belt
Developmental transitions	Psychosocial development	"The virus"
Generativity	Sandwich generation	Transitions of adulthood
"High blood"	Situational crises	Young adult
HIV/AIDS	Situational transitions	

LEARNING OBJECTIVES

1. Understand how culture influences adult development.
2. Explore how health-related situational transitions might influence adult development.
3. Analyze the influences of culture on caregiving in the African American culture.
4. Analyze the influences of culture on women's development in the African American family.
5. Evaluate cultural influences in adulthood that assist individuals and families to manage during health-related crises.
6. Assess the ways in which gender, religious views, and culture influence health–illness and/or situational transitions in adult development.

This chapter discusses transcultural perspectives of health and nursing care associated with developmental events in the adult years. Chapter 8 of the text discusses transcultural nursing care of older adults; therefore, this chapter will focus primarily on young and middle adulthood. The first section presents an overview of cultural influences on adulthood, with an emphasis on how **transitions of adulthood** might be influenced by cultural variations. The second section gives an example of problems faced by a middle-aged African American woman who is experiencing a situational crisis, as well as personal health problems. The situational crisis or transition begins when her young son develops HIV/AIDS, and he returns home to live with her. The influences of culture on individual and family responses to health problems, caregiving, and situational transitions are described. In this chapter, we will discuss developmental tasks, those transitions that occur in a normal successful adulthood. We will also refer to specific transitions, those points in life that indicate change or turmoil as individuals struggle to cope with various life events.

Overview of Cultural Influences on Adulthood

Developmental processes and how they relate to health during adulthood are of interest as development stages often influence responses to illness. In addition, adult development structures how individuals respond to health promotion and wellness by shaping lifestyles, including eating habits, exercise, work, and leisure activities.

The middle years are a time of physical and psychosocial change. These changes are usually gradual and reflect the processes of normal aging. **Physiologic development** is evident in the hormonal changes that take place in midlife in both men and women, whereas **psychosocial development** may be more subtle, but equally important. These changes, both physiologic and psychosocial, are influenced by cultural values and norms.

Physiologic Development During Adulthood

Women undergo menopause, a gradual decrease in ovarian function with subsequent depletion of progesterone and estrogen. While these physiologic changes occur, self-image and self-concept change also. The influence of culture is relevant because women learn to respond to menopause within the context of their families and culture. The *perception* of menopause and *aspects* of the experience of menopausal symptoms vary across cultures. It has sometimes been assumed that non-Western women do not experience the menopausal problems seen in Western society because their status increases as they age; however, this assumption has been challenged. Certainly the treatment of menopause differs, as Western medicine has tended to treat the symptoms of menopause with hormone replacement

therapy. This too is changing as studies are demonstrating the relationship between the use of hormone replacement therapy and the development of breast cancer. Although there are not many studies on the perimenopausal transition across cultural groups, there seems to be cultural differences in the reporting of symptoms associated with menopause and in the use of health care services, as well as prescribed treatments for menopausal symptoms. This reinforces an earlier statement that women (as well as others) learn to respond to menopause within the context of their families and culture.

Men also have physical and emotional changes from the decreased levels of hormones. Loss of muscle mass and strength and a possible loss of sexual potency occur slowly. However, developmental differences among both men and women have not been examined cross-culturally, and most existing theoretical and conceptual models of adult health do not provide insight into cultural variations. Recognition of the cultural belief that aging, however gradual, is a normal process and not a cause for medical and/or surgical intervention may be more culturally appropriate for persons of diverse cultural groups.

Psychosocial Development During Adulthood

Development in adulthood was termed the "empty middle" by Bronfenbrenner, (1977). A noted developmental psychologist, he implied that this term was an indication of Western culture's lack of interest in the adult years. Traditionally, these years were viewed as one long plateau that separates childhood from old age. It was assumed that decisions affecting marriage and career were made in the late teens and that drastic changes in developmental processes seldom occurred afterward. For many years, most developmental theorists saw adulthood as a period to adapt to and come to terms with aging and one's own mortality. Our thinking has changed a great deal in just a few years, and we are beginning to conceptualize middle age as a vigorous and changing stage of life involving importantly different eras and transformations.

Sociocultural factors in our society have precipitated tremendous changes, producing crises, changes, and other unanticipated events in adult lives. Divorce, remarriage, career change, increased mobility, the sexual revolution, and the women's movement have had a profound impact on the adult years. The middle-aged adult may be caught in the **sandwich generation**—still concerned with older children (and sometimes grandchildren) but increasingly concerned with the care of aging parents. Middle life can be a time of reassessment, turmoil, and change. Society acknowledges this with common terms such as *midlife crisis* or even *empty nest syndrome,* along with other terms that imply stress, dissatisfaction, and unrest. However, adulthood is not always a tumultuous, crisis-oriented state; many middle-aged persons welcome the space, time, and independence that middle age often brings. Midlife can be a time of challenge, enjoyment, and satisfaction for many persons.

Chronologic Standards for Appropriate Adult Behavior

Much of the work on adult development was done in the 1960s and 1970s by developmental psychologists such as Bronfenbrenner (1977), Neugarten (1968), and Havighurst (1974), all of whom proposed different theories about adult development. We still rely on some of this early work as we attempt to understand the complexities of adult development. Neugarten (1968) observed that each culture has specific chronologic standards for appropriate adult behavior and that these cultural standards prescribe the ideal ages at which to leave the protection of one's parents, choose a vocation, marry, have children, and in general, get on with life. The events associated with these standards do not necessarily precipitate crises or change. What is more important is the timing of these events. As a result of each culture's sense of social time, individuals tend to measure their accomplishments and adjust their behavior according to a kind of social clock. Awareness of the social timetable is frequently reinforced by the judg-

ments and urging of friends and family, who say, "It's time for you to..." or "You are getting too old to..." or "Act your age." Problems often arise when social timetables change for unpredictable reasons. An example is the recent trend of adult children, frequently divorced or unemployed or both, returning to live with their parents, often bringing along their own children. Grandparents caring for grandchildren are now a common phenomenon in our society. Being widowed in young adulthood or losing one's job close to retirement are other examples of events that are more likely to cause stress and conflict because they occur outside of our notions of social order.

Culture exerts important influences on human development in that it provides a means for recognizing stages in the continuum of individual development throughout the life span. It is culture that defines **social age**, or what is judged appropriate behavior in stages of the life cycle. In nearly all societies, adult role expectations are placed on young people when they reach a certain age. Several cultures have defined rites of passage that mark the line between youth and adulthood; in the United States, we tend to view the legal age to obtain a driver's license or to drink alcohol as markers of beginning adulthood.

Menarche is a milestone in women's development and a psychologically significant event, providing a rather dramatic demarcation between girlhood and womanhood. However, this is not an event that is celebrated openly in U.S. culture as most girls are too embarrassed to talk openly about it with anyone but their mothers or close friends. There are no definitive boundaries that mark adulthood for either young girls or young boys, although legal sanctions confer some rights and responsibilities at the ages of 18 and 21 years. Examples are the age requirements for obtaining a driver's license, for voting, and for purchasing alcohol and tobacco. Although the age of 21 years is often cited, there is no single criterion for the determination of when young adulthood begins, given that different individuals experience and cope with growth and development differently and at different chronologic ages.

Adulthood as such is usually divided into young adulthood (late teens, 20s, and 30s) and middle adulthood (40s and 50s), but the age lines can be fuzzy. Generally, a young adult in his or her late teens and early 20s struggles with independence and issues related to intimacy and relationships outside the family. Role changes occur while the young adult is pursuing an education, experiencing marriage, and starting a family while establishing a career. A middle adult most often concentrates on career and family matters. However, as previously mentioned, adulthood is not necessarily an orderly or predictable plateau. Experiences at work have a direct bearing on the middle-aged adult's development through exposure to job-related stress, levels of physical and intellectual activity, and social relations formed with coworkers. "Re-careering" or changing careers during middle adulthood is also becoming more common and can be a source of change. At home, family life can be chaotic, with role changes and other transitions occurring with dizzying frequency. Often adults are faced with the realization that they are getting older and feel like they have made the wrong choices or have left many things still undone. This realization can lead to developmental and/or situational crises. How well individuals cope with and manage the challenges and transitions required in adulthood are influenced by their cultural values, traditions, and background.

Developmental Tasks

Throughout life, each individual is confronted with developmental tasks: responses to life situations encountered by all persons experiencing physiologic, psychologic, spiritual, and sociologic changes. Although the developmental tasks of childhood are widely known and have long been studied, the critical experiences of adulthood are less familiar to most nurses.

Several theorists have studied and defined the developmental *or midlife* tasks of adulthood. Many personality theorists, for example, Freud, Erikson, and Fromm, cite maturity as the major criterion of adulthood. These various theories have implications for how we define "development," "maturity," and "wisdom". According to

Erikson (1963), the developmental task of middle adulthood is the attainment of generativity versus stagnation. Generativity is accomplished through parenting, working in one's career, participating in community activities, or working cooperatively with peers, spouse, family members, and others to reach mutually determined goals. Mature adults have a well-developed philosophy of life that serves as a basis for stability in their lives. Individuals in adulthood assume numerous social roles, such as spouse, parent, child of aging parent, worker, friend, organization member, and citizen. Each of these social roles involves expected behaviors established by the values and norms of society. Through the process of socialization, the individual is expected to learn the behaviors appropriate to the new role. It is important to note that many developmental theories have connotations of stability and blandness associated with adulthood, although this is not necessarily the case.

In many ways, the early theorists' views of what occurs in adulthood are the biases of "White" middle-class values and experiences. This constellation of characteristics has been attributed to predominantly White, Anglo-Saxon, Protestant (WASP) views and behaviors. For many cultural groups in Western society, the mastery of mainstream developmental tasks is not easily managed, and in some cases, it may even be undesirable. For some groups, developmental tasks may be accomplished through culturally defined patterns that are different from or outside of the norm of what is expected in the dominant culture. In Evidence-Based Practice Box 7–1, we examine how women who have been abused and left their husbands manage to regain strength, transition to a new life, and reintegrate their families. Promoting the health of their families and teaching children ways of behaving that do not include violence or aggressive behavior were priorities of the women in this nursing study. From an ideal and "model" developmental perspective, marriage partners are expected to love each other and care for their children, but this is not always the case. Unfortunately, nurses have many opportunities to intervene in cases where children and women are at risk to violence

Evidence-Based Practice 7–1:

Regenerating Family: Strengthening the Emotional Health of Mothers and Children in the Context of Intimate Partner Violence

This study suggests that concern for their children's well-being is pivotal in mothers' decisions to leave abusive partners. Seldom do mothers suggest that single-parent family life after leaving abusive spouses will be beneficial for the children's emotional health. This feminist-grounded theory study of family health promotion in the aftermath of intimate partner violence shows that families strengthen their emotional health by purposefully replacing previously destructive patterns of interaction with predictable, supportive ways of getting along in a process called *regenerating family*. This process describes how the mother and children purposefully work towards replacing previous destructive behaviors with new behaviors that establish predictable, respectful environments that enhance family members' emotional health.

Clinical Application

- Recognize that "traditional" families can be unhealthy.
- Acknowledge that single-parent families can promote the health of each family member.
- Assist the mother in creating a safe climate that promotes the health of all the family members.
- Help single mothers develop protective measures for their children.
- Understand that helping families "regenerate" is a health promotion process that strengthens the entire family.

Wuest, J., Merritt-Gray, M., & Ford-Gilboe, M. (2004). Regenerating family: Strengthening the emotional health of mothers and children in the context of intimate partner violence. *Advances in Nursing Science, 27*, 257–274.

and the situation is contrary to what is depicted in developmental norms. Helping individuals regain strength, transition to new roles, and promote their recovery and health are important nursing goals that facilitate resolution of situational crises in adulthood.

Early studies on the developmental experiences of women have led several authors (Belenky, McVicker, Clinchy, Goldberger, & Tarule, 1997) to suggest that developmental stages and the associated developmental tasks of adulthood have been derived primarily from studies of men; thus women may experience adult development somewhat differently. Women's traditional location of responsibility was in the home, nurturing children and husbands as well as parents. This view is changing, prompted by societal changes and informed by scholars who are addressing

women's psychosocial development in new ways. Some of these differences are described in the next section.

Adulthood has been conceptualized as step-by-step phases of development, but more recent theories (McCrae & Costa, 2003; Demick & Andreoletti, 2003) suggest that development is an evolutionary expanse involving different eras and transitions. These life transitions have triumphs, costs, and disruptions. Within nursing, Meleis, Sawyer, Im, Hilfinger Messias, and Schumacher (2000) proposed a framework to study life transitions. They suggest that transitions can be developmental, situational, health–illness, and/or organizational. The next section discusses several important adult life transitions and examines how culture and life events influence adult growth and change during these transitions.

These life transitions or successful progression through a developmental task occur slowly over many years, but they are important in terms of quality of life and life satisfaction. Culture influences these transitions, and it is important that nurses be able to evaluate their adult clients and to help them adjust and change in culturally appropriate ways.

Culture and Adult Transitions

DEVELOPMENTAL TRANSITION: ACHIEVING SUCCESS IN ONE'S CAREER

Some Americans define a "successful career" as financial success, while others may see it as a way to provide service or make a contribution to the lives of their fellow citizens. It is important to recognize that women as well as men now achieve success in their chosen careers. Other "new" Americans may find that the goal of a successful career is not possible for them. The United States, as other countries in the world, has experienced a tremendous influx of immigrants and refugees from Southeast Asia, Latin America, Eastern Europe, Africa, and other areas. While immigrants and refugees may aspire to a good job, that may be a difficult goal to attain. They may have difficulty with the language, with the skills and educational level required, and other factors necessary to holding a good job in the United States. Furthermore, many more women, including immigrants and refugees, are working outside of the home, and there may be a different division of time of energy for both spouses.

In many immigrant and refugee families, role conflict and stress occur within the family as gender roles begin to change during contact with American culture. For example, sometimes the male head of household is unable to find employment; if he was a professional in his former country, he may be reluctant to accept the menial jobs that are traditionally filled by immigrants or refugees when they first come to this country. Frequently, low-status jobs are more available to immigrant women, yet their traditional roles are closely tied to the home and family. When an immigrant woman begins to work outside of the home, her role changes and alters

the power structure and the roles within the family. The lack of adequate social supports, such as affordable day care and adequate compensation for work, and the additional physical and emotional stress result in an unacknowledged toll on immigrant and refugee families. Box 7–1 lists some characteristics of immigrant and refugee families.

At present, to expect members of certain groups, such as poor or ethnic minorities, newly arrived immigrants or refugees, the homeless, the

---

BOX 7-1

Some Characteristics of Immigrant and Refugee Families

1. Traditional family values are evident; for example, roles of men and women are differentiated. Women's role is in the home, with the family. Men are heads of the household and family providers.
2. Families tend to be extended; if members do not actually live in the same household, they visit and contact each other frequently.
3. Many immigrants come to the United States because they already have family members here.
4. Most immigrants and refugees are poor and struggle to earn an adequate income. Often men in refugee communities have been professionals in their home country but are unable to be employed in the same capacity in their new host country. Women are often more easily employed outside of the home and they often find employment as domestic or service workers.
5. Refugees may be fleeing war and political persecution. Many may experience symptoms of post-traumatic stress syndrome.
6. Traditional health and illness beliefs may influence behavior. Immigrant and refugee families may combine traditional health practices with modern Western health care. The use of traditional practices is fairly common in some groups.
7. Language is a significant barrier for the first few years that immigrants and refugees live in the United States and Canada. Children tend to learn English and become acculturated faster than their parents.

mentally ill, or the unemployed, to achieve satisfaction from jobs that interest them or from status derived from succeeding in a career is unrealistic and indicates a lack of sensitivity to the problems faced by these groups. Thus, although the work role is valued in American society, the attainment of a successful career may not be realistic for some minority groups, immigrants, or even certain individuals within the majority culture, some of whom are returning to school in the hope of preparing for a second career.

DEVELOPMENTAL TRANSITION: ACHIEVING SOCIAL AND CIVIC RESPONSIBILITY

Social and civic responsibilities are in part culturally defined. Whereas members of the dominant North American culture may value achieving an elected office in the local Parent Teacher Association (PTA) or Rotary Club, other cultures may find these goals baffling and emphasize other activities within the cultural group. For example, in some groups, religious obligations may be given priority over civic responsibilities. Usually, traditional religious groups have not encouraged the emergence of women in leadership roles within the church structure or the wider society, although this is being challenged by women within several religious groups.

Sometimes within traditional cultures, women who seek roles outside the family are criticized because recognition and acknowledgment outside the family group may conflict with the traditional role of women. Some religious and ethnic or cultural groups believe that a woman's place is in the home, and women who attempt to succeed in a career or in activities outside the home or group are frowned on by other members of the group. Civic responsibilities that relate to children or domestic matters may be viewed as appropriate for women to assume, whereas civic activities may be viewed as more within the province of men. Middle Eastern and Southeast Asian cultures emphasize responsibilities and contributions to the extended family or clan rather than to the wider society. Lipson and Miller (1994) reported that Afghan women in the United States continue to socialize almost exclusively with other Afghan women, usually extended family members. They do not talk with male strangers, no matter how unusual the circumstances. J. Lipson (personal communication, November 2000) described an experience of an Afghan woman during a recent San Francisco earthquake. The woman was hurrying along a street on her way to visit her sister at the time the earthquake occurred. She was thrown to her knees with the shaking of the ground underneath her. A man had been walking along on the other side of the street and he hurried over to help her, attempting to take her arm to help her up. The Afghan woman shrunk back in horror at the thought of a strange man so close to her and attempting to touch her. In spite of her shock from the earthquake and her trauma of falling, she jumped to her feet and scurried away, pulling her scarf over much of her face. The gentlemen who helped her was puzzled by her behavior and wondered why she had not thanked him for his concern and helpfulness.

DEVELOPMENTAL TRANSITION: MARRIAGE AND RAISING CHILDREN TO ADULTHOOD

The age at which young persons marry and become independent varies by custom or cultural norm as well as by socioeconomic status. Generally speaking, adults of lower socioeconomic status leave school, begin work, marry, and become parents and grandparents at earlier ages than middle-class or upper-class adults. It is relatively common in North American society for an 18-year-old, for example, to marry and move away from home or to leave home to pursue higher education or find employment. Indeed, many American families encourage early independence, or "leaving home," although this trend decreases when the economy declines. Other cultural groups, such as those from the Middle East and Latin America, place more emphasis on maintaining the extended family. Even after marriage, a son and his new wife may choose to live very close to both families and to visit relatives several times each day. Families from some cultural groups, such as Hispanics, or traditional religious groups, such as the Hutterites or the Amish, may be reluctant to allow their young daughters to leave home until they marry. In many Muslim families, girls do not leave home until they are married.

Increased mobility in American society has impacted family life as many young families now live far away from grandparents, and the traditional influences of grandparents on young grandchildren is decreasing. Sometimes because of geographical distance, grandparents barely know their grandchildren, although digital photos via home computers and cell phones are helping to keep grandparents up-to-date with the growth and activities of their grandchildren.

Caring for and launching their own children and caring for their own aging parents place some middle-age adults between the demands of caregiving from parents and those from children. Primarily, caregivers have been women, and the stress resulting from the demands of caregiving places them at increased risk of health problems (Teel & Leenerts, 2005). In cultures that value and maintain extended family networks, the responsibilities of caring for both children and older parents can be shared. Many American families still maintain very close and extended family networks (Figure 7–1) .

Adjusting to aging parents and responsibilities, as well as finding appropriate solutions to problems created by aging parents, are challenges created by situational, developmental and even health–illness transitions. Placing an aged mother or father in a nursing home may be a decision made with reluctance and only when all other alternatives have been exhausted. Such actions may be totally unacceptable to some members of other cultural groups, in which family and community structures would facilitate the complex care required by an aged ill person. Such cultural norms would exert a great deal of social pressure on an adult son (or especially a daughter) who failed in this obligation.

DEVELOPMENTAL TRANSITION: CHANGING ROLES AND RELATIONSHIPS

The relationship of wife and husband is often enhanced in middle adulthood, although divorce at this time is not infrequent in the United States. The frequent need for both spouses to work may conflict with traditional roles and cause feelings of guilt on the part of both the husband and wife. Some women continue to assume all responsibility for domestic chores while working outside the home, and they experience considerable stress and fatigue as a result of multiple role demands. If either or both spouses are working in low-paying jobs and still struggling to make ends meet, adulthood may not be a time of enjoyment and leisure activities.

An emphasis on an emotionally close interpersonal relationship between a husband and wife

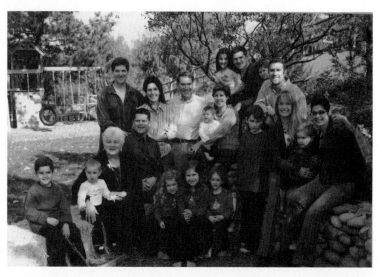

FIGURE 7-1. American families, such as the extended family of Teresa and Neil Cooper of Carlsbad, California, are multiethnic in each generation, yet maintaining close family ties is a priority. This emphasis on family has continued through three generations. The children look forward to seeing each other. Their parents and grandparents believe that this is the beginning of the fourth generation of close family ties.

may be a culturally defined value. In some Hispanic cultures, women develop more intense relationships or affective bonds with their children or relatives than with their husbands. Latin men, in turn, may form close bonds with siblings or friends—ties that meet the needs for companionship, emotional support, and caring that might otherwise be expected from their wives. Touch between men (walking arm in arm) and between women is acceptable in many societies. Gender roles and how men and women go about establishing personal ties with either sex are heavily influenced by culture. In North American society, women are more likely to have intimate, self-disclosing friendships with other women than men have with other men. A man's male friends are likely to be working, drinking, or playing "buddies." In southern Europe and the Middle East, men are allowed to express their friendship with each other with words and embraces. Such expressions of affection between men are uncommon in North American culture and might be attributed to homosexuality.

Affiliation and friendship needs in adulthood and the satisfaction of these needs are facilitated or hindered by cultural expectations. Social support, family ties, and friendship needs can be met through the extended family and kinship system or through other culturally prescribed groups such as churches, singles bars, work, and civic associations. Something new for many single adults are the various Internet sites where one can meet others who are single and interested in starting new relationships. An individual's health may be affected by these social ties: persons who have a reliable set of close friends and an extensive network of acquaintances are usually healthier—both emotionally and physically—than persons without supportive networks and close friends.

Changing cultural values also influence professional health care roles and relationships. How individuals are approached and greeted as well as the kind and type of relationship established may be closely tied to cultural expectations and norms. A casual, first-name basis has become the norm in many health care situations, with

medical receptionists (and often other health professionals as well) calling patients by their first names. This can be inappropriate in many instances. Health care professionals should inquire about the appropriate manner to use in approaching clients and their family members. Table 7-1 provides some suggestions and guidelines to use in approaching clients and using their names in interpersonal relationships.

Health-Related Situational Crises

The preceding section described developmental tasks, transitions, and some cultural variations influencing adulthood. This section contains an in-depth case study of a middle-aged African American woman who experienced health–illness **situational** and **developmental transitions.** Transitions often occur because of a serious illness in middle age. Leading causes of death in middle adulthood are heart disease, cancer, cerebrovascular disease, and accidents (Centers for Disease Control and Prevention [CDC], National Center for Health Statistics, 2004). These conditions affect individuals, but they also occur within a family system and affect children, spouses, aging parents, or other close relatives. Because middle-aged adults may be responsible for aging parents or ill adult children as well as for grandchildren, the illness of any one individual must be evaluated carefully for the myriad of ways in which it affects all members of the family.

Health care professionals need a better understanding of how families influence the health-related behavior of their members because definitions of health and illness and reactions to them form during childhood within the family context. Yet, there are many gaps in our knowledge. Cultural beliefs and values influence health promotion, disease prevention, and the treatment of illness. When the illness has social and/or cultural connotations, the issues become more complex. Medical treatment and nursing care must take into account the cultural history, values, beliefs, and practices that influence the client's and family's ability to cope with the ill-

TABLE 7-1 Guidelines for Names

Arab	Both male and female children are given a first name. The father's first name is used as the middle name; the last name is the family name. Usually, a person is called formally by the first name, such as Mr. Mohammed or Dr. Anwar.
Chinese	The family name is stated or written first and then the given name, just opposite of European and North American tradition. Only very close friends use the given name. Politeness and formality are stressed; always use the whole name or family name. Use only the family name to address men, e.g., if the family name is Chin and the man's given name is Wei-jing, address the man as Chin. Many Asians take an English name that they use in their North American host country. Use the title Mr. or Mrs. preceding the English name because the use of only the first name is considered rude. Some Asians switch the order of their names to be like Western names, and this can be very confusing to outsiders.
	Women in China do not use their husband's name after marriage. If the woman has lived in Hong Kong, Taiwan, or a Western country for a long time, her name may be the same as her husband's name.
Latin American	The use of surnames may differ by country. Many Latin Americans use two surnames, representing the mother's and father's sides of the family. "Maria Cordoba Lopez" indicates that her father's name is Cordoba and her mother's surname is Lopez. When Maria marries, she will retain her father's name and add the last name of her husband. Thus, Maria becomes Maria Cordoba de Reclnos. Many Latin Americans drop their mother's surnames after they immigrate to the United States. In approaching clients of traditional Latin cultures, it is appropriate to use the Spanish terms *Señor* or *Señora*, followed by the primary surname (the husband's), if the nurse is comfortable with those terms.
Native North American	Native North American names differ by tribal affiliation. Many tend to follow the dominant cultural norms. In the Navajo culture, a health care provider may call an older Navajo client "grandfather" or "grandmother" as a sign of respect. In the past, some tribes have tended to convert traditional names into English surnames. Thus, there are names like Joe Calf Looking and Phyllis Greywolf.

The above-mentioned examples are very general. If in doubt, always ask because it can be embarrassing for the nurse and the client if the nurse uses a name in an inappropriate manner. Members of cultures that adhere to traditional values might be confused by our current practice of using Ms. as a designation for women. Generally speaking, it is *always best and most appropriate* to be formal and to use the surname with the appropriate title of Mr. or Mrs. preceding the name.

Adapted from Purnell, L. D., & Paulanka, B. J. (2003). *Transcultural health care: A culturally competent approach* (2nd ed.). Philadelphia: F.A. Davis.

ness, as well as assessing whether the interventions are congruent with their culture.

Caregiving and African American Women

African American women, like all women, receive and provide health care in the context of the families in which they perform multiple caregiving roles: as wives, mothers, daughters, widows, single childless women, and so on. Women's assumption of the caregiving role is in line with traditional expectations of women's domestic role, and the majority of caregivers are women; therefore, it is not surprising that the caregiving roles of women often predispose them to interrupted employment and limited access to health care insurance and pension and retirement plans. Shambley-Ebron & Boyle (2006a, 2006b) have documented that these general problems and characteristics of caregivers are compounded for African American women by the special circumstances of their lives and the lives of the men and children for whom they care. In the case of African American caregivers, prejudice, discrimination, and poverty all interact to increase stress and pose challenges that frequently result in poor health.

Caregiving, as used in this chapter, implies the provision of long-term help to an impaired family member or close friend. Caregiving usually is labor intensive, time consuming, and stressful, although the exact effects on the physical and emotional health of caregivers are still being documented. Although positive outcomes, such as feelings of reward and satisfaction, do occur for caregivers, they still experience negative psychological, emotional, social, and physical outcomes (Wright, Hickey, Buckwalter, Hendrix, & Kelechi, 1999). When caregiving for other family members takes place during middle adulthood, the roles and challenges for both the caregiver and the recipient may change. In addition, culture and ethnicity influence beliefs, attitudes, and perceptions of what is normal and what is sickness, as well as what caregiving actions should be taken. Culture and ethnicity may influence how often individuals engage in self-care versus seeking formal health services, how many medications they take, how often they rest and exercise, and what types of foods they consume when ill. Yet we know very little about caregiving in diverse cultural groups. Wright observed that "caregiver research is based predominantly on White subjects, and ethnic differences are rarely analyzed" (1997, p. 277).

Studies of African American caregivers have found that they tend to use religious beliefs to help them cope with the stress of caregiving. Boyle, Hodnicki, and Ferrell (1999) described Black caregivers' belief in a personal God and their intense relationship with Him provided them with support during the illness of a family member and helped them cope with death and loss. Poindexter, Linsk, and Warner (1999) also found that a major source of support for Black caregivers was their personal relationships with "Jesus," "God," or "the Lord". Poindexter, Linsk, and Warner suggest that spirituality is both personal and empowering for some African Americans and is related to the deepest motivations in life. Spirituality is often expressed in the context of the daily life of Black caregivers, not necessarily by formal attendance at religious events. The specific nature of the religion–health connection among African Americans is of great interest to health professionals as it holds promise for integration into church-based health promotion interventions (Holt & McClure, 2006).

African American women also face a special situation in relationship to **HIV/AIDS.** African American women are especially hard hit by HIV/AIDS. From 2001–2004, African American women accounted for 68% of HIV/AIDS diagnoses for women in the 33 states that have confidential, named-based HIV reporting, and three-fourths of the HIV/AIDS cases in African American women were caused by heterosexual contact (CDC, U.S. Department of Health and Human Services, 2007). Shambley-Ebron and Boyle (2006b) studied African American women who were diagnosed with HIV/AIDS and who were caring for children who were also HIV positive. These mother–caregivers relied on spiritual traditions and religious practices to help deal with the pressures of living and mothering with HIV/AIDS.

Although several studies show the positive results of caregiving in African American caregivers, these caregivers pay a high emotional and physical price for their care. Caring for a family member who has HIV disease can be an intensively personal event; it brings the caregiver closer to the loved one but involves sadness and grief (Poindexter & Linsk, 1999). There is also some indication that African American caregivers may solve problems of caregiving differently and that these differences may result from social and cultural factors. For example, African American mothers who care for adult children with HIV disease may not always exhibit a proactive, problem-solving approach to effects of the disease (Boyle, Bunting, Hodnicki, & Ferrell, 2001). This is not because African American caregivers are uninterested in their adult children's health or cannot understand the complexity of medical regimens. Such behavior may be related more to the racial discrimination and racism that have remained significant factors in the health care of African Americans over time. In addition, there may be cultural influences that shape human behavior in such a way that problems arising from illness and caregiving are solved by different approaches.

The Context of HIV/AIDS and the African American Community

HIV/AIDS disproportionately affects African Americans and has had a devastating effect on African American communities. The CDC points out that at every stage—from HIV diagnosis through the death of persons with AIDS—the hardest-hit racial or ethnic group is African Americans. Even though African Americans make up only approximately 13% of the U.S. population, one-half of the estimated new cases of HIV/AIDS diagnoses in the United States in 2004 were for African Americans (CDC, U.S. Department of Health and Human Services, 2007a).

Prevention Challenges

From a public health standpoint, preventive education about HIV/AIDS has been hindered by an unwillingness to talk frankly about sexual and drug use behaviors, and this has been a substantial barrier in effective HIV preventive programs. In essence, the AIDS epidemic has forced society to examine and attempt to alter cultural behaviors and values that were largely ignored in the past.

Over the past 2 decades in the United States, the practice of high-risk HIV behaviors has changed from selected populations of White homosexual men with no history of drug use to heterosexuals having multiple sex partners and using drugs. HIV/AIDS disproportionately affects selected groups, especially Blacks and His-

panics, and risk patterns are different for men and women. *African American women*, a term that includes both adolescents and adults, are especially at risk. More than three-fourths of the HIV/AIDS cases diagnosed for African American women from 2001–2004 were caused by heterosexual contact. Injection drug use accounted for almost one-fifth of all cases. In 2004, the rate of AIDS diagnoses for African American women was 23 times the rate for White women and 4 times more than that for Hispanic women (CDC, U.S. Department of Health and Human Services, 2007a).

Most researchers and public health officials generally agree that preventive efforts and other interventions should match the social, cultural, linguistic, psychologic, developmental, and behavioral characteristics of the targeted risk group of interest (Sumartojo, Carey, Doll, & Gayle, 1997). However, implementing such interventions has proven extremely difficult. The CDC points out that the African American community faces numerous barriers that impact HIV prevention efforts.

Barriers to HIV Preventive Efforts in African American Communities

Poverty: African Americans, generally speaking, often have lower incomes than other Americans. Accessing health care services is a problem if an individual does not have health insurance. In addition, for many African Americans, day-to-day living activities often take precedence over whether an individual has access to educational information about HIV and AIDS. Poverty or lack of money and health insurance influence access to HIV testing and state-of-the art treatment if they are diagnosed with HIV.

Denial: Many African Americans still believe that HIV/AIDS is mostly a White, gay male disease and that it is a problem in Newark or New York, or even in Florida, but not in rural Georgia or Alabama. Homosexuality is a very sensitive topic in many African American communities as is drug use; therefore talking about HIV/AIDS may be met with disapproval or disdain. Talking frankly about sexual behavior with new partners and insisting on the use of condoms may be very difficult for African American women. They may be afraid to ask a male partner about his sexual history or his use of or experience with drugs for fear of abruptly ending their relationship.

Drug Use: Injecting drugs is the second leading cause of HIV infection for African American women and the third leading cause of HIV infection for African American men. In addition to the danger from contaminated needles, syringes, and other works, persons who use drugs are more likely to take other risks, such as unprotected sex, while under the influence of drugs (CDC, U.S. Department of Health and Human Services, 2007b).

Culturally Competent Nursing Care of an African American Woman Experiencing a Situational Crisis

A phenomenon that is becoming more common is that of HIV-affected caregivers, either mothers or grandmothers, who are caring for family members who are also HIV positive. Some caregivers are caring for one or more family members who need care and attention in addition to the person(s) diagnosed with HIV, and such caregivers are often caught between multiple sets of caring responsibilities. In the past decade or so, the nature of caregiving has changed with the impact of the AIDS epidemic because AIDS affects a much younger population. At first, caregivers to persons with AIDS often were men; however, mothers and other family members have become more involved as the incidence of HIV disease has changed from White homosexual men to the heterosexual population. Many African Americans living in the rural South first learned about HIV/AIDS from television programs, and many thought of AIDS as a disease that was common in large cities; few thought it was something that could happen in small Southern towns or to a member of their own family. Like many other Americans, most African Americans thought AIDS was a disease of White homosexual men, so it was something of a shock when rural African American families learned that one of their own

family members had HIV disease. HIV/AIDS still carries a tremendous stigma in African American communities. Many African Americans, especially younger adults or teenagers, now commonly refer to HIV/AIDS as **"the virus."** Case Study 7–1 provides an example of a middle-aged African American woman who provides care to her developmentally delayed sister and to her 26-year-old son with AIDS. Culturally appropriate ways in which the nurse might implement nursing care are suggested. The use of traditional family and religious systems is encouraged because these ties are of particular significance in rural African American culture.

CASE STUDY 7-1

Mrs. Ernestine Pollard, a 52-year-old Black woman, lives in a small town in rural South Carolina. Mrs. Pollard cares for an older sister, who is now 65 years old. Mrs. Pollard explains that her sister "can't talk, and her mind's not good."

Her sister has always lived with her and her husband. Mr. Pollard died a few years ago. Recently the sister's health has been deteriorating because of a series of "little strokes." Then, just a few months ago, Mrs. Pollard's 26-year-old son, Steve, returned home to live with her. Steve was living and working in Florida, where he became very ill. He was taken by friends to the emergency room and then admitted to the hospital. During this hospitalization, the results of a test for HIV disease were positive. After discharge from the hospital, he decided to return home to live with his mother. Mrs. Pollard welcomed this move because she worried about Steve living so far away from her.

Mrs. Pollard explains that sometimes with the stress of caregiving and worrying about Steve, her "pressure goes sky high." She has had "high blood" for several years. Her physician prescribed medication for her blood pressure, and she tries to take it on a regular basis, but sometimes she forgets. Lately, as Steve has become more ill, Mrs. Pollard is not sleeping well, and she is very worried about Steve's condition. She told her doctor that she has "bad nerves" and explained that she was unable to sleep at night. The physician prescribed sleeping pills for her, but Mrs. Pollard is unwilling to take them because she fears that she will not hear Steve during the night if he needs her. In addition to her worry about Steve, she is concerned about her sister's health. Mrs. Pollard has two daughters who are older than Steve, and they try to help their mother with her caregiving activities.

Health Promotion Strategies and Nursing Interventions

African American women are at high risk for cardiovascular diseases, particularly hypertension and stroke. Mrs. Pollard lives in that area of the South known as the **stroke belt** because morbidity and mortality from cardiovascular diseases (especially among African Americans) are so prevalent in this region (Graham-Garcia, Raines, Andrews, & Mensah, 2001). The nursing management priorities for Mrs. Pollard will be to support her caregiving role and provide health promotion strategies to control her blood pressure and help reduce the stress she is currently experiencing. In terms of blood pressure management, a nurse might advise Mrs. Pollard to lose weight and incorporate changes in eating habits and regular exercise into her lifestyle. However, social and cultural factors as well as the caregiving situation may compromise these health goals. Nurses can become more culturally sensitive to cultural norms and values of clients like Mrs. Pollard by listening carefully, being empathetic, recognizing the client's self-interest and needs of her family members, being flexible, having a sense of timing, appropriately using the client's and family's resources, and giving relevant information at the appropriate time.

Although Mrs. Pollard does have a private physician and tries to seek care when appropriate, she considers her sister's and Steve's needs before her own. Steve is the only member of the Pollard family who is receiving regular health care. He attends an infectious disease clinic about 50 miles from where his mother lives. His medications are provided through Ryan White legislation, a state and federal cooperative agreement that was passed in 1990 to provide care for persons with AIDS. The act fills gaps in care faced by those with low incomes and little or no health insurance (U.S. Department of Health and

Human Services, HIV/AIDS Bureau, n.d.). Mrs. Pollard does not accompany Steve when he visits the clinic because she does not wish to leave her sister alone. The nurses at the clinic wonder if anyone in Steve's family really cares about him because he always comes alone to the clinic appointments.

Mrs. Pollard is primarily concerned about Steve's appetite because she believes that the proper food will promote and enhance his health. She worries constantly about Steve's appetite. Like many other adults, Mrs. Pollard has fairly definite preferences about food and the way it is prepared and served. The Pollard family frequently eats foods that are high in fat; for example, they enjoy servings of bacon or fatback for breakfast once or twice during the week. They prefer their vegetables cooked with bacon for flavoring. One morning, Steve told his mother that he thought he would like a steak. Mrs. Pollard hurried to the grocery store to buy a steak and cook it for him, and he obviously enjoyed eating it. Symbolism is attached to food in every culture, and Mrs. Pollard believes that Steve will gain strength by eating healthful foods. In her concern for Steve and the time she spends with her sister, she neglects her own diet or eats whatever is convenient, often "fast foods" or those high in carbohydrates and sodium. Mrs. Pollard needs to be gently reminded by the nurse that it is important for her to pay some attention to her own nutrition also.

Clark (2003) suggested that food could have many meanings as well as being nourishing. For example, food can serve as a means of enhancing interpersonal relationships or as a means of communicating love and caring. Being able to prepare food that her son and sister will eat and enjoy is a source of satisfaction for Mrs. Pollard and a reinforcement of her successful role as caregiver. It is an act of caring and love for her to prepare a meal for her family. At the same time, she must maintain her own health to continue to provide care for Steve and her sister. A priority is that she take her medication on a regular basis to control her blood pressure. Taking her medication regularly, resting as often as she can, and avoiding foods that are high in fat and/or sodium or eating them only in small or moderate amounts may be realistic goals for Mrs. Pollard.

Nurses providing care to clients like Mrs. Pollard will need to consider other cultural factors that ultimately influence the nursing goals. Rural African Americans often have cultural ways to view health and illness. **"High blood"** is an illness condition that is associated with African Americans in the rural South. Many health care professionals make the wrong assumption that "high blood" is the same as high blood pressure, and although there are similarities, the cultural explanation of "high blood" is different from the biomedical explanation of high blood pressure. "High blood" is conceptualized in terms of blood volume, blood thickness, or even elevations of the blood in the body (e.g., "blood rushes to your head").

"High blood" is believed to be caused primarily by factors that "run blood up," such as salt, fat, meats, and sweets. This condition results in an increased "pressure" or high blood pressure. Sometimes "high blood" leads to a feeling of faintness that may cause the afflicted person "to fall out" or faint. Other causal factors that result in "high blood" are emotional upsets or prolonged stress. Sometimes it is thought to be caused by a falling out with God or by eternal forces such as enemies putting a "hex" on someone. Many older African American clients believe that eating slightly acidic foods, such as greens with vinegar or dill pickles, will lower "high blood." Thus, although there are similarities between "high blood" and high blood pressure, the explanations and treatments are not always the same in the cultural prescriptions as in the biomedical model. Mrs. Pollard tries to be conscientious about taking her blood pressure medication, but she sometimes forgets to take it and sometimes does not get around to promptly renewing the prescription, so she might go without her medication for several days or a few weeks. The nurse should acknowledge Mrs. Pollard's active involvement in her own health promotion, encourage her to take her blood pressure medication as prescribed, and remind her to renew it promptly before she is completely out of medication.

"Nerves" or even **"bad nerves,"** while not unique to the rural South, are commonly described by many Southerners. "Bad nerves" are often equated with anxiety and worry but may refer to something as serious as a "mental breakdown" or severe emotional disorder. Mrs. Pollard uses the term to refer to her worry, concern, and anxiety about Steve's health status and her anticipation of the loss of him and her sister. Sometimes she has "crying spells" that she describes as "just crying and crying, and not being able to stop." She gets up several times at night to answer her sister's call or to check on Steve and make certain that they are all right. Lack of sleep and continued worry and anxiety accelerate her psychological distress. Again, recognition from the nurse that she is providing excellent care for her sister and her son is reassuring for her. She should be encouraged to rest and should be assured that crying and feeling sad are normal reactions to her sister's deteriorating condition and Steve's HIV/AIDS.

Because of a lack of economic resources, African American midlife women are likely to be subjected to many stressful life events, such as job and marital instability, lack of male companions as heads of households, erratic income, and frequent changes and relocations. Because she has worked for self-employed businesses most of her life, Mrs. Pollard lacks health insurance. She has experienced many life stresses that were related to the lack of economic resources. When Steve first came home and told his mother that he had HIV/AIDS, Mrs. Pollard continued working as a clerk in a local dry cleaning establishment. However, as Steve's illness progressed and he became increasingly unable to care for himself, Mrs. Pollard quit her job to stay home and take care of him. She faces numerous situational crises: Steve's illness and worsening condition, the poor health and aging of her sister, and economic hardship because she is the family provider and is not working at the present time.

Stress and anxiety are normal reactions in the lives of middle-aged adults like Mrs. Pollard.

However, limited resources, lack of access to high-quality health care, and discrimination during a severe illness of a family member compound the stress and complicate a situational crisis. Mrs. Pollard's physician prescribed sleeping medication for her, assuming that would take care of her inability to sleep. Unfortunately, this reaction is fairly common: Physicians sometimes tend to prescribe medications for the symptoms reported by clients rather than probing more deeply into the situation. The nurse can reinforce Mrs. Pollard's decision not to take this medication and explore with her how to set aside time during the day when she might be able to take a nap. In addition, Mrs. Pollard's anxiety and inability to sleep well are directly related to the stress of caregiving. This can be dealt with in a more culturally acceptable manner than the routine prescription of sleeping medication. Some ways to support and help Mrs. Pollard deal with stress and anxiety may be family support, participation in religious activities, and coping through traditional spirituality.

Close family and spiritual ties within the African American family and community support the caregiving role. Extended and nuclear family members willingly care for sick persons and assume these roles without hesitation. Mrs. Pollard's two daughters try to help their mother and Steve as much as possible. They visit daily and bring their children with them. Steve enjoys being with his nieces and nephews, and he enjoys reading to the younger ones. The teenagers can help him with small tasks such as folding his clothes when they have helped with the laundry. Even Mrs. Pollard's sister tries to help out as best she can by sweeping the floor and wiping the dishes. After a family discussion that involved Steve, Mrs. Pollard, and his two older sisters, it was decided to disclose Steve's HIV/AIDS diagnosis to his older teenaged nieces and nephews. Steve felt strongly that he could help his nieces and nephews acknowledge the value of prevention of HIV/AIDS. By preventing others from contracting HIV/AIDS, Steve can find that his life and potential death will assume meaning and purpose.

Many individuals with HIV disease and their close family members are reluctant to disclose the diagnosis to others outside the family because the stigma of disclosure in a small community can affect all members of the family. Shambley-Ebron and Boyle (2006b) report that in spite of its prevalence in African American communities, HIV/AIDS continues to be a highly stigmatized condition. Mrs. Pollard's minister is aware of Steve's condition, as are a few members of Mrs. Pollard's "church family." One of the primary stressors of women during the midlife years is the loss of relationships and friendship networks, often because of competing demands on time. Caregivers have very little time for their own needs. It is extremely important for Mrs. Pollard's health and coping abilities that she continue to participate in church activities and to maintain those friendships and networks.

Spiritual beliefs form a foundation for Mrs. Pollard's daily life. Like other African Americans who live in the same rural community, Mrs. Pollard attends a small Protestant church whose membership is exclusively African American. Many, but not all, African Americans strongly believe in the use of prayer for all situations they may encounter. They use prayer as a means of dealing with everyday problems and concerns. Mrs. Pollard relies a great deal on prayer, and her religious beliefs and practices provide her with support and strength in her caregiving role. Encouraging Mrs. Pollard to take even 15 minutes each day to read her favorite biblical verses might be one of the most helpful interventions the nurse could suggest.

Mrs. Pollard has a lifetime of experience with her church; she attended church services as a child and has continued this pattern in her adult years. The role of the church in the African American community has always been important; the church was the center of activities for African Americans for decades (Poindexter, Linsk, & Warner, 1999). Mrs. Pollard's religious beliefs are integrated into her daily life as a caregiver, and her belief in God enhances her ability to care for Steve. She, like many other African Americans, has a personal relationship with God and is able to share her worries and concerns through prayer. Her traditional spirituality and church support provide a foundation for an active approach to coping with problems (see Evidence-Based Practice 7–2).

A Situational Crises and Nursing Interventions

An important priority of nursing care for Steve and his family members is to help them understand and adjust to the impact of HIV disease. The diagnosis of HIV/AIDS precipitated a situational crisis for the Pollard family. Such a situation can best be resolved by the provision of culturally relevant health-promotion and risk-reduction strategies. The health teaching and nursing interventions provided to the Pollard family should focus on wellness and health promotion. The nurse can continue this emphasis by helping Mrs. Pollard successfully manage the situational crises as well as the developmental transitions she is facing that are common to adulthood.

An important American cultural value is success in one's career, and over the past several decades, this has become as important to women as it had traditionally been for men. Mrs. Pollard has worked outside the home most of her adult life; yet, rural African American culture does not place the kind of emphasis on work and career that the wider American society does. Mrs. Pollard's ties of affection to Steve and her sister are reinforced by African American cultural values. Family ties and the lifelong attachments, as well as the extension of the maternal role to an adult child, are highly valued in African American culture (Boyle, Hodnicki, & Ferrell, 1999). These values are emphasized over women's careers outside the home. In a historical study of African American women in America, Hine and Thompson (1998) suggested that Black women have always been the financial providers in Black families and that women's work roles have been culturally viewed as an inherent part of Black motherhood, not as individual careers.

Many African American women of Mrs. Pollard's generation obtain meaning in their lives by caring for family members. Their feelings, behavior, and attitudes go beyond a simple sentiment of affection or of family ties. In explaining why she cares for her older retarded sister, Mrs. Pollard says, "We were little girls together. I always knew that I was going to take care of her." In many societies, women disproportionally provide caregiving services and social policies, and home-based programs are organized around the assumption of women's availability and willingness to provide care. At the same time, it is important to understand that Mrs. Pollard values the traditional caregiving role, and she needs support and assistance in providing the care she believes her family members need.

It is important for the nurse to assess and acknowledge that Mrs. Pollard is valued, recognized, and respected for her competence and expertise as a caregiver. The nurse could begin by including Mrs. Pollard, Steve, and his sisters in developing mutual goals for his care. Mrs. Pollard should be encouraged in her role of providing help and care to family members and in promoting the health of her son and others. It is also important that her attention be directed toward her own needs on occasion, considering she tends to focus on meeting the needs of Steve and her sister before her own. Of particular concern is the timing of Steve's serious illness. A terminal condition in a young, previously healthy adult child will cause unique trauma and conflict because of society's expectations that young adults will outlive their older parents.

Social and civic responsibilities among rural, older African Americans in the South are met almost entirely at the level of the extended family and the African American church. These ties and associations are very strong, are often complex, and are not readily understood by outsiders. African American pastors are key players in the lives of their congregations and in their communities. Mrs. Pollard should be encouraged to attend church services and to seek the help and support available to her through this important cultural resource. Mrs. Pollard sings in the church choir and tries to attend choir practice every Wednesday evening. One of her daughters

Evidence-Based Practice 7–2:

Faith and Feminism: How African American women from a storefront church resist oppression in healthcare

It is well documented within the health profession that racism and discrimination negatively affect health care. These factors impede access to and acceptance of care by poor African American women. Unfortunately, a historical pattern of dehumanization of Black people is mirrored in contemporary experiences with the medical profession and health care system. However, women of color are not unknowingly victims, and over the years they have developed ways of combating racism and discriminatory objectification that they encounter in health care.

This article describes a group of African American women and their church leaders, who attended the Morning Sun Missionary Baptist Church (a pseudonym), a small storefront church in the Pacific Northwest. The church's pastor defines a storefont church as a building that was originally meant for another purpose; in this case, the church had once been a small white-frame house in a residential area of the city. Through interviews and life histories, the women described how they interpreted their day-to-day experiences in clinical encounters as well as health beliefs about how to survive and create healing lifeways. The women related that through their experiences, the best action anyone could take when ill was to pray. Prayer was a healing force in the women's lives and brought about an altered consciousness that occurred in times of intensely spiritual moments and through the social action that was engendered as a result of the power of prayer. The women employed multiple strategies in preparing themselves to take control of the health interactions. They learned to be prepared, to take the initiative, and to ask questions. The women also made a point of taking the most assertive family member with them, especially if there was any procedure planned. They supported one another with discussions during church social times and reinforced the notion that they could redefine the dominant views of their experiences. Placing their trust in the Lord, believing that prayer had the power to change things, they were able to resist the dominant ideology of the health care system.

Clinical Application

- Read some of the sources cited in this article about Black feminism as they are enlightening about both institutional and individual racism in health care.
- Acknowledge the support and assistance that African Americans receive from their participation in religious activities.
- Incorporate the spiritual beliefs that strengthen and sustain African American women in your nursing care.
- Encourage the development of church-based and community-based educational efforts and support services for HIV-affected individuals and their family members.

Abrums, M. (2004). Faith and feminism: How African American women from a storefront church resist oppression in healthcare. *Advances in Nursing Science, 27* (3), 187–201.

comes by to stay with Steve and his aunt while Mrs. Pollard is away for the evening. The Black church has been a traditional source of support, and congregations are frequently made up of middle-aged or older adults. Coping strategies such as prayer or reading the Bible and resources such as family and church support may help mediate Mrs. Pollard's reaction to stressful situations. A culturally competent nurse understands that spirituality is a traditional cultural value that can be supportive to African Americans during a health crisis. Not all traditional values and traditions are beneficial during illness. Evidence-Based Practice Box 7-3 describes how traditional values in Mexican Americans can present barriers to the use of home health services. Culturally competent strategies are discussed that can help to overcome such barriers.

Mrs. Pollard's life revolves around her family and church. The nurse must understand the importance of cultural ties with kin and others. The support provided by these ties is crucial when an illness develops and is necessary to successful health promotion and maintenance in care-giving activities. Although social support is very important in situations like Mrs. Pollard's, some researchers have found that that many African American caregivers of persons with HIV

Evidence-Based Practice 7–3:

Cafecitos and Telenovelas: Culturally Competent Interventions to Facilitate Mexican American Families' Decisions to use Home Care Services

This study explored how selected cultural values such as *familialism* can be a barrier to elders' use of home health services. *Familialism* may promote the expectations in elders and caregivers that family members should be able to provide all of the care that is needed, that family caregivers can provide better care than outsiders, and that elders are safer being cared for by their children than by home health care providers. This pilot study tested the use of two culturally competent strategies, *cafecitos* and *telenovelas*, in affecting Mexican American elders' and caregivers' attitudes toward the use of home care services. In the *cafecitos*, Mexican American elders and caregivers participated in traditional, small get-togethers over coffee and pastries where informal visiting took place. During the *cafecitos*, elders and caregivers discussed barriers, attitudes, and needs related to whether home care services should be used to assist the elder and support the caregiver. In the telenovelas, dramatization lasted 8 minutes and was staged in 4 acts about an elder with uncontrolled diabetes who is cared for by her daughter. A home care nurse visits the family and uses culturally competent ways to get to know the elder, leading to acceptance of the nurse and improvement in the health of the elder.

Comparisons on pre-tests and post-tests showed a trend toward increased knowledge about the value of home health care. *Cafecitos* and *telenovelas* are promising, culturally competent strategies for increasing Mexican American elders' and caregivers' knowledge and willingness to consider using home health services. Although no definitive conclusions were provided, culturally competent ways of increasing elders' and caregivers' knowledge were described and may improve Mexican American elders' use of home care services. This study helps nurses think about how to use culturally appropriate ways to impart information and change attitudes.

Crist, J. (2005). Cafecitos and telenovelas: Culturally competent interventions to facilitate Mexican American families' decisions to use home care services. *Geriatric Nursing, 26*, 229–232.

illness have not disclosed the presence of HIV in the family to anyone outside the immediate family, including church members and ministers (Poindexter, Linsk, & Warner, 1999). When asked where they obtained help and support, these caregivers answered, "Jesus," "God," or "the Lord." It is not uncommon for older African Americans to cope without the amount of social support that would usually be expected in such a crisis, relying instead on internal spiritual resources (Poindexter, Linsk, & Warner, 1999, p. 231). Mrs. Pollard's daughters are crucial to support and assistance during this stressful time. The nurse should encourage them and acknowledge their contributions. In addition, they should be involved in planning Steve's home care and the support of their mother.

The nurse can continue to encourage Mrs. Pollard to attend church services because her social life is derived from her participation in the activities of her church. Arranging for one of Steve's sisters to stay with him and his aunt while Mrs. Pollard attends church services and choir practice would be appropriate. It will be the church family who will be instrumental in providing emotional support and help as Steve's condition continues to decline. If Steve should die, the church will offer spiritual support as well as the opportunity for Mrs. Pollard to find meaning and to cope with her loss and grief.

Summary

All individuals are confronted with life transitions or changes that we term *developmental tasks*. All cultures have acceptable and defined ways of responding to these life situations. There is a need to create new paradigms of adult development that reflect a more holistic picture of adult life. A situational crisis or transition was presented: an African American woman, Mrs. Pollard, who cared for her developmentally delayed sister and her 26-year-old son who had HIV/AIDS. Mrs. Pollard's own health problems were exacerbated by this situational transition, and her normal development through adulthood was disrupted. How nurses can understand such situations and provide culturally appropriate care was described.

REVIEW QUESTIONS

1. List and describe the types of transitions proposed by Meleis et al. (2000) and discussed in this chapter. Can you describe examples of these kinds of transitions in your family members and friends? Do you think it is helpful to think of "transitions" as opposed to "developmental tasks"? Why?

2. How does culture influence transitions or developmental tasks of adulthood? For example, explain how a woman from a traditional culture such as those in the Middle East might experience adulthood differently.

3. Discuss how gender might influence adult development in White "mainstream" North American culture.

4. Describe how social factors such as mobility, increased education, and changes in the economy have influenced adult development in mainstream North American culture.

5. How might caregiving for a family member bring about a situational transition for a middle-aged adult? Would this differ for cultural groups such as Chinese Americans or Mexican Americans? How?

6. Describe how culture influences the role of the caregiver in some African American cultures. What can you find in the literature about caregiving in other cultural groups?

CRITICAL THINKING ACTIVITIES

1. Interview a middle-aged colleague, a client, or a person from another cultural group. Ask about family adult roles and how they are depicted. How are these role descriptions typical of traditional roles that are described in the literature? If not, how are they different? What are some of the reasons why they have changed?

2. Interview a middle-aged client from another cultural group. Ask about the client's experiences within the health care system. What were the differences the client noted in health beliefs and practices? Ask the client about his or her health needs during middle age.

3. Using the cultural assessment guidelines provided in Appendix A, conduct a cultural assessment of a middle-aged client of another cultural group. Critically analyze how the client's culture affects the client's role within the family and the timing of developmental transitions. How might the assessment data differ if the client were older? Younger?

4. Review the literature on Mexican American culture. Describe the traditional Mexican American family. What are the cultural characteristics of Mexican Americans to consider in assessing the developmental tasks of adulthood in this group?

5. You are assigned a new patient, a 24-year-old man from El Salvador named Jose Calderon. At morning report you learn that he has been a gang member in El Salvador, and because he wanted to stop all gang-related activities, his life was threatened. He fled to the United States and has been granted political asylum. You are told that he has extensive tattoos on his body. What do you know about gang membership in Central America? How does membership in a gang address the needs of adolescents? What are the cultural factors that are important to consider when you are planning nursing care for a patient like Jose? For example, how does our culture view body tattoos? What are the issues related to political asylum, immigration, etc.? How might you assist Jose to meet his developmental needs? What might be the problems he will encounter in U.S. society or in our health care system?

REFERENCES

Abrums, M. (2004). Faith and feminism: How African American women from a storefront church resist oppression in healthcare. *Advances in Nursing Science, 27*(3), 187–201.

Belenky, M. F., McVicker, B., Clinchy, B. M., Goldberger, N. R., & Tarule, J. M. (1997). *Women's ways of knowing: The development of self, voice, and mind.* New York: Basic Books.

Boyle, J. S., Bunting, S. M., Hodnicki, D. R., & Ferrell, J. A. (2001). Critical thinking in African American mothers caring for adult children with HIV/AIDS. *Journal of Transcultural Nursing, 12*(3), 193–202.

Boyle, J. S., Hodnicki, D. R., & Ferrell, J. A. (1999). Patterns of resistance: African American mothers and adult children with HIV illness. *Scholarly Inquiry for Nursing Practice, 13*, 111–133.

Bronfenbrenner, U. (1977). Toward an experimental ecology of human development. *American Psychologist, 32*, 513–531.

Centers for Disease Control and Prevention, National Center for Health Statistics. (2004). *Fast stats A to Z: Deaths—Leading causes.* Retrieved December 21, 2006, from http://www.cdc.gov/nchs/fastats/lcod.htm

Centers for Disease Control and Prevention, U.S. Department of Health and Human Services. (2007a). *HIV/AIDS and African Americans.* Retrieved December 21, 2006, from http://www.cdc.gov/hiv/topics/aa/

Centers for Disease Control and Prevention, U.S. Department of Health and Human Services. (2007b). *Prevention challenges.* Retrieved December 22, 2006, from http://www.cdc.gov/hiv/topics/aa/challenges.htm

Clark, M. J. (Ed.). (2003). The cultural context. In M. J. Clark (Ed.), *Community health nursing: Caring for populations* (pp. 101–139). Upper Saddle River, NJ: Prentice Hall.

Crist, J. (2005). Cafecitos and telenovelas: Culturally competent interventions to facilitate Mexican American families' decisions to use home care services. *Geriatric Nursing, 26*(4), 229–232.

Demick, J., & Andreoletti, C. (Eds.). (2003). *Handbook of adult development.* New York: Kluwer Academic/Plenum.

Erikson, E. (1963). *Childhood and society* (2nd ed.). New York: Norton.

Graham-Garcia, J., Raines, T., Andrews, J., & Mensah, G. (2001). Race, ethnicity, and geography: Disparities in heart disease in women of color. *Journal of Transcultural Nursing 12,* 56–67.

Havighurst, R. J. (1974). *Developmental tasks and education.* New York: David McKay.

Hine, D. C., & Thompson, K. (1998). *A shining thread of hope: The history of Black women in America.* New York: Broadway Books.

Holt, C. L., & McClure, S. M. (2006). Perceptions of the religion–health connection among African American church members. *Qualitative Health Research, 16,* 268–281.

Lipson, J. G., & Miller, S. (1994). Changing roles of Afghan refugee women in the United States. *Health Care for Women International, 15,* 171–180.

McCrae, R. R., & Costa, P. T. (2003). *Personality in adulthood: A five-factor theory perspective* (2nd ed.). New York: Guilford Press.

Meleis, A. I., Sawyer, L. M., Im, E. O., Hilfinger Messias, D. K., & Schumacher, K. (2000). Experiencing transitions: An emerging middle-range theory. *Advances in Nursing Science, 23*(1), 12–28.

Neugarten, B. (1968). *Middle age and aging: A reader in social psychology.* Chicago: University of Chicago Press.

Poindexter, C. C., & Linsk, N. L. (1999). "I'm just glad that I'm here": Stories of seven African-American HIV-affected grandmothers. *Journal of Gerontological Social Work, 32,* 63–81.

Poindexter, C. C., Linsk, N. L., & Warner, R. S. (1999). "He listens...and never gossips:" Spiritual coping without church support among older, predominantly African-American caregivers of persons with HIV. *Review of Religious Research, 40,* 231–243.

Purnell, L. D., & Paulanka, B. J. (2003). *Transcultural health care: A culturally competent approach* (2nd ed.). Philadelphia: F.A. Davis.

Shambley-Ebron, D., & Boyle, J. S. (2006a). In our grandmothers' footsteps: Perceptions of being strong in African American women with HIV/AIDS. Advances in Nursing Science, 29(3), 195–206.

Shambley-Ebron, D., & Boyle, J. S. (2006b). Self-care and the cultural meaning of mothering in African American women with HIV/AIDS. *Western Journal of Nursing Research, 28,* 42–60.

Sumartojo, F., Carey, J. W., Doll, L. S., & Gayle, H. (1997). Targeted and general population interventions for HIV prevention: Towards a comprehensive approach. *AIDS, 11,* 1201–1209.

Teel, C. S., & Leenerts, M. H. (2005). Developing and testing a self-care intervention for older adults in caregiving roles. *Nursing Research, 54,* 193–201.

U.S. Department of Health and Human Services, HIV/AIDS Bureau. (n.d.). *The Ryan White HIV/AIDS Program.* Retrieved January 3, 2007, from http://hab.hrsa.gov/history.htm

Wright, L. K. (1997). Health behavior of caregivers. In D. S. Gochman (Ed.), *Handbook of health behavior research III: Demography, development, and diversity* (pp. 267–283). New York: Plenum Press.

Wright, L. K., Hickey, J., Buckwalter, K., Hendrix, S., & Kelechi, T. (1999). Emotional and physical health of spouse caregivers of persons with Alzheimer's disease and stroke. *Journal of Advanced Nursing, 30,* 552–563.

Wuest, J., Merritt-Gray, M., & Ford-Gilboe, M. (2004). Regenerating family: Strengthening the emotional health of mothers and children in the context of intimate partner violence. *Advances in Nursing Science, 27,* 257–274.

8

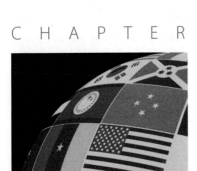

Transcultural Nursing Care of Older Adult Clients

Margaret A. McKenna

KEY TERMS

Case managers
Formal Support
Informal Social Support

Long-term care
Illness Behavior
Popular Health Care

Traditional Medicine
or Practices

LEARNING OBJECTIVES

1. Demonstrate knowledge of socioeconomic factors and community resources that influence the experiences of older adults in the health care system.
2. Apply concepts of cultural variation, life experiences, and acculturation to plan and implement nursing care for the older adults in community and institutional settings.
3. Integrate concepts of informal and formal support systems, patterns of caregiving, and available resources to plan appropriate nursing care of the older adult.
4. Develop nursing interventions for older adults, in a variety of caregiving contexts, that will be perceived as culturally acceptable

Nurses and health professionals will be caring for more older adults as there will be increased numbers of individuals aged 65 years or older in the years 2010–2030 (U.S. Department of Health and Human Services, Centers for Disease Control and Prevention [CDC], 2003). The median age of the world's population is increasing due in part to a decline in fertility and to a 20-year increase in the average life span during the second half of the 20th century (United Nations, 2002). In the United States, the proportion of older adults at least 65 years of age is projected to increase from 12% in 2000 to nearly 20% in 2030 (U.S. Census Bureau, 2005). Older adults are a heterogeneous sector of our population and as such will have a range of strengths as well as

various needs that require different levels of care, assistance, and support. The continuum of older adults' care needs will be met through a range of services that are provided in home-based care in community settings, retirement communities, congregate care facilities, assisted living centers, and long-term care facilities. Nurses will likely fill roles as long-term care case managers, direct care providers, discharge planners, and nursing consultants when caring for older adult clients.

Culture influences how individuals view aging; thus, groups of older clients vary in their adjustments to aging and in their health- and illness-related behaviors and practices. Culture is not the sole determinant of behavior but is a critical dimension in understanding the interactions of older clients in their families and in an encompassing societal context. When nurses give attention to the older client's cultural background, they will implement care that is more individualized to the strengths and needs of each client and most appropriate to each individual's circumstances.

To appropriately plan and implement care, nurses should assess the evolving socioeconomic, cultural, and family contexts that influence older adults and identify the relative impact of these factors on the individual. The available resources in the community as well as institutions, long-term care funding, and interventions at a societal level will affect any older client's options for care and will affect the individual's movement on a continuum of care. Understanding that the older adult is a participant in the culturally influenced patterns of care within a family, the nurse may consider the family as one resource for care. Nurses must assess cultural variations that should be included in planning and implementing nursing care of older adults. The older clients' cultural traditions and values will influence their preferences for their residence, their lifestyles, and their caregivers. Social and economic factors, including acculturation, influence the retention of traditional cultural values and practices. In assessing older adults, nurses must consider individuals in the contexts of society, of their cultural upbringing, and of their families who have varying strengths, resources, and capacities for care of aging family members.

To develop culturally appropriate care for older adults, nurses will first want to consider that the context for delivering care to clients is set by how available and affordable national, state, and local health care resources are for older adults. The U.S. Surgeon General's *Healthy People 2010* report (U.S. Department of Health and Human Services, 2000) states that the first goal is to help individuals to increase life expectancy and to improve their quality of life. States, and even rural and urban locations, differ in the range of information and referral sources, acute and extended care facilities, and community-based services that will be available to older

adults to support their quality of life. See Box 8-1 for highlights of multiple factors that will interact and shape the context for older adult clients who seek care or use health care services.

This chapter is organized in three sections that emphasize the dimensions that nurses will find relevant in planning care for older adults: (1) the encompassing social and economic factors that influence the older adult's help-seeking behavior and plans for long-term care, (2) the factors at the community level that include cultural values, practices, patterns of caregiving, and resources including informal and formal sources of help that are available to older clients, and (3) the interaction of needs and resources that impact older adults and their families who cope

---

BOX 8-1

Factors That Influence Older Adults' Responses in Seeking Health Care

At the Societal Level

- Social and economic factors and changes affect the experiences of older adults in the health care system.
- Interventions to control Medicare expenditures force shorter hospital stays.
- Gaps in health care services put greater burdens on older patients for home and community-based care.

Cultural Variation Within a Societal Context

- Different cultural traditions have values that influence patterns in caring for older adult family members as they require more assistance.
- Younger family members become acculturated and change traditional behaviors that may differ from older adults' expectations.

At the Individual Level

- Female family members who were considered primary caregivers for older family members are entering the work force.
- Families' economic situations, proximity to the older adult, and sources of formal support in the community will determine options for residence and care needs of the older adult.

with illness and make decisions in a continuum of care and services.

The Older Adult in Contemporary Society: Factors Impacting Health Care

This section addresses the encompassing context that surrounds and influences older adult clients: demographic factors of the aging population, economic factors, and social theories of aging that shape how older adults in Western society perceive growing older.

Changing Demographics

One of five Americans in 2030 will be 65 years or older, and individuals who are 85 years and older are the fastest growing sector, according to the last U.S. census. The American population aged 65 years or older will double between now and 2050 to 80 million (U.S. Census Bureau, 2005). Ethnic populations of color including Hispanic, American Indian, Eskimo, Aleut, Asian, Pacific Islander, and Arab American populations are expected to represent 25% of the elderly by 2030. Hispanic older populations are expected to grow the fastest from about 2 million in 2000 to 13 million by 2050 (U.S. Census Bureau, 2005). Improved living conditions, increasing life expectancies, and decreasing fertility rates are contributing to an increase in the proportion of older adults in the population of the United States and Canada, as well as in other developed countries.

Increased longevity may mean declining health and losses that increase isolation and loneliness for some older adults, different trajectories of relatively good health with a slow decline for some, or good health with recovery from illness episodes for others (Fonseca & Paul, 2004). There is evidence that disabilities associated with aging can be postponed through healthier lifestyles (Hubert, Bloch, Oehlert, & Fries, 2002). Disabilities measured by reduced instrumental activities of daily living among an older adult population have declined since 1980

(Freedman, Martin, & Schoeni, 2002), to the point that the majority of older adults in North American settings do not suffer from disabling conditions. Disability that affects independent activities of daily living in older adults living in the community ranges from 7% for those 65–74 years old to 24% for those aged 85 years or older (Hardy & Gill, 2004). This finding is true cross-culturally as well. In the United Kingdom, approximately 80% of the population 75 years and older are not disabled, which compares with 70% of the older adult population in Belgium and France that are similarly able (CDC, U.S. Department of Health and Human Services, 2003).

However, chronic illnesses affect a sector of older adults disproportionately and contribute to varying degrees of disability. In the United States, four of five individuals older than 65 years of age have one chronic condition, and 50% of older adults have at least two chronic conditions (CDC, U.S. Department of Health and Human Services, 2003). For approximately 20% to 25% of the older adult population, the care and management of chronic conditions becomes more problematic and costly with advancing age. A subgroup of the older adult population will experience significant aspects of physical decline or functional disability that requires extended use of hospital, community, or home-based personal health services. The health care systems in the United States, Canada, and other developed countries must face expanded demands of some older clients that include care for multiple chronic conditions.

Evidence indicates that older members of some racial and ethnic groups of color experience higher rates of several health conditions than do White populations. Strokes occur at a younger mean age for African Americans, American Indians/Alaska Natives, and Asian/Pacific Islanders than for Whites (CDC, U.S. Department of Health and Human Services, 2005). Hospitalization for congestive heart failure was higher in African Americans, Hispanics, and American Indians/Alaska Natives than in non-Hispanic Whites (American Heart Association, 2007).

Older adults who are African American, Hispanic (non-White), and American Indian/Alaska Native suffer a higher prevalence of cardiovascular disease and diabetes than do White (non-Hispanic) populations (American Heart Association, 2007). The rate of diabetes for American Indians/Alaska Natives is more than twice that for Whites. Hispanics are almost twice as likely to die from diabetes as are non-Hispanic Whites (U.S. Department of Health and Human Services, 2000). These disparities exist for interrelated reasons, including lower income levels, lack of insurance, lack of access to care, and lower quality of care for some health conditions even when the individual is insured and care is received (American Public Health Association, 2004).

Both ethnicity and income level affect the older adults' health status and need for care. Older White males with the highest incomes can generally expect to live more than 3 years longer than those in the lowest income levels. The percent of older adults in the lowest income families who report limitation in their activities of daily living caused by chronic disease is three times higher than for older adults in the highest income families (U.S. Department of Health and Human Services, 2000). Elderly African Americans often suffer functional declines at earlier ages than White Americans. Older African American women have a much higher proportion of disabling conditions than older African American men and older White adults. Thus, there is no simple correlation between the need for care and increased age because care needs and health status are affected by many dimensions in an older person's life, including socioeconomic level, ethnicity, and lifestyle (e.g., dietary habits).

To serve the growing proportion of older clients and their complex demands, nurses should consider that social and economic factors, cultural variation, and available support interact and impact the **illness behavior** and related help-seeking responses of older clients. As nurses prepare to care for older clients, they must assess the heterogeneity of the population as ethnicity, cultural traditions, social and economic situations, living arrangements, employment sta-

tus, and migration history of older adults are as varied as they are for younger adults. These background factors contribute to older adults' varied responses to the illness that brings them to the health care system.

Economic Factors

The cost of **long-term care** for older adults in the United States has contributed to growing Medicare expenditures for individuals aged 65 years and older as costs have shifted to management of chronic illness and not solely acute care episodes. Given that the numbers of older adults who may require long-term community-based or institutional care is likely to rise, financial burdens for health care at national, state, and local systems can only increase. The health care needs of older Americans, especially those who are 85 years or older and are referred to as the "old old" will place more burden on our health care system. These elderly Americans may have set aside resources for retirement, but they may not be sufficient to keep pace with their longer life spans. As the number of elderly who are 65 years or older increases, the elderly also continue to have the highest poverty level of adult Americans. Older adults who retire usually live on a fixed income, have increased health-related expenses, and may cope with the death of a spouse or life partner.

Among ethnic older adults, including Hispanics and African Americans, 40% have no private savings for their retirement and will look to state and federal reimbursement programs for health and social service needs. More than 20% of older Hispanics have incomes below the poverty level, compared to less than 10% of Anglo elderly. Poverty among a sector of the Mexican American elderly may be attributed to occupational history of low wage jobs, periods of unemployment, and lower educational levels as the proportion of Hispanic elderly with no formal education is eight times the rate for Anglo elderly. The reality is that many ethnic elderly of color have accumulated fewer financial assets; that is, they have a lower household income and have less income from private pensions than do elderly Whites. More ethnic elderly of color rely on Supplemental Security Income (SSI) as the primary source of income after age 65, while a much smaller number of elderly White clients (1 out of 20) relies on this source. One of the major problems that many ethnic older adults and their families face is that limited tangible assets and lower equity in their homes may limit possible care options because families cannot afford costly long-term care or community-based care of the older adult family member.

Social Health Maintenance Organizations (SHMOs) have Medicare and Medicaid funding to cover comprehensive services: homemakers, adult day care, transportation, personal care, and short-term institutional care. These organizations offer promising results that frail elderly who meet eligibility criteria and who are carefully assessed may receive community-based services at a cost savings from comparable nursing home care. This evidence may lead to broader implementation of similar services that will enable more elderly to reside longer in their preferred community residences.

The majority of older adults prefer to "age in place," that is, to stay in their homes and in their neighborhoods as long as possible. By considering the needs of the older adult and by designing health and social services programs, communities can be successful in meeting the older adults' needs. Demonstration projects to provide community-based services to older adults have proven success for several approaches: (1) Care of the elderly at home requires comprehensive services from a multidisciplinary team of providers along a continuum of care; (2) services provided at home in place of institutionalization may or may not be less costly and must include a broad spectrum of services, often using formal and informal networks of caregivers; and (3) nurses who provide primary care have a vital role to assess the older adults' physical, mental, and social well-being within the contexts of family, culture, and community. Providing community-based care has some limitations as frail older adults in very rural areas may have to enter nursing homes as a safe housing option when there

are too few community-based support services or assisted living centers to sustain the frail adult.

Nurses may be **case managers** for older adult clients in active retirement communities or other settings. An example from the caseload of a nurse who provides preventive health care and assessments in a low-income housing complex for older adults illustrates that individuals have different experiences using health care services and Medicare. An 82-year-old woman who worked as a housekeeper did not seek health care until she had a stroke related to untreated hypertension 4 years ago. She had limited contributions to Social Security owing to an episodic work history, and her illness depleted any savings. She received Medicare-funded services and continues to receive home health care through Medicaid, which is state-funded health care coverage for individuals with low income. This situation is representative of the experiences of many older adults who have lower socioeconomic status and are affected by the societal interventions, including Medicare, that provide health care coverage for older clients.

As a home health nurse, you may realize that older patients on your caseload would benefit from nursing assessments and medication monitoring, but you are informed that the patient's insurance and Medicare will not cover such services. Medicare pays only a small portion of home health care services, and the patient must be medically eligible to qualify. Older adults who have other insurance may have some coverage for additional home health services for a limited period of time.

The care that older adults may receive will be influenced and determined by economic necessity as well as environmental situations such as resources for nursing services and homemaker resources; rural and urban locations will affect resource availability. Older adults' needs for care, their requests for assistance, and the sources of caregivers are also dimensions that are culturally influenced. Within the United States, nurses and health care professionals see numerous variations in community caregiving support resources, both formal and informal, that are provided for older adults.

In addition to the demographic and economic factors that affect the older population, several theoretical assumptions underlie how people feel about aging adults and shape how resources are made available to care for older adults in communities.

Social Theories of Aging

How older adults are viewed as members of society varies, and these perceptions influence the experiences of older adults. The older adult clients' requests for services and the reactions of others to older adults are shaped in part by the prevailing social theories of aging:

- *Disengagement theory* focuses on the withdrawal of older adults who are forced into retirement or who incur disabilities.
- *Activity theory* supports the selective substitution of activities by retired individuals.
- *Continuity theory* focuses on the adaptation or continuation of patterns and behaviors from younger adulthood.

There are other cultural theories of aging, and these are Western theories that provide a framework for assessing how older clients respond to growing older and to making decisions about living arrangements and anticipated care needs. The theoretical frameworks are useful in working with older adults who were raised with Western values. In American society, the values of independence, self-reliance, and productivity contributed to the attitude that the aged, who no longer contribute to society as workers, had less self-worth. Traditionally, in mainstream American culture, retirement for many older individuals led to the loss of their occupations and status and to their disengagement from social interaction. However, researchers who study aging tend to promote a more current "active aging" paradigm. Active aging reflects the realities that industrialized nations have older populations who may remain engaged in economically and socially productive activities. Older adults are recognized not for imposing a financial burden, but for being involved in socially important activities: volunteering, providing household and child-care help, giving care to the disabled elderly, and supporting social service organizations. Under the newer active aging paradigm, industrialized societies are promoting social and economic integration of older people with respect for individuals' choices. The active aging paradigm and other theoretical perspectives are summarized in Box 8–2.

Accommodating Cultural Diversity at the Community Level: Older Adults in Different Ethnic and Cultural Contexts

This section describes intergroup and intragroup differences in how older adults' life experiences will shape their responses in seeking health care. Some older adults experienced living through the Depression; seeing the invention of television,

---

BOX 8-2

Theories of Reactions to Aging

Disengagement Theory

- A pattern of withdrawal is usually considered desirable by the older person
- Time is allocated for reflection and leisure activities

Activity Theory

- Substitute activities for the tasks, such as employment, that are regulated and have been withdrawn from the worker
- Maintain activity levels and resist changes that would mean withdrawal

Continuity Theory

- Continue lifelong activities that contribute to self-perceptions
- Find meaning in adapting behaviors from younger adulthood

Active Aging Paradigm Themes

- Improvements in active life expectancy
- Employment opportunities in an aging society
- Strengthened pension systems
- Role of caregiving and volunteerism
- Planning for age-related health and long-term care needs

computers, and video teleconferences; migrating to find employment; and fighting in an international conflict. European Americans in their 90s may have been young adults fleeing Poland or Czechoslovakia before World War II. Older Southeast Asian adults in their 60s may have fled Cambodia, Laos, or Vietnam when conflict and political unrest enclosed around them. Political refugees from countries in East Africa and immigrants from Eastern bloc nations who have lived through civil wars and political revolution could well have depleted their coping mechanisms as younger adults fleeing their homeland. As a newer wave of older adult immigrants, they may experience adjustment problems that warrant care in the health and mental health care system, but at the same time they may distrust the system or have no previous experience in seeking health care.

Nurses who are providing care to clients whose background differs from their own are usually sensitive to assessing the client's culture. Individuals who have immigrated from the same country or region will differ in their needs and in the ways that their cultural background influences their health- and illness-related actions. These differences are based on a number of factors:

- Regional or religious identity,
- Situation in their homeland that may have prompted them to emigrate,
- Length of time they have spent in the United States including degree of acculturation,
- Proximity to immediate family or extended family members,
- Network of friends and social support from their homeland, and/or
- Link with ethnic, social, and health-related institutions.

In the total Hispanic American population, persons of Mexican descent are most numerous (54%), Cubans represent 14%, Puerto Ricans 9%, and other Spanish-speaking countries represent 24%. Patterns of immigration and repatriation vary among these Hispanic groups and lead to substantial differences in the proportion of elderly Hispanic Americans. Cuban Americans have a higher proportion of elderly (13.3%) (Administration on Aging, 2005). This reflects that many educated and professionally well established Cubans immigrated to the United States in the 1960s and have remained here and are now retired. They probably experienced better socioeconomic conditions that resulted in longer life expectancies. In contrast, families leaving from Mexico have been younger, some older Mexican immigrants returned to their homeland, and older Mexican Americans do not have as long a life expectancy as their Cuban American peers. More attention should be given to understanding the diversity among Asian American, Native Hawaiian, and other Pacific Islanders as there are more than 40 distinct ethnic groups. Of the immigrant groups that have been represented in the United States for several generations (Chinese, Japanese, and Filipinos), the Chinese and Filipino elderly are the most numerous. Newer immigrants include Koreans and Thais, and among the refugees, the Vietnamese elderly are more numerous than Cambodians, Laotians, and Hmong.

Culture influences how individuals view aging, define health, manage interpersonal crises, and face alterations in health that accompany aging. Nurses should consider that for older adults, health has multiple dimensions: physical functioning, social and emotional well-being, plus quality of life measures including life satisfaction and happiness. Older adults differ in their perceptions of health but generally regard their physical activity and psychological well-being as indicators of health. In focus groups, older adults who were experiencing a chronic illness indicated that they worked at maintaining their current capacities that they termed "staying in control" so they could perform activities of daily living with the goal of "keeping what they had" (Loeb, Penrod, Falkenstern, Gueldner, Poon, 2003).

Older adults are inclined to seek health information and to make behavioral changes to maintain their independence into old age. Older adults who use self-help strategies to maintain their health generally report better psychological well-being and physical functioning than older adults who do not use these approaches. Older adults who decide to adopt positive health behaviors such as stopping smoking or starting exercise go through phases in making their decisions. The Transtheoretical Model encourages nurses to develop specific guidance to fit the individual's phase that may range from precontemplation through contemplation to maintenance (Spencer, Adams, Malone, Roy, & Yost, 2006). In applying this model, nurses usually provide information about the risks of not exercising as well as the benefits of increasing activity or stopping smoking or adopting healthy eating habits. Nurses may also ask older clients about the circumstances that lead to a lack of exercise and then help clients to take small steps such as seeing how others fit exercise in their lives. Nurses can prepare older adults to have peer support, to anticipate a possible setback in changing a behavior, and to use incentives through self-talk and rewards in order to make positive health changes.

In using a culturally sensitive approach, a nurse appreciates that older adults will have culturally-influenced values and experiences that will determine their behavior and any decisions they make. For example, the matriarch of an extended family who has always valued the social benefits that come from sharing meals with family members may be reluctant to stop that practice and substitute exercise and low-fat meals. Older adults will also have learned responses in their help-seeking behavior to cope with chronic illness and to assess new illness symptoms. Some older African-Americans have been more resourceful in their problem solving, planning, and coping that may be due in part to the lack of access to health care that they experienced over time.

Culture will influence the older person's expectations of what constitutes illness and will also influence whether the older adult maintains the use of traditional sources of health care in place of or in addition to the use of biomedical sources of care. Some older clients will prefer the use of traditional medicine from their native country or practices that they recall from their

childhood. The use of traditional sources of health care concurrently with or in place of the biomedical health care system is not limited to members of recently migrated cultural groups but is common to nearly all individuals. The lingering chronic conditions that often accompany age increase the likelihood that older adults will use traditional sources to treat their symptoms. The older adult may resort to an over-the-counter medication and may use other popular remedies before, during, or after the use of prescribed sources of care. Nurses can show an interest in the client and ask them about any actions they take to treat their conditions, in order to assess the older client's concurrent use of traditional practices, folk medicine, or popular medicine. Case Study 8–1 illustrates that assessing the client's use of alternative sources of treatment is useful in developing a care plan that the client will accept.

CASE STUDY 8-1

Mr. S.L. was a 78-year-old retired machinist who had degenerative joint disease that caused recurring pain in his elbows and knees. He referred to his condition as "arthritis" and attributed his pain to the wear and tear of his long career working around machinery, hauling parts, handling equipment, and standing for long intervals. He was raised in West Virginia and recalled that his mother used rubbing liniment and kerosene to relieve aching joints. He lived outside a major Northwest city when he was interviewed by a nurse researcher about his use of alternative sources of treatment for his joint pain. He said that in addition to over-the-counter pain medication, he regularly rubbed kerosene and sheep liniment on his affected joints. He explained that his joints were not well lubricated and that they felt like gears that were clashing. An oil-based rubbing compound penetrated the joints and relieved his discomfort.

Clinical Application
The nurse assessed that the use of the rubbing compound did not interfere with the prescribed medications. The patient's belief that rubbing compound improved his condition and decreased his pain allowed him to participate in a prescribed

exercise program. The nurse would continue to assess the treatment to determine whether the use of an alternative source of treatment would interfere with the prescribed care plan.

Older adult clients may also use **traditional medicine or practices** from their family of origin as a means to prevent illness. Preventive measures may combine a magical or religious element, such as burning a candle, offering cornmeal to the spirits, wearing an amulet, or reciting a prayer. The nurse may reinforce these preventive actions to prevent illness and maintain health. To assess the older adult's cultural beliefs and practices, the nurse can demonstrate a nonjudgmental attitude and ask questions that are similar in intent to the following:

- Have you eaten any foods that make you better?
- Have you used some herbs to make you feel better?
- Have you taken pills or medicine to help your problem?
- Did you talk to someone else and follow his or her advice about your problem?
- What do you expect your treatment to be?
- What would you like us to do to make you comfortable?

Older clients may use alternative sources of care and decide not to follow prescribed treatment plans. They do so based on their beliefs about the causes of their illness and their expectations for treatment. Older clients may blend some biomedical beliefs about the cause of illness with some traditional and popular notions about illness, so it follows that clients may adhere to some traditional practices and some biomedical treatments.

In planning nursing care, nurses should consider that older adults from different backgrounds might share experiences of migration, changing social and family structures, structural forces that include discrimination, and historical events that include political conflict. The hardships that older clients have endured may increase their striving for autonomy in later years

and push the client toward self-reliance. The older client may need time to reflect on decisions and may tend to regard health care cautiously. Some older clients will be fatalistic about many losses in life and weigh options about health care in relation to their fatalistic views.

Older clients may preserve their traditional values that connect them to their origins and give meaning to their lives. Nurses can provide culturally sensitive care when they identify that older clients retain traditional values or blend traditional values and practices with biomedical beliefs and practices. Many older clients could have grown up with limited preventive care and associate health care only with emergent conditions, so nurses should assess the older client's previous experiences in the health care system. Several examples of health care studies of older adults are highlighted in Table 8–1.

Understanding Culture Change in Older Adults

Some older adults have relocated to different regions of the country or have made a significant transition in their late adult years to be close to younger family members. Older clients may have the common experience of relocating or migrating, but the length of time that they have resided in one area may vary. Recent immigrants usually have a stronger family orientation and expectation of caregiving for parents by adult children.

Older immigrants may have lost their social positions and may be clinging to family roles in light of the stress of acculturation that reduces their status. The psychological stress related to cultural change is more intense for older refugees. Elderly ethnic Vietnamese, Chinese Vietnamese, and Laotians who resided with immediate family members had a higher sense of social adjustment compared to older refugees who shared a living space with many extended family members and non-kin. The older refugee has sometimes left behind a career and a status associated with that career.

Some examples will illustrate these factors. Mai Bliatout fled from Laos in the late 1970s and settled in the Pacific Northwest. She and her hus-

TABLE 8-1 *Highlights of Selected Cultural Studies of Older Adults, 2001–2005*

Study (Author, Date) and Group Studied	Cultural Values Relevant in Care of Older Adult Client	Implications for Nursing Care
Loeb, Penrod, Falkenstern, Gueldner, & Poon (2003): Caucasian older adults with chronic conditions in a Southern city in the United States	Nurses should negotiate models for working with individuals with chronic conditions to provide humanistic care.	Older adults described seven strategies for coping with the periods of gaining and losing their functioning capacities associated with experiencing chronic illness: relating with health care providers, medicating, exercising, changing dietary patterns, seeking information, relying on spirituality, and engaging in life.
Pincharoen & Congdon (2003): Older Thai persons living in an urban community in the United States	Spirituality and health coexisted and were linked to all of life.	Nurses working with older Thai clients in the United States may assess if the themes from this study emerge with other clients: A connection with spiritual resources provides comfort and peace; one can find harmony through a healthy mind and body; one values tranquil relationships with family and friends; and one can experience meaning and confidence in death.
Shellman (2004): Older African American adults in a Northeastern urban community in the United States	Few studies have included the life experiences of older African American adults to understand the relevance of such experiences to illness episodes.	Older African Americans expressed their experiences with discrimination and their coping strategies, which included lay remedies and spirituality. These older adults reinforced that nurses should elicit the client's views as these respondents expressed that "nobody ever asked me before" when their feelings and attitudes were elicited.
Zunker, Rutt, & Meza (2005): Older Mexicans living on the U.S.–Mexican border	Older adults' self-reported health care-seeking behavior was influenced by their life experiences, health status, family support, and socioeconomic status.	Participants perceived that the family was the primary source for providing care for older family members. Older adults' access and use of health services will be influenced by prior help-seeking behavior, and nurses interacting with clients will want to elicit this information to build an effective relationship with clients.

band had three daughters while they lived in Laos, and they had a fourth daughter in the United States. Mai and her family are Catholic as her family had been friends with missionaries, but some people from Laos follow Buddhism or animism. Since her husband's death, Mai has lived with her oldest daughter, son-in-law, and two granddaughters in an urban neighborhood where there are other Laotian families, Vietnamese, and some Korean families. The other three daughters live within 2 hours of Mai and visit her at least once a week. Mai travels with one of her daughters to a church that is in another part of the city to hear the mass in her native language, rather than hearing a native English speaker. She lives where she can shop in a market and buy Vietnamese noodles similar to what she used to have at home. She has contact with immigrants whose experience is similar to hers. Although Mai has lived in the United States for 30 years, she always preferred to speak her native language while at home with her husband. Mai and her husband are representative of approximately 85% of older Southeast Asian refugees who have traditional expectations of living with and receiving support from their children. In Case Study 8–2, an older immigrant parent assumes a new role and acquires a new source of status in the family.

CASE STUDY 8-2

Mrs. D.R. is a 79-year-old native of the Philippines. She moved to an urban area in California to be near her four children, who live in the same state. She had lived in the same town in the Philippines for her entire adult life and had stayed there to care for her husband and her sister, who both required care for chronic conditions. She is representative of Filipinos who migrate at a later age to join family members in North America. Although she was a much needed and highly esteemed member of her household in the Philippines, she, like many other immigrants, experienced role reversal when she lost the once dominant position within the family and became financially dependent on adult children during relocation. Mrs. D.R. was also like other older Filipino adults who had a more active social network before relocation. She, like many older Filipinos, spoke a dialect and did not speak Tagalog, the language spoken by many younger residents of the Philippines. After her relocation to the United States, her communication and interaction became restricted to her extended family because she did not feel confident using her limited English and did not find other speakers of her dialect. Mrs. D.R. found increasing comfort through prayer and attendance at the Roman Catholic Church to buffer the disequilibrium she felt as a result of her migration.

An older Filipino adult's status changes if he or she assumes child care or other duties within an adult child's home. Doing so maintains the older member's respect within the family, and this reciprocal relationship may lead to the perception of filial obligation between the generations of family members. After Mrs. D.R. assumed the care of her two daughters' children, her self-esteem, personal dignity, and pride in her family increased. The nurse who treated Mrs. D.R. in the emergency department after she fractured her wrist in a fall assessed that Mrs. D.R.'s injury would place a strain on the family because they would temporarily be without their child care provider. The nurse was able to involve her family members in the discharge plan for Mrs. D.R. so her recovery could be ensured, she would not lose respect, and she would not feel responsible to assume her usual duties until she felt better.

Clinical Application

The nurse caring for Mrs. D.R. assessed the following areas, which are relevant concerns for any older adult client:

- Dynamics of the family system
- Interaction of the older client within the family
- Environment to which the older client will return
- Adherence of the client and the family to traditional values
- Isolation of the older client associated with speaking native language

All of the above-mentioned factors may vary among older Filipino migrants, and nurses must assess the extent to which individuals retain their traditional practices and the related underlying values.

Under the current immigration policies, some recent immigrants do have a financial responsibility to their older family members. The older adult usually does not have an option to work, nor is public assistance an option, so the family must provide for the older adult members. Older family members may reciprocate services for younger family members. Nurses have described that in approximately one-third of Hispanic families; older clients provided child care to younger family members and actively assisted in family decisions. As part of a nursing assessment, the nurse notes if older adults are primary care providers for grandchildren or other family members and if an illness episode in the older adult disrupts the family.

Many immigrants who have migrated after the age of 50 years experience more depression associated in part with their increased dependence. Depressed older adults are more likely to have lower self-rated health (Han, 2002). In several studies of older adults, less satisfying relationships have been associated with more functional impairment, a greater number of depressive symptoms, and depression (Han, 2002; Speer & Schneider, 2003), which suggests that nurses should assess the quality of the older adult's relationships as well as their functioning status.

For many Mexican American older adults, low socioeconomic status could be a barrier to health care, especially for early diagnosis and treatment of chronic conditions. However, for many years, deaths from heart disease were found to be somewhat lower in Mexican Americans than in non-Hispanic White people. This is suggestive of protective aspects of traditional Mexican American culture that may include older adults' integration in the extended family and their care at home that contributes to a slightly better-than-expected health status. However, recent research found that heart disease deaths in Mexican Americans were as high as in non-Hispanic White people. The protective aspects of Mexican American culture may diminish over time among families as they become more acculturated. Older Mexican Americans and other older Hispanics may have chronic conditions that could respond to positive lifestyle changes if the messages to develop healthy habits are delivered in culturally appropriate programs.

Membership in a cultural group or the shared experience of immigrating from the same country does not imply that older adults are similar. The life experiences of the individuals, including their occupations and education, and their acculturation will affect their needs and expectations for care in their advancing years.

There are three cultural values—respect for the aging, intergenerational duty, and the primacy of family bonds—that are similarly held among many of the cultural groups that compose the large group that is referred to as Asian-Americans. In each group, the majority of individuals would likely expect and find that care for older adult family members is assumed by younger family members. Traditional Japanese culture offers us an example of the shared culturally influenced expectation that daughters and daughters-in-law would care for older family members as they face declines in personal health. However, while some families who are Japanese American may continue to uphold traditional values, there are increasing signs of conflicting traditional values and popular culture values.

While traditional values among Asian-American and Pacific Islander families may be desirable, other factors, including increasing education and career opportunities for women as well as economic necessity to enter the labor force, may influence the behavior of female family members to work outside the home and not to be full-time caregivers. There are other patterns that include the suburbanization of Japanese Americans and more varied geographic locations that reduce the relevance of traditional values in the lives of the Nisei (second-generation) Japanese Americans, which may impact lowered status and reduced authority for the Issei (first-generation) Japanese American elderly. Nurses may need to assess what could be disparities in what the older client expects for care and what the younger family members can realistically provide.

Caregiving of Older Adults by Family Members

Involving the family in the care of the older adult member is important because family members are participants in **informal social support** networks that often nurture and maintain older adults in their preferred community residences. It is also vital to consider the preferences of the older person and his or her family members, as well as the capacities of the older adult for self-care and the willingness and capabilities of the families to offer support and assistance with care. The type and duration of support that can be provided by family members must be considered in relation to sources of **formal support** that could be used to sustain the family care. This includes the skilled assessment, care, and evaluation of care that are provided by nurses and other health care professionals in different settings.

The contexts for formal support and health care for the older adult have evolved steadily over the last 2 decades. The image of care for older adults in skilled nursing facilities has given way to a continuum of services that includes self-care, supported self-care, assisted living communities, and skilled care. The roles that family members take in each of these levels of care vary according to cultural, socioeconomic, and demographic characteristics. We hear of adults who are "sandwiched between the layers" in the care of their own children and care of aging parents. While intergenerational caregiving is becoming increasingly common for families across the United States, families in other countries have values more consistent with caring for aging parents in extended families. All families have culturally influenced patterns of responsibility to care for older family members, but these patterns vary across cultures. Culture definitely influences the role that the family members will take in the care of older family members. Nurses and health care professionals must be increasingly aware of how social and economic factors may alter families' retention of traditional values that affect caring for older family members. One study of Filipino and Chinese immigrant caregivers living in a Western urban area indicated that the caregivers did see caring for their parents as a high calling, and they transformed the associated stress into some levels of satisfaction and personal well-being through accepting, mobilizing, and enduring (Jones, Zhang, Meleis, 2003). These caregivers were immigrants and may have had intensified feelings of family responsibility that have been similarly found in earlier research on children of Korean and Vietnamese parents. Nurses working with older adults should be sensitive to the evolving needs of family caregivers that will be influenced by the caregivers' acculturation and their time since immigration, two factors that place the caregiver between value systems. Evidence-Based Practice 8-1 refers to a study of female immigrant caregivers who integrated their caregiving roles with other demands and responsibilities.

While some Asian American women have a commitment to family caregiving, the increasing cultural diversity in North America calls for nurses to give more attention to assessing and understanding the cultural variations among individuals of Chinese, Japanese, Vietnamese, Hmong, or Cambodian heritage who may be expected to be caregivers.

The economic necessity that two adults in many households must work to provide adequate household income has contributed to a decline in the former taken-for-granted availability of adult female children as caregivers to parents and grandparents. The participation of women in the work place and the decline in the numbers of adult children in many families have contributed to families that are not available to provide personal care to the older adult family members. Adult children and other family members may be available to provide episodic assistance, emotional support through short visits, or some financial assistance to purchase in-home services. It is not possible to talk about older adults or their families as if they were a homogeneous group, in similar life situations. Rather it is necessary to consider that cultural diversity and lifestyle choices may actually influence and determine many different options for care of the older adult. Nurses working in acute, community, and long-term care settings will be asked to support family members who are involved and contributing to the care of older family members in different ways: tangible support, emotional support, financial assistance, personal caregivers, and relief caregivers.

Evidence-Based Practice 8–1:

Caregiving Experiences of Two Groups of Asian-American Women

A sample of Asian American women (Filipino-American and Chinese American) who cared for their elderly parents identified the cultural and role conflicts that may be experienced by caretakers. The women described that fulfilling filial values while also meeting the requirements of working women in contemporary Western society caused stress but they incorporated the caregiving into their lives out of respect for their families. Ethnicity was a factor that influenced the familial caregiving patterns and the support between generations that distinguished the Filipino-American and Chinese American women from their White peers who had similar access to resources and sources of assistance. The caregiving daughters mobilized and integrated their roles in patterns that were similar to other caregivers who were also immigrants and who arranged for their parents to follow them in immigrating. In an earlier study in Australia, two factors—cultural values and the length of time since immigration—determined the caregiving responsibility of immigrant female adult daughters.

Clinical Application

Nurses caring for older ethnic adults in the community will want to assess the capacities and preferences of the adult children in the family who may be immigrants who have invited their aging parents to live with them. The immigrant children who have assumed responsibility or are expected to assume responsibility for caring for a parent may be struggling with their own value conflicts and role conflicts. Nurses who are culturally competent will recognize that the older adult client and his or her family members will need to be consulted in developing a plan of care and in identifying personal, family, and community resources that may be accessed.

Jones, P. S., Zhang, X. S., & Meleis, A. I. (2003). Transforming vulnerability. *Western Journal of Nursing Research, 25* (7), 835–853.

In caring for older adults, community nurses may have to coordinate how families caring for older adult members can access and use formal support services (visiting nurse services, chore services, adult day care) and informal support services (family members, neighborhood volunteers, meal delivery). Nurses are giving increasing attention to assessing the caregiver's capacities, needs, and resources in planning for extended care of an older adult at home. A nurse needs to assess the caregiver's health and well-being as well as that of the older adult client, considering a caregiver may be a working mother sandwiched in the care of an older parent and adolescent children, or a caregiver may be a retired worker in her 60s with a chronic illness.

Nurses need to be increasingly aware of the growing cultural diversity and the increasing numbers of older adults who may require home care. Not only are clients more diverse, but their potential family caregivers vary widely in socioeconomic status, educational levels, and acculturation patterns. These factors will influence whether the caregivers, who are usually wives or daughters, will be expected to care for older family members. In a study of Hispanic caregivers in two Western states, the caregivers who were most positive about their roles (had large

Evidence-Based Practice 8–2:

Hispanic Families' Use of Support Services

Nurses need to be aware of intragroup differences among Hispanic families and should acknowledge that caregivers and care recipients will differ in income, level of education, degree of acculturation, and expression of traditional values. In a study of 53 Hispanic families in two Western states, the characteristics of the caregiver and the older adult care recipient influenced the use of formal support services. The adult children who felt most positive about their caregiver roles had larger family networks and were less acculturated; they were also less likely to use formal services. This finding is consistent with previous research that the presence of more family caregivers lessens the use of formal services in caring for a community-based older family member.

Clinical Application

Nurses can appreciate that older adult clients may have traditional cultural beliefs about long-term care but may have modified their expectations when they acquired new cultural views through their immigration or relocation. Nurses could assist older clients and their families by coordinating services for in-home care including medication management, assistance with activities of daily living, meal delivery, physical or occupational therapy, and health assessments.

Radina, M. E., & Barber, C. E. (2004). Utilization of formal support services among Hispanic Americans caring for aging parents. *Journal of Gerontological Social Work, 43*(2/3), 5–23.

family networks and were less acculturated) were least likely to use formal services (Radina & Barber, 2004). Evidence-Based Practice 8-2 highlights this study.

Dimensions of Social Support

Social support assumes special relevance for the older client, but many older clients sustain social deprivation from several sources:

- Separation from immediate family members because of geographic mobility
- Age-related segregation caused by increased nuclear families in neighborhoods
- Loss of spouse because of death or illness
- Loss of leisure pursuits or entertainment due to illness or loss of income

It is especially important for many older adults to have social, emotional, and physical sources of support to assist them to remain as

independent as possible. Understanding the patterns of support that older adults might need and assessing the cultural variations in these patterns of support is good preparation for nurses who may be working in acute, extended-care, or community settings. Social support has been delineated in three ways:

- Affective support: expressions of respect, love
- Affirmational support: receiving endorsement of one's behavior, perceptions
- Tangible support: receiving some kind of aid, physical assistance such as accompanying a person to an appointment

One implication is to identify the importance that an older adult places on types of social support. Nurses may assess what the older client identifies as his or her sources of affective, affirmational, and tangible supports. Sources of social support are described in Table 8-2.

TABLE 8-2 *Social Networks Common to Older Clients in Community Settings*

Network	Participants in Network	Characteristics of Network
Integrated support network with local support	Family members living nearby, friends, neighbors	Based on long-term local residence of the older adult, frequent contact with available kin, usually a large network; older client remains involved in community. Friends may offer tangible assistance, affirmational support. Family offers affective support.
Community-based support network	Family members do not live in proximity, friends may be available, neighbors more accessible	Family members accessible by phone for affective support, friends may not be in good health to help, younger neighbors who are available help as they can for tangible support.
Family-dependent network	Adult children, other relatives, minimal or no contact with friends, contact with neighbors for emergencies or occasional relief support	Adult children and other relatives provide most sources of support. Network may depend on a primary caregiver with planned relief. Would benefit from some formal source of support: homemaker, aide.
Restricted support network	Spouse or adult children of the older client are primary caregivers; friends do not maintain contact or are not available because of their own illness or distance	Older client may be out of touch with peers. Older client may live in the adult child's home. Usually frailer older adult. Network may fall apart if the one primary caregiver becomes ill or loses touch with peers. Older adult unable to provide support. Usually needs formal source of support to be maintained.

To understand that culture may influence the types of social support family members offer to older clients, nurses may assess the concept that the structure of families affects how informal support is provided. Some families, including the Yankee Americans, German Americans, and families of English heritage often have a linear structure. The expectation is that adult children will assume care responsibilities for aging parents, and grandchildren will assume caregiving for aging parents and grandparents when needed. Another family structure is collateral when the perceived bonds are more diffuse. Parents, aunts, uncles, grandparents, and family friends may be part of the collateral bonds of families. Among families with a collateral structure are those of Irish, Polish, and African American families, who expect to receive and to provide informal support among all collateral contacts. The expectation

for care among many Irish families is that relatives must assist each other when needed. Many Irish and Irish American families would agree with two assumptions that describe mutual support within kinship relations: (1) a person must act like a relative in order to be thought of as one, and (2) their relatives are obliged to enter into generalized reciprocity.

Research among African American families has indicated that church members may provide assistance that supports family members' care. Non-kin, or individuals who are friends but not related, may be significant helpers in the informal network for older African Americans.

In addition to cultural variation in patterns of giving help and support, it is not surprising that socioeconomic status will influence the amount and level of assistance that family members provide to older adult family members. It is important to identify the relative influence of two types of factors on patterns of family members providing support to their older members. These are (1) demographic factors such as family size, migration patterns, rural/urban residence, and (2) socioeconomic factors including income level and educational level. Both of these sets of factors may determine the availability of family members to offer assistance and may influence the type of support that is offered. Thus, nurses must assess the influence of these factors on the older adult's social support network and identify that demographic and socioeconomic factors may be blended with culturally influenced patterns of behavior.

There are sectors of the Native American elderly population who have lived in urban areas and have generally assimilated more than their rural peers who live on reservations. Elder Native Americans tend to socialize less outside of their extended families and expect that the needs of clan members and extended family members will come before those of the individual. Native American values support the care of older family members in the home, but the pool of available caregivers is diminishing because of declining fertility and employment mobility. Elder Native Americans living in multigenerational households are more likely than White peers to have significant disabilities. A pattern that has been seen in some Native American families is that each adult child, in birth order, assumes the burden of responsibility and cost of care for the aging parent, using up the son's or daughter's personal limited financial resources.

It is more likely that an older Mexican American or Chinese American in a traditional or immigrant family will live with an adult child and receive help from an adult child than an older European American. This suggests that economic necessity or the presence of larger families may lead to the observed pattern of residence and assistance for some families. Nurses and other health care professionals must also be cautious to identify the variations within groups and not just between groups. Nurses and health care professionals should certainly move beyond

generalizations and toward appreciating the cultural differences among groups of older adults who may indicate on the census or on required forms that they are "Hispanic" or "Asian." We should not assume that all Hispanic families are familistic, nor should we assume that this is a characteristic among only Hispanic families. We would find that other groups are just as familistic in their attention to older adults and that some Hispanic families are not demonstrating that characteristic to any greater extent than are other families.

Variations Among Members of Cultural Groups

Among the groups referred to as *Hispanic*, there are differences in patterns of older adults regarding daily contacts, church attendance, and socialization with friends. Older Cuban Americans are more likely than Mexican Americans and older Puerto Ricans to get together often with friends. Older Mexican Americans are more likely than either Cuban Americans or Puerto Ricans to attend church and to have daily contact with their children. There are also significant variations in other groups of older Asian Americans and Pacific Islanders. Older Korean Americans may have immigrated with their highly educated adult children, but a higher proportion of the older clients wish to live independently from the adult children. The Korean American elderly may socialize with their peers through Korean churches but are more likely to be lonely and isolated than Chinese, Japanese, and Filipino elderly.

The nurse may look for ways to support an older adult in making ties to his or her home country to enhance self-esteem and feelings of belonging. Nurses may ask if an older adult can talk to a group of children at an ethnic community center, such as the Ukraine Community Center, El Centro, or the Polish Association. The older adult can also tell the history of his or her immigration to adolescents who may be tracing their cultural heritage for an oral history project. Senior adults may also be connected to school-age children by walking them to and from school or tutoring them through an after-school project. Nurses who are working with ethnic elderly clients may want to look for resources in the local community to do outreach to these community members and to involve them in their care.

The Individual Level: Integrating Social and Cultural Factors In the Care of Older Adults

The purpose of this section is to identify that older adults will experience the interaction of socioeconomic factors at a societal level with their culturally determined values and practices. Social and cultural factors influence most older clients' progress in meeting the developmental tasks of aging. The developmental tasks that older adults achieve include the satisfaction of basic needs, such as safety, security and dignity, and the fulfillment of integrity and self-actualization. For the majority of older adults, these needs are intertwined with the lifestyle and the residence of the older adult. For that reason, this section focuses on the options that older adults have for community or institutional care as these options provide older clients with safety, security, and an opportunity to possess dignity and autonomy. The older adult also usually exerts some control over planning where he or she will live and exercises self-determination and self-esteem. Usually in conjunction with the community or institutional residence of the older client, the individual may find an outlet for individual or group activity, volunteer efforts, artistic activity, or socialization that are sources of self-esteem, give meaning to one's life, and contribute to positive fulfillment of the developmental tasks of aging.

Nurses are especially well prepared to work with older clients as they demonstrate a professional understanding that in all cultural groups aging is a developmental experience for individuals who are in a stage of reflecting on life experiences and finding meaning in their lives.

Older adults may have many transitions that are chosen or are inevitable with growing older. In mainstream American society, these include retirement, grandchildren, changed living arrangements, family mobility, declining health, and deaths of family members including spouse, siblings, or children. Older adults may assume new roles, and nurses who work with older adults in community settings can reinforce changing roles as opportunities for positive growth. Nurses often view the strengths and residual abilities that older clients possess rather than dwelling on the losses, and in doing so, the nurse promotes optimal functioning when the older adult may be experiencing unavoidable dependency.

Cultural factors, including the cultural group history, and life experiences, including immigration, will interact and determine the older client's efforts to achieve security, autonomy, and integrity. In achieving integrity, the older client has a need to bring closure to life and acceptance of eventual death. A nurse may assess this need in a client's family and be a sensitive listener when the client works through the steps of achieving integrity. Older clients need time for a purposeful life review. The older adult may relinquish some aspects such as paying bills to an adult child, so the older person is free to reflect on life successes and failures.

Faith and Spirituality in the Lives of Older Adults

The importance of religion, faith, and spirituality for older adults has been described in nursing and social work for residents in rural areas as well as individuals of African American or European American heritage. Religion may be a source of instrumental or emotional support, a psychosocial resource, or a coping mechanism for older adults who experience challenging health conditions. Among older adults in rural areas, which included areas in the Southern United States, some Native American, European American, and African American elders had integrated their religious beliefs in their health-related practices. Previous studies found that there were no significant differences in the use of religion that were related to gender or to race; rather, the members of all groups identified that religion had been a stable influence in their lives when there were numerous changes in living conditions, housing, and employment. Groups of rural African American older adults presented complex health belief systems with religion being one of the interrelated dimensions and God sometimes personalized as a "divine other." As many older adults possess religious or spiritual beliefs, all older clients require culturally sensitive communication and intervention that is specific to their backgrounds.

Decisions on a Continuum of Care

Many older adults will require three types of care that can be summarized as (1) intensive personal health service, depending on the presence of acute and chronic conditions; (2) health maintenance and restorative care, depending on chronic conditions; and (3) coordinated nursing, social services, and ancillary services that may be provided on an episodic basis for older clients in the community. Depending on the level of disability that an older person suffers, he or she may be faced with a decision to continue to live in one's home with assistance, with family members, in an assisted living residence, or in a skilled nursing facility. Nurses will observe that older clients express different attitudes that range from resignation to acceptance when they must change residences. The nurse can assess that the older client's attitudes about community or facility residence have been influenced by social and peer groups, and the nurse can be sensitive to the older client's reactions.

Researchers have found that the most consistent factor in determining the placement of the older person into a skilled nursing facility is the lack of an adequate informal network. Nurses who provide care to older clients and families from different cultural backgrounds will notice that families vary in their capacities to provide care for the older relative who declines in func-

tional abilities. Culture can influence the extent that functional disabilities will be perceived as disabling or merely annoying, and it will influence the extent that individuals seek help for their disabilities.

Families have often developed culturally influenced patterns of caregiving and social support. The nurse may assess the following: Does the family modify the environment and assist in home care so that the older adult remains at home? Do children and grandchildren share tasks, provide meals, and run errands so the grandparents can live alone? Do family members have a plan to have relatives share responsibility to provide support and supervision for an older family member? Does the older family member have caregivers and alternates who can provide care as needed if the older adult wishes to remain at home?

Some differences have been noted in the patterns of living arrangements according to ethnic background. Even when single older African Americans lost functional abilities, they were less likely than Whites with similar losses to enter skilled nursing facilities. That finding indicates that some older African Americans may be able to reside in the community with family assistance and informal and formal social support for a longer duration than White clients. In one study of Puerto Ricans in skilled nursing facilities in New York City, the residents had higher levels of disability than did a comparison group of other facility residents. That finding suggested that Puerto Rican family members might have been more inclined to care for family members with declining health status and for a period of time longer than other families. Older individuals with adequate support systems may maintain their health and remain in a community-based setting for a longer period of time before institutional care becomes necessary. Mexican-American institutionalized elderly were more physically and functionally impaired than their Caucasian peers that lends support to the theories that informal networks provided help with activities of daily living, transportation, nutrition, respite care, and social support that deferred the necessity of nursing home placement. Older Mexican Americans interacted more frequently with younger family members than their White counterparts, owing in part to closer geographic proximity. Nurses must also assess that the values of independence and self-reliance may be very strong for some older clients, and they may refuse any assistance from family members, so the nurse should evaluate clients' behaviors relative to underlying values.

Nursing facility admissions show that while 6% of Whites over the age of 65 years may reside in a nursing facility on a typical day, the percentage of Hispanics older than 65 residing in a nursing home is half that, or 3%. The census category subsumes many different cultural groups under a broad category of Asian Americans, and only 3% of those older than the age of 65 years would reside in a nursing facility on a representative day. White elderly clients aged 85 years and older make up 23% of the nursing home residents in the United States. Hispanic and Asian/Pacific Islander older adult clients make up 10% of the nursing home population aged 85 years or older.

Among different ethnic and cultural groups, cultural traditions may influence the perceived responsibility of adult children to care for their parents at home. Historically, a higher proportion of older adults from diverse cultures have been cared for in home environments than have elders who are White. The interaction of other factors including the availability, acceptability, and affordability of a skilled nursing facility that is in proximity to the ethnic populations also definitely impacts the overall residence patterns by members of cultural and ethnic groups.

Older foreign-born Chinese-American residents were asked about the desired residence for older adults with diminishing capacities for self-care, and the respondents indicated that a nursing home was a good choice for the older person to become healthy but was not preferred for the incapacitated person who would relinquish personal control in that setting. The elders' expectation was that adult children would care for them. In contrast, nearly one-third of elderly Korean respondents indicated that a nursing home was the best living arrangement for a chronically ill or disabled person. Although more elderly Korean respondents still preferred to remain in their own homes, they also expressed less willingness to be a burden to their adult children if they became incapacitated.

Older adults who for the majority, if not all, of their lifetime have spoken their native language and surrounded themselves with friends who also shared their customs could find it enormously difficult to enter a skilled nursing facility that would appear quite different in its practices. Much of the professionals' actions and behavior that occurs in health care facilities is the result of acculturation in the biomedical culture. Nurses and other health care professionals are not always aware that their behavior, such as an insistence on schedules, order, and cleanliness, would not be valued equally by older adults from different cultural groups. Thus, ethnic elders may feel especially uncomfortable if they do not understand why they are awakened at a certain time, required to be dressed, and asked to participate in group socialization. The ethnic elder may find the skilled nursing facility to be hostile and unfriendly.

Some older adults who have immigrated to North America from other nations may have negative perceptions of skilled nursing facilities based on their experiences in their native countries. Nurses can do much to ease the entry of ethnic elders into skilled nursing facilities when they assess each resident's cultural background, food preferences, choices for daily care and personal schedule, and interaction with family members. The individual's life experiences and personality will certainly shape the reaction to being in a skilled care facility. A nurse may ask questions on topics that were meaningful to the older client, for example, what was most important for them to maintain in their daily routines and what would they like to do so they could be as independent as possible. Older clients in long-term care facilities for care of their debilitating physical conditions have expressed their desires to maintain their quality of life by controlling personal care and making decisions about their personal affairs whenever possible.

Community Based Services for Older Adults

The skilled nursing facility represents only one option for extended care of the older adult. The current nursing facility resident is regarded by experts in the field as an individual who has generally exhausted the opportunities for care in the community. This individual usually only enters a facility after home care and levels of assisted living have been implemented. Long-term care nursing consultants and nurses working in ambulatory care settings often are asked to assess older clients to help determine the best care option. Criteria that the nurse often considers to recommend the level of care or residential placement that would be most appropriate for an older client include mental orientation, physical mobility restrictions (use of assistive devices and ability to walk unaided), degree of assistance needed to complete activities of daily living, frequency of incontinence, and level of risk for accident or injury if living independently.

Nurses can assess social and cultural factors that influence the care that older adults will need, the resources to meet those needs, and the locations for residence and care that are most acceptable to the client. Nurses must assess the physiologic status of the older adult and consider the safety of the client in a residential setting. The nurse must also consider medication management of the older client, and there are physiologic changes in aging that must be considered for every client. Additionally, a nurse should reduce potential misunderstandings caused by language differences in a care plan for any older client. The nurse should assess for the older clients' understanding of medication directions as the client's eyesight may be failing and consider directions such as "take with meals," which may be open to multiple interpretations. Other factors to assess include cultural values that affect the older adult's expectations for family member care. The cultural values held by the older client and his or her family will influence the available resources, including informal sources of support such as children and grandchildren who are called upon to provide personal care, assistance with activities of daily living, and financial support.

Nurses and health care professionals who are aware of the older adult client's preferences for in-home care or for residence in skilled nursing facilities realize that the client's economic resources may affect preferred care options. For the poor elderly person, purchasing part-time personal health care services or attendant care that would enable him or her to remain at home may not be an option, so the older adult manages in less-than-desirable or potentially unsafe living situations. Nurses who are working with individual clients and those who are assigned a caseload of groups of older adults in community settings, such as apartment complexes and assisted living centers, will assess the client's needs, available sources of support from the family, and formal sources of support that are affordable to the client in a total plan of care for each client. Local programs through the Division of Aging, Aging Services, or a comparable agency may leverage available state or federal funds in innovative programs to reduce rental costs to assist elderly clients so they can remain in the community.

Local or church affiliated agencies that recruit and train volunteer visitors and caregivers to the elderly may be used in conjunction with the aging agency programs to enable the fragile older adult to function at home with formal sources of support. These organized sources of support that may include a weekly visitor or a person to do chores for the elderly client may supplement the care and support that family members may provide. Nearly all older adults indicate their preferences for remaining in the community and in their homes rather than in institutional care. The desire to be independent is a cultural value that is highly regarded by many older adults who proudly proclaim how they have supported and cared for themselves for years. For the majority of older American adults, the long-held value to be independent is so strong that the person would rather live alone even in poor health than be a burden to his or her family.

Older individuals who are independent or self-sufficient in the previously mentioned areas are the most likely candidates for what are termed *continuing care retirement communities*. These are common residential locations that offer the older adult a comfortable apartment, a range of levels of assistance with activities of daily living, meals, social activities, and supervised exercise programs. Some residential communities have an attached facility for the skilled nursing care. Many of these communities have accommodations to move the client to higher and lower levels of care based on the older client's needs, which may change over time. Factors that could cause changes in the older client's condition that would warrant transfers from one level of care to another would include acute exacerbations of chronic illness, new illness episodes, surgical care, and declines in functional abilities associated with falls or accidents.

These continuing care retirement communities offer many older adults the security to summon health care assistance if needed, the opportunity to interact with peers, and the option to remain in a community setting with an increased likelihood of participating in community resources, including cultural events, shopping trips, or entertainment provided by younger adults or school children. But some older adults would feel stigmatized by residence in such a facility and would prefer to live in an independent location in the community. Other perspective residents might prefer the stimulation of intergenerational contact outside of an age-related residence and would prefer living on their own with other means of informal and formal support.

The challenge that the majority of older individuals will face is the high cost of paying for levels of care in residential communities or in skilled nursing facilities. Many older clients and their families assume that Medicare will be the means for paying for such care. However, Medicare is limited to reimbursement for posthospital acute nursing facility stays and does not cover what is termed custodial or maintenance care of the older client. Older individuals and their families may exhaust their personal resources to cover extended care needs and custodial care. Nurses working in ambulatory care are finding many new work experiences in caring for older adult clients for short-term posthospital care or for assessment of clients who need extended care.

In the last decade, there has been an increase in the development of day programs in communities that provide nursing assessment, physical or occupational therapy, group socialization, and nutrition to older adults. These programs may supplement the affective support and tangible assistance that families give, and the programs provide settings that affirm the older clients' dignity (Figures 8–1 and 8–2). The range of these services provided at each site varies according to the

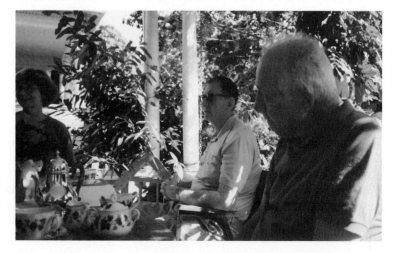

FIGURE 8-1. Opportunities to recall and share life experiences affirm the older client's identity and self-esteem (Elderwise in Seattle, Washington).

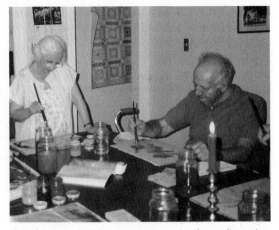

FIGURE 8-2. Creative expression stimulates discussion among participants in an older adult enrichment program (Elderwise in Seattle, Washington).

support of the local community, including volunteers and professional staff. Some sites provide group socialization and nutrition for a lunchtime meal. The older adults are usually ambulatory or able to be independent with assistive devices, so they may be transported to the sites by public or private transportation. In some Asian American communities, adult day centers offer programs and services for older adults who may be caregivers for their grandchildren. The grandparent may bring the grandchild for well child examinations and also access a health care provider for himself or herself, so two generations access health care at the same site.

The options are expanding for the older client to continue to reside in the community and to participate in an adult day program. On Lok Senior Health Services is an adult day-care program pioneered in Chinatown, San Francisco, which hires a multidisciplinary team to provide comprehensive services to the very frail elderly who would be at risk of nursing home placement. The Cherokee Nation of Oklahoma is adapting a culturally specific approach to provide a Program of All-Inclusive Care for the Elderly (PACE) for the frail elderly in rural Oklahoma communities that have a high Cherokee population. Salud Para Su Corazon has been a comprehensive outreach program using a culturally acceptable *pro-*

motora model to teach heart healthy behavior for the Hispanic elderly, their families, and their communities. Elderwise is a senior enrichment program in Seattle, Washington, with activities that include art, exercise, and discussion topics, so adults review events in their personal histories and they are validated as authorities on their lives and for their abilities (see Figures 8–1 and 8–2).

Nurses may want to assess the availability of enrichment programs in local settings and encourage attendance at such a program for older adult clients. Many mutual assistance associations or cultural affiliations, for example, the Khmer Community, Asian Counseling Services, Croatian Cultural Center, or the Eritrean Center may provide programs for older adults to interact with young people and to share cultural traditions. These cultural center programs and similar church-affiliated programs provide a means for older clients to receive affirmational peer support and to reinforce their cultural identity in a way that restores self-esteem and dignity.

Other intergenerational programs support older adults becoming involved within the community and the educational system. These types of program include the Older American Volunteer Program, the Retired Senior Volunteer Program, and the Foster Grandparents Program. There are also intergenerational child-care centers that are demonstrating that older volunteers are resources in the community, and the children and older adults benefit. Evaluations of multigenerational programs found that the older volunteers had a high level of life satisfaction, including psychosocial adjustment and self-esteem. Older adult volunteers experienced high life satisfaction prior to volunteering, so they appear to be successfully demonstrating the active aging theory.

Evaluating Services to Improve Delivery of Care

The nurse manager who evaluates the use of services by older clients can assess the cultural appropriateness and acceptability of services. Clients may be reluctant to use services for vari-

BOX 8-3

Barriers That Impede Service Delivery to the Older Adult Client

Internal barriers

Perception that there is no need for service

Lack of awareness of existing services

Inadequate knowledge needed to enroll in a service

Perception that one is not entitled to services

Desire to remain self-sufficient

Perception that providers are rude, address older clients in overly familiar terms, and interrupt the elderly

Contextual barriers

Space: lack of private space for most interactions that occur in clinical settings

Position: embarrassing position of the client in relation to the health care provider

Technology overload: presence of signs, contact with many personnel

Sensory overload: printed instructions, verbal messages, visual cues, video-tapes

Service barriers

Accessibility to care (transportation, hours of service)

Affordability of care (covered by insurance)

Availability of services (Practitioners, interpreters speak clients' languages)

ous reasons that include internal barriers, contextual barriers, and service barriers. These barriers are summarized in Box 8–3.

To overcome the barriers that are perceived by older clients, nurses can assume several approaches to interact effectively with older adults from diverse groups:

- Be sensitive to the life experiences and previous health care experiences of the older clients.
- Listen attentively to the older client's experiences, complaints, and recollections.
- Listen to related conversations to assess for underlying depression.
- Elicit information about the older client's preferences for care, including diet and use

of self-care remedies, and include them when appropriate.

- Identify available sources of informal support and confirm availability.

Summary

A cultural approach to the older client recognizes that individuals are the products of, as well as the participants in, an encompassing societal framework. Within the societal framework, the cultural backgrounds of the older clients will influence their variations in their perceptions, behavior, and practices. Culture serves as a guide to the older client to determine what choices and actions are appropriate and acceptable. Within cultural groups, individual variation is evident in response to the physiologic signs and the psychosocial demands of increasing age. Examples of older immigrant clients demonstrate that the clients' views and perceptions may differ from those of family members and from the views of the nurse. The different attitudes, practices, and behaviors among older clients result from their heritage, experiences, education acculturation, and socioeconomic status. Nursing care is not acceptable if it is based on assumptions that members of cultural groups are all the same. Instead, nursing care must be based on the assessment of individual differences in the variables that influence responses to illness and help-seeking behaviors. Nurses who are providing care in acute care settings or in the community often ask several questions as part of the nursing assessment:

1. Is the older adult isolated from culturally relevant supportive people, or is the older client enmeshed in a caring network of relatives and friends?

2. Has a culturally appropriate network replaced family members in performing some tasks for the older adult client?

3. Does the older adult expect family members to provide care, including nurturance and emotional support, which family members are unable to provide?

4. Does language create a barrier in the older client's receipt of services from formal resources?

Older adult clients have often developed their own systems including informal support for coping with illness and with changes associated with age. Nurses who are working with older clients in a variety of settings will want to assess who provides affirmation and tangible support that maintains the older client in an optimal level of functioning. Formal resources may be used to sustain the informal support systems to promote the lifestyle preferred by the older client. It is increasingly important for nurses to recognize the expanded roles that the older client may have

in his or her family as a caretaker of young grandchildren or another family member. Nurses caring for older adult clients should give attention to the client's family and social roles and develop care plans that maintain and restore the individual to his or her usual roles and patterns of activity. In the future, nurses will assess and work with more older clients as they progress along a continuum of services and through more than one type of residence in the community. By assessing the client's cultural background and available support resources, nurses will plan appropriate care that will help older clients to optimize their self-esteem and dignity based on the client's functional abilities, affective support, and affirmational support.

REVIEW QUESTIONS

1. What resources, needs, and limitations should the nurse assess to develop a care plan for a recently discharged 82-year-old chronically ill man who is returning to a single-room occupancy hotel in a crowded inner-city location?
2. As the nurse who does health assessments for frail older adults who attend a community comprehensive day program, what information should the nurse assess to

identify culturally appropriate care plans or service delivery plans for older Filipino and Chinese-American clients?
3. The short-term subacute unit where you are the nurse manager serves a multinational group of older clients who are admitted for orthopedic surgery. What cultural assessments do you teach the staff to use in identifying the needs of clients and their families?

CRITICAL THINKING ACTIVITIES

1. Many local communities offer adult day care for older adults with chronic health care problems who are residing alone or with family members. Services usually include health screening by a nurse as well as occupational health and/or physical activity sessions for these community-based older adults. Request permission to attend an activity as an observer and attentive listener. Through observation and, if possible, conversation with a participant, try to assess the levels of self-care that session participants possess and identify the types of assistance that these clients require to remain in the community.

2. As a case manager for a managed care organization, you receive many authorization requests for in-home nursing services to assist older adults who have been discharged home following hospitalization for acute illnesses or surgery. List the factors that you will

consider and the types of data that you need to make an informed decision about the nursing and health-related services and the duration of services that the older client should receive while at home.

3. In many communities, nurses provide hospice services to residents in long-term care facilities or to older adults living in other settings. Contact a community-based hospice nurse to request information about how the services meet older adults' needs for love and belongingness, as well as reflection and recollection that are expressed late in life.

4. With your awareness that cultural traditions and life experiences influence many older adults to prefer independent living, prepare a letter as a home health nurse to the appropriate official to request government-funded home health services for older adults.

REFERENCES

American Heart Association. (2007). *Statistical fact sheets.* Available from http://www.americanheart.org/presenter.jhtml?identifier=2007

American Public Health Association. (2004). *Racial/ethnic health disparities.* Available from www.nphw.org

Fonseca, A. M., & Paul, C. (2004). Health and Aging: Does retirement transition make any difference? *Reviews in Clinical Gerontology, 13,* 237–260.

Freedman, V. A., Martin, L. G., & Schoeni, R. F. (2002). Recent trends in disability and functioning among older adults in the United States: A systematic review. *JAMA, 288,* 3137–3146.

Han, B. (2002). Depressive symptoms and self-rated health in community-dwelling older adults: A longitudinal study. *Journal of the American Geriatrics Society, 50,* 1549–1556.

Hardy, S. E., & Gill, T. M. (2004). Recovery from disability among community-dwelling older persons. *JAMA, 291* (13), 1596–1602.

Hubert, H., Bloch, D., Oehlert, J., & Fries, J. (2002). Lifestyles habits and compression of morbidity. *Journal of Gerontology: Medical Sciences, 57,* A347–351.

Jones, P. S., Zhang, X. S., & Meleis, A. (2003). Transforming vulnerability. *Western Journal of Nursing Research, 25* (7), 835–853.

Loeb, S. J., Penrod, J., Falkenstern, S., Gueldner, S. H., & Poon, L. W. (2003). Supporting older adults living with multiple chronic conditions. *Western Journal of Nursing Research, 25* (1), 8–29.

Pincharoen, S., & Congdon, J. G. (2003). Spirituality and health in older Thai persons in the United States. *Western Journal of Nursing Research, 25* (1), 93–108.

Radina, M. E., & Barber, C. E. (2004). Utilization of formal support services among Hispanic Americans caring for aging parents. *Journal of Gerontological Social Work, 43* (2/3), 5–23.

Shellman, J. (2004). "Nobody ever asked me before": Understanding life experiences of African American elders. *Journal of Transcultural Nursing, 15* (4), 308–316.

Speer, J. C., & Schneider, M. (2003). Mental health needs of older adults and primary care: Opportunity for interdisciplinary geriatric team practice. *Clinical Psychology: Science and Practice, 10* (1): 85–101.

Spencer, L., Adams, T. B., Malone, S., Roy, L., & Yost, E. (2006). Applying the Transtheoretical Model to exercise: A systematic and comprehensive review of the literature. *Health Promotion Practice, 7* (4), 428–443.

United Nations. (2002, April 8–12). *Report of the Second World Assembly on Aging.* Presented at the United Nations, Madrid, Spain.

U.S. Census Bureau. (2005). International Database. Table 094: *Midyear population by age and sex.* Available from http://www.census.gov/ipc/www/idbagg.html

U.S. Department of Health and Human Services. (2000). *Healthy People 2010: Understanding and Improving Health,* 2nd ed. Washington, DC: U.S. Government Printing Office. Retrieved in 2006 from http://www.healthypeople.gov/

U.S. Department of Health and Human Services, Centers for Disease Control and Prevention, (2003). Trends in aging— United States and worldwide, *Morbidity & Mortality Weekly Report, 52* (6), 101–106.

U.S. Department of Health and Human Services, Centers for Disease Control and Prevention. (2005). Disparities in deaths from stroke among person aged less than 75 years— United States 2002. *Morbidity & Mortality Weekly Report, 54* (6), 477–481.

Zunker, C., Rutt, C., & Meza, G. (2005). Perceived health needs of elderly Mexicans living on the U.S.–Mexico Border. *Journal of Transcultural Nursing 16* (1), 50–56.

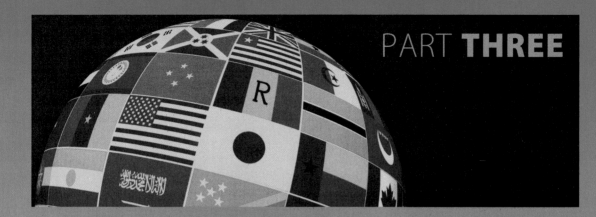

PART THREE

NURSING IN MULTICULTURAL HEALTH CARE SETTINGS

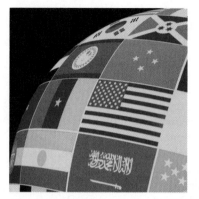

CHAPTER 9

Creating Culturally Competent Organizations

Patti Ludwig-Beymer

An individual's culture affects access to care and health-seeking behaviors, as well as perceived quality of care. In addition to understanding the culture of patients or clients, however, it is also essential to examine the culture of providers and organizations. The interplay of client, provider, and **organizational cultures** may create barriers, cause cultural conflicts, lead to a client's lack of trust or reluctance to access services, and may ultimately result in health care inequities.

Nurse leaders recognize the importance of transculturally based administrative practices in health care settings (Andrews, 1998). According to the American Nurses Association Council on Cultural Diversity in Nursing Practice (1991), "[n]urse administrators must foster a climate in which nurses and other health care providers understand that provider-patient encounters include the interaction of three cultural systems." These three systems are the culture of the health care providers, the culture of the client, and the culture of the organizational setting.

Leininger defines **transcultural nursing administration** as "a creative and knowledgeable process of assessing, planning, and making decisions and policies that will facilitate the provision of educational and clinical services that take into account the cultural caring values, beliefs, symbols, references and lifeways of people of diverse and similar cultures for beneficial or satisfying outcomes" (1996, p. 30). One very important role of nurse administrators is to ensure that organizational policies are culturally sensitive and appropriate and that they recognize the rights of individuals and families. Such policies should incorporate Leininger's (1991) decisions and actions of culture care preservation/maintenance, culture care accommodation/negotiation, and culture care repatterning/restructuring. Malone (1997) describes several strategies for improving organizational cultural competence. First, health care organizations must implement training that helps **corporate culture** to value and manage cultural diversity. Second, nursing administration must reward practice that values differences and is culturally appropriate and collaborative. Third, nursing should seek members who are culturally competent. Finally, nursing should recruit and hire members who are culturally diverse to better reflect the demographics of the country. Literature suggests that culturally diverse organizations outperform more homogenous organizations (Cox, 1994; Dreachslin, 1996).

This chapter serves to augment the current dialogue on creating **culturally competent organizations**. It defines a culturally competent organization, explains the need for culturally competent organizations, describes organizational culture, and provides a mechanism for assessing an organization's culture. Both the physical environment of care and the community context are considered. Finally, strategies for developing culturally competent initiatives and the role of health care providers in creating culturally competent organizations are described.

Defining a Culturally Competent Organization

Culturally competent health care, broadly defined as services that are respectful of and responsive to the cultural and linguistic needs of patients, is increasingly viewed as essential in reducing racial and ethnic disparities, improving health care quality, and controlling costs. The U.S. government considers cultural competence as a method of increasing access to quality care for all patients. The aim should be to develop systems more responsive to diverse populations. Managed care organizations view cultural competence as driving both quality and business. By embedding cultural competence strategies into quality improvement initiatives to make care more efficient and effective, clinical outcomes are improved while costs are controlled. Those in academic settings agree that cultural competency education is crucial for preparing future health care workers, although appropriate education on the topic is provided in only half of the medical schools in the United States (Betancourt, Green, Carrillo, & Park, 2005).

According to the Office of Minority Health, **cultural competence** refers to the ability of health care providers and organizations to understand and respond effectively to the cultural and linguistic needs of patients (U.S. Department of Health and Human Services, Office of Minority Health, 2001). Cultural competence encompasses a wide range of activities and considerations. It includes providing respectful care that is consistent with cultural health beliefs of the clients and family members. Providing competent interpreter services and programs to promote staff diversity are other ways in which health care organizations can increase cultural competence (Clancy & Stryer, 2001).

In the United States, a variety of organizations have addressed the need for culturally competent organizations. For example, the Joint Commission for the Accreditation of Hospitals and Healthcare Organizations (JCAHO) has set standards, outlined in Box 9–1, to ensure that patients receive care that respects their cultural, psychosocial, and spiritual values (JCAHO, 2005). As outlined in Box 9–2, the American Nurses Association (2001) and American Nurses Credentialing Center (2005) have also addressed the need for culturally competent care.

The U.S. government has also addressed culturally appropriate health care systems. For

BOX 9-1

JCAHO Standards that Address Culture

Ethics Rights and Responsibilities

Overview

The goal of this function is to improve treatment, services, and outcomes by recognizing and respecting the rights of each patient. Care, treatment, and services are provided in a way that respects and fosters dignity, autonomy, positive self-regard, civil rights, and involvement of patients. Care, treatment, and services consider the patient's abilities and resources; the relevant demands of his or her environment; and the requirements and expectations of the providers and those they serve. The family is involved in care, treatment, and service decisions with the patient's approval.

Specific Standards

RI.1.10 The hospital follows ethical behavior in its care, treatment, and services and business practices.
RI.1.30 The integrity of decisions is based on identified care, treatment, and service needs of the patients.
RI.2.10 The hospital respects the rights of patients.
RI.2.100 The hospital respects the patient's right to and need for effective communication.

Provision of Care, Treatment, and Services

Overview

The provision of care, treatment, and services is composed of four core processes or elements: assessing patient needs; planning care, treatment, and services; providing the care, treatment, and services the patient needs; and coordinating care, treatment, and services

Specific Standards

PC.4.10 Development of a plan for care, treatment, and services is individualized and appropriate to the patient's needs, strengths, limitations, and goals.
PC.6.30 The patient received education and training specific to the patient's abilities as appropriate to the care, treatment, and services provided by the hospital.

example, the Institute of Medicine (IOM) report *Health Professions Education: A Bridge to Quality* (Greiner & Knebel, 2003) identifies five core competencies for all health professionals: provide patient-centered care, work in interdisciplinary teams, employ evidence-based practice, apply

quality improvement, and utilize informatics. Providing patient-centered care includes sharing power and responsibility with patients and caregivers; communicating with patients in a shared and fully open manner; taking into account patients' individuality, emotional needs, values, and life issues; implementing strategies for reaching those who do not present for care on their own, including care strategies that support the broader community; and enhancing prevention and health promotion. In order to accomplish the goal of meeting patients' individuality, emotional needs, values, and life issues, the IOM report further indicates that clinicians must provide care in the context of the culture, health status, and health needs of the patient.

In addition, the Office of Minority Health in the U.S. Department of Health and Human Services developed the **National Standards for Culturally and Linguistically Appropriate Services (CLAS) in Health Care**, outlined in Box 9–3, to correct health care inequities that currently exist and to make health care services more responsive to the individual needs of all patients. All people entering the health care system should receive equitable and effective care in a culturally and linguistically appropriate manner. The CLAS Standards apply to all cultures and are especially designed to address the needs of racial, ethnic, and linguistic populations that experience unequal access to health services. Ultimately, the aim of the standards is to contribute to the elimination of racial and ethnic **health disparities** and to improve the health of all Americans.

The Need for Culturally Competent Organizations

Disparities in health have long been acknowledged. The National Institutes of Health (2000) define disparities in health as "differences in the incidence, prevalence, mortality, and burden of diseases and other adverse health conditions that exist among specific population groups in the United States." At the most basic level, disparities

BOX 9-2

Standards and Forces that Address Culture

Select standards from the Code of Nurses (American Nurses Association [ANA], 2001)

Standard 1
The nurse, in all professional relationships, practices with compassion and respect for the inherent dignity, worth, and uniqueness of every individual, unrestricted by considerations of social or economic status, personal attributes, or the nature of health problems.

Standard 2
The nurse's primary commitment is to the patient, whether the patient is an individual, family, group, or community.

Standard 3
The nurse promotes, advocates for, and strives to protect the health, safety, and rights of the patients.

Standard 8
The nurse collaborates with other health professionals and the public in promoting community, national, and international efforts to meet health needs.

Magnet Criteria Related to Providing Culturally Congruent Care (American Nurses Credentialing Center, 2005)

Force 2. Organizational Structure
- The organizational structure is responsive to changes in the health care environment.

Force 6. Quality of Care
- There is integration of the ANA Code of Ethics into practice at all levels of the organization.

Force 10. Community and the Health care Organization
- Collaboration with institutions, health care organizations, and other community-based organizations is apparent.
- Examples are provided of outcomes resulting from nursing collaborations/partnerships with other community nursing entities.
- Resources used, fiscal if indicated, in the process of collaborating/partnering with other community nursing entities are appropriate.

Force 11. Nurses as Teachers
- There is a patient education program that meets the diverse needs of patients in all of the care settings of the organization.

are evident in life expectancies. For example, the Centers for Disease Control and Prevention (CDC, 2005) report the U.S. life expectancy is 77.6 years. However, that age varies by race, with White males (75.4 years) and White females (80.5 years) living longer than African American males (69.2 years) and African American females (76.1 years).

Access to primary care is a key aspect of health care in the United States. Research suggests that having a usual source of care increases the chances that people will receive adequate preventive care and other important health services. However, 30% of Hispanic, 20% of African Americans, and 16% of Whites lack a usual source of health care. Hispanic children are nearly three times as likely as non-Hispanic White children to have no usual source of care. Both African Americans (16%) and Hispanic Americans (13%) are

more likely to rely on hospitals or clinics for their usual source of care than are White Americans (8%) (Agency for Healthcare Research and Quality [AHRQ], 2000).

Preventive services, such as infant immunizations, adult immunizations, and mammography, show disparities based on race and culture. Also, access to health care demonstrates variability in areas such as health insurance, prenatal care, doctor visits, and emergency department visits. African American, American Indian, and Puerto Rican infants have higher death rates than White infants. For example, the death rate for African American infants is 2.3 times greater than that of White infants. African American women are four times more likely and American Indian and Alaska Native women are nearly twice as likely to die of pregnancy-related complications as White women (CDC, 2006). Even in Canada, with its

BOX 9-3

National Standards for Culturally and Linguistically Appropriate Services (CLAS) in Health Care

Culturally Competent Care

Standard 1

Health care organizations should ensure that patients/consumers receive from all staff members effective, understandable, and respectful care that is provided in a manner compatible with their cultural health beliefs and practices and preferred language.

Standard 2

Health care organizations should implement strategies to recruit, retain, and promote a diverse staff and leadership at all levels of the organization, which are representative of the demographic characteristics of the service area.

Standard 3

Health care organizations should ensure that staff at all levels and across all disciplines receive ongoing education and training in culturally and linguistically appropriate service delivery.

Language Access Services

Standard 4 (Mandate*)

Health care organizations must offer and provide language assistance services, including bilingual staff and interpreter services, at no cost to each patient/consumer with limited English proficiency at all points of contact, in a timely manner, during all hours of operation.

Standard 5 (Mandate*)

Health care organizations must provide to patients/consumers both verbal offers and written notices in their preferred language informing them of their right to receive language assistance services.

Standard 6 (Mandate*)

Health care organizations must ensure the competence of language assistance provided to limited English proficient patients/consumers by interpreters and bilingual staff. Family and friends should not be used to provide interpretation services (except on request by the patient/consumer).

Standard 7 (Mandate*)

Health care organizations must make available easily understood patient-related materials and post signage in the languages of the commonly encountered groups and/or groups represented in the service area.

Organizational Supports for Cultural Competence

Standard 8

Health care organizations should develop, implement, and promote a written strategic plan that outlines clear goals, policies, operational plans, and management accountability/oversight mechanisms to provide culturally and linguistically appropriate services.

Standard 9

Health care organizations should conduct initial and ongoing organizational self-assessment of CLAS-related activities and are encouraged to integrate cultural and linguistic competence-related measures into their internal audits, performance improvement programs, patient satisfaction assessments, and outcome-based evaluations.

Standard 10

Health care organizations should ensure that data on the individual patient's/consumer's race, ethnicity, and spoken and written language are collected in health records, integrated into the organization's management information systems, and periodically updated.

Standard 11

Health care organizations should maintain a current demographic cultural and epidemiological profile of the community as well as a needs assessment to accurately plan for and implement services that respond to the cultural and linguistic characteristics of the service area.

Standard 12

Health care organizations should develop participatory, collaborative partnerships with communities and use a variety of formal and informal mechanisms to facilitate community and patient/consumer involvement in designing and implementing CLAS-related activities.

*Mandate—indicates the standard is a current Federal requirement for all recipients of Federal funds.

(Continued on following page)

BOX 9-3

National Standards for Culturally and Linguistically Appropriate Services (CLAS) in Health Care

Standard 13	Standard 14
Health care organizations should ensure that conflict and grievance resolution processes are culturally and linguistically sensitive and capable of identifying, preventing, and resolving cross-cultural conflicts or complaints by patients/consumers.	Health care organizations are encouraged to regularly make available to the public information about their progress and successful innovations in implementing the CLAS standards and to provide public notice in their communities about the availability of this information.

Source: U.S. Department of Health and Human Services, Office of Minority Health. (2001, March). *National Standards for Culturally and Linguistically Appropriate Services in Health Care: Final Report.* Washington, DC: Author.

National Health Insurance Model, many individuals experience similar disparities in access to preventative services. Such disparities are often rooted in culture, race, geographic location, and socioeconomic status.

Race and ethnicity influence a patient's chance of receiving many specific procedures and treatments. Medical management varies by gender and race (Hendrix, Mayhan, Lackland & Egan, 2005). Several studies suggest that members of minority racial and ethnic populations in the United States receive fewer invasive interventions related to cardiac disease, lung cancer, and renal transplants (Ayanian, Cleary, Weissman, & Epstein, 1999; Ayanian & Epstein, 2001; Einbinder & Schulman, 2000; King & Brunetta, 1999; Sheifer, Escarce, & Schulman, 2000). Compared to White women, the length of time between an abnormal screening mammogram and a follow-up diagnostic test is more than twice as long for African American, Asian American, and Hispanic women. African Americans with HIV infection are less likely to be on antiretroviral therapy, less likely to receive prophylaxis for *Pneumocystis* pneumonia, and less likely to be receiving protease inhibitors than other persons with HIV (AHRQ, 2000).

More than 90 million Americans live with chronic illness. Chronic diseases account for 75% of the nation's $1.4 trillion medical care costs annually, and chronic disease is a major cause of death in the United States (CDC, 2006). In fact,

five chronic diseases—heart disease, cancers, stroke, chronic pulmonary diseases, and diabetes—account for more than two-thirds of the deaths in the United States (CDC, 2004). Women and minority racial and ethnic groups bear a large burden in terms of chronic disease. Rates of death from cardiovascular disease are 30% higher for African Americans than for Whites. African American women are more likely to die of breast cancer than are women of other racial or ethnic groups. The incidence of cervical cancer is more than five times greater in Vietnamese women in the United States than White women. The prevalence of diabetes is 70% higher among African Americans and nearly 100% higher among Hispanics than among Whites. The prevalence of diabetes among American Indians and Alaska Natives is more than twice that of the total population, and the Pimas of Arizona have the highest known prevalence in the world (CDC, 2006).

Racial and ethnic disparities also exist in potentially preventable hospital readmissions. In patients with diabetes mellitus, Jiang, Andrews, Stryer, and Friedman (2005) found that African Americans and Hispanics had a higher risk for complications that were potentially preventable with effective postdischarge care. Non-Hispanic African Americans and Hispanics are also less likely to self-monitor blood glucose levels and have poor glycemic control (Harris, 2001). Among preschool children hospitalized for asthma, only 7% of African American and 2% of

Hispanic children are prescribed routine medications to prevent future asthma-related hospitalizations, compared to 21% of White children (AHRQ, 2000). Disparities in access to and quality of primary care may be partially responsible for differences in health status among members of minority groups, although many other complex factors are undoubtedly involved.

For African Americans, Asians, and American Indians/Alaskan Natives, disparities in quality of care exist but are narrowing. However, both quality and access disparities are widening for Hispanics (AHRQ, 2005). Disparities in measures of quality and access are observed in low-income people regardless of race or ethnicity. However, disparities in health cannot be explained wholly by disparities in income and health insurance coverage. For example, one study found that one-half to three-quarters of all disparities observed in 1996 would have remained even if racial and ethnic differences in income and health insurance had been eliminated (Weinick, Zuvekas, & Cohen, 2000). This implies that other factors may account for health disparities. Although these factors have not yet been identified, potential barriers that contribute to the disparities may be related to demographics, culture, and the health care system itself. Potential barriers are summarized in Box 9–4.

In addition to differences in health status and clinical outcomes, research suggests consumer ratings of care vary by race/ethnicity. Researchers (Weech-Maldonado et al., 2003) surveyed 49,327 adults enrolled in Medicaid-managed care plans in 14 states and found that racial/ethnic minorities tended to report receiving worse care than did Whites. Linguistic minorities, those who reported speaking a language other than English at home, reported receiving even worse care than the overall racial/ethnic minorities. Culturally competent organizations are needed to address disparities in health within racial and ethnic groups.

Approximately 18% of the U.S. population speaks a language other than English at home, and 8% of the population has **limited English proficiency (LEP)**. Recent research found that

BOX 9-4
Potential Demographic, Cultural, and Health System Barriers

Demographic Barriers

Age
Gender
Ethnicity
Primary language
Religion
Educational level and literacy level
Occupation, income, and health insurance
Area of residence
Transportation
Time and/or generation in the United States

Cultural Barriers

Age
Gender, class, and family dynamics
Worldview/perceptions of life
Time orientation
Primary language spoken
Religious beliefs and practices
Social customs, values, and norms
Traditional health beliefs and practices
Dietary preferences and practices
Communication patterns and customs

Health System Barriers

Access to care
Insurance and other financial resources
Orientation to preventive health services
Perception of need for health care services
Ignorance and/or distrust of Western medical practices and procedures
Cultural insensitivity and incompetence in providers
Lack of diversity in providers
Western versus folk health beliefs and practices
Poor doctor–patient communication
Lack of bilingual and bicultural staff
Unfriendly and cold environment

children of parents with LEP were more likely to be in fair or poor health when compared to parents proficient in English. LEP parents were also less likely to be insured and less likely to receive needed medical care because of cost, transportation, scheduling difficulties, and cultural barriers

(Flores, Milagros, & Tomany-Korman, 2005). Evidence-Based Practice 9-1 summarizes further details on the current status of national health care disparities.

While identifying disparities in care is important, it is not sufficient. Research is needed to focus on why these disparities exist and develop strategies to address them. Organizational culture is one area that is being investigated. A variety of projects are underway to develop tools to help eliminate racial and ethnic disparities.

How, then, does an organization move toward cultural competency? A culturally competent organization is extremely complex. Within the health care setting, practitioners must be aware of the effects of culture on individual behaviors. A culturally competent organization, however, goes beyond this awareness and calls for an understanding of the interplay among organizational culture, professional culture, and community culture.

Organizational Culture

Nurses, while familiar with the concept of culture, may be less familiar with the area of organizational culture. Yet organizational culture has emerged over the past 20 years as an important variable for behavior, performance, and outcome in the workplace. Leininger (1996) defines organizational culture as the goals, norms, values, and practices of an organization in which people have goals and try to achieve them in beneficial ways. Schein (1985) defines organizational culture as "a learned product of group experience" that develops wherever there is "a definable group with a significant history." Organizational culture encompasses an organization's preferred ways of accomplishing goals, determining priorities, and making decisions. These shared norms and expectations guide the thinking and behavior of the group members, and the shared values provide a sense of common direction and behavior.

Organizations are complex, with multiple and competing subcultures. For example, nurse specialties result in subcultures within hospitals

that impact nurse and patient outcomes (Mallidou, 2004). Organizations are subcultural systems with inherent values and beliefs, folklore, and language; these systems are organized in a hierarchy of authority, responsibilities, obligations, and functional tasks that are understood by members of the organization. Organizational culture affects not only people working in the institution, such as employees and volunteers, but also customers, such as physicians and patients. The social organization of hospitals and other health care facilities has a profound effect on patients, both directly through the care provided and indirectly through organizational policies and philosophy (Jones, Bond, & Cason, 1998). However, organizational culture has not been directly linked to patient or provider outcomes (Seago, 1997).

Theories of Organizational Culture

A variety of definitions, methods of measurement, and theories for organizational culture exist. However, there is reasonable consensus on the following points (Strasser, Smits, Falconer, Herrin, & Bowen, 2002):

- An organization's culture consists of shared beliefs, assumptions, perceptions, and norms leading to specific patterns of behaviors.
- An organization's culture results from an interaction among many variables, including mission, strategy, structure, leadership, and human resource practices.
- Culture is self-reinforcing; once in place, it provides stability and changes are resisted by organizational members.

Strasser, Smits, Falconer, Herrin, and Bowen (2002) describe four types of hospital culture: personal, dynamic, formal, and production oriented. A **personal hospital** is like an extended family. People share information about themselves. A **dynamic hospital** is entrepreneurial. People are willing to take risks. A **formal hospital** is structured. Bureaucratic procedures govern actions. A **production-oriented hospital** is concerned primarily with getting the job done. Peo-

Evidence-Based Practice 9–1:

Current Status of National Health Care Disparities

Disparities related to race, ethnicity, and socioeconomic status still pervade the American health care system.

Quality of Care

For sizable proportions of measures, minorities and the poor receive lower-quality care.

- African Americans and American Indians and Alaska Natives (AI/ANs) received poorer quality of care than Whites for 40% of quality measures. African Americans received better care than Whites for 11%, and AI/ANs received better quality care for 14% of measures.
- Asians received poorer quality of care than Whites for 21% of measures and better quality of care for 38% of measures.
- Hispanics received poorer quality of care than non-Hispanic Whites for 20 of 38 measures and better quality care for 16% of measures.
- Poor people (defined as those having a family income of less than 100% of the federal poverty level) received a lower quality of care than high-income people (defined as those having a family income of 400% or more of the federal poverty level) for 85% of the measures and better quality for 8% of measures.

Access to Care

- For many measures, minorities and the poor have worse access to care.
- African Americans and AI/ANs have worse access to care than Whites for 50% of measures and better access to care for no measures.
- Asians have worse access to care than Whites for 43% of measures and better access for 14% of measures.
- Hispanics have worse access to care than non-Hispanic Whites for 88% of measures.
- Poor people had worse access to care than high-income people for all measures.

Increasing Disparities

Health care disparities are increasing for many conditions.

Group	Measure
African American compared to White	Children with admission for asthma
	Children with recommended vaccines
	Elderly with pneumococcal vaccine
	Hospital treatment of pneumonia
Asian compared to White	Elderly with pneumococcal vaccine
American Indian/Alaska Native compared to White	Hospital treatment of heart attack
	High-risk nursing home residents with pressure sores
	Home health care patients admitted to hospital
	Dialysis patients on waiting list for transportation

(Continued on following page)

Evidence-Based Practice 9–1: (continued)

Current Status of National Health Care Disparities

Group	Measure
Hispanic compared to Non-Hispanic White	Persons who needed and received substance abuse treatment
	Persons with diabetes with three recommended services
	Persons needing mental health treatment for serious mental illness
	Adults with patient–provider communication problems
	People who need illness or injury care as soon as wanted
	Tuberculosis patients who complete treatment within 12 months
	Children with patient–provider communication problems
	Hospitalized smokers with advice to quit
	Elderly with pneumococcal vaccine
	Children with dental visit
	Patients needing hospital treatment of heart attack
	New AIDS cases
Poor compared to High-Income Patients	Hospitalized smokers with advice to quit
	People needing illness or injury care as soon as wanted
	Persons with diabetes with three recommended services
	Adults with patient–provider communication problems
	Children with all recommended vaccines

Clinical Application

Nurses should be aware of these issues and advocate for health care quality and access for all populations.

Source: AHRQ. (2005). *2005 National Healthcare Disparities Report.* Rockville, MD: U.S. Department of Health and Human Services, Agency for Healthcare Research and Quality. Retrieved March 2, 2006, from www.ahrq.gov

ple are not personally involved. Studies suggest that teams in cultures perceived as personal and dynamic have higher ratings of team functioning (Strasser et al.).

Bolman and Deal (1997) describe four organizational culture perspectives or "frames" that affect the way in which an organization resolves conflicts. The **human resource frame** strives to facilitate the fit between person and organization. When conflict arises, the solution considers the needs of the individual or group as well as the needs of the organization. The **political frame** emphasizes power and politics. Problems are viewed as "turf" issues and are resolved by developing networks to increase the power base. The

structural frame focuses on following an organization's rules or protocols. This culture relies on its policies and procedures to resolve conflict. The **symbolic frame** relies on rituals, ceremony, and myths in determining appropriate behaviors.

To understand how these four perspectives will result in different outcomes, consider typical responses to the following situation. Hospital A is located on the border of two communities. One community is primarily African American. The other community is primarily Hispanic. The hospital has traditionally provided care to African Americans and is well regarded by that community. The hospital has noted, however, that few members of the Hispanic community use its services. The hospital's board of directors realizes that to survive, the hospital must expand its patient base. The approach to this challenge will vary based on the organization's culture.

Hospital leaders in a human resource perspective culture are likely to approach the situation by assessing the needs of both communities and the staff. For example, a hospital with a human resource perspective culture may convene focus groups with members of the Hispanic community to identify why that community does not use the hospital's services. At the same time, the hospital will assess the African American community's perspective on the hospital's expanding its services and becoming a more inclusive organization. The hospital will also provide opportunities for staff members to provide input and to express their feelings about the goals of the organization. In the end, the hospital with a human resource perspective culture will reach a decision that balances the needs of all of these groups while enhancing the goal of expanding the patient base.

Hospital leaders in a political perspective culture will take a different approach. They will identify key "power" leaders in the Hispanic community. Perhaps they will invite a Hispanic leader to join their board of directors or serve in another advisory capacity or ask a priest from a Hispanic congregation to serve as a hospital chaplain. In addition, they will actively recruit Hispanic physicians and other clinician leaders. They will build a Hispanic power base within the hospital and use it to reach out to the larger Hispanic community and expand the patient base.

Hospital leaders in a structural perspective culture will develop policies and procedures to attract more Hispanic patients. For example, they may make certain that all signage appears in both English and Spanish or develop a policy that requires all patient educational materials to be available in both Spanish and English. They may require all staff to attend a session on Hispanic culture, and they may strongly encourage or mandate Spanish-language training for key personnel.

Finally, hospital leaders in a symbolic perspective culture will use ceremony to meet their goal.

They will make physical changes to the environment to attract more Hispanics. For example, they may create or alter a chapel, inviting a priest from a Hispanic congregation to say mass. They may display other religious symbols, such as a crucifix or a statue of Our Lady of Guadalupe, or alter their artwork to be more culturally inclusive. They may also include Hispanic stories and rituals in their internal communications. These leaders will draw on symbols and rituals that will make persons of Hispanic culture more comfortable in the hospital environment and that will attract a larger Hispanic patient base.

None of these organizational cultures are inherently good or bad, just different. Each presents both strengths and weaknesses, and more than one culture may exist in an organization. For example, an organization may be guided primarily by both human resource and symbolic perspectives.

Schein (1985) uses a tree analogy to describe organizational culture as having leaves, a trunk, and roots. Leaves represent the artifacts of the institution: what is seen and heard in the institution. Signage, statues and other decorations, pictures, décor, dress code, traffic flow, medical equipment, and visible interactions are all part of the visual "leaves." Audible "leaves" include languages spoken, stories, myths, and other conversations. The trunk represents an organization's values: what is good, what is right, and what is true. The roots represent an organization's assumptions. Assumptions define the culture of the organization, but because they are invisible, they may not be recognized. At times, the assumptions of an institution are ambiguous and self-contradictory, especially when an institutional merger or acquisition has occurred.

The basic premises of an organization, reflected in its mission statement, provide insight into the presence or absence of a commitment to providing culturally competent care. Organizations are well aware of the need to identify a consistent vision and a set of values to guide their organizational culture. As seen in Table 9-1, the values may address behaviors demonstrated both toward clients and colleagues.

TABLE 9-1 *Vision and Values*

We will...

Vision ...be *the* premier health care provider where patients choose to come for services, physicians choose to practice, and employees choose to work.

Values

We will...	**Together, we will...**
Commitments to our Customers:	Commitments to Each Other:
Welcome you	**Work as a team**
We will welcome you immediately, introduce ourselves, and call you by name.	We will support each other's individuality and value differing experiences, skills, and ideas.
We will tell you our role and what we'll do for you.	We will treat each other kindly.
We will offer you a personal escort to your destination.	We will warmly welcome new employees to Edward Hosptial and Health Services.
	We will help each other succeed.
Care for you	**Communicate openly**
We will be caring and treat you as an individual.	We will compliment and recognize each other.
We will coordinate your services among our coworkers.	We will approach our work in an honest and professional manner.
We will ensure your privacy and confidentiality.	We will keep our sense of humor.
Promote safety	**Promote a safe environment**
We will ask you to speak up with questions and concerns.	We will speak up about errors and potential safety concerns.
We will listen and work with you to find the answers.	We will work together to resolve safety concerns and prevent future errors.
We will explain your plan of care.	We will focus on solutions rather than blame.
We will involve you in decisions about your care.	We will use safe practices in our work.
We will provide a clean, safe environment.	**Strive to be the best**
Provide great service	We will ensure quality and timeliness of work.
We will provide on-time service or inform you promptly about any delays.	We will base our decisions on what is best for the customer.
We will do everything reasonably possible to make you comfortable and relieve your pain.	We take pride in our work and celebrate each other's success.
We will answer your calls and requests promptly.	We will use Edward's resources efficiently and protect them against loss, theft, or misuse.
	We will foster an environment of optimal health and well-being.

Courtesy of Edward Hospital & Health Services. (2004), Naperville, IL: Author.

Organizational Culture and Employees

There is a significant relationship between race/ethnicity and beliefs about the quality of workplace relationships and career opportunities. For example, research suggests that African Americans feel less accepted within an organization, perceive they have less job discretion, receive lower performance ratings, are less frequently promoted, and are less satisfied with their careers

(Greenhaus, Parasuraman, & Wormley, 1990) Health care organization leaders are called upon to implement strategies to make diversity work in health care organizations.

Many organizations are aware of the impact of organizational culture on its employees. When filling positions, recruiters consider the "fit" between the organization and the potential employee, because a good "fit" results in better retention and satisfied employees. Nurses and other health care professionals also learn how to determine whether an organization will match their personal values. For example, a nurse who wants to provide care in a culturally competent manner to lesbians and homosexuals will not be happy in a setting that openly engages in "gay bashing."

Culturally caring organizations are needed for nurses and other staff members, and humans need care to survive, thrive, and grow. Historically, however, organizations have made few attempts to nurture and nourish the human spirit. According to Leininger (1996), organizations need to incorporate universal care constructs, including respect and genuine concern for clients and staff.

An inclusive workplace is characteristic of a caring organization. Such a workplace, however, is not satisfied simply by a diverse workforce. An inclusive workplace reaches out beyond the organization by encouraging members of the workforce to become active in the community and participate in state and federal programs, working with the poor and with diverse cultural groups (Mor Barak, 2000). Rather than espousing the golden rule (treat others as you wish to be treated), an inclusive workplace treats others as they wish to be treated, in what is sometimes called the platinum rule (Carnevale & Stone, 1995). Organizations with inclusive workplaces draw staff members who are committed to cultural competence and who value diversity and mutual respect for differences.

Although the impact of organizational culture on employees has been acknowledged, the impact of organizational culture on the community being served has received less attention. For years, hospitals and other health care organizations have espoused the view that "If we build it, they will come" (i.e., all that is needed is to offer the services). Now, there is a growing recognition that health care services should be structured in ways to appeal to and meet the needs of various members of the community. Health care leaders recognize that cultural competence in organizations is essential if organizations are to survive, grow, satisfy customers, and achieve their goals. Image is critically important for an organization's survival. A variety of factors are needed to move an organization toward cultural competence.

Assessing the Organizational Culture

Organizational culture may be assessed in numerous ways. Two instruments frequently used to measure hospital culture or work group culture are the Organizational Culture Inventory (OCI) (Cooke & Lafferty, 1987) and the Nursing Unit Cultural Assessment Tool (NUCAT-2) (Coeling & Simms, 1993). Dansky, Weech-Maldonado, De Souza, and Dreachslin (2003) describe a 64-item tool that measures the breadth and degree of diversity management practices. The Magnet Hospital Recognition Program for Excellence in Nursing Services also evaluates organizational climate or culture (American Nurses Credentialing Center, 2005) and is used by many organizations as a blueprint for achieving excellence (Schaffner & Ludwig-Beymer, 2003). Evidence-Based Practice 9–2 outlines the original research that resulted in the creation of **magnet designation** and defines the 14 forces of *magnetism*.

Roizner (1996) identifies a checklist for culturally responsive health care services. Health care services are considered for their availability, accessibility, affordability, acceptability, and appropriateness. When the organizational culture is assessed by this model, it is important to consider these "five A's":

- Are the health services that are needed by the community readily available? In a community with rampant illicit drug use, for example, one should expect to find a variety

Evidence-Based Practice 9–2:

Magnet Research and the Forces of Magnetism

The Magnet Recognition Program for Excellence in Nursing Services grew out of a 1982 descriptive study conducted by the American Academy of Nursing's Task Force on Nursing Practice (McClure, Poulin, Sovie, & Wandelt, 1983). The study began by asking fellows from the American Academy of Nursing to identify hospitals that attracted and retained professional nurses who experienced professional and personal satisfaction in their practice. The fellows nominated 165 institutions. These institutions were viewed as "magnets." The task force then began narrowing the list based on specific criteria and the hospitals' willingness and availability to participate in the study.

Data were then collected from staff nurses and nursing directors in 41 hospitals. Nurses identified and described variables that created an environment that attracted and retained well-qualified nurses and promoted quality patient care. Nurses were asked nine questions, which remain valuable for structuring nursing input even today:

1. What makes your hospital a good place to work?
2. Can you describe particular programs that you see leading to professional/personal satisfaction?
3. How is nursing viewed in your hospital, and why?
4. Can you describe nurse involvement in various ongoing programs/projects whose goals are quality of patient care?
5. Can you identify activities and programs calculated to enhance, both directly and indirectly, recruitment and retention of professional nurses in your hospital?
6. Could you tell us about nurse–physician relationships in your hospital?
7. Describe staff nurse–supervisor relationships in your hospital.
8. Are some areas in your hospital more successful than others in recruitment and retention? Why?
9. What single piece of advice would you give to a director of nursing who wishes to do something about high RN vacancy and turnover rates in his or her hospital?

Staff nurses identified a variety of conditions that made a hospital a good place for nurses to work, specifically related to administration, professional practice, and professional development. Clustered together, these conditions from this descriptive study revealed a clear culture of nursing.

Based on findings from the original magnet study, the Magnet Recognition Program was developed in 1990. The program was created to advance three goals:

- Promote quality in a milieu that supports professional practice
- Identify excellence in the delivery of nursing services to patients/residents
- Provide a mechanism for the dissemination of "best practices" in nursing services

The 14 forces of magnetism (American Nurses Credentialing Center, 2005), derived from the 1982 study, are used to assess organizational culture. The forces are presented in Box 9–5.

Clinical Application

As they rotate to different facilities for their clinical experiences, nursing students are in an ideal position to evaluate organizational climate. Nurses and nursing students are encouraged to use the magnet framework, presented in Box 9–5, to assess nursing subcultures and determine organizational fit.

of types of drug abuse prevention and treatment programs offered that are readily available to the local population.

- Are health care resources accessible? A pediatrician's office, for example, might need to expand its hours of operation to accommodate the schedules of working parents. Geographic location should be considered in terms of proximity to public transportation, traffic patterns, and available parking. Structural changes may also be needed to accommodate specific types of clients, such as those who use wheelchairs.

- Are the services affordable? Partnerships between public and private organizations may be needed to ensure that services are affordable. A sliding scale might be developed to accommodate the needs of people with diverse financial resources.

- Are the services acceptable? Providers need to carefully consider this question: Do community members who use the services perceive the services to be of high quality? Do community members value the services? Are the waiting rooms stark, dimly lit, or untidy? Is the furniture worn or the reading material frayed and outdated? Providers need to understand what makes services acceptable to the community they seek to serve. Community members may avoid a particular agency or institution because services are delivered in an uncaring and patronizing fashion.

- Are the services appropriate? Community members may not use services if they do not perceive that these services meet their needs. For example, community members who struggle with day-to-day survival with limited financial and social resources may not use fitness classes. Programs that are disconnected from the daily life of community members constitute a recipe for failure.

Andrews (1998) provides an assessment tool for cultural change that examines demographic/descriptive data; strengths; community resources; continued growth; perspectives of patients, families, and visitors; institutional perspective; and readiness for change. This tool allows organizational leaders to assess the needs of the community they serve and to use their findings to guide strategic planning for the future.

Leininger's (1991) Theory of Culture Care Diversity and Universality is also helpful in assessing the culture of an institution. **Leininger's Culture Care Model** may be used to conduct a cultural assessment of the organization, with dominant segments of the Sunrise Model identified. An example of such an assessment is provided in Table 9–2. Other cultural care assessment tools are available to assess the culture of an institution. This assessment is then compared with the values and beliefs of the groups who use the health care organization.

The 14 forces of magnetism may also be helpful in assessing the culture of an organization. Several questions to assess each force are listed in Box 9–5.

Barriers to Creating Culturally Competent Health Care Organizations

Standards for providing culturally and linguistically appropriate health care services have been clearly articulated. Regulatory bodies, such as JCAHO, and certification groups, such as the prestigious Magnet Award, require adherence to several mandates related to culturally competent health care organizations. Regardless, a variety of barriers exist.

Prejudice, racism, stereotyping, and ethnocentrism are present in all health care settings. The dominant subgroup is often ignorant of its own privilege. For example, services may be organized for the convenience of providers, and providers may be completely oblivious to the fact that inconvenient hours or locations are affecting the community members who seek services.

The identity of a group or organization is based on phenotype, culture, or any other characteristic that a group shares that sets it apart from others. The professional values espoused by nurses, for example, set us apart from other health care providers. Numerous boundaries

TABLE 9-2 *Example of Leininger's (1991) Culture Care Model Used to Conduct an Organizational Assessment in a Hypothetical Hospital*

Factor	Types of Questions	Assessment Findings
Environmental context	What is the general environment of the community that surrounds the organization? Socioeconomic status? Race/ethnicity? Emphasis on health? Living arrangements? Access to social services? Employment? Proximity to other health facilities?	Hospital A is in a low-income urban setting. The majority of residents in the area are Black, with a few Asians and Whites. A public housing complex is located within a few blocks of the hospital. The economy is depressed, and many are out of jobs. Drug abuse and alcoholism are rampant. Families are challenged to survive, and they tend to view disease prevention as unimportant. There is a short-term perspective on health, which is defined as being able to do normal activities. Several social agencies nearby provide assistance with food pantries. There are no other hospitals within a 5-mile radius.
Language and ethnohistory	What languages are spoken within the institution? By employees? By patients? How formal or informal are the lines of communication? How hierarchical? What communication strategies are used within the institution? Written? Poster? Electronic? Oral? "Grapevine"? How did the institution come to be? What was the original mission? How has it changed over the years?	Patients primarily speak English. Employees typically speak English, although Polish and Russian are heard, particularly among the housekeepers. The grapevine is alive and well at Hospital A. Although memos are circulated, verbal communication is prized throughout the institution. The president/chief executive officer, chief nurse executive, and chief medical offi cer all maintain an open-door policy in their offices. Posters are also used to communicate, especially in the elevators. Electronic communication via e-mail has not been successful because computer workstations are in short supply throughout the institution. Hospital A was founded by a Roman Catholic religious order of nuns in 1885. The original mission was to provide care to immigrants and the poor. Immigrants from many nations, including Ireland, Poland, Hungary, and Russia, originally inhabited the area. The mission is still to provide the highest quality of care to the poor and underserved, although that is becoming increasingly difficult financially.
Technology	How is technology used in the institution? Who uses it? Is patient documentation electronic? Is electronic order entry in place? Is cutting-edge technology in place in the emergency department, critical care units, labor and delivery, radiology, surgical suites, and	There are a few computer work-stations on each nursing unit, which are primarily used by the clinical secretaries. Nurses do not document electronically, and physicians do not use electronic order entry. Hospital A received external funding several years ago to renovate their old emergency department (ED). The new ED has state-of-the art equipment, as do the critical care units. The labor and delivery area is cramped and overcrowded. Equipment is well worn. Similarly,

(Continued on following page)

TABLE 9-2 *Example of Leininger's (1991) Culture Care Model Used to Conduct an Organizational Assessment in a Hypothetical Hospital* (continued)

Factor	Types of Questions	Assessment Findings
	similar units? Is electronic mail used? Is Web-based technology embraced?	the surgical suites are dated. The radiology department is scheduled for a major capital investment next year.
Religious/ philosophical	Does the institution have a religious affiliation? Are religious symbols displayed within the facility? By patients? By staff? Is the institution private or public? For-profit or not-for-profit?	Founded by a religious order, Hospital A is very clearly viewed as Roman Catholic. Outside, the hospital is marked with a large cross on its roof. Inside, a crucifix hangs in each patient room. A large chapel is used for daily mass. A chaplain distributes communion to patients and staff every evening. Nurses demonstrate a variety of religious symbols. One nurse is seen wearing a cross; another wears a Star of David. Patients adhere to a variety of faith traditions, including Southern Baptist and Black Muslim. Chaplains come from a variety of faith traditions and attempt to meet the needs of diverse groups.
Kinship and social factors	What are the working relationships within nursing? Between nursing and ancillary services? Between nursing and medicine? How closely are staff members aligned? Is the environment emotionally "warm" and close or "cold" and distant? How do employees relate to one another? Do they celebrate together? Turn to one another for support? Do employees get together outside of work?	RNs at Hospital A tend to be White and are often the children of immigrants. They are most often educated in associate degree or diploma programs. LPNs and aides tend to be Black. There is tension between the two groups, especially as the role of the aide has expanded. Nurses tend to be somewhat in awe of physicians. Physicians' attitudes toward nurses range from respect to disrespect. Many physicians are angry about the erosion of their own careers. Units tend to be tight knit, with celebrations of monthly birthdays and recognition provided when staff members "go the extra mile." Nurses rarely socialize with one another outside of work. Staff nurses are middle-aged (mean age 42). Most of them commute from the suburbs to the hospital and are anxious to return home after their shift. On the other hand, many of the aides are from the immediate community, know each other, and socialize outside of work.
Cultural values	Are values explicitly stated? What is valued within the institution? What is viewed as good? What is viewed as right? What is seen as truth?	The institution clearly identifies its mission and strives to fulfill it in economically difficult times. Its stated values are collaboration and diversity. Although diversity training has been provided to managers, tensions still exist between work groups, particularly because the workforce tends to be racially divided.

(Continued on following page)

TABLE 9-2 *Example of Leininger's (1991) Culture Care Model Used to Conduct an Organizational Assessment in a Hypothetical Hospital* (continued)

Factor	Types of Questions	Assessment Findings
Political/legal	How politically charged is the institution? Where does the power rest within the institution? With medicine? With finance? With nursing? Is power shared? What types of legal actions have been taken against the institution? On behalf of the institution?	Historically, Hospital A has been politically naïve. It has gone about its mission without regard to the external environment. Recently, the hospital has begun to lobby for better reimbursement for care provided under Medicaid. Institutional power rests with the strong medical staff and department chairs. Because the hospital is not academic, nurses are less likely to have advanced degrees.
Economic	What is the financial viability of the institution? Who makes the financial decisions? How do the salaries and benefits compare with those of competitors in the immediate environment?	Hospital A has a very low margin: 0.5%, compared with an industry standard of more than 2%. This means that little money is available for capital improvements, which results in less technology and some units being cramped. Community needs are considered, along with all financial decisions. People are valued, and salaries are kept competitive.
Educational	How is education valued within the institution? What type of assistance (financial, scheduling, flexibility) is provided for staff seeking advanced degrees? Does the institution provide education for medicine, nursing, and other professions? Are advanced-practice nurses utilized? What is the educational background of staff nurses? Nurse managers? Nursing leaders? How does this compare with education of other professional groups? With competing organizations?	Nurses tend to be educated at the associate and diploma levels. Although flexible scheduling and limited tuition reimbursement are provided, many nurses do not take advantage of the benefits because of the need to work extra shifts to ensure staffing and competing personal and family priorities. All nurse managers are required to have a BSN, and directors are required to have a master's degree. Nursing students from five different programs rotate through the institution. In addition, Hospital A has developed a relationship with one school of nursing and provides a summer preceptor program to those students. Faculty members are also employed during summers and holidays.
		Medical education is also provided at Hospital A: 150 residents and many third-year and fourth-year medical students rotate through the facility. The residents, while learning, also provide important service to the community, particularly through their clinic rotations.

exist in the health care professions; they may be based on gender, ethnic differences, class and hierarchy, licensure and certification, history, and tradition (Dreachslin, 1999).

Institutional racism may also exist in health care. The *MacPherson Report* (2001) defines **insti-**tutional racism as "the collective failure of an organization to provide an appropriate and professional service to people because of their colour, culture or ethnic origin." In contrast with individual behaviors, institutional racism occurs when systematic policies and practices disadvan-

BOX 9-5

Using the forces of magnetism to assess organizational culture

Quality of nursing leadership

- What are the mission, vision, values, and philosophy for the organization? For nursing?
- How does the chief nursing officer (CNO) advocate for nurses? For patient care?
- How are nurses involved in the budget process?
- How satisfied are nurses? What actions are taken to increase satisfaction?

Organizational structure

- How influential is the CNO within the organization?
- How does decision making involve all nurses?
- How has the organizational structure been modified to accommodate internal or external forces?

Management style

- How is feedback obtained from direct care nurses? How is the feedback used in decision making?
- How is communication fostered horizontally and vertically?
- How do direct care nurses initiate changes to improve patient care, nursing practice, and the work environment?

Personnel policies and program

- What workplace policies and procedures safeguard employee rights and promote a safe and healthy work environment?
- How does the organization foster a climate where care is delivered in a manner that is sensitive to diversity?
- How does the organization address workforce diversity?
- How are data used to formulate staffing plans and acquire necessary resources?

Professional models of care

- How does the model of care address patient needs, patient population demographics, number of nursing staff members, and ratio of nurses serving in various roles and levels?
- How do direct care nurses implement the model of care and meet the needs of specific patient populations?
- What nursing theorists underpin the professional model of care?

Quality of care

- How are nurses involved in assessing and improving the quality of care they deliver?
- What programs, services, and initiatives have been developed and implemented to meet the cultural, ethical, and demographic needs of diverse patient populations?
- How are nurses involved in using research to change clinical practice and conducting research studies?

Quality improvement

- How do all stakeholders receive quality data?
- What changes in practice have resulted from analysis of financial and human resource data, clinical outcomes, and satisfaction survey scores?
- How are nurses involved in evidence-based quality initiatives to improve coordination and delivery of care across the continuum of services?

Consultation and resources

- What internal and external resources are available to nurses at all levels to support professional nursing practice?
- How are nurses involved in health care and community organizations?

Autonomy

- How do nurses function autonomously and in accordance with national professional nursing standards?
- How do direct care nurses use professional standards, literature, and research findings to support their nursing practice, independent decision making, and assertiveness/leadership in patient care management and practice?
- How do direct care nurses exercise independent judgment to resolve patient care issues?

Community and hospital

- What partnerships and programs have been established by nursing with community-based entities to meet the health care needs of the populations served?
- How are nurses engaged in community volunteer activities?
- What programs and outcomes have resulted from nursing collaboration and partnerships with other nursing entities in the community or region?

(Continued on following page)

BOX 9-5 (continued)

Using the forces of magnetism to assess organizational culture

Nurses as teachers

- How are the educational needs of nurses assessed, planned for, organized, implemented, and evaluated?
- What types of mentoring activities exist within the organization for nurses at all levels?
- What process is used to assess, plan for, organize, implement, and evaluate the educational needs of patient populations, reflecting concern for cultural differences and languages?

Image of nursing

- How does the CNO influence organizational decision making and strategic planning?
- How does the organization recognize the contribution of nurses toward the accomplishment of strategic priorities?
- How does the community perceive the organization, the nurses, and the care provided within the organization?

Interdisciplinary relationships

- How are nurses at all levels involved in interdisciplinary activities?
- What types of interdisciplinary collaboration occur within the organization and across multiple settings?
- How is interdisciplinary conflict managed within the organization?

Professional development

- What types of professional development programs exist?
- How is the development of cultural competence in the professional health care staff promoted and supported?
- What education is provided on ethics, nursing research, evidence-based practice, patient rights, and leadership development?

Adapted from: American Nurses Credentialing Center. (2005). *Magnet Recognition Program. Recognizing excellence in nursing service* [Application Manual]. Silver Springs, MD: Author.

tage certain racial or ethnic groups. Institutions may be overtly racist, as when they specifically exclude certain groups from service. More often, institutions are unintentionally racist. For example, a dress code that requires everyone to wear the same hat would institutionally discriminate against Sikh men, who are expected to wear turbans, and Muslim women, who wear the hijab or veil. Institutions don't necessarily adopt such policies with the intention of discriminating and often revise their practice once the discrimination is pointed out to them.

This is an international concern. In Australia, for example, a government report in the 1990s identified that the exclusionary culture of the health care system was a major impediment to equity and access for people of non-English speaking background. Health care providers tend to use their own cultural frameworks as the normative reference point and may view people of

culturally and linguistically diverse backgrounds as a problem. Blackford (2003) found that a hospital in Melbourne, Australia, was designed to deliver care to an Anglo-Saxon population rather than meeting the needs of the surrounding multicultural population. Blackford suggests that the interactions that occur between health professionals and non-English speaking patients may result in systems of exclusions and repressions. For example, Blackford found that families were defined from an Anglo-Saxon perspective. This resulted in a physical environment that could not accommodate large family groups, policies that limited visitors to two at any time, and parental expectations that were culturally incongruent with non–Anglo-Saxon cultures.

In some cases, organizations may fail to correctly collect race and ethnicity data. Research conducted in California (Gomez, Le, West, Santariano, & O'Connor, 2003) suggests that while

85% reported consistently collecting data on race, 55% reported never collecting ethnicity data. Approximately half of the hospitals obtained data on race by observing a patient's physical appearance. In addition, only 12% of the hospitals reported having a procedure for recording the race and/or ethnicity of a patient with mixed ancestry. Similar results have been reported elsewhere. According to a report from the Commonwealth Fund and the American Hospital Association's Health and Research Educational Trust (2004), fewer than 80% of hospitals collect data on race and ethnicity. Most often, data are collected because of a law or regulatory requirement. However, the information that is collected may not always be accurate or valid. Frequently, the admitting clerk collects the data by asking questions of the patient and/or by observing patients. The report recommends that hospitals standardize procedures defining who provides the information, when it is collected, which racial and ethnic categories should be used, and how the data are stored.

The Institute of Medicine (2002) reports that 51% of providers believe that patients do not adhere to treatment because of culture or language. At the same time, nurses and other health care workers report having received no language or cultural competency training (Baldonado et al, 1998; Park et al., 2005). Many medical residents feel unprepared to treat patients who have religious beliefs that may affect treatment (20%), have limited English proficiency (22%), are new immigrants (25%), use complementary medicine (26%), or distrust the U.S. health system (28%) (Weissman et al., 2005). Similarly, while both nurses and baccalaureate nursing students perceive an overwhelming need for transcultural nursing, only 61% report confidence in their ability to provide care to culturally diverse patients (Baldonado et al., 1998). Providing care to non–English-speaking patients is especially problematic.

Large health care organizations may have resources to secure trained professional interpreters and bilingual providers. Regardless of setting, however, Youdelman and Perkins (2005)

suggest the following eight-step process for developing appropriate language services:

1. Designate responsibility
2. Conduct an analysis of language needs
3. Identify resources in the community
4. Determine what language services will be provided
5. Determine how to respond to LEP (limited English proficiency) patients
6. Train staff
7. Notify LEP patients of available language services
8. Update activities after periodic review

The Physical Environment of Care

Organizational leaders must assess the physical environment of care to determine barriers and potentially negative messages. A flowchart is a helpful tool for determining such barriers. For example, in an effort to provide comprehensive women's health programs in a caring fashion, organizational leaders may examine the steps for admission to a particular hospital for the delivery of a baby. To determine this, staff members may walk through this care process at their site and then create a flowchart that outlines the steps. Staff members may be particularly alert for possible sources of confusion for parents at this highly stressful time. The flowchart can then be used to design changes in the environment that can be implemented to decrease barriers and improve services.

The physical environment should also be assessed. Approaching this assessment as a potential client is helpful, and a variety of factors should be considered. What message does organization send through its physical surroundings? How is the facility organized physically? How does the entryway present the culture of the organization to the public? Is the entrance warm and inviting? Is the signage prominent? What languages are presented on signs? Is the patient at a loss for where to go to give or receive information? Are amenities available to patients and their family members? Are the doors open or closed? Do people talk with one another, and what language(s) are spoken? What is the traffic pattern, and what is the general flow of traffic? Does the environment appear calm or turbulent? Are the staff members attentive and courteous?

A physical environment may send unintentional messages. Several years ago, I visited a birthing unit in a city hospital. The hospital's service area was undergoing tremendous changes, with a large influx from the African American, Hispanic, Indian, and Polish American communities. The birthing unit was beautifully and tastefully decorated with oak furniture and pastel prints. Every picture on the walls, however, showed a Caucasian family. This clearly sent a message of exclusivity rather inclusiveness. When I brought this to the attention of the nurse manager, she was completely dumbfounded and quickly took steps to rectify the situation. Ethnocentrism and stereotyping were in play here, but it took an outsider to recognize this and bring it to recognition and resolution.

Community Context

Understanding what culturally competent health care means from the standpoint of patients is an important first step in building culturally competent organizations. Researchers (Napoles-Springer, Santoyo, Houston, Perez-Stable, & Stewart, 2005) conducted 19 community focus groups to determine the meaning of culture and what cultural factors influenced the quality of their medical visits. Culture was defined in terms of value systems, customs, self-identified ethnicity, and nationality. African Americans, Latinos, and non-Latino Whites all agreed that the quality of health care encounter was influenced by clinicians' sensitivity to complementary/alternative medicine, health insurance discrimination, social class discrimination, ethnic concordance between patient and provider, and age-based discrimination. Ethnicity-based discrimination was identified as a factor for Latinos and African Americans. Latinos also described language issues and immigration status factors. Overall,

participants indicated greater satisfaction with clinicians who demonstrated cultural flexibility, defined as the ability to elicit, adapt, and respond to patients' cultural characteristics.

Health care institutions exist to provide care. A variety of factors, summarized in Box 9-6, contribute to mortality in the United States and Canada. Confronting these factors will require individual behavioral change, community change, social change, and economic change. Health care organizations cannot confront these complex factors in isolation but must partner with their communities to build trust in their institutions and meet the needs of their local communities.

Community partnerships may be configured in a variety of ways. Hospitals and health care systems usually articulate their desire to improve the health of the communities they serve. Historically, hospitals have fulfilled this mission through charity care, health care provider education, research in health care, community education programming, and community outreach (Pelfrey & Theisen, 1993). Recognition is growing that true improvements in the health of a community require the focused efforts of the entire community. Such improvement may occur only in partnerships with community members and other community organizations.

An ethnographic study of community (Davis, 1997) revealed five themes related to the experi-

---

BOX 9-6

Major Contributors to Mortality in the United States and Canada

Tobacco use
Poor diet and physical inactivity
Microbial agents
Toxins
Firearms
Sexual behaviors
Motor vehicle accidents
Illicit drug use
Poverty
Lack of access to medical care

ence of community caring. Of particular significance to this chapter are three themes: (1) reciprocal relationships and teams working together are central to building healthy communities; (2) education with a focus on prevention is key to enhancing health; and (3) understanding community needs is a primary catalyst for health care reform and change. The healthy communities program, with partnerships between communities and hospitals, is one example of this trend in health care. In a healthy communities program, health care professionals collaborate with surrounding communities to conduct community health assessments. In community mapping,

staff collect a variety of data, including demographics, health status, community resources, barriers, and enablers. Both strengths and needs are identified from the perspective of the community. All these data are then used collaboratively with communities to set priorities (an example of such a community assessment is provided in Box 9–7). Data from these assessments are used to set priorities and guide the planning and implementation of key initiatives. These initiatives are most well accepted when they are sponsored by a variety of community organizations rather than by a single health care organization such as a hospital.

BOX 9-7

Community Assessment Example

By using the assessment of the communities served by Advocate Lutheran General Hospital, one of Advocate Health Care's hospitals, and by analyzing data from clinical practice, staff members realized that Hispanics made up an increasing proportion of the population and were the most frequently underserved population. As a result, a family practice physician initiated the idea for a community center for health and empowerment. A coalition composed of individuals from social services, health care agencies, schools, police, churches, businesses, city government, and other community services also identified the Hispanic community as underserved. This group provided an etic, or outsider, view of the Hispanic community.

To provide a local, or emic (insider), view, community members worked with health care personnel to design and conduct a door-to-door community assessment. As described elsewhere (Ludwig-Beymer, Blankemeier, Casas-Byots, & Suarez-Balcazar, 1996), Leininger's Theory of Culture Diversity and Universality served to guide the assessment. The assessment process involved 2 focus groups, 15 community interviewers, and 220 door-to-door interviews. In addition, 5 meetings, attended by 180 community members, were held to report the findings to community members and solicit their input into the causes and retention of strengths or resolution of needs. As a result, numerous task forces were formed to preserve strengths or mediate needs.

Major strengths were identified as access to friends and families to socialize and get support, prenatal and postnatal care, and pediatric care. Major needs were identified as affordable housing, programs to help immigrants, Spanish-speaking dentists, and activities for youth.

The community was involved in key decision making from the beginning, including selecting the site for the center, choosing the name for the center, and establishing a sliding scale for fees. The bilingual center provides primary health care services, a Women, Infants, and Children (WIC) program run by the county health department, and a community empowerment program. A salaried community outreach worker coordinates the community empowerment program. In collaboration with businesses, churches, and city services, community members have undergone training in group work and priority settings. Recently, monthly dental services through a dental van were added at the center.

Activities for youth were identified as concerns in the community assessment. As a result, community members and center personnel have actively partnered with the park district, schools, churches, and the police to provide recreational activities for youth. The community also uses this as an opportunity to celebrate its cultural heritage. Health promotion materials and activities are also provided through collaboration.

Focus groups may assist an organization in assessing how well they are meeting the needs of the populations they serve. For example, the Boston Pain Education Program worked collaboratively with community representatives to develop a culturally sensitive, linguistically appropriate cancer pain education booklet in 11 languages and for 11 ethnic groups. Focus groups were used to develop materials that would empower patients and families to more effectively partner with health care professionals and manage pain in culturally competent ways (Lasch et al., 2000). To ensure valid focus group results, the organization must understand racial identity development theory, models of communication style differences, cultural archetypes, and ethnic markers (Dreachslin, 1998).

Conducting community assessments requires cultural awareness and sensitivity. Interpreting the data requires knowledge of the cultural dimensions of health and illness. Using the data to develop and implement programs in conjunction with the community requires the ability to plan and implement culturally competent care. The skill of a transcultural nurse or other culturally competent health care professional is invaluable in these situations.

Developing Culturally Competent Initiatives

Once the basics, as previously outlined, are in place, it is possible to develop culturally competent initiatives. Many important factors must be considered in planning programs across cultural groups. Before a program is planned, a cultural assessment of the target population should be a routine component of the needs assessment process (Huff & Kline, 1999). In many cases, cultural competence must be demonstrated with multiple cultures simultaneously. For example, one hospital in the Chicago area provides care for individuals who speak 64 different languages. This calls for much effort and creativity on the part of patients, health care providers, and interpreters. Culturally competent initiatives must

reach out to multiple cultural groups. The case study that follows describes the development and implementation of a culturally competent initiative.

CASE STUDY 9-1

Caring Hospital is a not-for-profit hospital that serves clients who differ in multiple ways, including socioeconomic status, education, race, ethnicity, religion, language, and culture. Organizational leaders embrace Leininger's Theory of Culture Care Diversity and Universality. In particular, nursing leaders believe that nursing care must be congruent with the client's culture if nursing intends to promote the client's health and satisfaction.

Through its Healthy Community Program, the hospital remains grounded in the reality of its clients. The Healthy Community Program, developed and staffed by two nurses with community health backgrounds, is responsible for broadly defining community-based health promotion initiatives that address individual, social, and community factors. Their goal is to establish partnerships with community members and governmental and community organizations to ensure that everyone has access to the basics needed for health; that the physical environment supports healthy living; and that communities control, define, and direct action for health.

The nurses in the Healthy Community Program bring together resources from settings both within and outside their hospital. For example, they work closely with other community-focused staff members, such as home care and parish nurses. They also work with multiple external organizations, such as local health departments, government, religious institutions, community businesses, schools, and other health care entities. These nurses work specifically with the communities surrounding their facility. In this way, they acknowledge the specific needs of diverse groups.

The Healthy Community Program nurses use Leininger's Culture Care Diversity and Universality model in their practice. They use data gathered from cultural assessments to assist them in understanding the communities they serve. They consider environmental context, ethnohistory, language, kinship, culture values and lifeways, the political and legal system, and technologic, economic, religious, philosophic, and educational factors. They understand the interactions among the folk system, nursing care, and the professional systems. They also understand the importance of using the three culture care modalities: preservation/maintenance, accommodation/negotiation, and repatterning/restructuring.

Because of their community health backgrounds, the nurses are knowledgeable about disparities in health. The nurses use data from a variety of sources, including hospital-specific data, census tract data, and health department data, to help them understand health and access disparities in their area. They also talk to community members and to health care providers to identify competing priorities. Using these processes, they discover that their communities have not achieved the Healthy People 2010 goal of 90% full immunization for children by the age of 2 years (U.S. Department of Health and Human Services, 2000).

To address the lack of immunizations, the nurses acknowledge that the issues that affect immunizations are multifaceted. The immunization schedule changes frequently and is quite complex. Even health care providers have difficulty interpreting it. Communication with parents has been sketchy and has been complicated by controversy. Parent may not view immunizations as essential until they are mandated for entry into elementary school. Immunizations may not be easily accessible, available, and affordable. Parents may make decisions based on misinformation, rumor, or hearsay. The nurses know, however, that community members want to keep their children healthy and that immunizations have contributed greatly to reduced illness in individuals and better overall health for the community. They also know that community members prefer to have their children immunized in a consistent place as part of an overall "medical home."

Because the childhood immunization levels are suboptimal in the communities served by the hospital, childhood immunization is selected as a quality initiative. A group of clinicians is convened to implement a program with the goal of increasing immunization to the Healthy People 2010 goal of 90%. There is much discussion on the best way for increasing immunization rates by using a broad-based program. Both telephoned and mailed reminders are known to be effective in increasing immunizations in adults and children (Szilagyi et

al., 2000). Because reminders by telephone are substantially more expensive than mailed reminders, the hospital opts to use mailed reminders.

Various materials are developed in both English and Spanish, and incentives are put into place to assist parents. Babies are automatically enrolled in the program when they are born in the hospital. Mailings occur at regular intervals and include a personalized letter indicating what vaccines are due, a vaccine record, vaccine information statements, and a growth and development newsletter. Additionally, incentives are mailed to help keep the parents motivated to use preventive services. Materials are written at a sixth-grade level. All materials are reviewed for cultural congruity, and the illustrations include babies from various ethnic groups.

New materials are developed as needed, based on a continuous assessment of the needs of the parents. For example, reproducing all the materials in all the languages used by patients is too expensive, so a multiple-language brochure is developed in the 11 most common languages. The brochure explains the program and asks that non–English-speaking and non–Spanish-speaking families obtain help in translating the materials. In addition, after families express a major concern about the multiple injections required to keep their babies fully immunized and their babies' resultant distress and crying, a "calming strategies" flyer is developed.

Because financial barriers still exist among parents seeking immunizations for their children, the Healthy Community Program nurses implement several additional strategies. First, they work with physicians and help them enroll in the Vaccines for Children program, making vaccines available at no cost or low cost right in their offices. They also work with the staff in physicians' offices to enhance their role in fostering childhood immunizations. In addition, they work with the health department to provide monthly immunizations on site at the hospital.

This case study focuses on one culturally competent program provided to a community. Additional programs, targeting the needs of other age groups, may also be envisioned. For example, adult immunizations are also an issue for many communities, so a program might be developed that focuses specifically on older adults and their immunization needs. Similarly, programs might be instituted to deal with other health issues of concern to community members. The case study demonstrates the importance of incorporating an understanding of culture in every aspect of an initiative. To design and implement an effective program, the cultural values of patients must be understood and addressed.

The Role of Individual Health Care Providers in Creating Culturally Competent Organizations

All of us play a role in creating culturally competent organizations. Individual health care providers are at the core of helping an institution attain cultural competence. If they listen and attend carefully, health care providers have a valuable window directly into the world of their patients. They can take what they learn and escalate it as needed to improve the cultural responsiveness of their organization. Speaking the language can also be an advantage.

When health care providers fail to take the patient's culture seriously, they misinterpret the patient's value system and, by doing so, elevate their own value systems. This posture is culturally destructive (Dana, 1993) because it minimizes the other person's culture. A better approach is to take time to ask questions about patient preferences and to listen attentively. In the end, this will increase understanding, trust, collaboration, adherence, and satisfaction.

Even when serving a diverse patient base, health care providers can make a difference. At the University of California in San Diego, the assistant nurse manager of an oncology transplant unit created a special program that addresses the spiritual needs of terminally ill patients. She collected a variety of objects to bring comfort to the critically ill. In large wicker baskets, referred to as "love baskets," she places a variety of items, including spiritual texts that reflect individual patients' belief systems (Buddhist teachings, the Koran, Hindu prayers, the Torah, and the Bible translated into many different languages), CDs of ethnic music, religious items, aromatherapy products, and massage lotions. Nurses and family members can quickly use these items to provide a comforting atmosphere for patients. Patients, families, nurses, and physicians have given the baskets a positive evaluation (Gabriel, 2001).

Summary

As with individuals, the quest for organizational cultural competence is a lifetime journey. There is always room for improvement. To be truly effective in improving patient care for all, health care services and social services that take cultural diversity into account must make an organizational commitment to cultural competence. Cultural competence cannot live in one or two nurses; it must be systemic. It must involve all layers of the organization: the policy-making level, the administrative level, the management level, and the provider level. In addition, an organization must have a mutually beneficial relationship with the community it serves to achieve cultural competence. As such, organizations must reach out to community members.

REVIEW QUESTIONS

1. What types of access, health care, and health outcome disparities exist in the United States?
2. How does the culture of an organization affect the quality of care provided?
3. What tools or models are helpful for assessing organizational culture?
4. How does an organization's culture influence or affect its employees?

CRITICAL THINKING ACTIVITIES

1. An excellent way to understand a culturally competent organization is to assess the organizational culture by using the "five A's" described in this chapter. With some of your classmates, compare and contrast the availability, accessibility, affordability, acceptability, and appropriateness of the organization. Discuss what actions could be taken by the organization to increase its cultural competency.

2. Then use a different approach to assess the cultural competency of the same organization. Use Leininger's Theory of Culture Care Diversity and Universality (1991) to assess the culture of the organization. Table 9–2 in this chapter provides an example of how Leininger's Culture Care Model can be used. Compare and contrast the values and beliefs of the organization with the values and beliefs of the groups using the health care organization's services. What areas would be most problematic and why?

3. Many members of ethnic or minority communities lack adequate access to care because they do not have adequate health insurance. Often these individuals use the emergency departments (EDs) of city hospitals for episodic care. Visit a busy ED. What types of patients do you see? Assess the physical environment to determine potential barriers to culturally competent care. Develop a flowchart that outlines the steps a patient takes when he or she seeks care in an emergency room. Identify the changes that would decrease barriers and improve services if they were implemented.

REFERENCES

AHRQ. (2000). *Fact sheet: Addressing racial and ethnic disparities in health care.* Retrieved March 2, 2006, from http://www.ahrq.gov/research/disparit.htm

AHRQ. (2005). *2005 national healthcare disparities report.* Rockville, MD: U.S. Department of Health and Human Services, Agency for Healthcare Research and Quality. Retrieved March 2, 2006, from www.ahrq.gov

American Nurses Association. (2001). *Code of ethics for nurses with interpretive statements.* Washington, DC: Author.

American Nurses Association, Council on Cultural Diversity in Nursing Practice. (1991). *Cultural diversity in nursing practice* [Position statement]. Washington, DC: Author.

American Nurses Credentialing Center. (2005). *Magnet Recognition Program. Recognizing excellence in nursing service* [Application Manual]. Silver Springs, MD: Author.

Andrews, M. M. (1998, October). A model for cultural change. *Nursing Management, 66,* 62–64.

Ayanian, J. Z., Cleary, P. D., Weissman, J. S., & Epstein, A. M. (1999). The effect of patients' preferences on racial differences in access to renal transplantation. *New England Journal of Medicine, 341*(22), 1661–1669.

Ayanian, J. Z., & Epstein, A. M. (2001). Racial disparities in medical care. *New England Journal of Medicine, 344,* 1443–1349.

Baldonado, A., Ludwig-Beymer, P., Barnes, K., Starsiak, D., Nemivant, E. B., & Anonas-Ternate, A. (1998). Transcultural nursing practice described by registered nurses and baccalaureate nursing students. *Journal of Transcultural Nursing, 9*(2), 15–25.

Betancourt, J. R., Green, A. R., Carrillo, J. E., & Park, E. R. (2005). Cultural competence and health care disparities: Key perspectives and trends. *Health Affairs, 24*(2), 499–505.

Blackford, J. (2003). Cultural frameworks of nursing practice: Exposing an exclusionary healthcare culture. *Nursing Inquiry, 10*(4), 236–244.

Bolman, L. G., & Deal, T. E. (1997). *Reframing organizations: Artistry, choice, and leadership* (2nd ed.). San Francisco: Jossey-Bass Publishers.

Carnevale, A. P., & Stone, S. C. (1995). *The American mosaic: An in-depth report on the future of diversity at work.* New York: McGraw-Hill.

CDC. (2004). *The burden of chronic diseases as causes of death, United States.* Retrieved March 2, 2006 from http://www.cdc.gov/nccdphp/burdenbook2004/Section 01/tables.htm

CDC. (2005). *Deaths: Preliminary data for 2003.* Retrieved March 2, 2006 from http://www.cdc.gov/nchs/pressroom/05facts/lifeexpectancy.htm

CDC. (2006). *Chronic disease prevention.* Retrieved March 2, 2006 from http://www.cdc.gov/nccdphp/overview.htm

Clancy, C. M., & Stryer, D. B. (2001). Racial and ethnic disparities and primary care experience. *Health Services Research, 36*(6), 979–986.

Coeling, H. V. E., & Simms, L. M. (1993). Facilitating innovation at the nursing unit level through cultural assessment: How to keep management ideas from falling on deaf ears...Part 1. *Journal of Nursing Administration, 23*(4), 46–53.

Cox, T. (1994). *Cultural diversity in organizations.* San Francisco, CA: Berrett-Koehler Publishers.

Dana, R. H. (1993). *Multicultural assessment perspectives for professional psychology.* Boston: Allyn & Bacon.

Dansky, K. H., Weech-Maldonado, R., De Souza, G., & Dreachslin, J. L. (2003). Organizational strategy and diversity management: Diversity-sensitive orientation as a moderating influence. *Health Care Management Review, 28*(3), 243–253.

Davis, R. N. (1997). Community caring: An ethnographic study within an organizational culture. *Public Health Nursing, 14*(2), 92–100.

Dreachslin, J. L (1996). *Diversity leadership.* Chicago, IL: Health Administration Press.

Dreachslin, J. L. (1998). Conducting effective focus groups in the context of diversity: Theoretical underpinnings and practical implications. *Qualitative Health Research, 8*(6), 813–820.

Dreachslin, J. L. (1999). Diversity leadership. *Journal of Nursing Administration, 29*(6), 3–4, 21.

Einbinder, L. C., & Schulman, K. A. (2000). The effect of race on the referral process for invasive cardiac procedures. *Medical Care Research and Review, 57*(Suppl. 1), 162–180.

Flores, G., Milagros, A., & Tomany-Korman, S. C. (2005). Limited English proficiency, primary language spoken at home, and disparities in children's health and healthcare: How language barriers are measured. *Public Health Reports, 120*(4), 418–430.

Gabriel, B. A. (2001, October). When physicians and patients "speak a different language": The difficult quest for cultural competency. *Association of American Medical Colleges Reporter, 11*(1), 8–9. Retrieved July 8, 2002, from http://www.hssc.gc.ca/fnihbdgspni/fnihb/chp/publications/second_diagnostic_fni.pdf

Gomez, S. L., Le, G. M., West, D. W., Santariano, W. A., & O'Connor, L. (2003). Hospital policy and practice regarding the collection of data on race, ethnicity, and birthplace. *Journal of Public Health, 93*(10), 1685–1688.

Greenhaus, J. H., Parasuraman, S., & Wormley, W. M. (1990). The effects of race on organizational experiences, job performance evaluations and career outcomes. *Academy of Management Journal, 3391,* 64–86.

Greiner, A. C. & Knebel, E. (Eds.), Institute of Medicine. (2003). *Health professionals education: A bridge to quality.* Washington, DC: The National Academies Press.

Harris, M. I. (2001). Racial and ethnic differences in health care access and health outcomes for adults with type 2 diabetes. *Diabetes Care, 24,* 454–459.

Hasnain-Wynia, R., Pierce, D., & Pittman, M. A. (2004, May). *Who, when, and how: The current state of race, ethnicity, and primary language data collection in hospitals.* The Commonwealth Fund and the American Hospital Association's Health Research and Educational Trust. Retrieved March 20, 2006, from www.cmwf.org

Health Canada. (1999). *A second diagnostic on the health of First Nations and Inuit People in Canada.*

Hendrix, K. H., Mayhan, S., Lackland, D. T., & Egan, B. M. (2005). Prevalence, treatment, and control of chest pain syndromes and associated risk factors in hypertensive patients. *American Journal of Hypertension, 18*(8), 1026–1032.

Huff, R. M., & Kline, M. V. (1999). The cultural assessment framework. In *Promoting health in multicultural populations: A handbook for practitioners.* Thousand Oaks, CA: Sage Publications.

Institute of Medicine. (2002). *Unequal treatment: Confronting racial and ethnic disparities in health care.* Washington, DC: National Academies Press.

JCAHO. (2005). *Comprehensive accreditation manual for hospitals: The official handbook.* Oakbrook Terrace, IL: Author.

Jiang, H. J., Andrews, R., Stryer, D., & Friedman, B. (2005). Racial/ethnic disparities in potentially preventable readmissions: The case of diabetes. *American Journal of Public Health, 95*(9), 1561–1567.

Jones, M. E., Bond, M. L., & Cason, C. L. (1998). Where does culture fit in outcomes management? *Journal of Nursing Care Quality, 13*(1), 41–51.

King, T. E., & Brunetta, P. (1999). Racial disparities in rates of surgery for lung cancer. *New England Journal of Medicine, 341*(16), 1231–1233.

Lasch, K. E., Wilkes, G., Montuori, L. M., Chew, P., Leonard, C., & Hilton, S. (2000). Using focus group methods to develop multicultural cancer pain education materials. *Pain Management Nursing, 1*(4), 129–138.

Leininger, M. (1991). *Culture care diversity and universality: A theory of nursing care.* New York: National League for Nursing Press.

Leininger, M. (1996). Founder's focus: Transcultural nursing administration: An imperative worldwide. *Journal of Transcultural Nursing, 8*(1), 28–33.

Ludwig-Beymer, P., Blankemeier, J. R., Casas-Byots, C., & Suarez-Balcazar, Y. (1996). Community assessment in a suburban Hispanic community: A description of methods. *Journal of Transcultural Nursing, 8*(1), 19–27.

MacPherson report. (2001). Retrieved December 29, 2006, from http://news:bbc.co/uk/vote2001

Mallidou, A. A. (2004). The impact of hospital nurse specialty subcultures on nurse and patient outcomes. Unpublished doctoral dissertation. University of Alberta, Canada.

Malone, B. L. (1997). Improving organizational cultural competence. In J. A. Dienemann (Ed.), *Cultural diversity in nursing: Issues, strategies, and outcomes.* Washington, DC: American Academy of Nursing.

McClure, M. L., Poulin, M. A., Sovie, M. D., & Wandelt, M. A. for the American Academy Task Force on Nursing Practice in Hospitals. (1983). *Magnet hospitals: Attraction and retention of professional nurses.* Kansas City, MO: American Nurses Association.

Mor Barak, M. E. (2000). The inclusive workplace: An ecosystems approach to diversity management. *Social Work, 45*(4), 339–353.

Napoles-Springer, A. M., Santoyo, J., Houston, K., Perez-Stable, E. J., & Stewart, A. L. (2005). Patients' perceptions of cultural factors affecting the quality of their medical encounters. *Health Expectations, 8,* 4–17.

Park, E. R., Betancourts, J. R., Kim, M. K., Maina, A.W., Blumenthal, D., & Weissman, J. S. (2005). Mixed messages: Residents' experiences learning cross-cultural care. *Academic Medicine, 80*(9), 874–880.

Pelfrey, S., & Theisen, B. A. (1993). Valuing the community benefits provided by nonprofit hospitals. *Journal of Nursing Administration, 23*(6), 16–21.

Roizner, M. (1996). *A practical guide for the assessment of cultural competence in children's mental health organizations.* Boston: Judge Baker's Children's Center.

Schaffner, J. W., & Ludwig-Beymer, P. (2003). *Rx for the nursing shortage.* Chicago, IL: Health Administration Press.

Schein, E. H. (1985). *Organizational culture and leadership.* San Francisco: Jossey-Bass.

Seago, J. A. (1997). Organizational culture in hospitals: issues in measurement. *Journal of Nursing Measurement, 5*(2), 165–178.

Sheifer, S. E., Escarce, J. J., & Schulman, K. A. (2000). Race and sex differences in the management of coronary artery disease. *American Heart Journal, 139*(5), 848–857.

Strasser, D. C., Smits, S. J., Falconer, J. A., Herrin, J. S., & Bowen, S. E. (2002). The influence of hospital culture on rehabilitation team functioning in VA hospitals. *Journal of Rehabilitation Research and Development, 39*(1), 115–125.

Szilagyi, P. G., Bordley, C., Vann, J. C., Chelminski, A., Kraus, R. M., Margolis, P. A., et al. (2000). Effect of patient reminder/recall interventions on immunization rates. *Journal of American Medical Association, 284*(14), 1820–1827.

U.S. Department of Health and Human Services. (2000). *Healthy people 2010.* Washington, DC: Author.

U.S. Department of Health and Human Services, Office of Minority Health. (2001, March). *National standards for culturally and linguistically appropriate services in health care: Final report.* Washington, DC: Author.

Weech-Maldonado, R., Morales, L. S., Elliott, M., Spritzer, K., Marshall, G., & Hayes, R. D. (2003). Race/ethnicity, language, and patients' assessments of care in Medicaid managed care. *Health Services Research, 38*(3), 789–808.

Weinick, R. M., Zuvekas, S. H., & Cohen, J. W. (2000). Racial and ethnic differences in access to and use of health care services, 1977 to 1996. *Medical Care Research and Review, 57*(Suppl. 1), 36–54.

Weissman, J. S., Betancourt, J. R., Campbell, E. G., Park, E. R., Kim, M., Clarridge, B., et al. (2005). Resident physicians' preparedness to provide cross-cultural care. *Journal of the American Medical Association, 294*(9), 1058–1067.

Youdelman, M., & Perkins, J. (2005). *Providing language services in small health care provider settings: Examples from the field.* Retrieved October 17, 2005, from the Commonwealth Fund Web site: www.cmwf.org

10

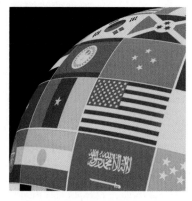

Transcultural Perspectives in Mental Health Nursing

Kathryn Hopkins Kavanagh

The two largest consumer groups of mental health care today are the chronically, seriously mentally ill and the aged. Nurses are increasingly involved in rehabilitative training, resocialization programs, partial hospitalization centers, and support groups in addition to one-to-one relationships. Hospital admissions have become increasingly brief despite increased acuity and the management problems that it presents. Most clients with diagnoses of chronic schizophrenia and other major psychiatric illnesses can receive maintenance care psychotropic drugs in community and ambulatory settings. Psychiatric/mental health nurses function as liaisons among clients, health care facilities, and families. As such, they can facilitate effective integration of multiple belief systems, or they can impose preset expectations that lead to interventions oriented toward the practitioner's and health care system's values and goals rather than the client's (Nelson, 2004).

New care management and case management strategies are making significant inroads with both the mentally ill and the aged. Often the two populations overlap as aging becomes a major category of diversity in Western societies. While the field of geropsychiatric nursing will require more and more skilled psychiatric nurses in the future for work with both the elderly and their caregivers, those nurses will be ever more challenged by the cultural diversity also characterizing their aging clients.

Nurses sometimes question how they can learn all the relevant characteristics of the clients they care for (they cannot, and they should not try) and why they should know about group patterns when it is individuals with whom they work. The important task is to ascertain a client's cultural orientation and what it means to him or her (or them, given that many nurses work with families or other groups). It is not a matter of matching clients to their reference groups, but of learning about and understanding the actual relationships involved. It is, for example, more useful and accurate to ask "How is this client Norwegian or Lutheran?" than to ask "How Norwegian or Lutheran is this client?" (see Figure 10-1).

The former question allows comparison of the answer against the expectable patterns (that is, generalizations about Norwegians and Lutherans), whereas the latter question seeks a match between the client and stereotypic standards for his or her reference groups. Always, easy stereotypes should be avoided: "Chinese do this, and Latinos do that" or "old people usually want things this way." Stereotypes simply cannot be depended on to work effectively. Although every group has discernible patterns that help distinguish it from other groups, most individuals also express beliefs or traits that do not match the group norm. What is more, most people cross categories, that is, they identify with an ethnic group, a religious affiliation, an age set, a gender, and multiple other categories. One may also be traditional in one aspect and modern in others. When people are ill, they sometimes become more traditional in their expectations and thinking, but not always. There is also the fact that significant variation exists not only between groups, but within them. Knowledge of the group is valuable inasmuch as it provides a set of realistic expectations. However, only by learning about the individual or family at hand can the clinician understand in what ways the group patterns are meaningful.

Before 1950, psychiatric services in the United States were provided primarily at state hospitals. Today, most patients hospitalized in the United States with a primary psychiatric diagnosis are treated in general hospitals, and many of them occupy beds scattered throughout various areas rather than in designated psychiatric units. Likewise, many of Canada's large tertiary care psychiatric facilities have closed, and psychiatric patients now receive care in alternative institutional and/or community-based settings. This means that many nurses who do not particularly identify with care of the mentally ill are exposed to that population.

Another reason it is important for nurses to be culturally sensitive, knowledgeable, and skillful is that they are instrumental in the export of mental health concepts to other societies. Nurses educated in the United States and Canada work

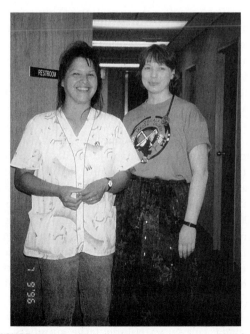

FIGURE 10-1. Traditional peoples bring cultures together in contemporary life in many ways. Ideally, individuals with more than one cultural affiliation can bring parts of each culture together without conflict. Tipis at a Lakota Nation Powwow, Pine Ridge, South Dakota.

throughout the world, as well as with people who come to North America from elsewhere. We must be aware of our potential as communicators of more than we intend.

Given the fact that illness (unlike disease, which is physiologically based) is always socially constructed, there was a time when mental illness did not exist as a separate conceptual category. That statement may sound extreme, but it is not when the difference between disease and illness is understood. People have always had problems, and some were psychotic. But whether tolerated, pitied, shunned, or punished, and whether they lived out their years or died, the "mad" were more likely to be viewed as fools or "possessed" than ill. Eventually, with growing social consciousness, the mentally deranged were given refuge in asylums, where, isolated and in large part gratefully forgotten by society, they received at least a modicum of care and shelter.

Today, persons who are mentally ill are, for the most part, living in the community. The same people, a few generations ago, would have been institutionalized. Community programs tend to emphasize basic, comprehensive, and preventive care (Oakley & Potter, 1997), as well as crisis intervention and care management specific to client needs. At the same time, the aspects of health care systems that relate most closely to mental health tend to suffer from chronic neglect and lack of funding and support, largely because mental health care is not based firmly enough in biology or science to give it a high status in the culture of medicine. Most mentally ill individuals are not psychotic and therefore do not receive diagnoses of psychiatric diseases. Overall, other problems affecting **mental health** are far more numerous in today's society, such as severe stress, violence, anxiety, anger, mood disturbances (for example, depression, suicidal thoughts, or intense and prolonged grieving), confusion (related to aging, drug use, or other issues), and substance abuse. In a culture that tends to be oriented more toward consumerism than social interaction, people often have problems relating to each other, whether it is about sex, food, work, pain, chronic illness, or physical health problems. Spiritual distress also comes under the rubric of mental health.

The interrelatedness of mental health phenomena in everyday life with physical illness means that most mentally distressed and ill people encountered in health care settings, both inpatient and outpatient, are not always labeled "psychiatric" or "mental health" patients. This is particularly true in rural areas, where mental health resources may be scarce. Wherever they occur today, nearly all services that support mental health are short term. Meanwhile, the mentally ill often confront ongoing, severe social and economic strains, while mental health needs and care resources are minimal and in flux (Oakley & Potter, 1997).

The challenge in providing appropriate and adequate psychiatric/mental health care is complicated by **diversity**. Each person learns one or more languages from those around him or her; ethical, religious, or other guidelines for living; and other meaningful and systematic ways of relating to a cultural orientation within society. That culture, in sum, is learned, transmitted, shared, and integrated—both ideal and real, and it is constantly changing (Leininger, 2002c). Traditionally, ethnicity was the basis of such an orientation, but human diversity exists everywhere. There are differences in age, sex, experience, socioeconomic status, social view, gender preference, race, and so on. Increasingly, in these postmodern times, traditional meanings of social categories give way to affinities for and allegiances to groups, meanings, and activities based on personal interest and preference (Kottak, 2000), rather than those passed along through family enculturation. It is important to keep in mind that transcultural nursing is limited to neither health care nor culture in the sense of ethnicity; it involves all human diversity in virtually all imaginable contexts.

The populations of the United States and Canada currently include large numbers of refugees and immigrants. Furthermore, both populations are changing continuously. The "browning of America" alludes to projections that by the middle of the 21st century, the average resident (as defined by U.S. Census Bureau statistics) will trace his or her ancestry to Africa, Asia, the Pacific Islands, or the Hispanic or Arab worlds—or to a blend of widely disparate cultures—rather than to European roots. By 2050, one of every five Americans will be Hispanic (U.S. Census Bureau as cited by the U.S. Department of Health and Human Services, 2001).

Given the complexity generated by such diversity, these nations are moving away from stereotyped "one-size-fits-all" expectations of medical treatment and nursing care. Themes related to diversity in mental health care continue to develop, such as advocacy, participatory decision making, pluralism, multiculturalism, mind/body holism, and increased emphasis on psychosocial issues in health and illness (Siegrist, 2000). Health care providers as well as clients are increasingly committed to recognizing the rights of individuals and affiliate groups (that is, the groups with which people identify or to which they reference themselves) as well as being involved in health care. This means that care is expected to meet the standards of the groups with which people are affiliated. Culturally competent nurses learn the effective use of cultural sensitivity, knowledge, and skills in meaningful cultural encounters and culturally competent care (Andrews, 2003).

This chapter discusses transcultural nursing as it relates specifically to psychiatric/mental health nursing. It presents a practical and flexible framework based on a balance of cultural awareness, sensitivity, knowledge, and skills (Figure 10-2). This model is premised on the value of respectful, open, mutual communication and collaborative relationships between nurses and clients. The medium for both collaborative treatment and **diversity management** is mutual communication. This approach portrays the client as someone more expert about his or her situation than the health care provider is, and from whom the nurse can learn to understand the situation as the client does. The culturally competent transcultural nurse has the ability to manage diversity effectively, when management of diversity is defined as helping each person to

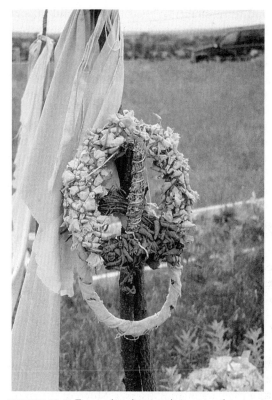

FIGURE 10-2. Transcultural nurses bring together sensitivity, knowledge, and skill to promote health and care for the mentally ill in culturally congruent ways.

reach his or her full potential—however that might be defined by individuals and cultural groups. The key to managing diversity lies in understanding the perspective of the patient and the ways it is grounded in his or her culture.

A balance of cultural awareness, sensitivity, knowledge, and skills in the context of meaningful interaction allows nurses to link receptivity and sensitivity with knowledge of typical, expectable group patterns. Awareness, sensitivity, and knowledge, in combination with cultural assessment, communication, and other mental health nursing skills, can produce respectful, culturally acceptable, and effective nursing interventions for diverse peoples in specific, individual situations.

Cultural sensitivity is never enough. Limiting attention to awareness of issues and differences, and to sensitivity to their meaning and import, leaves the nurse powerless because he or she still lacks the knowledge and skills required to act knowingly on the issue. Knowledge of expectable cultural patterns provides starting places against which the reality of a given situation can be tested. Such knowledge differs from stereotypes, which lock out real evidence through acknowledgment of only that which was expected. Lack of sensitivity, knowledge, and skill may be involved when people are labeled "noncompliant," "problem patients," or too resistant or defensive to benefit from treatment or to recognize the value of the care being offered. It may be that the client's ideas (and his or her expression) about care and caring simply differ from those of the nurse.

Mental Illness and Mental Disease

In many ways, health and illness are more central to transcultural psychiatric/mental health nursing than are mental diseases. Much of the counseling, therapy, and other care given by mental health professionals focuses on illness prevention and improvement of everyday life. The distinction between illness and disease is important. **Illness** emphasizes subjective behavioral, psychological, sociocultural, and experiential dimensions of disorders. **Disease**, by contrast, pertains to chemical, physiologic, and other organic and objective phenomena related to sickness (McElroy & Jezewski, 2000). Biological disorders of memory, perception, and feeling surely exist, as do compensatory processes of rationalization and action that are strongly influenced by social and cultural factors (Kleinman & Seeman, 2000). The rates of mental illness and mental diseases do not seem to vary much among groups when social and economic factors are controlled. There is no conclusive evidence that mental illness and disease rates vary with race or other intrinsic human characteristics, although they are clearly associated with low socioeconomic status, low educational level, separation, and loss.

Psychiatric Resources

Four-fifths of the global population lives in non-Western, partially industrialized countries (Kottak, 2000), whereas most psychiatric resources are in Western and industrialized societies. The schizophrenias, manic-depressive disorders, major depressions, and anxiety disorders are thought to occur throughout the world, although diagnosis is difficult because the expression of symptoms varies so much with cultural differences (Jenkins & Barrett, 2004). Depression anxieties and somatiform disorders (that is, the expressions of problems in physical rather than psychological signs and symptoms) are probably most prevalent in the non-Western world (Janzen, 2002). However, despite international epidemiologic and research efforts, at present there are no international centers focused on mental health treatment programs comparable to, for example, the World Health Organization. The global emphasis has been on physical health (and only some aspects of that [Garrett, 2000]), although somatic disorders are interwoven with culture and with mental distress and illness (Kleinman & Seeman, 2000).

Every society has systems of beliefs and practices related to health care, and specific persons trained as healers. There are many places where biomedicine is not widely available and where most people depend on traditional healers, although they also exist (and are depended on) in modern Westernized societies. Whereas shamans and traditional healers are often not very effective in treating chronic mental disorders, the outcome for some conditions tends to be more positive in societies where clients are not negatively stigmatized and are not alone with their problems. Where persons with mental illness are devalued, they are more likely to be demoralized and isolated, to feel dehumanized, and to curtail the development of potential support systems (Kleinman & Seeman, 2000). The North American values of individualism and self-reliance further reinforce a tendency toward social isolation and alienation. Additionally, many individuals cross cultures, which requires special psychoso-

Diagnosis: Problems with Normality and Abnormality

cial resilience and adaptation (e.g., McEwen, 2005), both in everyday living and in health care.

There is probably more variation among etiologic beliefs of mental health care professionals than is commonly acknowledged, but belief in relatively impersonal, environmental, and natural causation generally prevails. For a variety of reasons or simply by chance, parts, systems, families, or individuals take on characteristics that are assessed as dysfunctional. By contrast, members of many cultural groups believe illness is caused by a supernatural being (a deity or god), a nonhuman being (such as an ancestor, a ghost, or an evil spirit), or another human being (a witch or sorcerer) (Janzen, 2002). The sick person in such a case is viewed as a victim who is not responsible for his or her condition or its resolution.

The division of sickness into physical and mental categories is Western, although every society labels some behaviors as abnormal. The cultural assumption that mind and body are somehow separate, which is now increasingly challenged in terms of relationships between healing and the mind (Dossey, 2004–2005), has for several centuries strongly swayed Western ideas about normality and abnormality. What is considered "normal" and what is "abnormal" is always based on cultural perspective. Culture influences (that is, it shapes but does not determine) expression, presentation, recognition, labeling, explanations for, and distributions of mental illnesses (Evidence-Based Practice 10-1).

Interpretations of health and even of the overt signs of physical disease vary widely. Mental health and mental illnesses are more difficult than physical disorders to delineate because of the lack of readily observable, discrete, and organic phenomena. The symptoms of mental illness, dependent as they are on behavioral expression, vary because they depend on social definitions rather than physical measures.

Assessment is based on the appropriateness of behaviors (for example, dress, posture, odor, gestures, speech, nonverbal communication, facial expression, and physical activity) that lack fixed standards and depend on context and social relationships to differentiate what is considered normal from what is viewed as abnormal. Although psychiatry is part of Western biomedicine, it deals with ambiguous areas of life, such as self and symbolic behavior, deviance and marginality, and power and control (Frank, 2000).

Diagnoses involve social competence, which to be sensitively evaluated must be assessed against culture-specific criteria. Many cultures do not dichotomize normality and abnormality as rigidly as Western societies tend to, or even distinguish health from illness. These may be viewed as multidimensional, continual, and perhaps overlapping, with ideas about mental health and mental illness mixed with those about health and medicine in general (Janzen, 2002). To members of such societies, concepts such as mental health have little meaning. The distinction between illness and health may be based on the ability to perform one's normal roles in society. A health care provider's diagnosis, prognosis, and treatment, based on imprecise and unobservable phenomena, may seem ludicrous.

The pattern used by a client to express concern or disorder is referred to as a **language of distress**. Close examination of how people interact and express themselves is essential in understanding relationships between psychiatric and social factors. The same phenomena (for example, visions and dream states, trance states, hallucinations, delusions, belief in spirits, speaking in "tongues," drug or alcohol intoxication, or suicide) may be judged normal or abnormal according to the settings and circumstances in which they occur (Janzen, 2002). At times, cultural groups encourage altered states of consciousness that others may view as mental disturbances. However, because addictive substances (such as alcohol, tobacco, and opiates) in most societies were traditionally reserved for use during special times or rituals, widespread related health problems seldom occurred. Today, by contrast, the Western redefinition of addiction as disease (rather than as a primarily social, moral, or legal issue) has helped make this a primary mental health concern (Singer, 2006).

How symptoms are expressed and how they are perceived and treated by others vary widely. Although psychotic disorders occur in every society, and the primary symptoms (that is, social

Evidence-Based Practice 10–1:

The Challenge of Living in New Worlds

Although most immigrants and refugees adjust well to new circumstances, many immigrant and refugee groups have relatively high incidences of psychological and psychiatric disorders when compared with the general population. No one disorder predominates, but posttraumatic stress disorder (PTSD) and major depressive disorders, in addition to various organic causes of mental health problems, are the most numerous. Acculturating to a new culture and society is challenging in the best of times; when serious mental diseases or illnesses interfere, or an individual's history includes great loss and worry, the circle of failure to both cope and acculturate may become desperate. This may lead to either development of mental health problems or exacerbation of old problems. Consider, for example, the older person who migrates to a new land, retains traditional cultural values and social norms (which may include beliefs that mental illness is rooted in spiritual or preternatural origins), and struggles to learn even the rudiments of the new language. Increasing interpersonal stress may lead to accusations of witchcraft and even threatened violence.

Clinical Application

The first step is negotiating appropriate acculturation goals. Acculturation occurs through involvement in the new culture—learning some of the language. Television helps many immigrants but cannot do it all. For an older person, learning fluent English is often not a realistic goal. However, many other goals are, such as learning the local currency, shopping in nearby stores, using the telephone to contact friends (perhaps even e-mail in some circumstances), using public transportation to access ethnic groups or associations of age-mates.

Many health professionals avoid traditional and "alternative" healing approaches, but it may also be helpful to encourage consultation with traditional healers (who, of course, also immigrate when other people do) for both the client and the nurse attempting to understand how to help the client. Most traditional healing ways are not harmful and lead to a sense of well-being that modern pharmaceuticals and other curative techniques do not. The healer (shaman, spirit healer, or herbalist, among others) is usually especially helpful in diagnosing ("naming") the problem from the point of view of the culture with which the client identifies, suggesting a resolution or at least respite (often a ritual) that matches the way the problem is understood, makes the support of the family and immigrant community apparent, and brings people together in their concern and care for the individual. In some societies, traditional healing can be expensive and pose an extra burden for the family, as well as blame the family or client for the client's failure to improve in health. On the other hand, the potential for benefit is well worth an open-minded investigation and negotiation.

(Continued on following page)

Evidence-Based Practice 10–1: *continued*

The Challenge of Living in New Worlds

Refer to *Healing by heart: Clinical and ethical case stories of Hmong families and Western providers* (Culhane-Pera, Vawter, Xiong, Babbitt, & Solberg, 2003) for an excellent ethics-focused, ethnography-based set of culture-specific clinical stories of Hmong families and Western providers. In addition, *The spirit catches you and you fall down: A Hmong child, her American doctors, and the collision of two cultures* (Fadiman, 1999) is a rich but heart-wrenching description of a case in which professional biomedicine failed to understand the cultural contingencies inherent in cross-cultural treatment and care.

Other References:

Helsel, D., Mochel, M., & Bauer, R. (2005). Chronic illness and Hmong shamans. *Journal of Transcultural Nursing, 16*(2), 150–154.

Westermeyer, J. (2003). Cultural interpretations of psychosis. In K. A. Culhane-Pera, D. E. Vawter, P. Xiong, B. Babbitt, & M. M. Solberg, (Eds.), *Healing by heart: Clinical and ethical case stories of Hmong families and Western providers* (pp. 241–250). Nashville, TN: Vanderbilt University Press.

and emotional withdrawal, auditory or visual hallucinations, general delusions, flat affect, mood changes, and insomnia) occur across cultures, the secondary features of these disorders are highly influenced by culture (McElroy & Jezewski, 2000). For example, in some groups, guilt and suicidal ideation do not accompany depression; in others they frequently do. For some peoples, suicide is an acceptable escape from problems ranging from marital dissension, illness, sorcery, loneliness, and hopelessness to criticism from others (Armstrong, 2000).

Analogously, among many groups, somatic (physical) rather than psychological symptoms are prominent among depressed individuals; in others, such as middle-class European North Americans, psychological "blues" prevail (Kleinman & Seeman, 2000). **Somatization** pertains to a preoccupation with physical symptoms that are thought to have a psychological rather than a physical cause (Janzen, 2002). Somatic symptoms that express psychological distress occur at high rates, for example, among clients who are Hispanic or Chinese (McElroy & Jezewski, 2000). It is

not unusual for nurses to encounter clients who deny being depressed but describe having headaches, backaches, stomachaches, and other physical phenomena prompted by (and sometimes consciously associated with) sorrow and suffering.

The content of delusions and hallucinations also reflects cultural patterns. For instance, the content may be primarily psychological, religious or spiritual, moral or social, naturalistic or supernatural, or physical or medical. Cultural comparisons of the meanings of psychotic delusions to those who experience them find those meanings highly reflective of the cultural repertoires in which they occur. For instance, some people tend to have religious delusions, while others might focus on persecution or delusions about scientific phenomena. Likewise, some may associate sex with guilt, whereas others do not (Fine, Weis, Weseen, & Wong, 2000). For example, middle-class European American criticism of sex and pregnancy outside of marriage among Blacks does not take into account the social history that made many women of color vulnerable to unwanted sexual activity and that, over time, helped some to redefine extramarital sex and pregnancy as events apart from moral apprehension. Despite considerable research evidence that married persons generally experience more positive mental health than the unmarried, too little research attention has been paid to Blacks to allow generalization to that group (Roche, Neaigus, & Miller, 2005). Both "normal" and "abnormal" are interpretations that often become confounded with moral ideology.

Some conditions, such as posttraumatic stress disorder, can occur in various forms anywhere. Others, known as **culture-bound syndromes**, exist within specific cultural groups. Some conditions may represent labeling differences, as in China, where the term "neurasthenia" is widely used for symptoms produced by social stressors and may correspond to what Western medicine refers to as depression (Janzen, 2002). Conditions fall into categories of folk illnesses that defy Western psychiatric identification, although they are very real to the persons experiencing them (McElroy & Jezewski, 2000). Examples of folk illnesses include fright or soul loss (Bliatout, 2003), which may be associated by Hispanics with a sudden start or sneeze. Various conditions thought to result from the evil eye ("mal ojo") are believed to occur unintentionally when, for instance, a nurse fails to touch a child he or she has noticed or examined. Herbal remedies, rubbing, massage, and other physical manipulations by *curanderos* (*curanderas*, if they are women) are typical treatments. These may be used with home remedies (such as teas) or prayers and trips to religious shrines or charismatic folk healers to alleviate distress.

The United States and Canada have numerous folk illnesses, such as "nervous breakdown," that occur throughout the society. There are also culture-bound syndromes. Anorexia nervosa, for example, occurs only where food is abundant, although even then it takes various forms. Other culture-bound syndromes are seen more often in traditional, nonindustrialized societies and in immigrants from those societies. Despite the exotic nature of many of the classic culture-bound syndromes, it is useful to know of the existence of these conditions. Several culture-bound syndromes are described in Box 10-1.

Misdiagnosis (for example, the overdiagnosis of antisocial disorders and psychoses and underdiagnosis of depressions [Trafzer & Weiner, 2001]) is a major problem among members of groups that differ from those upon which many of the standards for behavior have been based and with which others are compared. It is often assumed that, by default, that standard represents the European North American, middle-class, Christian, and male orientation that dominates North American culture and medicine (Kleinman & Seeman, 2000; McElroy & Jezewski, 2000). The fact is, however, that there is great diversity within groups, as well as between them, and that includes Western males. Consequently, misdiagnosis is always possible, particularly when cultural influences are not adequately taken into consideration. An example of a commonly misdiagnosed folk illness is "falling out," a stress-relieving pattern of shaking and falling that typically occurs when sympathetic others are present; it is seen among Blacks, Haitians, Whites, and other Southern U.S. ethnic groups (Leininger, 2002c). Adding to the complexity of psychiatric diagnosis is that despite the influence of culture in patterned psychological and physical conditions, there are individual or idiosyncratic explanations and expressions of behavior.

Like any other field, psychiatry is not completely homogeneous. Sociocultural and cross-cultural approaches exist that extend the thinking of many psychiatric and mental health care providers to allow for cultural, social, and increasingly more holistic explanations of clients' behavior (National Center for Complementary and Alternative Medicine, 2000). However, at the same time, the widely used series of *Diagnostic and Statistical Manuals of Mental Disorders* (American Psychiatric Association [APA], 1994)—the *DSM–IV* and the subsequent text revised version (APA, 2000), as well as earlier versions (APA, 1980, 1987)—requires the surrender of many cultural insights (Kleinman & Seeman, 2000). Works such as the *DSM–IV* (and now the *DSM–IV–TR*) organize symbolic and instrumental evidence of the forms of deviance that are now

BOX 10-1

Culture-Bound Syndromes and Variants

Amok: an acute reaction resulting from hostility and dissociative amnesia after a period of brooding (American Psychiatric Association, 1994). The term "running amok" comes from the frenzied lashing out associated with this syndrome.

Anorexia nervosa: an eating disorder associated in Western societies and industrialized cultures, but not in societies without a high degree of individualization and in which food is not abundant. It involves fear of obesity (Tseng & Streltzer, 1997).

"Ataque de nervios" is reported among Latinos from the Caribbean, Latin Americans, and Latin Mediterranean groups as attacks of crying, uncontrollable shouting, trembling, and sensations of heat rising to the head from the chest. Associated with stressful events, it also involves dissociative experiences, seizure-like or fainting episodes, and sometimes suicidal gestures (American Psychiatric Association, 1994).

Attention deficit hyperactivity disorder (ADHD), which was virtually unknown in the United States' past before recent decades or is not recognized in many other places in the world, suggests the possibility that ordinary variations in human physiology can be reinterpreted as "disease" as cultural conditions change. While many American children spend hours being inactive in front of televisions or computers, and many schools have curtailed recess, diminished periods of unstructured play, or lack playgrounds, large numbers of children are treated pharmaceutically for being hyperactive or hyperkinetic (Moerman, 2002).

Falling out or blacking out occurs primarily in peoples from the Southern United States and the Caribbean. It is characterized as a sudden collapse that occurs without warning or after a swimming sensation in the head. Typically the eyes remain open, although the afflicted person claims he or she cannot see. Hearing is unimpaired, but a sense of powerlessness prevents movement (American Psychiatric Association, 1994).

Ghost sickness (sometimes called ghost infection) is found among members of many American Indian nations and tribes, such as the Navajo. It is characterized by a preoccupation with death and the belief that a person who has died releases a ghost at death. The symptoms are fainting, loss of consciousness, hallucinations, anxiety and feelings of danger, loss of appetite, bad dreams about evil spirits, and fear of the night (American Psychiatric Association, 1994). The treatment is a traditional ceremony and ghost medicine (Hirschfelder & Molin, 2001).

Magical death is the term given to the phenomenon of a person dying when and because he or she believes the death is going to occur. Such sociocultural death that has been explained as a result of a "flight-or-fight" response, belief in the power of threat and suggestion, and the acceptance of hopelessness. The existence of such occurrences are tributes to the power of belief and persuasion (Ember & Ember, 2003).

Rootwork involves several cultural illnesses associated with hexing, spells, voodoo, witchcraft, sorcery, or the evil influence of another person. The symptoms include generalized anxiety, dizziness, and fear of being harmed (especially poisoned or killed). A "root doctor" releases the victim from the problem. Rootwork is found in the Southern United States among both Black and White populations and in Caribbean societies (American Psychiatric Association, 1994). It is known as *"mal puesto"* or *"brujeria"* in Latino societies.

Susto (also known as fright or soul loss) is a traumatic, anxiety-depressive state with psychophysiologic changes; "fright sickness" results from stimuli such as a fall, a thunderclap, meeting some threat, or other frightening experiences. Susto causes anxiety, insomnia, listlessness, loss of appetite, and social withdrawal. This folk illness occurs throughout Latin America (American Psychiatric Association, 1994). It is believed that the soul (or spirit) leaves the body and cannot return with the help of a healer. Susto is usually interpreted as a type of depression.

Trance dissociation is a set of possession syndromes occurring in various parts of the world with varying degrees of social sanction. This differs from primary schizophrenic reactions and is believed to be caused by disease, the loss of one's soul, or the invasion of a benign or evil spirit. In some circumstances it is viewed as a mystical state (Harvey, 2003). Some American Indian vision quests result in altered states of consciousness similar to this.

considered medical concerns and provide the medical community with administratively useful classifications for diagnosis and record keeping. However, despite varying cultural expressions of psychiatric problems, in less affluent countries than the United States and Canada, where library funds are particularly limited, the *APA Diagnostic and Statistical Manuals of Mental Disorders* standards tend to be used as the ultimate text on psychiatric diagnoses and categories. This seems contradictory to the evidence that although medical involvement in "madness" has been recorded for at least 2,000 years, the aspects of treatment and care that foster transcultural understanding emerge more as humanitarian reform than as biomedical accomplishment.

Socioeconomic Factors Influencing Mental Health

Social and environmental conditions often lead to mental health problems. Children and adolescents are vulnerable to the mental health effects of current social and economic conditions. Parenting styles vary greatly. Some parents, for example, may view "good parenting" as keeping a child safe, fed, and clean, without including activities that stimulate cognitive, affective, and physical development. Substantial numbers of children and adolescents live in poverty, with severe mental health effects (Dodgson & Struthers, 2005). Children and adolescents of every social class and ethnic background are vulnerable to sexual and physical abuse (Freund, McGuire, & Podhurst, 2003). In the United States, children are likely to be exposed at a tender age to adult sexual roles and to violence through the mass media. High rates of depression are associated with problems in areas of family and personal relationships, finances, and general living conditions. Crime, drug use, and suicide are prevalent problems that may be associated with perceived limitations on hope (Trafzer & Weiner, 2001).

Poverty and lack of social support also have implications for mental health. Although disorganized and dysfunctional families are not specific to poor people, the poor often have higher

mortality and morbidity rates (Janzen, 2002) and access to relatively few treatment resources. Lower birth rates mean that elders have fewer adult children and kin as potential caregivers. Increased geographic mobility and separate living styles result in loose social networks and increased social alienation. Parents, particularly those who are single, are more alone with child-rearing responsibilities in industrialized societies than is the case where extended families are more common and socialization responsibilities are shared with other adults. Immigration, globalization, and geographic change can lead to conflict between traditional and modern roles (Helsel & Mochel, 2002) and prompt new health concerns (Culhane-Pera, Vawter, Xiong, Babbitt, & Solberg, 2003; Dundes, 2003). Similarly, increased divorce rates often disrupt the flow of personal support. Today, many members of groups that were traditionally cohesive find themselves isolated from culturally relevant support persons (Tom-Orme, 2002) and are challenged to establish meaningful ties in merged, blended, or widely disparate families or support systems. Rapid increases in the populations of older adults have led to ethnogerontology: the study of relationships between culture and age and their impact on physical and mental well-being as elders' contexts, roles, prestige, and patterns of social interaction change (Culhane-Pera & Xiong, 2003).

Traumatic societal and personal events also affect mental health. Painful separations, torture, loss, sudden death, bereavement, uncertainty, and violence have made posttraumatic stress syndrome a general diagnostic category for persons of any age and any traumatic background (Lyfoung, 2003; Mouanoutoua, 2003). Noninvasive expressive therapies such as storytelling and therapeutic writing are increasingly used for treating posttrauma problems (Draucker & Hessmiller, 2002; Roche, Neaigus & Miller, 2005; Singer, Scott, Wilson, Easton, & Weeks, 2001). Although approaches to self-disclosure vary widely with cultural orientation, the results have been positive among diverse groups. There is also increasing evidence that techniques borrowed from traditional Chinese medicine are useful in circumstances (such as treatment of drug addiction and intractable pain) in which Western biomedicine has not proven adequate to resolve mental health problems (Baer, 2001). Hypnosis is another form of treatment that is sometimes found valuable in treating hard-to-manage psychosomatic conditions, such as obesity (Wickramaseker, 1999), as well as increased emphases on self-reflection (Rew, 2000) and spirituality (Burkhardt & Jacobson, 2000).

Mental Health Beliefs and Practices of Specific Cultural Groups and Subpopulations

In the early part of the 20th century, the goal was to Americanize the many peoples already in the United States, along with those who came from all over the world to make their homes in this country. They were expected to learn English and to become as much a part of the dominant culture as they could, which often meant compromising or even giving up their original cultures (Patterson, 2001). During this time, many minority groups in Canada also experienced similar pressures to assimilate. For example, to promote the incorporation of Indians into mainstream Canadian society, the Indian Act of 1876 defined nearly every aspect of Indian life and placed many restrictions on their activities. Furthermore, until as recently as 1962, Canadian immigration policy favored European immigrants over those from Asia and other developing countries. This favoritism was based on the notion that immigrants from European countries could assimilate with greater ease and speed into mainstream Canadian society (Li, 1999). Times have changed. As the 21st century unfolds, people from diverse ethnic and other backgrounds are expecting, demanding, and considered deserving of opportunities to preserve their various lifestyles, beliefs, and practices. Ethnicity and ethnic identity are viewed as relational and dialogic, multilayered and multifaceted, and dialectic in terms of the historical tension in the United States and Canada between cultural **assimilation** and cultural pluralism (Winkelman, 2001). Some people find the trend toward increased diversity (particularly recognition of ethnic, racial, and gender-oriented groups) threatening. Others view it as an opportunity to help North American society live up to its democratic ideals. In any event, this transition is occurring, and nurses must be prepared to care for this diverse population.

Many differences in mental health care needs are attributable to ethnic variation (Westermeyer, 2003), although it must be remembered that there is significant diversity within each group as well as between groups and that many people cross groups, identifying with and belonging to several. Another important factor is that some peoples are traditional in their views, whereas others are more acculturated and modern. There can be great variation within groups and even within families. Despite the limitations imposed because ethnic categories are not mutually exclusive in a diverse society, it is useful for transcultural nurses to be aware of the generalized patterns associated with those aggregates, who represent increasingly large proportions of the total population—but it must be remembered that the variability within each group is tremendous.

Blacks

It must always be remembered that great diversity exists within groups, as well as between them. For example, in distinguishing African Americans from others who come to the United States from the Caribbean islands, Africa, or other parts of the world, it is obvious that people of color, sometimes collectively called "Blacks," are very diverse. Centuries of discrimination in a predominantly "White" culture has perpetuated a focus on differences and leaves "Blacks" and "Whites" artificially divided and many people of color without access to culturally congruent mental health resources. Various ethnopsychiatric innovations have helped fill the need (Kess-Gardner, 2004). More recent and more respectful mainstream mental health efforts have drawn attention to Black resilience and strengths and away from association of difference with psychopathology (Hartmann, 2002). Contemporary

Blacks often remain enthusiastic about religion and spirituality, are characterized as adaptable and bicultural (that is, able to function in two worlds, one Black and one White, which requires considerable effort and energy), and typically value work and education despite a history of limited opportunity to acquire or use those institutions. Traditionally, strong networks extended beyond households to multiple collateral relationships. Expectations for culturally congruent care among Blacks usually include general concern for one another (the "brothers and sisters") (Kess-Gardner, 2004; Miller, Serner, & Wagner, 2005). In a society in which dark skin rendered people socially invisible for centuries (Kavanagh, 2005), genuine respect and acknowledgment are essential to acceptable care (Evidence-Based Practice 10–2).

Black folk medicine, traditionally not separated into mental and physical components, contains elements of various origins (Baer, 2001). In addition to a strong and adaptive knowledge of the use of herbs, early 19th-century Haitian slaves rebelling against French masters brought with them a form of voodoo (a blend of European Roman Catholicism and African tribal religions with modified aspects of humoural pathology). This spread through the Protestant American South and assimilated practices from 17th- and 18th-century European occultism, probably because of the insistence on using English rather than African languages. Reflecting its multiple origins, Black folk medicine today provides widely varied terms and methods, including, for example, "root" medicine, "rootwork," "mojo," "conjuring," "voodoo," and "hoodoo." There remains a tendency to bring to the health care situation a mixture of somatic, psychological, and spiritual problems (Baer, 2001).

In traditional Black belief systems, diseases may stem from causes that are natural or spiritual in nature (e.g., punishment for sins or violation of sacred beliefs). The causes of disease may be viewed as natural (such as failure to protect the body against inclement weather) or unnatural (for instance, divine punishment for sin) and tend to represent a perspective that holds the world to be a dangerous and hostile place. The individual is traditionally viewed as being vulnerable to outside attack and dependent on outside help (Harvey, 2003). This perspective was reinforced by nearly 3 centuries of slavery and then another century of struggle for full rights.

North American Indians

There are more than 500 different Native American and Alaskan Native tribes and nations, and tremendous diversity among those. Thus, generalizing "the American Indian culture" is no more realistic than stereotyping a culture as "Black." Members of various groups may share aspects of history, language, or culture yet may be notably different from each other in significant ways. It is never safe to stereotype groups or individuals on the basis of presumed similarities.

Also referred to as American Indians, First Nations, Amerindians, or Indigenous Americans, and variously including or excluding Native Hawaiians, some indigenous groups in the United States are recognized by the federal government and others at only the state or local level (Oswalt, 2006). Similarly, in Canada there are many different categories and titles applied to native peoples. For example, aboriginal peoples, North American Indians, and status and nonstatus Indians are terms commonly used in Canada to identify native peoples in both legal and social terms (Li, 1999). It is important to know individual and group preferences for being called Native American or North American Indian; there is no one correct label. Most native peoples with tribal affiliations identify with tribal names (for instance, Cree, Cherokee, Lakota, Mi'kmaq, or Navajo) rather than with the pan-Indian collective terms (Native American, Native Canadian, or North American Indian).

Most indigenous populations in the Americas shared a traditional orientation to being in the present (rather than to doing and to the future, which is more typical of European North Americans), to cooperation rather than competition, to giving rather than keeping, and to respect age rather than youth (Oswalt, 2006; Reyhner & Eder, 2004). Traditionally, the life cycle emphasizes rhythmic, natural phenomena aimed at a

Evidence-Based Practice 10–2:

Race and the History of Race Continue to Influence Relationships Today

Centuries of slavery, discrimination, and the experience and fear of unequal treatment by members of the dominant culture result in a collective psychology that requires special sensitivity, knowledge, and skills. Known as historical hostility, this phenomenon may be expressed as hostility, hopelessness, and a paranoid perception of discrimination in cross-racial encounters with health care providers. Members of Black and other groups may manifest such a response pattern, particularly if they are from cultures that were formerly oppressed by colonization. Consider the case of a patient who identified herself strongly as African American but found out, after many months of hospitalization, that her hospital chart erroneously labeled her "White." While someone may have felt they were doing her a favor by such recharacterization, the patient was extremely angry at what she interpreted as denial of an essential part of who she was. When persons are stressed with serious illness, such seemingly small things may have mighty meanings and ramifications.

Managing historical hostility starts with recognition that a client is both a unique individual and a member of a historically oppressed group. Although everyone deserves equal opportunities for culturally congruent care, this care must also be specific to patterns of reaction and outlooks on reality. In psychiatry, as in the rest of health care, one size does not fit all! It is important to remember that there is a wide variation within any group. The effective transcultural psychiatric nurse realizes that the defensiveness known as historical hostility may or may not be manifested by clients. If it is anticipated, it can be recognized and managed. However, if it is expected, the nurse may project defensiveness that generates client resistance.

Clinical Application

Accept and work with the fact that some Black clients will be hostile toward White, middle-class health care professionals who are likely to be perceived (and to inadvertently behave) as privileged.

Recognize that although the client is a unique person with special attributes, he or she may also have patterns of reaction and outlooks that reflect a historical oppression. If hostility is recognized, it can be recognized and managed in the milieu of the therapeutic relationship.

Mental health professionals must be accepting and sensitive to cultural variations in their clients, and willing to explore clients' perceptions of "White" culture.

Cultural influences on stress and coping constitute important information for dealing with mental health problems, and the culturally competent nurse should understand these influences.

Kavanagh, K. H. (2002). Neither here nor there: The story of a health professional's experience with getting care and needing caring. In N. L. Diekelmann (Ed.), *First do no harm: Power, oppression, and violence in healthcare* (pp. 49–117). Madison, WI: University of Wisconsin Press.

Vontress, C. E., & Epp, L. R. (1997). Historical hostility in the African American client: Implications for counseling. *Journal of Multicultural Counseling and Development, 25*, 170–184.

balance between living and working toward achieving Indian goals; self-development is never completed. Noninterference is valued, and behaviors that imply manipulation or control may be offensive (Biolsi, 2001; Adams, 2000) (Figure 10–3). The astute clinician makes sure that the North American Indian client is aware of the consequences of behavior but then leaves it to the individual to decide how to proceed. Silence and a conservative show of interest (including, for example, minimizing eye contact) are respectful, caring behaviors.

The potential for personal confusion is obvious in a situation where mainstream society devalues most of the concepts integral to traditional Native North American philosophies and ideologies. North American Indian ideas about health and illness place less emphasis on dysfunction of the body than is typical of biomedi-

cine and more on relationships within society. For many Indians, health typically denotes a special, balanced relationship between humankind and its physical, relational, and supernatural environment. Illness implies having fallen out of balance and harmony with the world (Melton, 2005).

Traditional self-care prevention measures may include religious or traditional magical elements (for example, singing special songs, burning herbs or candles, wearing amulets, reciting prayers, or making offerings) (Tom-Orme, 2002). Although the prevalence of alcohol and drug use varies by tribe and by age within tribes (as it does within other groups, such as European North Americans, Latinos, and Blacks [Singer, 2001]), Native North Americans tend to have higher rates of alcoholism than those experienced by other groups. Associated phenomena include high suicide rates among the young, domestic (spouse and child abuse) violence, and homicide (Christie, 2001). However, many tribes today pride themselves on their increasing social pride, their tribal stability and sovereignty, and their rates of sobriety that are markedly higher than in the past when their peoples were more oppressed (Lowe, 2002; Struthers & Lowe, 2003).

Stress-producing socioeconomic situations accompanied by psychological, cultural, and spiritual stressors lead to perceptions of loss and depression. Those who are least acculturated to White society and who have strong tribal identities often tend to have the fewest problems, whereas those living in two seemingly contradictory societies are greatly challenged. Group therapies with an emphasis on society have been found to be especially useful for treatment (Schwarz, 2001). Often they are family-network therapy, traditional Indian group talking (such as talking circles), and purification therapies such as ritual sweats (Adams, 2000; Steeler, 2001).

Hispanic Americans

Generally, the terms *Latino* and *Hispanic* refer to Spanish ethnicity, language skills, and ancestry, but, as is true with other groups, they also imply

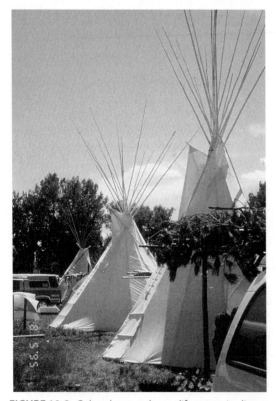

FIGURE 10-3. Cultural groups honor life stages in diverse ways. Here tobacco ties and sage, circular in form to reflect unity, mark a traditional Lakota grave.

significant cultural variation. Some common themes among Hispanic Americans include Roman Catholicism (although increasing numbers of Hispanics are turning to Protestant religions and Pentecostal sects), orientation toward extended family systems (which may include godparents [*compadres*] and other nonbiologic kin), distinctly different roles for men and women, a high value of respect for self and others, the priority of spiritual and humanistic over commercial values, clear hierarchy and patriarchy, and fairly common reliance on folk systems of medicine. Because Hispanic Americans tend to value being listened to and having time spent with them, task-oriented hurrying about is viewed as uncaring. Involvement, loving, and empathy are valued caring behaviors (Berry, 2002). There is a wide variability in levels of **acculturation** (that is, integration into the mainstream European American system) (Baer, Weller, Garcia, & Rocha, 2004; McEwen, 2005). Although the average Mexican American was born in the United States, and many members of other Hispanic groups are American by birth, numerous others are immigrants.

Hispanic, Latin American, and Puerto Rican traditions of folk medicine, despite some variation by place and group, clearly reflect their humoural antecedents as well as Roman Catholic ritual and beliefs about supernatural influences (Baer, 2001). Many illnesses, whether predominantly physical or mental, are "hot" or "cold," based on a long tradition of humoural theory. These qualities do not refer to temperature but to symbolic properties. Ill persons are treated with medicines and foods of opposite characteristics. By understanding the hot/cold interpretations to which specific patients or groups ascribe, care and treatment regimens can be negotiated with patients within that framework.

Many Americans fear that large numbers of immigrants, for example, peoples of Hispanic origin, in the United States may lead to division of the country into two languages and two cultures (Grossman, 2004). America's history is, in large part, one of immigration, but over time, the offspring of earlier immigrants generally dropped their original languages and accul-

turated (that is, while retaining some traditional ways, learned to get along in Euro-American culture), or even assimilated wholly into the English-speaking, European-based cultural mainstream. Today's multiculturalism demands more adaptation on the part of the host country's populace, parts of which resent what it sees as economic erosion at the hand of people from other places. As with the other groups discussed, generalizing and stereotyping fail to do justice to the needs of the people encountered in the mental health system, both on an individual basis and as a group.

Asian North Americans

North Americans of Asian ancestry represent numerous diverse cultures from Japan, China, Korea, India, the Philippines and other Pacific islands, and Southeast Asia, along with many others whose families have lived in the United States for generations. Education and hard work have paid off for many Asian immigrants, although the "Asian success story" and assumptions of an extension of "White privilege" to Asian immigrants (Goode, 1998) fail to take into account that there are many poor Asian North Americans (despite relatively low rates of dependence on public assistance and welfare) and that a notable discrepancy between education level and income persists.

Strong Asian values generally involve harmonious interpersonal relationships, webs of obligation, and fear of shame (which is a social concept, in contrast to the Westernized notion of guilt, which is more individualized) (Mull, Nguyen, & Mull, 2001). The family and its honor are of great importance, and family sharing is a major construct in care. Respect—especially for family, elders, and those in authority—is seen as vital. Respect is expressed through recognition of family members and in listening to and valuing their input (Leininger, 2002a). Reciprocity and generosity are highly valued; disruptive and conflict situations are viewed as uncaring (Basuray, 2002).

Traditional Asian health care practices include such varied preventive strategies as worshipping gods and ancestors and striving for balance in all aspects of life. The goal of balance also permeates all culturally congruent treatments. Asian societies share a tradition of Chinese medicine (which is more general than Western medicine because it has a single unifying theoretic basis and has been around for more than 4,000 years) as well as of shamanism. There is a strong reliance on Chinese medicine for specific problems and for prevention (Kaptchuk, 2000). Traditional healers draw on biologic, psychological, social, and ecologic evidence to diagnosis conditions arising from disruptions in the client's life. For example, the patient's brain and body may be out of balance, and the patient's relationships with past lives, ancestors, and destiny may be disturbed in some way (Ratanakul, 1999). Inappropriate behavior may leave the patient vulnerable to problems stemming from traditional categories of brain collapse, ancestral vengeance, and interference from evil spirits and people. Communication is viewed as fundamental to the healer–patient relationship.

Traditional Chinese have characteristic ways of dealing with mental illness in the family, starting with a protracted period of intrafamilial coping with even serious psychiatric illness, followed by recourse to friends, elders, and neighbors in the community; consultation with traditional specialists, religious healers, or general physicians; and finally treatment from Western specialists. Although it may conflict with Western practices of multiple dosage in tablet or capsule form, many Asians prefer to use over-the-counter drugs that come in liquid form as well as in single doses, as was typical of liquid preparations in Chinese folk practices. Others believe that only injections will be effective.

India, like many other nations in Asia, is greatly diverse in cultures, languages, levels of technology, and ideological traditions (Basuray, 2002). Like traditional Chinese medicine, with which it has much in common, classic Ayurvedic medicine is rooted in the mists of antiquity in the Indian subcontinent. Yoga, an important aspect of Ayurvedic medicine, promotes a balanced flow of energy that has great appeal to members of diverse groups, not only those from Asia.

For many Asian North Americans, the forces of tradition, with their holistic and complete (including mental health and stability) therapeutic systems, are entangled with those of modernization (Meleis & Im, 2002). Traditionally, most care has been provided within families despite the shame associated with mental illness; the strains and changes of recent urbanization and industrialization have led to increasingly diverse lifestyles and a need to discard stereotypes of well-satisfied, well-cared for, and respected ill persons and elders (Evidence-Based Practice 10-3).

Middle Eastern Cultural Groups

In recent decades, the United States and Canada have experienced an influx of peoples from Middle Eastern and Northern African cultures. This has increased the traditionally Judeo-Christian North American awareness of the complex cultural beliefs, values, and lifeways of members of predominantly (but not exclusively) Islamic societies. Since 2001, ethnic diversity and immigration have confronted renewed turmoil in terms of stigma, homeland security, and terrorism. Headlines proclaim potential for terror and lament missed opportunities to foil deadly attacks without addressing the effect of perceived threat and risk on the people. Stories of torture evoke far greater political than social fervor (Rudmin, 2004). With the United States' boundaries being protected as never before, many Americans cast a benign eye on the impact 9/11 has had on Americans of Middle Eastern background (Haasoun, 2004)—or those who merely look like they might be. At the same time, interestingly, Islam is one of the fastest growing religions in the United States (Miller, 1999). Its tenets (including views on race) are diverse.

Similar things can be said about nearly every religious, ethnic, and other cultural group in America. There is great diversity within, as well as between, categories. Despite considerable cultural diversity among Middle Eastern peoples, generally shared value orientations include Moslem (Muslim or Islamic) submission and obedience to God and prescribed rituals of prayer and washing. Strict concepts of what is allowed

Evidence-Based Practice 10–3:

Mental Health Care for Asian and Pacific Islander Americans

Care and consideration in how people are represented are among the major challenges of health care today. This may be even more important in mental health contexts. Demographically, the category "Asian and Pacific Islander Americans" includes more than 40 different cultural groups. What they share in common is either ancient or recent roots in Asia. Asians are so often described as "model" or "successful" minorities that actual problems experienced by individuals, families, and subgroups may be overlooked or minimized. Levels of acculturation vary widely. The families of some Asian Americans have been in the United States for four or more generations; others may be new immigrants. Generally, more acculturated peoples tend to have higher levels of mental health-seeking behaviors. Ancestral values and language patterns also differ greatly. Training to increase cultural competence is important for mental health practitioners.

Clinical Application

Explore with the client just how he or she views himself or herself culturally. For example, how does the individual client "name" his or her culture?

Ask the client to describe his or her culture for you and to explain cultural characteristics for your benefit.

Understand that by the act of seeking mental health care, your client is probably more acculturated than others of the same cultural group.

Organize a training session at your work site, and invite members of the local Asian and Pacific Islander communities to come and talk with you about themselves and their cultures.

Kavanagh, K. H. (2005). Representing: Interpretive scholarship's consummate challenge. In P. M. Ironside (Ed.), *Beyond method: Philosophical conversations in healthcare research and scholarship* (pp. 58–110). Madison, WI: University of Wisconsin Press.

Sandhu, D. S. (1997). Psychocultural profiles of Asian and Pacific Islander Americans: Implications for counseling and psychotherapy. *Journal of Multicultural Counseling and Development, 25,* 7–22.

and forbidden (that is, clean and unclean, good and bad) impose important dietary and other rules that should be verified and accommodated as much as possible in health care situations. Class, status, education, modesty, and emotional expression are generally valued. Patriarchy and the centrality of religion typify Middle Eastern social and familial organizations. Elders are honored, gain in status, and, interestingly, tend not to experience the senility common in more youth-oriented cultures (Luna, 2002).

Oriented traditionally to the present, some Middle Easterners may not value making plans because the future is seen as neither uncertain nor preordained but as something that one accepts with fatalistic grace. Nursing research suggests that immigrants who are more traditional in social integration, cultural attitudes, and family orientation tend to face more difficult challenges of morale than those who are more acculturated (Luna, 2002).

Since the terrorist attacks on the World Trade Center in New York City and the Pentagon in Washington DC, on September 11, 2001, many Arab Americans have experienced a backlash of bias, distrust, and hate crimes. Such a backlash can negatively affect their mental health. In response, many Arab Americans have been active in helping dispel negative images of their culture and in educating the public about Islam and the contributions of Arab Americans to American life. Other Americans have also shown an increased interest in learning about Islam, its tenets, and its history. There is also increased concern for and activism toward social healing (Thompson & O'Dea, 2005).

The Appeal of Alternative Systems

Folk and popular systems of health care continue to serve, to a greater extent than is often recognized by mental health (or other health) personnel, to smooth harsh cultural gaps between traditional societies and the predominant North American systems. They are available in every North American city (and many other areas), do not require going to unfamiliar places or being seen by people who are strangers, and are readily understandable to someone socialized to the group. Folk systems are also simply organized, compared to biomedical health care systems, and relatively devoid of intimidating and invasive testing, technology, lengthy history taking (which often seems irrelevant to patients and families), and dubious diagnostic procedures designed to rule out rather than ascertain specific phenomena. Interpersonal, social, and kinship relationships are emphasized in traditional or folk systems of healing, rather than the isolated individual. Traditionally, a focus on groups has minimized the discomfort associated with unaccustomed attention to individuals outside the context of the family.

Traditional systems of understanding illness and healing are experienced as more humanistic than scientific, and are usually less mechanized, less urbanized, and less intellectualized than is biomedicine, with its focus on fixing dysfunctional components, limits in access, expectations regarding use, and dependence on rationality and efficiency to such an extent that emotional needs may be overlooked. For example, in some traditional cultures, the person who is mentally ill is labeled as "possessed by the devil." Because this disturbance and society's labeling are associated with the culture's religious system, the appropriate healing or "cure" is to include the religious leader in an attempt to cast out the devil through the use of prayer or other religious intervention, such as exorcism.

The use of psychiatric resources may be discouraged by professionals' intolerance for magical and religious orientations and practices, which is common when science and systems of symbolic beliefs and faith compete. However, multiple systems of healing may be used while the professional system is simply not aware of the pluralistic practices. Interest in traditional healing beliefs and practices is in no way limited to immigrant or indigenous groups. Today, North Americans of every ethnic heritage are expressing an increased interest in alternative or complementary health and healing traditions.

Culturally Competent Nursing Care for Clients with Mental Health Considerations

Transcultural nurses use many ways of understanding to move beyond the rigidity of trying to fit diverse experiences, interpretations, and expectations into a few ready-made (but culture-bound) categories. All cultural groups share time-honored systems of health beliefs and practices; it is often nurses who can interpret expectations within and between groups. Sensitive cultural interviews are required to know who clients are. Nursing, to provide culturally congruent care, attends to relationships between the self and others; between mental illness and such phenomena as poverty, suffering, violence, chronic illness, and aging; between the cultures of nursing and psychiatry and those of our clientele; and between nursing ethics and the provision of appropriate care. When nurses and clients come from different cultural backgrounds, accurate diagnosis, treatment, and care depend on time-consuming special knowledge and skills (Kavanagh, 2005).

Transcultural nursing may involve collecting information about specific cultures; acquiring a culturally acceptable ally or advocate for the client and/or a cultural consultant for the nurse; working with a translator; learning clients' behavioral, attitudinal, and cognitive norms; or ensuring that only culturally fair psychometric tests and functional measures are used. Standardized tests are appropriate only when they are properly modified to fit a client's cultural heritage and experiences. Some transcultural nurses view culture brokering (bridging, linking, or mediating between groups that differ in background or orientation) as part of their roles (McElroy & Jezewski, 2000). Ideally, this is done with information from the client's perspective; the nurse serves merely to facilitate the opportunity to be heard. Other transcultural nurses define their responsibility more in terms of expediting situations in which clients can do their own negotiating.

Because psychopathology and mental illnesses occur at roughly the same rate in all societies, despite a multitude of expressions of such distress (Turner, 2000), it stands to reason that a transcultural perspective is essential to appropriate mental health and psychiatric nursing care. The value of psychiatry is questionable if cultural relevance is limited to middle-class Europeans and European North Americans. In its current thinking, ethnopsychiatry, which involves culture-specific constructions of psychiatric systems, attempts to move beyond the assumption that Western ways of understanding and treating psychiatric conditions are universally applicable. Instead, mental health and mental illness are understood within the cultural contexts in which they develop (Knowlden & Kavanagh, 2004; Tseng & Streltzer, 1997). Nursing faces the same challenge; ethnonursing methods foster understanding of care-related phenomena from the perspectives of the people who experience the culture and the phenomena (Leininger, 2002b).

It is essential for clients to feel accepted if they are to share with health care providers what they believe and practice outside the biomedical system. This will not happen if clients are left to assume that their beliefs and activities are not of interest to health care providers or will be rejected by them. It may be important, however, to know what the patient or client believes and does to minimize the possibility of harm from treatments or medicines that interact disadvantageously with those of the alternative systems. Although it is dangerous to assume that all indigenous approaches are innocuous, many practices are harmless, whether or not they are effective cures. Often treatments (and the contexts in which they are experienced) provide valuable psychological support and, because of that contribution, should not be discouraged.

Assumptions that coping patterns of clients and patients are or should be similar to those of nurses (and others socialized to the health care system) can simplify care. However, differences may be overlooked in efforts to avoid time-consuming complications. The risk involved in such behavior is that clients and health care providers may work with different strategies or toward dissimilar goals. The nurse, for example, may hurry to include all items relevant to health promotion for high-risk clients, when it is the nurse's presence and the time spent with them that the clients value, rather than the information.

Assessment

The realization that perspectives are shaped by specific values and beliefs rooted in specific cultures and subcultures allows objective assessment of diverse practices that people use to promote health and cope with illness. Whether or not they are understood, people have reasons for their behavior. They may, for example, refuse to have blood drawn because of a belief that it could be used for sorcery or, as was traditionally believed in Asian societies, that blood contains the personality. It does not make sense to risk personality loss or disruption through exchange of blood or other organs. On the other hand, it may make sense for clients to alter their medication dosages when they believe that the "big" European North American physicians who prescribe medicines are likely to order too large a dose for someone of smaller stature (Janzen, 2002). Likewise, the appreciation that one person's "superstition" may be someone else's firmly held explanation or belief allows the culturally competent nurse to objectively consider the behavior associated with

that belief for its own merit, neutrality, or harm. Automatic discrediting of ideas or practices because they are unfamiliar, "old-fashioned," or not scientific risks the alienation of clients as well as the loss of potentially useful resources (Evidence-Based Practice 10–4).

Evidence-Based Practice 10–4:
There Are Many Views of the History of Psychiatric and Mental Health Care

Oral histories have been collected as data for several books on the history of psychiatric and mental health nursing. Interviews of staff or former staff reveal opinions, attitudes, feelings, and practices of care. One wonders why the recollections of former patients are not collected as well as those of the staff. However, it is race and ethnicity that the author addresses, noting that "Differences of ethnic origin, surprisingly, do not seem to have been much discussed, in spite of the many different nationalities of nurses working at various times in the hospital" (Russell, 1997, p. 493). Russell speculates that the notable racial mix among both nurses and physicians may have facilitated tolerance and acceptance within the setting. Although that may be the case, other research has suggested that race, ethnicity, and gender issues may actually be avoided in psychiatric settings (Kavanagh, 2005). Culturally competent nurses realize that diversity-related issues can play important parts in communication, relationships, mental health, and mental illness. It is questionable, therefore, whether a care setting can truly be therapeutic if such issues are not openly and comfortably discussed. Discourse is essential to manifesting power relations, hidden agendas, and dogma. Its critical use is important.

Clinical Application

Issues related to diversity, such as race, ethnicity, and gender, must be identified, and health care professionals must make an effort to move beyond such issues. They can best do this by openly identifying the issues and discussing them with colleagues. Such a discussion calls for openness and sensitivity with other health care providers as well as with clients.

Estefan, McAllister, and Rowe (2004) offer useful suggestions for nurses in clinical practice when working across cultures. Rather than posing questions from a "problem orientation," a solution orientation tends to be far more positive. Here are some examples (adapted from p. 56):

Problem orientation	Solution orientation
Asking what is wrong and why	Asking what he or she wants to change and how
Searching for underlying "causes"	Inviting clients to clarify their main issues and priorities for health care
Assuming client is deficient, resistant, misguided, or naive	Assuming client is competent, resilient, and resourceful

Estefan, A., McAllister, M., & Rowe, J. (2004). Difference, dialogue, dialectics: A study of caring and self-harm (pp. 21–61). In K. H. Kavanagh & V. Knowlden (Eds.), Many voices: Toward caring culture in healthcare and healing. Madison: University of Wisconsin Press.
Russell, D. (1997). An oral history project in mental health nursing. Journal of Advanced Nursing, 26, 489–495.

Cross-Cultural Communication

The crux of transcultural psychiatric/mental health nursing is communication, the style of which varies greatly with the culture involved. Some of these differences are quickly evident, as is the contrast that appears when mental health practitioners expect a degree of openness, verbosity, self-disclosure, emotional expression, and insight that reflect the dominant Western culture rather than the client's orientation, which may be very different. Groups also vary widely in their ideas about appropriate stance, gestures, language, listening styles, and eye contact. Traditional Asian, Black, Native North American, and Appalachian people typically consider direct eye contact inappropriate and disrespectful (Andrews, 2003).

With the increasingly complex variety of languages used in the United States and Canada (Urciuoli, 2001), the creation of linguistic boundaries is often prompted by the belief that there is a single standard English that should be used. Because language differences can cause mental health treatment to take much longer and be more complicated than treatment for English-speaking patients, it is sometimes tempting to use the most readily available person to facilitate the process. However, dependence on family members (or unprepared others, such as a passing janitor or available food handler) to translate may only complicate the situation, particularly when the patient and translator are not of the same sex, class, or age. The use of inappropriate translators may result in new problems being fabricated to avoid stating the real ones in front of the individual solicited to translate. It is important when using a translator to communicate with the client with a mental health condition that extra time be allowed to discuss the client's responses. For example, the nurse might want to ask the translator to be alert to nonverbal cues, such as body language, eye contact, or other behavior that would provide helpful information. Although linguistic assistance is vital, further difficulties arise when some translators interpret rather than directly translate what the

client says. The nurse, unfamiliar with the language, may not realize whose views are being expressed (Box 10-2).

Transcultural nursing care of mental health patients requires primary transcultural communication skills (Crowe, 2000; McAllister & Walsh, 2003) (Figure 10-4). The first skill is the ability to understand and state an issue or problem as it is perceived from the client's perspective. It is important that sincere (not patronizing) interest be taken in the client's views and experiences and that they be taken seriously. The second and third skills involve recognizing and reducing resistance and defensiveness, which directly impede the development of productive relationships between nurses and clients and further

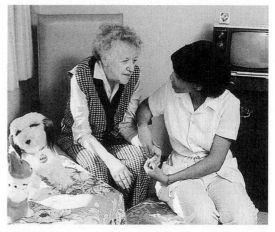

FIGURE 10-4. Effective cross-cultural communication skills are particularly important when caring for mental health patients. Developing lasting meaningful relationships across potential social barriers such as race contributes to improved communication.

contribute to the basis for negative attitudes and labels such as "noncompliance." The fourth transcultural communication skill involves the recognition that everyone makes interactive mistakes from time to time (Kavanagh & Kennedy, 1992).

Communicating with culturally diverse mental health patients requires testing stereotypes against reality. If one stereotypes all psychiatric patients as dangerous, for example, the generalization does not accurately represent the high proportion of patients who are not (Evidence-Based Practice 10–5). When cognition and affect are impaired by mental illness, communication can be especially time-consuming and complex, although it is no less important. Assumptions must be avoided. Unusual use of language may, for example, represent cultural differences rather than thinking or hearing impairments, although those explanations might also be valid. The skilled communicator learns how to identify and bridge differences.

Mutual communication involves awareness and knowledge of social process, and sensitivity to and recognition of barriers to acceptance and sharing, as well as skill in communication techniques. Whereas the functional utility of words and gestures has communicative value to all involved, most important is the ability to empathize—that is, to understand others' beliefs, assumptions, perspectives, and feelings (Kavanagh, 2005). The effective communicator learns to acquire and to understand, to the greatest extent possible, multiple perspectives. Tolerance and acceptance of others' attitudes, beliefs, and behaviors, and the willingness to expose one-

Evidence-Based Practice 10–5:

"Lunatics" and the Moon: Nature and Madness, or Just a Phase?

For centuries (at least since Hippocrates posited the relationship some 2,500 years ago) people have associated increases in violence and aggression in psychiatric patients with the full moon. Over time, this came to be known as the Transylvanian effect. Research examined the use of seclusion in various phases of the moon as a way of investigating the relationship (if any) between the moon and madness. Seclusion, in various forms, is used universally for disturbed patients and in psychiatric settings for the control and management of violence and aggression. If the Transylvanian effect actually occurs, there should be a demonstrable relationship between lunar cycles and the use of seclusion. Although staff members may use seclusion when they fear that they or others may be in danger and thus may be hypervigilant during the full moon (whether or not the moon has any effect on patients' behavior), no such correlation was found between the full moon and use of seclusion for the mentally ill.

Clinical Application

Seclusion, in various forms and used universally for centuries, may be used appropriately when mental health professionals believe they are in danger from a client's violent and aggressive behavior.

Violent behavior in clients is sometimes triggered by such factors as noncompliance with medication, stress, or other events in the clients' environment, rather than the full moon.

Mason, T. (1997). Seclusion and the lunar cycles. *Journal of Psychosocial Nursing, 35*(6), 14–18.

self as interested but still learning sensitivity, knowledge, and skills are important strategies.

Self-Reflection and Awareness

Learning to understand the cultures of clients requires learning about your own cultural orientation and about yourself. The culture of the nurse interacts with those of clients. It is important to realize that culture includes the values and norms learned in the process of becoming a nurse (or a member of any other group), as well as those associated with ethnicity, age, class, or gender background. Understanding who you are requires close examination of your own orientation to recognize where your own sense of personal and social identity comes from and how it was formed. Ask yourself what kind of person you were socialized to be, and how your social identity has changed and is changing. Culture is never static.

Such self-knowledge is critical to realizing which cultures or groups one tends to favor or avoid, and which groups one negatively or unrealistically positively stereotypes. Such blind spots (that is, biases) can keep one from considering, for example, that a "nice, middle-class grandmother" might also be a much conflicted lesbian woman who is addicted to cocaine. Each of us has attitudinal limitations that obscure facts from our consideration and vision. With whom do you feel strange and uncomfortable, and why? How do your concerns and biases affect who gets care and what type of care you give? It is well known that there are cultural preferences among mental health care providers for clients who are young, attractive, verbal, intelligent, and successful (also known as YAVIS) (Kavanagh, 2003b), whereas those who are considered quiet, unattractive, old, indigent, different, and stupid (that is, the QUOIDS) often get less attention.

Commitment to transcultural nursing assumes the recognition and value of human dignity, cultural relativism (that is, the idea that all perspectives deserve respectful consideration) as an acceptable and preferred philosophy, willing-

ness to alter personal behavior in response to the cross-cultural interactive process, and willingness to monitor personal resistance and defensiveness. Consider how you feel about those criteria.

People may avoid professional mental health care because of incompatible values and beliefs, poverty, social stresses that occur among special populations but are not well understood by professionals, language barriers, lack of education, social isolation, stigma, bureaucratic barriers, and the unequal distribution of services. It is crucial that the nursing process be examined from the cultural perspectives of health care providers and consumers to maximize appropriate use and quality of care. Then informed practitioners can provide care in ways that are perceived as both acceptable and appropriate (Evidence-Based Practice 10–6).

Culture-Specific Care

It may be tempting to avoid close examination of basic values and beliefs because they seem amorphous, complex, or too intimate. However, a grasp of the concepts of normality, abnormality, ethnocentrism, relativism, pluralism, stereotyping, prejudice, and discrimination provides a basis for understanding how society handles differences in attitude and behavior. Social ranking (that is, social stratification) and its consequence, social inequality, affect human experience, opportunities, and the availability, acceptability, and use of mental health care resources.

It is a myth that treating people differently because of racial, religious, ethnic, cultural, gender, or other characteristics implies prejudice and discrimination. That is an overused excuse to avoid dealing with issues that are part of social process. On the other hand, treating everyone the same in the name of justice is equally insensitive because it too denies differences that matter to people. Failure to acknowledge diversity denies meaningful variations in real-life experience. It is not necessarily irrational for the individual who has been discriminated against because of his or

Evidence-Based Practice 10–6:

Urban/Rural Differences Are Important Too

When major depressive disorders occur in rural areas where few professional mental health treatment resources exist and clients may be hard to access and treat, effective psychosocial interventions must be adapted for specific populations. A primary care setting providing screening, diagnostic care, brief treatment, and follow-up care can produce a significant reduction in symptoms, improved functional ability of clients, and programs of relapse prevention. This was done in the rural Piedmont area of the South by training generalist nurses with psychoeducational skills to work with a culturally competent advanced practice psychiatric nurse and by designing a program for specific care needs. Field testing and evaluation of the program for rural women in the area studied indicated that a combination of self-care skills (including self-assessment, stress reduction, and health behavior modification) and minimum psychiatric resources can create a promising and powerful partnership.

Clinical Application

Rural clients can be treated effectively in primary care settings in their own communities. These services should include screening and diagnostic and brief treatment services. Follow-up services can be provided as needed. This model has been shown to improve the functional ability of clients and reduce their symptoms.

Nurses can be trained to provide culturally competent psychiatric services in rural areas. Their partnerships with each other, other professionals, community groups, and clients are essential, particularly when resources are sparse.

Self-care skills that can be taught to rural women include self-assessment, stress reduction, and health behavior modification. These practices can decrease symptoms in clients who live in hard-to-access rural areas.

Feller, L. M., Hunsley-McTighe, A., Ray, A. L., & Schliessmann, L. A. M. (2005). Rural South Dakota: The power of education and care delivery partnerships. *Home Health Care Management & Practice, 15*(X), 1–4.
Hauenstein, E. J. (1997). A nursing practice paradigm for depressed rural women: The women's affective illness treatment program. *Archives of Psychiatric Nursing, 1,* 37–45.

her skin color or language, or the woman who has been raped, to feel paranoid. On the other hand, it is painful to have one's experience (including the identity affiliations that help us understand who we are) discredited or made to seem unimportant, and situations do not go away simply because they are ignored or avoided. The sense of distancing and pain remain, and aspects of the issues may eventually surface.

In trying to satisfy the basic needs of his or her client, the transcultural nurse asks, in essence,

"How do you want to be cared for?" Culturally congruent nursing care decisions and actions have the potential to intervene in three ways: cultural care preservation, accommodation, and repatterning (Leininger, 2002b).

The need for cultural maintenance or preservation is demonstrated in Case Study 10-1. The second mode of nursing intervention involves assisting clients to negotiate or adapt to new cultural ways (Leininger, 2002b). As nurses become sensitive to the complex factors that influence clients' responses to care, they learn to negotiate. This mode of intervention is illustrated in Case Study 10–2. A third approach to intervention involves culturally acceptable and appropriate care that enables change to new or different behavioral patterns that are meaningful, satisfying, and beneficial (Leininger, 2002b). Changing a person's view of events requires altering the meaning of the situation. However, the need for such restructuring is less common than that for cultural preservation and negotiation, and it involves only partial behavioral repatterning. Those cultural attributes that are useful are preserved, as described in Case Study 10–3.

CASE STUDY 10-1

A student from New Zealand came to a university mental health clinic describing chronic headaches, sleeplessness, and inability to focus on his school work. He explained that the onset of these symptoms coincided with his father's death, about which he did not learn until it was too late to return for the burial rites. Owing to his failure to be there when his mother especially needed his support, a relative "pointed a bone" at him, and that action, he believed, resulted in his present problems. A thorough assessment did not produce additional reasons for the young man's somatic complaints, decreased academic achievement, and social discomfort.

Fortunately, a clinician was located who had previously worked in the South Pacific, and she made herself available to work with both the clinic staff and the disturbed student. Together they delineated the problem, worked to understand what it would take to alleviate it, and participated in an adapted ceremony that allowed the client to believe that the effect of the bone-pointing had been neutralized. The student was at peace with the knowledge that no fault of his had caused him to miss his father's funeral. He knew that further amends for the social transgression could wait until after the successful completion of his studies. This would allow him to serve his affiliation group more effectively than would his premature return as an academic failure.

CASE STUDY 10-2

Maria, a 15-year-old Mexican American girl, was referred to the mental health clinic after a suicide attempt. Her school attendance was sporadic, her grades were poor, and she was depressed. Both parents worked outside the home, and her older brothers had moved out, leaving her as primary caretaker for several young siblings. Although she had been dating a boy for several months, her parents planned to send her to Mexico to marry a man they knew there. Soon after she argued with her family about her household chores and her future, her boyfriend ended their relationship, and the school threatened to suspend her for nonattendance. Maria cut her wrists. Verbalizing her identity and role confusion, guilt over her rejection of her family's expectations, and anger at their rejection of her viewpoint, she intensely resented her parents' and the school authorities' expectations and her limited choices.

Individual and family therapy with mental health clinical nurse specialists helped negotiate a realistic and acceptable plan that would keep Maria in school (thus increasing her life choices later) while helping her bridge the gap between traditional and more modern ways. In a group with other young women, Maria was empowered by sharing and learning that there were aspects of her culture and her circumstances that she could accept, reject, ignore, and change. She had a voice and choices that she could learn to affirm.

CASE STUDY 10-3

In an urban program designed to strengthen family processes, families were encouraged to spend social time in the program's community center. When parents were confronted in writing (as well as with oral reprimand) with the program's expectation that there would be no hitting on the premises, several families stopped coming. It was not until the staff realized the parents' need to learn alternative ways to set limits for children that those families began to feel comfortable at the center.

For many program participants, physical recourse was the only mode of discipline with which they were familiar; the no-hitting policy had been interpreted as meaning "no discipline." Parents had to learn alternative ways of dealing with disciplinary issues and with stress, and children eventually learned that their parents would be consistent in their nonphysical limit setting, that punishments would correlate with the transgression, and that the expression of caring was not limited to physical evidence. With repatterning over time, meaningful verbal and other nonphysical ways of disciplining were modeled, learned, and implemented.

Ideologic Conflict in Psychiatric/ Mental Health Nursing

A growing awareness of the changing and complex nature of illness, the influence of social context, and the importance of holistic perspectives can leave nurses in a quandary when the dominant model in psychiatry focuses on organic and genetic factors as underlying causes of mental disease (Duster, 2003). For some, psychiatry's realignment toward biology, high-tech brain scans, and powerful new drugs, along with a reorientation away from staff–patient relationships and toward objective observation and documentation, threatens to minimize the importance of the patient as a person or at least to risk the sacrifice of communication and understanding to cold, hard documentation (Kavanagh, 2005; Wagner, 2005). This substitution of psychiatric materialism for humanism may lead nurses who are surrounded by others who think differently to question their ability and worth, to resent psychiatry's role in social control, or to accuse mental health nursing of a lack of critical examination of its own ideology and of those hegemonic psychiatric beliefs and practices imposed on their practice from medicine (Morgan & Maskovsky, 2003; Rylko-Bauer & Farmer, 2002).

Ideologic conflict is not new in psychiatric/ mental health care and continues to shadow nurse–physician and nurse–client relationships (Estefan, McAllister, & Rowe, 2004; Kavanagh, 2003a, 2005). Continued frustrations with a plethora of phenomena, many of them (such as poverty and discrimination) beyond the scope of conventional medical treatment, confront public psychiatric/mental health systems. Despite the medicalization of mental health, nurses often feel that they must balance structural requirements (which may conflict) with operationalizing knowledge of care and therapy (which may be ambiguous), all the while communicating with persons who may communicate not only in culturally diverse ways, but also abnormally (Estefan, McAllister, & Rowe, 2004). All of this occurs in a society that is ambivalent toward individuals who exhibit unpopular differences. Nurses must continue to explore diverse models of caring and attend closely to the practices they actually use (Figure 10–5).

Implications for Transcultural Mental Health/Psychiatric Nursing Practice

As a practical science of caring, nursing strives to use strategies that lead to positive outcomes. How does the nurse incorporate cultural beliefs and practices into daily practice? Key points for

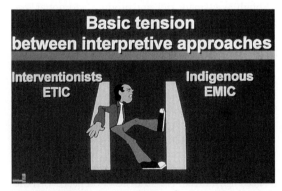

FIGURE 10-5. Being an applied profession with a humanistic ethic, nursing grapples with tension between the outsider (etic) values of the nursing and medical subcultures (which neglect the dominant society) and an insider (emic) view reflecting the values of individuals, families, communities, and other affiliation and cultural groups for whom nurses advocate. Transcultural nursing helps bring emic perspectives together with the etic.

the transcultural mental health nurse are summarized here, using Diekelmann's (1995, 2005) framework of "concernful practices" (Kavanagh, Absalom, Beil, & Schliessmann, 1999).

Welcoming, Gathering, and Accepting

Welcoming, gathering, and *accepting* involve creating effective relationships and establishing open communication. The nurse's role is to suggest illness prevention and health maintenance practices, as well as treatment strategies that fit with and reinforce clients' cultural beliefs and practices. Understand clients' desire to please and their motivations to comply or not to comply. Often "noncompliance" occurs because clients are trying to preserve their own priorities (Kavanagh, 2005; Knowlden & Kavanagh, 2004). Understand relationships between clients and authority, health care institutions and bureaucracies. Whenever possible and appropriate, involve significant others and leaders of relevant local groups. Confidentiality is important, but ethnic and other leaders know the issues and can often suggest acceptable interventions. Try to make the setting comfortable. Consider colors, sound, atmosphere, scheduling expectations, seating arrangements, pace, tone, and other environmental variables. Be prepared for the fact that children go everywhere with members of some cultural groups, as well as with families who do not have options because of economic limitations; include them.

Knowing, Connecting, and Staying

Knowing, connecting, and *staying* involve finding meaningful ways in which clients, families, and others can contribute their own cultural input and goals while both patterns and variations are recognized. As nurses become more mindful of managing their own diversity, questions initiated by "Why don't they ...?" are gradually balanced with "Why do we ...?"; this often prompts ongoing discussion of various approaches and perspectives. Becoming more aware of the potency of cultural expectations as well as personal choices, all participants in cross-cultural relationships find themselves consciously setting priorities and considering options regarding what to accept, reject, ignore, or try to change.

Presencing, Attending, and Staying Open

Presencing, attending, and *staying open* are confounded with time, which continually frustrates modern health care and nursing. Routinization and efficiency are valued by the dominant culture, whereas caring, connecting, and learning take time. Visiting, sharing stories, and many other simple encounters are useful strategies for learning what care and caring mean to the client and family. Understand what members of the cultural or subcultural group consider "caring," both attitudinally and behaviorally. Ask what they would like and expect to have happen. Acquire basic knowledge about cultural values, health beliefs, and traditional health-related practices common to the group with which you are working. Learn about expectations for personal hygiene, rest and sleep, ideas about health and illness, and communicating and eating. Language and food are important symbols; respect and use them. Also know the folk illnesses and remedies common to the cultural group with which you are working. Inquire about over-the-counter and folk remedies being used; research indicates that most treatments used by clients are not reported because health care professionals do not ask about them (Knowlden & Kavanagh, 2004; Mull, Nguyen, & Mull, 2001). Build on cultural practices, reinforcing those that are positive; do not discredit any beliefs or practices unless you know for sure that specific practices are harmful.

Creating a Place and Keeping Open Possibilities

Creating a place and *keeping open possibilities* entail working to establish caring relationships and increasing sensitivity to our own implicit understandings and expectations. Present yourself with confidence. Shake hands if it is appropriate. Ask how clients prefer to be addressed. Allow them to choose seating for comfortable personal space and culturally appropriate eye contact.

Avoid assumptions about where people come from; let them tell you. Most people are pleased when others show sincere interest in them. Strive to gain the other's trust, but do not resent it if you do not get it. Avoid body language that may be offensive or misunderstood—which may involve some research and surprises. Determine the patient's level of fluency in English, and arrange for an interpreter if one is needed. Speak directly to the client, even if an interpreter is present. Choose a speech rate and style that promotes understanding and demonstrates respect for the client. Avoid jargon, slang, and complex sentences. Do not expect clients to share your medical orientation. Use open-ended questions or questions phrased in several ways to obtain information, but be aware that some groups do not consider direct questions to be polite. Invite individuals to tell you stories about themselves and their problems. Determine the patient's English reading ability before using any written materials.

Safeguarding, Preserving, Advocating and Protecting

Safeguarding, preserving, advocating, and *protecting* guide awareness that people tend to see what they expect to see and that stereotypes narrow vision by ignoring variations that occur naturally. Learning about diversity and caring involves recognizing and replacing stereotypes with informed, expectable patterns that serve merely as starting points for inquiry and comparison. Advocacy roles require cultural sensitivity, knowledge, and skill—including a willingness to examine personal values and those of the subcultures of nursing and biomedicine, as well as those of other individuals and cultural groups. Negotiate goals that are explicit and realistic. Check for the client's understanding and acceptance of recommendations. Be patient; do not expect rapid change. Be sensitive when describing or writing about groups. Present a generally comprehensive perspective that emphasizes the positive over the negative. Relate social organization, structure, and process to each group's unique history.

Acknowledge the diversity that occurs within as well as between and among groups. Beware of literature that uses models of deviance or pathologic conditions rather than unbiased and fair information about groups. There is much of value to be found in both classic and modern literature, but it must be used critically, owing to the propensity for bias.

Engendering Mutuality and Community

The need for *engendering mutuality and community* reflects ways in which health care providers and clients come together, get to know and value differences as well as commonalities, and form flexible, open, and creative relationships and caring communities. Avoid stereotypes by sex, age, race, ethnicity, socioeconomic status, and other characteristics. Remember that cultural generalizations may not differ much from stereotypes and may lead to prejudice if they are not open to being revised, that some people do not like having ethnic labels attached to them and wish to "be treated like everyone else," that culture is not restricted to people of color, that differences within groups may be greater than differences between groups, and that our own attitudes and blind spots may be more important than those of clients in terms of outcome. Understand your own cultural values and biases. Emphasize the positive points and strengths of health beliefs and practices. Be respectful of values, beliefs, rights, and practices. Express interest in and understanding of other cultures without being judgmental. Some ideas may conflict with your own or with your determination to make changes, but every group and individual wants respect above all else. Show respect, especially for male clients, even if it is the female clients or children in whom you are particularly interested. Men are often decision makers about health care.

Letting Be and Letting Go

Transcultural mental health nursing also necessitates an additional genre of practices that constitute *letting be* and *letting go* to expedite openness to learning. Learn to appreciate the richness of diversity as an asset rather than viewing it as a hindrance to communication and effective intervention. Honor the uniqueness of clients and their dignity and worth. Attempt to establish caring relationships that can overcome any cultural misstep, and strive to help clients obtain their self-determined goals, to learn how clients understand and explain their experiences, and to get to know yourself as an effective transcultural nurse.

Summary

Mental health nursing might almost be defined as crossing cultures. Unlike other aspects of nursing, both psychiatric and transcultural care is based upon sensitivity, knowledge, and skills that emphasize beliefs and behaviors, rather than physical or biomedical issues. In that sense, the premises underlying both transcultural and mental health are also relevant to other aspects of caregiving.

REVIEW QUESTIONS

1. How has the interpretation of mental health and mental illness changed with time?
2. Describe three ways in which diversity influences mental health and mental illness.
3. How are culture and mental health integrated into other aspects of living?
4. Describe ways in which interactive processes and communication facilitate effective transcultural mental health care. How might interactive processes and communication erect barriers to effective transcultural mental health care?
5. Describe seven strategies that nurses can use to facilitate effective transcultural mental health care.

CRITICAL THINKING ACTIVITIES

1. Write a story or a narrative about a personal experience you have had or observed in which a cultural misunderstanding occurred. Critically evaluate and discuss how you felt as an observer and how you suppose the others involved in the situation felt. Discuss how the situation might have been managed more effectively.

2. Having a family member with a severe mental illness poses a strain on the entire family. Ask someone who has a family member with a psychiatric diagnosis to share his or her story. Critically analyze what the situation has been like for the family. An excellent model or example for this is *Imagining Robert: My Brother, Madness, and Survival: A Memoir* by J. Neugeboren (1997).

3. A great activity for pulling together cultural sensitivity, knowledge, and skills for effective transcultural mental health nursing involves interviewing someone from a culture significantly different from your own. After getting to know the person and some background, practice your communication skills to ask about ideas and practices related to mental health and illness. Then delve into the literature about that person's affiliation or cultural group(s). Whether your interviewee is from Tibet, gay, or a century old,

consider (and discuss with classmates) how your reading material fails to represent (or successfully represents) the individual that you interviewed.

4. Compile a list of the groups that you affiliate with and in which you feel you are an "insider." Then list several groups with which you are not affiliated and where you would feel an "outsider." As honestly and comprehensively as you can, critically analyze why you are comfortable with some groups and not with others. If possible, get an insider's perspective of the group(s) to which you do not belong. Critically analyze the traits and attributes with which you might be comfortable (or uncomfortable). Evaluate the strengths and vulnerabilities of each group.

5. Psychiatric symptoms typically reflect the cultural orientation of the mentally ill individual. How would you manage the following situation? You realize that your next-door neighbor, a retired European North American electrical engineer, has lined the interior walls of his house with aluminum foil to protect himself against the "beams" from the neighbors on the other side of him, who are immigrants from another country and speak little English. What assessment strategies would you use to distinguish the mental health issues from confounding social and cultural issues?

6. Role play is an effective strategy for developing cultural competence. With three colleagues, simulate a cultural encounter in which each of you takes a different role: One is the client, one is the nurse who does not know what the client's cultural background is, one is a backup for the client and can say the things that the client is thinking but might hesitate to articulate, and one is the backup person for the nurse and provides ideas for questions or approaches when the nurse is stumped. Each person can see and hear each of the others as they role-play encounters that are as realistic as possible (adapted from Kavanagh & Kennedy, 1992).

7. Effective communication involves listening attentively to people, accepting and acting on what they say, ensuring that all communication can be understood by everyone, being trustful and sincere, acting in socially and culturally appropriate ways, and regularly advising others about what is happening (Knowlden & Kavanagh, 2004). Discuss with someone you consider culturally competent how each of these criteria contributes to understanding in mental health settings.

8. The terrorist attacks in September 2001 and devastation of Hurricane Katrina in August 2005 left a lasting impact on America's mental health. Ongoing challenges, such as the wars in Iraq and Afghanistan and increasingly hostile weather associated with global warming add new risks and new opportunities. Discuss, in both societal and personal terms, how threats such as terrorism, violence, and threats pose hazards to positive mental health and challenge effective coping. In what ways has society been positively as well as negatively affected?

REFERENCES

Adams, A. (2000). The road not taken: How tribes choose between tribal and Indian Health Service management of health care resources. *American Indian Culture and Research Journal, 24*(3), 1–19.

American Psychiatric Association. (1980). *Diagnostic and statistical manual of mental disorders* (3rd ed.). Washington DC: Author.

American Psychiatric Association. (1987). *Diagnostic and statistical manual of mental disorders* (3rd ed., rev.). Washington DC: Author.

American Psychiatric Association. (1994). *Diagnostic and statistical manual of mental disorders* (4th ed.). Washington DC: Author.

American Psychiatric Association. (2000). *Diagnostic and statistical manual of mental disorders* (4th ed., text rev.). Washington DC: Author.

Andrews, M. M. (2003). Culturally competent nursing care. In M. M. Andrews & J. S. Boyle (Eds.), *Transcultural concepts in nursing care* (4th ed., pp. 15–35). Philadelphia: Lippincott Williams & Wilkins.

Armstrong, D. (2000). Social theorizing about health and illness. In G. L. Albrecht, R. Fitzpatrick, & S. C. Scrimshaw (Eds.), *The handbook of social studies in health and medicine* (pp. 24–35). London: Sage.

Baer, H. A. (2001). *Biomedicine and alternative healing systems in America: Issues of class, race, ethnicity, and gender.* Madison: University of Wisconsin Press.

Baer, R. D., Weller, S. C., Garcia, J. G. de A., & Rocha, A. L. S. (2004). A comparison of community and physician explanatory models of AIDS in Mexico and the United States. *Medical Anthropology Quarterly, 18*(1), 3–22.

Basuray, J. (2002). India: Transcultural nursing and health care. In M. Leininger & M. R. McFarland (Eds.), *Transcultural nursing: Concepts, theories, research, and practice* (3rd ed., pp. 477–491). New York: McGraw-Hill.

Berry, A. (2002). Culture care of the Mexican American family. In M. Leininger & M. R. McFarland (Eds.), *Transcultural nursing: Concepts, theories, research, and practice* (3rd ed., pp. 363–373). New York: McGraw-Hill.

Berry, A. B. 1999. Mexican American women's expressions of the meaning of culturally congruent prenatal care. *Journal of Transcultural Nursing, 10*(3), 203–212.

Biolsi, T. (2001). Contemporary Native American struggles. In I. Susser & T. C. Patterson (Eds.), *Cultural diversity in the United States: A critical reader* (pp. 175–189). Malden, MA: Blackwell.

Bliatout, B. T. (2003). Social and spiritual explanations of depression and nightmares. In K. A. Culhane-Pera, D. E. Vawter, P. Xiong, B. Babbitt, & M. M. Solberg (Eds.), *Healing by heart: Clinical and ethical case stories of Hmong families and Western providers* (pp. 209–215). Nashville, TN: Vanderbilt University Press.

Burkhardt, M. A., & Jacobson, M. G. N. (2000). Spirituality and health. In B. M. Dossey, L. Keegan, & C. E. Guzzetta (Eds.), *Holistic nursing: A handbook for practice* (3rd ed., pp. 91–121). Gaithersburg, MD: Aspen.

Leininger, M., & McFarland, M.R. (2002). *Transcultural Nursing: Concepts, theories, research, and practice* (3rd ed., pp. 415–428). New York: McGraw-Hill.

Christie, S. (2001). Renaissance man: The tribal "schizophrenic" in Sherman Alexie's "Indian Killer." *American Indian Culture and Research Journal, 25*(4), 1–19.

Crowe, M. (2000). The nurse–patient relationship: A consideration of its discursive context. *Journal of Advanced Nursing, 31,* 962–967.

Culhane-Pera, K. A., Vawter, D. E., Xiong, P., Babbitt, B., & Solberg, M. M. (2003). *Healing by heart: Clinical and ethical case stories of Hmong families and Western providers.* Nashville, TN: Vanderbilt University Press.

Culhane-Pera, K. A., & Xiong, P. (2003). Hmong culture: Tradition and change. In K. A. Culhane-Pera, D. E. Vawter, P.

Xiong, B. Babbitt, & M. M. Solberg (Eds.), *Healing by heart: Clinical and ethical case stories of Hmong families and Western providers* (pp. 11–68). Nashville, TN: Vanderbilt University Press.

Diekelmann, N. L. (1995). *Narrative pedagogy: Caring, dialogue, and practice.* Madison, WI: Advanced Nursing Institute for Heideggerian Hermeneutical Studies, University of Wisconsin-Madison.

Diekelmann, N. L. (2005). *Narrative pedagogy: Caring, dialogue, and practice.* Fairfax, VA: Advanced Nursing Institute for Heideggerian Hermeneutical Studies, George Mason University.

Dodgson, J. E., & Struthers, R. (2005). Indigenous women's voices: Marginalization and health. *Journal of Transcultural Nursing, 16*(4), 339–346.

Dossa, P. Narrative mediation of convertional and men "mental health" paradigms: reading the stories of immigrant and Iranian women. *Medical Anthropology Quarterly, 16*(3), 341–359.

Dossey, L. (2004–2005). The unsolved mystery of healing. *Shift: At the Frontiers of Consciousness,* December–February, 25–26.

Draucker, C. B., & Hessmiller, J. M. (2002). Telling stories of suffering and survival: Women and violence. In N. L. Diekelmann (Ed.), *First do no harm: Power, oppression, and violence in healthcare* (pp. 204–250). Madison: University of Wisconsin Press.

Dundes, L. (Ed.). (2003). *The manner born: Birth rites in cross-cultural perspective.* Walnut Creek, CA: AltaMira Press.

Duster, T. (2003). *Back door to eugenics.* New York: Routledge.

Estefan, A., McAllister, M., & Rowe, J. (2004). Difference, dialogue, dialectics: A study of caring and self-harm. In K. H. Kavanagh & V. Knowlden (Eds.), *Many voices: Toward caring culture in healthcare and healing* (pp. 21–61). Madison: University of Wisconsin Press.

Fadiman, A. (1999). *The spirit catches you and you fall down: A Hmong child, her American doctors, and the collision of two cultures.* New York: The Noonday Press, Farrar, Straus and Giroux.

Feller, L. M., Hunsley-McTighe, A., Ray, A. L., & Schliessmann, L. A. M. (2005). Rural South Dakota: The power of education and care delivery partnerships. *Home Health Care Management & Practice, 15*(X), 1–4.

Fine, M., Weis, L., Weseen, S., & Wong, L. (2000). For whom? Qualitative research, representations, and social responsibilities. In N. K. Denzin & Y. S. Lincoln (Eds.), *Handbook of qualitative research* (2nd ed., pp. 107–131). Thousand Oaks, CA: Sage.

Frank, G. (2000). *Venus on wheels: Two decades of dialogue on disability, biography, and being female in America.* Berkeley: University of California Press.

Freund, P. E. S., McGuire, M. B., & Podhurst, L. S. (2003). *Health, illness, and the social body: A critical sociology.* Upper Saddle River, NJ: Prentice Hall.

Goode, J. (1998). The contingent construction of local identities: Koreans and Puerto Ricans in Philadelphia. *Identities, 5,* 33–64.

Grossman, R. (2004, July 6). A nation divided by language? *The (Baltimore) Sun,* p. 4A.

Haasoun, R. (2004, September). Impact of US occupation in the Middle East on Arab Americans. *Anthropology News, 45*(6), 18–19.

Hartmann, S. M. (2002). Pauli Murray and the "Juncture of women's liberation and Black liberation." *Journal of Women's History, 14*(2), 74–77.

Harvey, G. (Ed.). (2003). *Shamanism: A reader.* London: Routledge.

Hauenstein, E. J. (1997). A nursing practice paradigm for depressed rural women: The women's affective illness treatment program. *Archives of Psychiatric Nursing, 1,* 37–45.

Helsel, D. G., & Mochel, M. (2002). Afterbirths in the afterlife: Cultural meaning of placental disposal in a Hmong American community. *Journal of Transcultural Nursing, 13*(3), 282–286.

Janzen, J. M. (2002). *The social fabric of health: An introduction to medical anthropology.* Boston: McGraw-Hill.

Jenkins, J. H., & Barrett, R. J. (Eds.). (2004). *Schizophrenia, culture, and subjectivity: The edge of experience.* Cambridge, UK: Cambridge University Press.

Kaptchuk, T. J. (2000). *The web that has no weaver: Understanding Chinese medicine.* Chicago: Contemporary Books.

Kavanagh, K. H. (2002). Neither here nor there: The story of a health professional's experience with getting care and needing caring. In N. L. Diekelmann (Ed.), *First do no harm: Power, oppression, and violence in healthcare* (pp. 49–117). Madison, WI: University of Wisconsin Press.

Kavanagh, K. H. (2003a). Mirrors: A cultural and historical interpretation of nursing's pedagogies. In N. L. Diekelmann (Ed.), *Teaching the practitioners of care: New pedagogies for the health professions* (pp. 59–153). Madison: University of Wisconsin Press.

Kavanagh, K. H. (2003b). Transcultural perspectives in mental health nursing. In M. M. Andrews & J. S. Boyle (Eds.), *Transcultural concepts in nursing care* (4th ed., pp. 272–314). Philadelphia: Lippincott Williams and Wilkins.

Kavanagh, K. H. (2005). Representing: Interpretive scholarship's consummate challenge. In P. M. Ironside (Ed.), *Beyond method: Philosophical conversations in healthcare research and scholarship* (pp. 58–110). Madison: University of Wisconsin Press.

Kavanagh, K. H., Absalom, K., Beil, W., & Schliessmann, L. (1999). Connecting and becoming culturally competent: A Lakota example. *Advances in Nursing Science, 21*(3), 9–31.

Kavanagh, K. H., & Kennedy, P. H. (1992). *Promoting cultural diversity: Strategies for health care professionals.* Newbury Park, CA: Sage.

Kess-Gardner, J. (2004). *The incredible journey: The Jermaine Gardner story.*

Baltimore: Incredible Journey Productions. *in healthcare and healing* (pp. 62–104). Madison: University of Wisconsin Press.

Kleinman, A., & Seeman, D. (2000). Personal experience of illness. In G. Albrecht, R. Fitzpatrick, & S. Scrimshaw (Eds.), *The handbook of social studies in health and medicine* (pp. 230–242). London: Sage.

Knowlden, V., & Kavanagh, K. H. (2004). An introduction: Caring and culture in interpretation and practice. In K. H. Kavanagh & V. Knowlden (Eds.), *Many voices: Toward caring culture in heathcare and healing* (pp. 3–20). Madison: University of Wisconsin Press.

Kottak, C. P. (2000). *Anthropology: The exploration of human diversity.* Boston: McGraw-Hill.

Leininger, M. M. (2002a). Japanese Americans and culture care. In M. Leininger & M. R. McFarland (Eds.), *Transcultural nursing: Concepts, theories, research, and practice* (3rd ed., pp. 453–464). New York: McGraw-Hill.

Leininger, M. M. (2002b). The theory of culture care and the ethnonursing research method. In M. Leininger & M. R. McFarland (Eds.), *Transcultural nursing: Concepts, theories, research, and practice* (3rd ed., pp. 71–98). New York: McGraw-Hill.

Leininger, M. M. (2002c). Transcultural mental health nursing. In M. Leininger & M. R. McFarland (Eds.), *Transcultural nursing: Concepts, theories, research, and practice* (3rd ed., pp. 239–252). New York: McGraw-Hill.

Li, P. S. (Ed.). (1999). *Race and ethnic relations in Canada* (2nd ed.). New York: Oxford University Press.

Lyfoung, P. (2003). Changing gender roles and domestic violence in the Hmong community: A feminist perspective. In K. A. Culhane-Pera, D. E. Vawter, P. Xiong, B. Babbitt, & M. M. Solberg (Eds.), *Healing by heart: Clinical and ethical case stories of Hmong families and Western providers* (pp. 234–238). Nashville, TN: Vanderbilt University Press.

Lowe, J. (2002). Balance and harmony through connectedness: The intentionality of Native American nurses. *Holistic Nursing Practice 16*(4), 4–11.

Luna, L. J. (2002). Arab Muslims and culture care. In M. Leininger & M. R. McFarland (Eds.), *Transcultural nursing: Concepts, theories, research, and practice* (3rd ed., pp. 301–311). New York: McGraw-Hill.

Mason, T. (1997). Seclusion and the lunar cycles. *Journal of Psychosocial Nursing, 35*(6), 14–18.

McAllister, M., & Walsh, K. (2003). C.A.R.E.: A framework for mental health. *Journal of Psychiatric and Mental Health Nursing, 9,* 39–48.

McElroy, A., & Jezewski, M. A. (2000). Cultural variation in the experience of health and illness. In G. Albrecht, R. Fitzpatrick, & S. Scrimshaw (Eds.), *Handbook of social studies in health and medicine* (pp. 191–209). London: Sage.

McEwen, M. M. (2005). Mexican immigrants' explanatory model of latent tuberculosis infection. *Journal of Transcultural Nursing, 16*(4), 347–355.

Meleis, A. I., & Im, E. O. (2002). Grandmothers and women's health: From fragmentation to coherence. *Health Care for Women International, 23*(2), 207–224.

Melton, A. P. (2005). Tradition and transition. *Shift: At the Frontiers of Consciousness,* June–August (7), 32–35.

Miller, L. (1999, July 9). Son of Elijah Muhammad preaches gentler Islam in tune with the times. *Wall Street Journal,* p. B2.

Miller, M., Serner, M., & Wagner, M. (2005). Sexual diversity among Black men who have sex with men in an inner city community. *Journal of Urban Health, 82*(Suppl. 1), i26–i34.

Morgan, S., & Maskovsky, J. (2003). The anthropology of welfare "reform:" New perspectives on U.S. urban poverty in the post-welfare era. *Annual Review of Anthropology, 32,* 315–338.

Mouanoutoua, V. L. (2003). Depression and posttraumatic stress disorder: Prevailing causes and therapeutic strategies with Hmong clients. In K. A. Culhane-Pera, D. E. Vawter, P. Xiong, B. Babbitt, & M. M. Solberg (Eds.), *Healing by heart: Clinical and ethical case stories of Hmong families and Western providers* (pp. 216–221). Nashville, TN: Vanderbilt University Press.

Mull, D. S., Nguyen, N., & Mull, J. D. (2001). Vietnamese diabetic patients and their physicians: What ethnography can teach us. *Western Journal of Medicine, 175*(5), 307–311.

Oakley, L. D., & Potter, C. (1997). *Psychiatric primary care.* St. Louis: C. V. Mosby.

Oswalt, W. H. (2006). *This land was theirs: A study of native North Americans* (8th ed.). New York: Oxford University Press.

National Center for Complementary and Alternative Medicine. (2000). *Expanding horizons of healthcare: Five year strategic plan, 2001–2005* (NIH Publication No. 01-5001). Washington DC: U.S. Government Printing Office. Retrieved from http://nccam.nih.gov/about/plans/fiveyear/fiveyear.pdf

Neugeboren, J. (1997). *Imagining Robert: My brother, madness, and survival: A memoir.* NY: William Morrow & Co.

Patterson, T. C. (2001). Class and historical process in the United States (pp. 16–28). In I. Susser & T. C. Patterson (Eds.), *Cultural diversity in the United States: A critical reader.* Malden, MA: Blackwell.

Ratanakul, P. (1999). Buddhism, health, disease, and Thai culture. In H. Coward & R. Ratanakul (Eds.), *A cross-cultural dialogue on healthcare ethics* (pp. 17–33). Waterloo, ON: Wilfrid Laurier University Press.

Reyhner, J. A., & Eder, J. (2004). *American Indian education: A history.* Norman: University of Oklahoma Press.

Rew, L. (2000). Self-reflection: Consulting the truth within. In B. M. Dossey, L. Keegan, & C. E. Guzzetta (Eds.), *Holistic nursing: A handbook for practice* (3rd ed., pp. 407–423). Gaithersburg, MD: Aspen.

Roche, B., Neaigus, A., & Miller, M. (2005). Street smarts and urban myths: Women, sex, work, and the role of storytelling in risk reduction and rationalization. *Medical Anthropology Quarterly, 19*(2), 149–170.

Rudmin, F. W. (2004, September). Torture at Abu Ghraib, and the telling silence of social scientists. *Anthropology News, 45*(6), 9.

Russell, D. (1997). An oral history project in mental health nursing. *Journal of Advanced Nursing, 26,* 489–495.

Rylko-Bauer, B., & Farmer, P. (2002). Managed care or managed inequality? A call for critiques of market-based medicine. *Medical Anthropology Quarterly, 16*(4), 476–502.

Sandhu, D. S. (1997). Psychocultural profiles of Asian and Pacific Islander Americans: Implications for counseling and psychotherapy. *Journal of Multicultural Counseling and Development, 25,* 7–22.

Schwarz, M. T. (2001). *Navajo lifeways: Contemporary issues, ancient knowledge.* Norman: University of Oklahoma Press.

Steeler, C. W. (2001). *Improving American Indian health care: The Western Cherokee experience* (R. L. Bashur & G. W. Shannon, Eds.). Norman: University of Oklahoma Press.

Struthers, R., & Lowe, J. (2003). Nursing in the Native American culture and historical trauma. *Issues in Mental Health Nursing, 24*(3), 257–272.

Thompson, J., & O'Dea, J. (2005). Social healing for a fractured world. *Shift: At the Frontiers of Consciousness,* June–August, (7), 10–13.

Tom-Orme, L. (2002). Transcultural nursing and health care among Native American peoples. In M. Leininger & M. R. McFarland (Eds.), *Transcultural nursing: Concepts, theories, research, and practice* (pp. 429–440). New York: McGraw-Hill.

Trafzer, C. E., & Weiner, D. (Eds.). (2001). *Medicine ways: Disease, health, and survival among Native Americans.* Walnut Creek, CA: AltaMira Press.

Tseng, W., & Streltzer, J. (1997). Integration and conclusions. In W. Tseng & J. Streltzer (Eds.), *Culture and psychopathology* (pp. 241–252). New York: Brunner/Mazel.

Turner, B. S. (2000). The history of the changing concepts of health and illness: Outline of a general model of illness categories. In G. L. Albrecht, R. Fitzpatrick, & S. C. Scrimshaw (Eds.), *The handbook of social studies in health and medicine.* London: Sage.

Urciuoli, B. (2001). The complex diversity of language in the United States. In I. Susser & T. C. Patterson (Eds.), *Cultural diversity in the United States: A critical reader* (pp. 190–205). Malden, MA: Blackwell.

U.S. Department of Health and Human Services. (2001). *Healthy people 2000.* Arlington, VA: CACI Marketing Systems.

Vontress, C. E., & Epp, L. R. (1997). Historical hostility in the African American client: Implications for counseling. *Journal of Multicultural Counseling and Development, 25,* 170–184.

Wagner, W. G. (2005). Confronting utilization review in New Mexico's Medicaid mental health system: The critical role of "medical necessity." *Medical Anthropology Quarterly, 19*(1), 64–83.

Westermeyer, J. (2003). Cultural interpretations of psychosis. In K. A. Culhane-Pera, D. E. Vawter, P. Xiong, B. Babbitt, & M. M. Solberg (Eds.), *Healing by heart: Clinical and ethical case stories of Hmong families and Western providers* (pp. 241–250). Nashville, TN: Vanderbilt University Press.

Wickramaseker, I. (1999). Hypnotherapy. In W. B. Jonas & J. S. Levin (Eds.), *Essentials of complementary and alternative medicine* (pp. 120–138). Philadelphia: Lippincott Williams & Wilkins.

Winkelman, M. (2001). Ethnicity and psychocultural models. In I. Susser & T. C. Patterson (Eds.), *Cultural diversity in the United States: A critical reader* (pp. 281–301). Malden, MA: Blackwell.

11

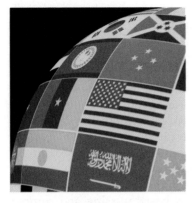

Culture, Family, and Community

Joyceen S. Boyle

Acculturation
Aggregates
Alternative therapies
Assimilation
Asylees
Community-based nursing
Community-based services
Community health nursing
Community nursing

Community settings
Cultural assessment
Cultural health care
    systems
Cultural knowledge
Enmeshment
Epidemiologic model
Immigrants
Kinship

Levels of prevention
Primary prevention
Refugee
Secondary prevention
Subcultures
Tertiary prevention
Traditional health beliefs
    and practices
Worldview

1. Use cultural concepts to provide care to families, communities, and aggregates.
2. Understand the necessary components of a cultural assessment of an aggregate group.
3. Explore interactions of community and culture as they relate to concepts of community-based practice.
4. Analyze how cultural factors influence health and illness of groups.
5. Critically evaluate potential health problems and solutions in refugee and immigrant populations.
6. Assess factors that influence the health of diverse groups within the community.

An understanding of culture and cultural concepts enhances the nurse's knowledge and facilitates culturally competent nursing care in **community-based settings**. Currently, many nurses practice in community settings with clients from a wide variety of cultural backgrounds, and this trend is expected to increase with more nurses moving from acute-care institutions to community settings. The care of clients in the community can be extremely complex, calling for a high level of nursing skill. In addition, it is predicted that cultural diversity will increase in the United States. Trends in the health care delivery system as well as an increased emphasis on health promotion and disease prevention have influenced nurses to make changes in their practice as well as the setting in which care is delivered. Concepts such as partnership, collaboration, empowerment, and facilitation now form the basis for community-based nursing practice with individuals, families, and **aggregates** in the community. For some time, national nursing associations, including the National Institute of Nursing Research (NINR), have urged a community focus in both nursing research and practice. For example, NINR defines community-based services as those services requiring "active involvement of clients and communities in assessing the needs for care, designing service programs, implementing interventions, and evaluating outcomes" (NINR, 1995, p. 2). While it is possible to provide community-based nursing services to individuals and families in communities as well as to provide community-oriented nursing care to either the community or groups within the community, for culturally relevant care to be provided, clients and populations must be involved in all aspects of the care or services.

Community-based services that are culturally relevant to the people served are built on collaboration and partnerships between community leaders, health consumers, and health care providers. When community residents or health consumers are involved as partners, community-based services are more likely to be responsive to locally defined needs, are better used, and are sustained through local action. The NINR *Strategic Plan on Reducing Health Disparities* provides leadership in emphasizing the inclusion of cultural and ethnic considerations, as well as collaborative efforts among federal, state, and local agencies for broad-based public and private collaboration and partnerships as prerequisites for funding of community-based research and services (Flynn, 1997; NINR, n.d.) This implies a sustained collaboration between the public and private sectors as well as those persons most directly affected by health concerns or health problems.

Community-based services are complex and often fragile. They require a high level of nursing knowledge and skill in working with and relating to different individuals and groups. In many instances, the complexity is increased when clients and their families come from diverse cultures. Nurses must understand how to help persons from various cultures work with community leaders and health care providers to form partnerships that are responsive and can structure nursing care in ways that are culturally sensitive and appropriate. It is often the cultural factors that determine whether a particular population or group will choose to participate in community-based health services. There is always a need for continuing communication among health care providers and community residents that is characterized by mutual understanding and respect. It is this understanding and respect that forms the basis for culturally relevant and competent nursing care.

In this chapter, the terms **community nursing, community-based nursing,** and **community health nursing** are used interchangeably, even though they have different meanings in some settings and in different contexts (Williams, 2006). Whether the nurse is employed as a community health nurse in a health department or practices in a community-based setting, he or she needs the knowledge and skills to provide culturally competent care. The practice of nursing in a community setting requires that nurses be comfortable with clients from diverse cultures and the broader socioeconomic context in which they live. In the current health care climate of economic restraints, the health care industry has focused on cost-effectiveness, and sometimes this has been misguided. Care that is not congruent with the client's value system is likely to increase the cost of care because it compromises quality. Furthermore, members of diverse cultural groups, such as the officially designated minority groups in the United States, tend to experience greater health disparities than do members of the general population. This was the impetus for targeting the four ethnic minority groups in *Healthy People 2000* (U.S. Department of Health and Human Services, 1990) and *Healthy People 2010* (U.S. Department of Health and Human Services, 2000) because cultural diversity must be respected and taken into account by health care professionals. Equally important, we must address the stark disparities that exist in health status between minority groups and the wider American society.

Overview of Culturally Competent Nursing Care in Community Settings

Nurses practice in many settings within the community, including work sites, schools, physicians' offices, health care program sites, churches, and the community itself (Figure 11–1). The use of **cultural knowledge** in community-based nursing practice begins with a careful assessment of clients and families in their own environments. Cultural data that have implications for nursing care are selected from clients, families, and the environment during the assessment phase and are discussed with the client and family to develop mutually shared goals.

Community nurses are particularly challenged when they frequently encounter clients and families who must change behaviors and living patterns to maintain health or promote wellness. Nursing interventions based on cultural knowledge help clients and families to adjust more easily and assist nurses to work effectively and comfortably with all clients, especially those from different cultural backgrounds.

Cultural data are important in the care of all clients; however, in community nursing, they are a prerequisite to successful nursing interventions. Community nursing is practiced in a community setting, often in the home of the client, and frequently requires more active participation by the client and family. Usually, the client and family must make basic changes in lifestyle, such as changes in diet and exercise patterns. Cultural competence requires that the nurse understand the family lifestyle and value system, as well as those cultural forces that are powerful determinants of health-related behaviors. Nurses often work closely with clients with chronic diseases or other health problems over a long time, and nursing interventions must include aspects of counseling and education as well as anticipatory guidance directed toward helping clients and families adjust to what may be lifelong conditions. Nursing care must take account of the diverse cultural factors that will motivate clients to make successful changes in behavior because improvement in health status requires lifestyle and behavioral modifications.

Transcultural nursing practice has the potential to improve the health of the community as well as the health of individual clients and families. An additional consideration of the nurse who is involved in community-focused planning is the health needs of populations at risk. Special at-risk groups can be found in all communities: the homeless, the poor, persons with HIV/AIDS and/or tuberculosis, refugees, prison populations, and even the elderly are groups at risk for decreased health status. From a community standpoint, an understanding of culture and cultural concepts will increase the skill and abilities of the nurse to work with diverse groups within the community. Identification of high-risk groups and appropriate community-based strategies to reduce health risks requires considerable knowledge about cultural and ethnic groups and their place in the community.

Consider, if you will, what problems might arise if one were to design a health program for a

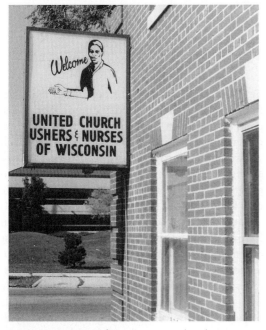

FIGURE 11-1. Some African American churches are organized to meet health, social, and emotional needs of church members.

community composed primarily of Vietnamese people who recently arrived in the United States. They may have spent years in refugee camps in other countries and lost many family members, or their family members may be still in Vietnam and they are now making a life for themselves in a strange country. Certainly language would be a major problem, but so could many other cultural differences, from nuances in communication to differences in beliefs of what constitutes health and illness, as well as treatment and cure. A failure to understand and deal with these differences would have serious implications for the success of any health or nursing intervention. Nurses who have knowledge of, and an ability to work with, diverse cultures are able to devise effective community interventions to reduce risks that are consistent with the community, group, and individual values and beliefs of community members.

A Transcultural Framework

A distinguishing and important aspect of community-based nursing practice is the nursing focus on the community as the client (Nies & McEwen, 2007; Stanhope & Lancaster, 2006). Effective community nursing practice must reflect accurate knowledge of the causes and distribution of health problems and of effective interventions that are congruent with the values and goals of the community. An **epidemiologic model** can be used by the community nurse to collect, organize, and analyze information about high-risk groups that are encountered in community practice.

An epidemiologic model emphasizes human biology, environment, lifestyle, and the health care system; however, with modifications, the nurse can use this model to collect cultural data that influence the health of the community (Clark, 2003). The epidemiologic model focuses on the community or on aggregate groups rather than on individuals or families. Using a cultural overlay with the epidemiologic model enhances nurse–community interactions in numerous ways.

Identifying Subcultures and Devising Specific Community-Based Interventions

A transcultural framework for nursing care helps the nurse to identify subcultures within the larger community and to devise community-based interventions that are specific to community health and nursing needs. For example, in the multicultural societies of the United States, it is common to speak of "the Black community," "the Hispanic community," or "the Francophone community." We might also speak more broadly of "the immigrant community" or the "refugee community" or of other unique groups within or near a local community. A cultural focus allows this variety and facilitates data collection about specific groups based on their health risks. A cultural/epidemiologic framework facilitates a view of the community as a complex collective yet allows for diversity within the whole. Interventions that are successful in one subgroup may fail with another subgroup of the same community, and often the failure can be attributed to cultural differences or barriers that arise because of these differences.

Identifying and Analyzing Various Components of the Community

Transcultural concepts often are useful in identifying and analyzing various components of the community, such as social structure and religious and political systems. A cultural approach allows the nurse to identify **cultural health care systems**, which are made up of individuals who experience illness as well as those who provide care for them. Anderson and MacFarlane (2004) suggest that each cultural health care system can have as many as three recognized sectors, most commonly referred to as popular, folk, and professional. We often forget that alternative systems and **alternative therapies** exist side by side with the professional system. How individuals organize themselves to meet group and individual needs within the cultural health care system is important information for community and transcultural nurses. An assessment of whether social institutions such as churches and schools meet the health, social, and emotional needs of their members, and whether the health and political systems are responsive to the needs of all citizens, can sometimes pinpoint critical needs and identify gaps in care. Cultural traditions within a community often determine the structure of community support systems as well as how resources are organized and distributed.

Identifying the Values and Cultural Norms of a Community

A transcultural framework is essential to the community nurse's identification of the values and cultural norms of a community. Although values are universal features of all cultures, their types and expressions vary widely, even within the same community. Values often serve as the foundation for a community's acceptance and use of health resources or a group's participation in community-based intervention programs to promote health and wellness. Just as nurses share data and collaborate with clients and families to establish mutually acceptable goals for nursing care, the community-based nurse works with the community or aggregates within the community to plan community-focused health programs. In addition to forming partnerships with communities, the community nurse considers the influences of social, economic, ecologic, and political issues. Larger policy issues directly and profoundly affect many, if not all, community health issues. These larger policy issues are, in turn, influenced by the wider national and/or international culture. An example of this can be seen in the recent emphasis on bioterrorism, now a focus and concern of local and state health departments as well as national.

Cultural Issues in Community Nursing Practice

The need for nurses to be sensitive to clients who are culturally different is increasing as we become more aware of the complex interactions between health care providers and clients and how these interactions might affect the client's health. The material in this chapter will assist nurses to be aware of cultural factors that affect health, illness, and the practice of nursing in community settings. Several cultural assessment tools or guides are available that provide comprehensive frameworks to guide the nurse in the assessment of cultural factors in the care of individuals, families, and groups. The Andrews/Boyle Transcultural Nursing Assessment Guide (see Appendix A) provides an outline for the nurse to collect and assess cultural data relevant to individuals, families, and communities. The majority of cultural assessment guides are oriented to individuals and occasionally to families. Only a few have the comprehensive view necessary for assessing cultural factors for intervention at the community level. Because individual clients and their families constitute larger communities, nurses who work in community settings must understand cultural issues as they relate to individuals and families as well as communities. We shall begin with a discussion of cultural influences on individuals and families before moving to a discussion of cultural factors within communities.

Cultural Influences on Individuals and Families

When assessing individuals and families, the community health nurse should carefully examine the following:

1. Family roles, typical family households and structure, and dynamics in the family, particularly communication patterns and decision making
2. Health beliefs and practices related to disease causation, treatment of illness, and the use of indigenous healers or folk practitioners and other alternative therapies
3. Patterns of daily living, including work and leisure activities
4. Social networks, including friends, neighbors, kin, and significant others, and how they influence health and illness

5. Ethnic, cultural, or national identity of client and family, e.g., identification with a particular group, including language
6. Nutritional practices and how they relate to cultural factors and health
7. Religious preferences and influences on well-being, health maintenance, and illness, as well as the impact religion might have on daily living and taboos arising from religious beliefs that might influence health status or care
8. Culturally appropriate behavior styles, including what is manifested during anger, competition, and cooperation, as well as relationships with health care professionals, relationships between genders, and relations with groups in the community

A cultural assessment of individuals and families includes all the preceding factors. This list is by no means exhaustive; rather, it is presented as a guide for community nurses as they assess cultural aspects of individuals and families.

Cultural values shape human health behaviors and determine what individuals and families will do to maintain their health status, how they will care for themselves and others who become ill, and where and from whom they will seek health care. Most importantly family members are often the ones who decide on the course of treatment. Families have an important role in the transmission of cultural values and learned behaviors that relate to both health and illness. It is in the family context that individuals learn basic ways to stay healthy and to ensure the well-being of themselves and their family members.

One commonality shared by members of functioning families is a concern for the health and wellness of each individual within the family because the family has the primary responsibility for meeting the health needs of its members. The nurse not only must assess the health of each family member, but also define how well the family can meet family health needs. Just how well families function in relation to this will determine how, when, and where interventions will take place; by whom; and what the specific approach to the family will be. A cultural orientation assists the nurse in understanding cultural values and interactions, the roles that family members assume, and the support system available to the family to help them when health problems are identified.

The family is usually an individual's most important social unit and provides the social context within which illness occurs and is resolved and within which health promotion and maintenance occur. Most **traditional health beliefs and practices** promote the health of the family because they are generally family and socially oriented. Frequently, traditional beliefs and practices reinforce family cohesion. Some values are more central and influential than others; given a competing set of demands, these central values will typically determine a family's priorities. In families that adhere to traditional cultural values, the family's (or tribe's or community's) needs and goals often will take precedence over an individual's needs and goals. The culturally competent nurse can recognize and use the family's role in promoting and maintaining health. This requires an appreciation of the family context in health and illness and how this varies among diverse cultures. Box 11–1 provides some ideas on how to develop the cultural competence and sensitivity that is necessary for successful health promotion programs for diverse cultural groups.

Cultural Factors Within Communities

In addition to identifying and meeting the cultural needs of clients and families, the community health nurse must consider social and cultural factors on a community level to respect cultural values, mobilize local resources, and develop culturally appropriate health programs and services. Important cultural factors include demographics in the United States, with detailed data on specific states and cities; cultural diversity in communities; subpopulations in the United States; refugee and immigrant populations, with special consideration given to newly

BOX 11-1

Developing Cultural Competence to Promote Health in Diverse Cultural Groups

- Learn about the history of the cultural group or diverse population with which you are working. For example, an understanding of African American culture would not be complete without considering the effect of slavery on this group of Americans.
- Make an effort to understand the cultural values beliefs and ways of life of the community. Read some of the works of noted African American authors such as James Baldwin, Malcolm X, Langston Hughes, etc.
- Incorporate as many of the traditional values, beliefs, and ways of life into the design and use of any educational materials. Whereas Chinese American teenagers might prefer a comic book or video in English, their grandparents might prefer a health magazine or a news article in the Chinese language.
- Become familiar with the appropriate verbal and nonverbal communication patterns within the group as well as many of the communication nuances that are contextual in nature. An example might be that a traditional Afghan woman would never speak to a strange man outside of her own kinship circle.
- Become familiar with beliefs and practices related to religion, gender, food preferences, and other related

cultural differences that might lead to the quick success or failure of a health program. Be aware that the most effective health programs are those that foster community ownership and involvement. This implies that they must be planned with community input.
- Spend as much time as possible within the community, attending local events. Examples might be churches, school programs, fairs, and meetings with leaders. Taking an intervention into the community rather than having the community come to the intervention might be more effective over time. See Evidence-Based Practice Box 7–3, "*Cafecitos* and *telenovelas: Culturally competent interventions to facilitate Mexican American (MA) families' decisions to use home care services.*" This article describes the importance of community involvement on the part of nurses.
- Seek the community's input and feedback for any health program that is planned for the community. Be aware that the use of peer educators, such as *promotoras* from within the community, has been found to be effective in delivering health promotion programs to diverse communities.

Adapted from Huff, R. M., & Kline, M. V. (1999). *Promoting health in multicultural populations*. Thousand Oaks, CA: Sage.

arrived refugee communities; maintenance of traditional cultural values and practices; and access to health and nursing care for diverse cultural groups.

Demographics and Health Care

During the 21st century, the United States and many other countries will face enormous demographic, social, and culture change. North America is becoming more diverse, not less so, and thus it is incumbent on nurses to be prepared to respond appropriately. Since the 1990s and 2000s, there has been a steady growth in cultural diversity in the United States. The health status of individuals in the United States differs dramatically across cultural groups and social classes. Certain population groups in the United

States face greater challenges than the general population in accessing timely and needed health care services, and national goals have been adopted in *Healthy People 2010* to address these health disparities (U.S. Department of Health and Human Services, 2000). Major indicators such as morbidity and mortality rates for adults and infants show that the health status of minority Americans in the United States is substantially worse than that of White Americans. The same holds true for differences in social class: Health status is worse among those who live in poverty. Similarly, older people, the unemployed, welfare recipients, single women supporting children, and minorities and immigrants have a higher chance of experiencing poor health (U.S. Department of Health and Human Services,

2000). Lack of economic resources predisposes individuals, families, and communities to major difficulties in accessing appropriate health care. Thus, community nurses must assess groups within the community in a very sensitive manner; often those characteristics that we assume are related to the group's culture may be caused by poverty instead.

Cultural Diversity Within Communities

The United States has many diverse cultures as a result of the history of immigration to this country by a variety of cultural and ethnic groups and because of the indigenous populations of Native Americans, Native Alaskans, and Native Hawaiians. If current immigration trends continue, the United States will consist of an even greater variety of cultural groups. In 2005, minority groups accounted for 33% of the population. Assuming that current trends continue, the U.S. Census Bureau News (2004, March 18) projects that by the middle of the 21st century, minorities will account for more than 50% of the total population. Although most people in this country share broad cultural values, a rich diversity of cultural orientations does exist, including those with considerable variations in health and illness practices.

Subcultures in the United States

Subcultures are aggregates of people that establish certain rules of behavior, values, and living ways that are different from mainstream culture. Leininger described subcultures as having "distinctive patterns of living with sets of rules, special values and practices that are different from the dominant culture" (1995, p. 60). Many newcomers to the United States are actually relatives of citizens or are new immigrants, adding numbers to the original subculture. Obviously, there can also be diversity within each subculture. Hispanic culture as a group includes Mexican North Americans, Puerto Ricans, Cubans, and Central and South Americans, as well as undocumented individuals, and there is diversity within each of these groups.

Certain geographic areas of the country, such as Appalachia, can be singled out as containing subcultures. Persons born and reared in the South or in New York City can often be identified by their language and mannerisms as members of a distinct subculture. We used to believe that the United States had a "melting pot" culture in which new arrivals gave up their former languages, customs, and values to become Americans. It is now agreed that the "melting pot" or "blending" concept may not be appropriate, at least not for everyone. A more accurate metaphor would be to view the U.S. population as a rich and complex tapestry of colors, backgrounds, and interests (Figure 11–2).

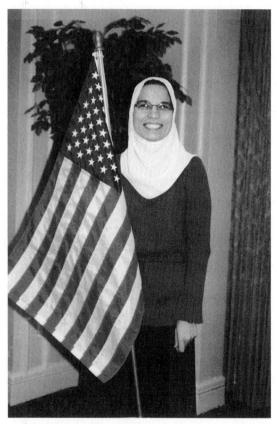

FIGURE 11-2. Communication between people from different cultures can help to break down misunderstandings, stereotypes, and other cultural barriers. Immigrants from other cultures have contributed much to enrich American culture.

Refugee and Immigrant Populations

Immigrants are persons who voluntarily and legally immigrate to the United States to live. Immigrants come of their own choice, and most plan to eventually become citizens of their new host country. Of course, many persons also come to the United States, Canada, and Western Europe illegally or without the proper documentation. Although terms differ for these persons, in the United States they usually are referred to as "undocumented" or, perhaps in a more pejorative sense, "illegal immigrants." Evidence-Based Practice 11-1, the Lost Boys of the Sudan, discusses health issues and coping strategies used by unaccompanied refugee youth from the Sudan. Under international law, *refugee* is a special term that describes a person who is outside of his or her country of nationality or habitual residence and who has a well-founded fear of persecution if he or she returns to his or her own country.

By definition then, refugees are persons escaping persecution based on race, religion, nationality, or political stance (United Nations Economic Commission for Europe, n.d.). Table 11–1 shows other terms that are used to refer to persons who are in the process of moving to another country or leaving their birthplace or a country in transition. Currently, immigration is a contentious issue in the industrialized nations of the world, and many of the key issues in the debate on immigration policy are economic (Friedberg & Hunt, 1995).

Perhaps the most well-known group of refugees is made up of persons who came to the United States from Southeast Asia after the Vietnam War. In more recent times, refugees have come to the United States from the Sudan, Somalia, Eastern Europe, the Middle East, and other countries undergoing violent transitions; refugees are fleeing war, famine, and other social upheavals. They are fleeing for their lives and safety rather than personally choosing to leave their homeland. The term *refugee* and the status of an individual who is a refugee have legal meanings and designations that differ from those of ordinary immigrants. Another classification of newcomers is that of **asylees**—persons who come to a particular country seeking political asylum from some sort of persecution in their home country. These various types of classification—immigrant, refugee, asylee, or undocumented or illegal immigrant—often determine the rights of individuals (e.g., the granting of work permits or residency status, or the types of social and health services that newcomers may access). In addition, those who are undocumented, or without appropriate residency status may face arrest and deportation to their country of origin.

The United States has grown and achieved its success as a nation of immigrants and foreigners. Immigration is a continuing phenomenon in our countries. Many recent immigrants and refugees are not acculturated to prevailing Western norms of health beliefs or behaviors. Many arrive with scant economic resources and must learn English and become economically self-sufficient as quickly as possible. Certain factors such as settlement patterns or living near friends or family, communication networks, social class, and education have helped many immigrants maintain their cultural traditions. In writing about the transitions that immigrants face, Meleis (1997) noted that immigrant or refugee communities provide support for newcomers and opportunities for cultural continuity because these ethnic communities reflect the identities of the home countries. At the same time, belonging to such a community tends to set immigrants and refugees apart and isolate them from the larger community. For example, newcomers from Mexico realize that they need to learn English to get better jobs, but they often join expanding Latino communities where most residents speak Spanish. Learning English well enough to obtain employment in the English-speaking world is difficult, and it is to their credit that most immigrants and refugees do learn English and make significant contributions to their new country. Nevertheless, where immigrants live and how they participate should remain individual choices and privileges rather than prescribed options.

In addition to the legal entrance of immigrants and refugees, many other persons seeking

Evidence-Based Practice 11–1:

The Lost Boys of the Sudan

Refugee children, those who are unaccompanied by a parent or relative, are at highest risk because of the interplay between traumatic experiences and separation from significant others. In the late 1980s, during the civil war in the Sudan, an estimated 17,000 children fled their homes when their parents and families were killed and their villages burned. Most of these children were boys from the Dinka and Nuer tribes of southern Sudan, and many were as young as 3 or 4 years old when they fled. They spent many months traveling by foot over large distances in hostile territory inhabited by rebel troops, rebel recruitment squads, slave traders, and rival tribes. They finally stumbled into a large refugee camp where they spent the next 8 years in mud huts that they built, subsisting on rations of corn and lentils, raising themselves and each other. In 1999, the United Nations High Commissioner for Refugees (UNHCR) recommended 3,600 of these unaccompanied refugee youth for resettlement in the United States. The study reported here explores how unaccompanied minor refugee youths, who grew up amidst violence and loss, coped with trauma and hardships. While their stories were replete with tales of horrors and sufferings of young children caught up in war and famine, four themes were identified that reflected coping strategies: (a) collectivity and the communal self, (b) suppression and distraction, (c) making meaning, and (d) emergence from hopelessness to hope.

Clinical Application

1. The Sudanese youth had a strong sense of communal identity with their fellow Sudanese refugees. The Sudanese youth saw themselves as a part of a "collective," telling stories with the words *we* and *us*. Strong social networks were evident.
2. The youth kept busy with school and resettlement in the United States to protect themselves from feelings that they felt powerless to handle. The strategy of not thinking about traumatic events was effective with the immediate situation but not necessarily effective in the long term. Mental health workers must be available to help unaccompanied youth refugees.
3. Storytelling is an effective method of coping for refugees who have undergone such trauma and violence.
4. Children's or youth's responses to traumatic situations cannot be understood by focusing only on individual mediating factors; the mediating factors of social, political, and ecological contexts must also be considered.
5. The importance of hope is significant for refugee youth.
6. Because developmental changes influence coping and resilience, questions remain about how the strategies the boys used to cope with difficulties will play out in their development.

Goodman, J. H. (2004). Coping with trauma and hardship among unaccompanied refugee youths from Sudan. *Qualitative Health Research, 14*(9), 1177–1196.

"Terms"	"Description of Terms".
TABLE 11-1 *Terms Used for Indiviuals Residing in a Country Who are not Citizens*	
Illegal immigrant	A person who is in a country without the appopriate documentation and permission
Immigrant	A person who comes to a country to take up permanent residence
Refugee	A person who is escaping persecution based on race, religion, nationality, or political persuasion
Emigrant	A person departing from a country to settle elsewhere
Émigré	A person forced to emigrate for political reasons
Asylee	A person seeking political asylum from persecution in his or her home country
Temporary stay migrant	A person who moves to another country with the intention of staying there for only a limited time, usually for occupational reasons
Undocumented	A person without the required documents that provide evidence of status or qualification, such as nationality or specified length of time a person may legally reside within a country

political asylum have entered the United States from all over the world. Often those seeking asylum or those who enter the country both legally and illegally are at considerable risk for health and social problems (Aroian, 1993; Yount, McEwen, & Boyle, in press). Table 11–1 shows terms commonly used for individuals residing in a country where they are not citizens. In addition to language and employment barriers, they have few economic resources, some have experienced rapid change and traumatic life events, their coping abilities have been overwhelmed, and few resources are available to assist them. Immigrants in general, whether they are here legally or illegally, have special health risks. Health care along the U.S.–Mexico border poses special problems and challenges for residents who live there.

Special Considerations: Cultural Factors Affecting an Afghan-American Community

*Afghans fled their country beginning in 1978 after a coup d'etat by the communist faction of the Afghan government, which was followed by an invasion from the Soviet Union. Although the Soviets left Afghanistan in 1989, continued fighting between political groups and the deprivations of war reduced Afghanistan's population from 15.5 million to 8 or 9 million people (Lipson, 1991). Lipson (1991) pointed out that a

decade ago, Afghans, who had fled the Soviet-Afghan war, were the largest group of refugees in the world. Pakistan was host to 3.4 million, Iran had 2.2 million, and a third group of countries, including the United States, hosted 100,000 Afghans. Then, a radical fundamentalist Islamic group, the Taliban, gained control of the Afghan government in 1996 and imposed its harsh view of Islamic law on the population (McGeary, 2001). This included the severe repression of women, including seclusion and veiling as well as other extreme measures, such as forbidding the education of women and prohibiting them from occupational pursuits or working in public places. Several years of famine and natural disasters have further worsened the conditions in this country, long one of the poorest in the world. The number of Afghans fleeing their country has once again greatly accelerated after the September 11, 2001, terrorist attack in the United States and the subsequent antiterrorist campaign focused on the Taliban forces in Afghanistan.

In particular, Afghan refugees and immigrants have undergone stressful, traumatic, and

*The author thanks Juliene G. Lipson, RN, PhD, FAAN, for her assistance and contributions to the sections in this chapter about Afghan refugees.

even catastrophic experiences such as war, torture, refugee camps, death of family members, and loss of homeland. Obviously, under such circumstances, the experiences associated with fleeing one's country of birth can produce psychologic stress (Lipson, 1993). However, trying to make a new life in their host country can also be very stressful. Factors such as unemployment, decreased family income, changes in lifestyle, lack of ability to speak English, culture conflict, and separation from family and loved ones continue to add to stress and decrease the quality of life for many Afghan refugees (Lipson & Omidian, 1997).

Studies have indicated that many Afghan refugees experience posttraumatic stress disorder, which follows a psychologically traumatic event outside of the range of usual human experiences. The symptoms may include nightmares, depression, withdrawal, hopelessness, sleep disorders, and other somatic complaints (American Psychiatric Association, 1987). The terrorism attack of September 11, 2001, and its association with Afghanistan has only added to the stress faced by Afghan refugees living in the United States, such as coping with biases against them and hate crimes and dealing with pain at the further destruction of their country. However, Afghan activists are redoubling their efforts on behalf of women's rights and in educating the public about Afghanistan and Islam.

TRADITIONAL AFGHAN CULTURE

Traditional culture in Afghan was strongly patriarchal and has been divided among tribal, political, social class, and ethnic lines. These political divisions continue after Afghans leave their country and are often intensified by the high levels of stress as they attempt to cope with life in the United States. Traditional customs include arranged marriages, often between first cousins; polygyny when affordable (as many as four wives); and a patriarchal family system (Lipson & Omidian, 1992). Women are usually fairly young when they marry and have less education than men. Marriage and childbearing have traditionally been the only acceptable roles for women. There are considerable variations, given that

Afghan family life is in transition. Women do not usually socialize with men outside the family. Afghan women remain in the home and primarily socialize with other women within the extended family; however, many women work to help support the family, and some educated women are activists in the community, both here in the United States and back home in Afghanistan. Despite social class and generational variations, family life is the core of Afghan culture. A key difference between Afghan and American culture is family interdependence versus individualism. For traditional Afghans, family obligations always come before anything else. Lipson and Omidian (1992) reported that culture conflict is central to the difficulties that Afghans face in adjustment to a new life in the United States.

CHARACTERISTICS OF AN AFGHAN AMERICAN COMMUNITY

A community assessment of an Afghan community within the United States requires that the nurse assess cultural factors such as **kinship**, religious practices, family roles and patterns, language use, and cultural health beliefs and practices. Obviously, other parameters of a community assessment such as population trends, environment, industry, education, recreation, and health care services are important also. However, the composition of refugee and other immigrant communities requires that nurses study and interpret cultural data and understand how these data influence health and wellness. DeSantis has observed "that interventions that are not built on an understanding of the concept of culture will always limit the effectiveness of nursing" (1997, p. 184).

Although Afghans share nationality and religion, the community is strongly heterogeneous and divisive in politics, social class, ethnicity, and region as well as urban or rural origin in Afghanistan (Lipson, 1991). Afghans, even when living in the United States, often appear to be divided and disorganized along the traditional lines of politics, social class, and urban or rural origin. Lack of community cohesion is not unusual because Afghans are organized by kinship and the extended family. Barth

(1987) observed that these divisions reflect Afghanistan's traditional tribal social structure. Tribal structure is often difficult for Americans to understand. Lipson and Miller (1994) and Lipson and Omidian (1997) found that the Afghan community is further divided along gender and generational lines—the experiences of men, women, and the children who have grown up in the United States are strikingly different from those of their elders. Thus, any attempt to bring health care services to the community or to address some of the community's health problems must take into account the tremendous diversity within the whole community. This obviously requires flexibility and ingenuity on the part of health care professionals. Further complicating this situation are several languages. Most Afghans speak Pashto or Dari (Farsi/Persian), but other languages are also spoken. Elderly women, in particular, are illiterate (not able to read or write) in their own language (Lipson, Omidian, & Paul, 1995).

THE AFGHAN FAMILY

Family life is at the core of Afghan culture. Although many health care professionals are familiar with strong family systems among the family groups that they care for, they still may have difficulty comprehending the differences and the profound influence of Afghan family life on psychologic well-being. Lipson & Miller (1994) reported that what Western psychiatrists call **enmeshment** (and is labeled as abnormal by American culture) is normal family behavior for Afghans. Afghans tend to socialize almost exclusively with extended family members, and this can cause cultural conflict when they live in the United States because there may be geographic distances between the family members, thus making frequent visiting difficult. Afghan culture supports dependence on family members, whereas North American culture emphasizes independence and individualism. Extended family obligations, especially to parents and older siblings, take precedence over all other responsibilities, including affiliation with one's spouse, work responsibilities, and certainly one's own preferences and needs. Extended families may

average 50 to 70 individuals and are contained within a tribal unit of 1,000 or more. The main social events are related to family obligations such as engagement parties and weddings. In traditional families, these parties can be very elaborate and occur over several days and nights.

Afghan Women's Roles

Most Afghans are staunch Muslims. Although the role of women is changing, women tend to socialize almost exclusively with other women. They experience conflict over women's freedom, conflict between maintaining traditional values and becoming Americanized, role overload from adding new American roles to Afghan roles, a lack of suitable spouses for single women, and parenting difficulties.

Lipson and Miller (1994) reported that there are generational differences in changes in women's roles. For example, elderly women, who are often widows, appear the most stressed and unhappy. They are socially isolated because their grown children and grandchildren work outside the home or are at school. Many women, especially if they are of late middle age or older, do not speak English and are essentially homebound; they miss the constant visiting and support from kin that they experienced back home in Afghanistan. Traditionally, the status of women in Afghanistan increased with age, but this has not been the case in the United States, and elderly women tend to dwell on past traumatic experiences, to be depressed, and to experience numerous psychosomatic symptoms (Lipson & Miller, 1994). There are variations in Afghan family life after families have relocated to the United States. Thus, it is important to carefully assess each situation rather than making assumptions based on stereotypes.

Middle-aged Afghan women, like other women refugees, have experienced profound role changes. In traditional Islamic culture, a woman's proper place is in the home. However, in the United States, it has been necessary for many Afghan women to work outside the home. Many professional Afghan women at first have had difficulty obtaining employment in their accustomed profession, and often they have been able to find only low-status jobs in the United States. As women's roles have changed, their husbands have often reacted with frustration. Some men have begun to drink heavily or abuse family members, increasing the stress and pressure on women and families.

Single status is viewed as unnatural. As previously stated, women marry at a fairly young age. However, finding an appropriate spouse has been difficult for some young Afghan women. Many Afghan men believe that women who have lived in the United States have been contaminated by American ideas and thus are not properly submissive to their husbands. Unmarried women live with parents or siblings; it would be extremely rare for a young woman to live alone. There are no role models for single women. Teenage girls are also caught in a bind. Daughters who do not maintain modest behavior are perceived as destroying the family's reputation. Traditional Afghans perceive the dress, makeup, behavior, speech, and freedom of American teenagers as improper and even immoral. Young Afghan women who have spent several years in the United States, exposed to a culture that views women in quite a different way, are not always willing to marry traditional Afghan men.

Afghan parents frequently worry about their children as they are exposed to American culture at school and on television. Sex, violence, and other controversial aspects of American life are pervasive and difficult to avoid. Children tend to acculturate more rapidly than their parents, learning English more quickly and, in general, adapting to new social roles and gender identities as well as establishing roots in American culture. This does not imply that Afghan childhood is free from conflict. On the contrary, the cultural clash between generations can be profound, given that Afghan parents are often adamantly opposed to many of the American cultural beliefs and behaviors their children have acquired. This is often a source of great conflict and dissension.

In his book, *Come Back to Afghanistan: A California Teenager's Story*, Said Hyder Akbar (Akbar & Burton, 2005), who came to the United States from Afghanistan when he was 2 years of age,

answers the question: Do you feel more Afghan or more American? He writes, "My identity itself isn't intrinsically interesting; it's the perspective it gives me that's compelling. I probably don't totally understand either world, but I understand more of both than most."

HEALTH CARE FOR AFGHAN REFUGEE COMMUNITIES

Case Study 11-1 describes an Afghan refugee family struggling with the difficulties of adjusting to a new and different life. The case study serves as the basis for this discussion on health care for Afghan refugee communities.

CASE STUDY 11-1

Afghan Family Health
The Abdul family came to the United States in 1990 after an extended stay in a refugee camp in Pakistan. Like other Afghan refugees, they experienced difficulty fleeing Afghanistan and lost family members in the war and turmoil that engulfed their home country. They came to California because they had relatives in the San Francisco Bay area and knew of the Afghan community there. Even though they have lived in the United States for more than 10 years, they still struggle with the difficulties of adjusting to a new and different life. Resettlement and adjustment in the United States have not been easy for them. Although they appreciate the safety they have experienced in this country, they believe that the quality of life was better in Afghanistan, where they had fresher food, more exercise, social support, and no pollution (Lipson, Omidian, & Paul, 1995).

Many of the health problems experienced by both Mr. and Mrs. Abdul can be traced to significant stressors of migration. Mr. Abdul was a successful businessman in Afghanistan. He has worked only intermittently in the United States and, as could be predicted, he has experienced considerable stress related to work problems, loss of property, and loss of status. Like many Afghans in the United States, the Abduls have received welfare assistance, and Mr. Abdul was reluctant to forfeit this income for a minimum-wage job with few or no benefits. Mr. Abdul has struggled to learn English, and as his English-language ability has improved, he has been able to find more satisfactory employment. Mr. Abdul is not aware that he is hypertensive because he has not seen a physician for several years. Like all refugees and immigrants, Mr. Abdul has experienced difficulties with access to health care, insurance problems, and the need for translation and transportation.

Mrs. Abdul has been relatively isolated at home with the children. In Afghanistan, she would have lived very close to family members, and she would have spent a great deal of time visiting with them. Without the social support and interaction of her family, she feels lonely and has experienced some depression, which is not uncommon in refugee women. Like many other Afghan refugee women, Mrs. Abdul would seek and accept health care only from a woman physician or nurse. Cultural barriers often inhibit such health practices as breast self-examination and Papanicolaou smears. Mrs. Abdul does not talk about such intimate matters with her husband or even with another woman. The lack of social interaction with other women relatives makes her vulnerable not only to social isolation, but also to the lack of health information that would be shared among women in a traditional culture. She is reluctant to make friends with strangers, even if they are other Afghan women. She misses the constant visiting and social interaction characteristic of life back in Afghanistan. Although many Afghan men and women had horrific experiences in the war and the escape from Afghanistan, many others like the Abdul family are adjusting to life in the United States and are coping as well as possible with their past experiences. Their lives are not stress free by any means, but the Abduls and other refugees have demonstrated considerable strength in adjusting to traumatizing experiences and the stress of adapting to life in the United States.

Mr. and Mrs. Abdul worry a great deal about their children, a boy aged 16 years and a girl aged 14 years. They are worried about raising their children in American society. The parents are distressed by what they see on television and are shocked by the explicit sex and violence portrayed in the media. They are offended by public demonstrations of affection between men and women. And, like other Afghan refugees, the Abduls are concerned because their children are served pork in school lunchrooms and are exposed to poor role models (Lipson, 1991). The Abduls fear that schools often teach disrespect for parents and encourage sexual freedom through sex education.

The teenage girl, Rahima, like other young Afghan girls, is torn between traditional values, which emphasize socializing only with families, and behaving like her American peers. Although her father is pleased that she can receive an education in the United States, he is worried that she might wear lipstick and short skirts like her American classmates. Rahima sometimes is resentful because her brother has more freedom than she does to visit friends, play sports, and participate in other activities outside the home and away from parents.

News from Afghanistan through the media, the telephone, and direct communication with friends and family members is a source of great stress for Afghans in the United States. Many Afghans have cable television and can monitor television news from Middle Eastern countries. The powerful effect of news and the events in Afghanistan in the wake of the terrorist attacks on the United States cannot be overstated. The Abdul family is upset and distressed about the news from their country and the family members who remain there. They are equally worried about what might happen to them as Afghans living in the United States, and they fear repercussions and stigmatization related to their cultural and ethnic identity.

Careful assessment of cultural backgrounds and individual factors can help nurses anticipate and work with difficulties experienced by refugees and immigrants with regard to seeking health care. The Andrews/Boyle Transcultural Nursing Assessment Guide for Individuals and Families used in this text is recommended for use with clients and their families as well as communities. Because this assessment is quite comprehensive, the following topics, adapted from Lipson & Meleis (1983), are suggested to provide minimum information for the nurse to plan culturally competent care.

- Length of time the client and family have been here, and where the client was raised. Not only is the country important, but rural and urban differentiation may also be important, as well as social, political, and economic levels.
- Language spoken in the home and language skill in English

- Nonverbal communication style
- Religious practices
- Ethnic affiliation or identity
- Family roles and how they are influenced by the resettlement experience
- Social support or networks, especially relatives or family members in the new country

Assessment of these factors would assist the nurse in planning health care for the Abduls and other Afghan families. Mental health services, preventive care, and health education needs were identified as important in an Afghan community health survey conducted by Lipson, Omidian, & Paul (1995). Stress is a significant problem for the Abdul family and is not uncommon in other Afghan families. Stress is related to the refugee experience and also to inadequate income, work-related problems, and loss of culture and tradition. Lipson, Omidian, & Paul (1995) reported in their community survey of Afghan health that many Afghans were reluctant to seek mental health services because of fear of stigma—of "being crazy"—as well the lack of health insurance and the existence of few Dari/Pashto-speaking therapists. The lack of mental health services is a grave concern in refugee and immigrant communities and should be addressed by creative and innovative solutions. Afghan men like Mr. Abdul are reluctant to seek mental health services. He is reluctant to admit that he needs such services, his income is limited, and even if he had health insurance, most likely it would not pay for psychiatric services even if they were available from a professional who spoke his own language.

Preventive care in the areas of dental health, breast self-examination, mammography, and Papanicolaou (Pap) smears are important for Mrs. Abdul. Surveys have shown that many Afghans are not aware of the risks of smoking, obesity, and hypertension (Lipson, Omidian, & Paul, 1995). Many barriers to good preventive care are environmental and social rather than cultural. Constraints are based on Afghan refugees' language, economic, occupational, and transportation problems. Mrs. Abdul is not likely to seek these personal health care services on her own initiative and would not be likely to talk about them with other women unless they were family members. Health care professionals must learn sensitive ways of broaching these subjects and helping Afghan clients access culturally appropriate care. Health care professionals, especially women physicians and nurses, should design outreach programs that consider problems in access to and lack of language-appropriate and culturally sensitive health care for women. Many Afghan women would not be comfortable with a male physician; thus female nurse practitioners and/or midwives could be used in culturally specific settings.

Health education, including information about access to care, is always important in planning services for refugee and immigrant communities. Many Afghans do not use health education services, not necessarily because of cultural barriers but because of difficulties with access, the need for translation and transportation, and the desire for women health care providers, as well as other barriers. Lipson, Omidian, & Paul (1995) reported that Afghans wanted information on dealing with stress, heart health, nutrition, child raising (particularly adolescents) in the United States, aging in the United States, and diabetes. They requested that health education be delivered in lectures via television or through face-to-face meetings, written brochures, or videotapes in their own language.

Health services, from the beginning, should include bicultural health care providers on their staff. Community health workers could be trained to serve as interpreters and translators. Lipson (1991) cautions against using family members as interpreters because of divisions along age and gender lines. The health care provider's gender is especially important for Afghan women, who will not feel comfortable with male doctors or nurses and probably will avoid health care altogether if female care providers are not available. Obviously, non-Afghan care providers must be knowledgeable about the refugees' or immigrants' experiences and background, cultural and social factors, and other unique aspects of this population. Health education is especially important for this community; however, barriers to care are often environmental and social. Afghans need access to language-appropriate and culturally sensitive health care; according to one study (Lipson, Omidian, & Paul, 1995), they prefer to receive such information in a group or social setting.

The traditional or classic definition of community tended to use a geographic boundary, such as a village, town, or urban settlement such as a city. This sense may be conveyed somewhat in terms such as Little Havana, Little Kabul, and Little Saigon, but such designations do not really convey the nature or quality of the immigrant experience, which tends to cross geographic boundaries and does not remain the same as in the home country. The sense of shared displacement or uprootedness that serves to unite and distinguish immigrant or refugee communities from other groups or communities is quite profound and cannot be ignored (DeSantis, 1997).

Immigrant communities have often been reduced to a psychoemotional phenomenon. Immigrants are seen as dominated by the psychoemotional experiences and consequences of relocation. Indeed, much of the literature on immigrants and refugees focuses on posttraumatic stress syndrome. While certainly many immigrants and refugees have endured horrific experiences, this focus alone is not holistic. This view, according to DeSantis (1997), focuses on the primacy of the individual rather than the community and thus prescribes psychiatric treatment rather than addressing the sociocultural and economic barriers at the macro level. It is at the macro level that transcultural health care providers must be engaged if they are to be effective participants in building healthy refugee and immigrant communities.

Maintenance of Traditional Cultural Values and Practices

An important aspect of transcultural nursing is the collection of cultural data and the assessment of traditional values and practices and how they are maintained over time. The processes of **assimilation** and **acculturation** can be briefly defined as those ways in which individuals and cultural groups adapt and change over time. Yet, at the same time, both individuals and groups may be resistant to some changes and retain many traditional cultural traits. Hispanics are the largest cultural/ethnic group in the United States, and in several large American cities, they constitute large percentages of the population. Obviously, in these ethnic communities, it is easier to speak Spanish and to maintain other traditional cultural practices. Because traditional health beliefs and practices influence health and wellness, it is important for the nurse to understand the degree to which clients, families, and communities adhere to traditional health values and how nursing practice should reflect those values. Spector (2003) suggests that a person's health care and behavior during illness may well have roots in that person's traditional belief system. Unless community health nurses understand the traditional health beliefs and practices of their clients and communities, they may intervene at the wrong time or in an inappropriate way.

Many factors influence the likelihood that clients, families, and communities will maintain traditional health beliefs and practices. For example, the length of time a person lives in the new host country will influence factors such as language and the use of media such as radio and television. Teenagers may quickly adjust to American culture and prefer headphones with a CD player. The ability to speak English and to communicate with members of the majority culture is crucial to acculturation. The size of the ethnic or cultural group is also important; obviously, if the group is small, individuals from that group are more likely to be exposed to outsiders and will not spend all their time within their own group or community.

Generally, children acculturate quicker because they are exposed to others through schooling and learn cultural characteristics through that association. The need to work outside the household often exposes women from traditional cultures to others of the majority culture; thus, they learn English more quickly than if they remain isolated at home. When individuals from other cultures seek health care in their Western host country, they become familiar with its health care system. This does not necessarily mean that they comply with all health advice, but contact with the system decreases anxiety and confusion, and individuals are more likely to seek care again. In addition, if individuals or groups have distinguishing ethnic characteristics such as skin color, they may be more isolated because of discrimination and thus retain traditional values, beliefs, and practices over a longer time. Some factors that influence the likelihood that clients, families, and communities will maintain traditional health beliefs and practices are shown in Box 11–2, Factors Influencing Traditional Beliefs and Practices.

Access to Health and Nursing Care for Diverse Cultural Groups

Members of diverse cultural groups, especially those who are poor, face special problems in accessing health and nursing care. Access to care is often determined by economic and geographic factors. Community nurses who focus on the care of aggregates face the challenge of promoting the health of populations with new causes of mortality (such as HIV/AIDS) and underserved populations who are more likely to experience health problems. Certain cultural groups have faced discrimination and poverty, and their ability to access care has been compromised. Sensitivity to cultural factors has often been lacking in the health care of traditional communities and identified minority groups. In addition to economic status and discriminatory factors that limit access to care, geographic location plays an important role. Many rural areas lack medical personnel and the variety of health facilities and services that are available to urban populations. For example, Native Americans, living in sparsely settled and isolated reservations in the western part of the United States, must travel long distances over primitive roads to obtain health care services. Many individuals from culturally diverse backgrounds seek the services of health care professionals who speak their language. When this is not possible, they are reluctant to seek care or may not understand the importance of following medical advice.

Another common and significant factor that limits access to health services is a lack of under-

---

BOX 11-2

Factors Influencing Traditional Beliefs and Practices

1. Length of time in the new host country.
2. Size of the ethnic or cultural group with which an individual identifies and interacts.
3. Age of the individual. As a general rule, children acculturate more rapidly than adults or seniors.
4. Ability to speak English and communicate with members of the majority culture.
5. Economic status. For example, if the family economic situation necessitates that a Salvadoran woman work outside the home, she may learn English more quickly than if she remains within the household and speaks only Spanish with her family members.
6. Educational status. In general, higher levels of education lead to faster acculturation.
7. Health status of family members. If individuals and their families seek health care in their host country, they begin to "learn the system," so to speak. This does not mean that they comply with all health advice by any means, but contacts with the system should decrease anxiety and confusion.
8. Individuals and groups who have distinguishing ethnic characteristics, such as skin color. These individuals may be more isolated because of discrimination and thus may retain traditional values related to health beliefs and behavior.
9. Intermarriage. Ethnic intermarriage is associated with a greater loss of traditional ethnic identity.
10. Rigidity or flexibility of the host society. This refers to the extent to which the host society is willing to allow members of different ethnic groups, along with their traditions and practices, into their structure, culture, and identity.

---

standing by clients of how to use health resources. This lack of understanding may be due in part to cultural factors. Often this lack of understanding means that members of diverse cultural groups are less able to adequately cope with health problems than are other members of the community. Nurses can develop sensitivity to diverse groups within communities and reach out to them with culturally specific health programs. Box 11–3 lists some important factors

---

BOX 11-3

Factors to Consider in the Nursing Care of Culturally Diverse Groups

1. Lack of employment opportunities and finances for health care services
2. Different traditional belief systems as well as different norms and values
3. Lack of cultural sensitivity on the part of social service and health care workers
4. Lack of bilingual personnel or staff members or the lack of interpreters to assist clients and care providers
5. Rapid changes in the U.S. health care system, where clients are "lost" in the gaps between agencies and services
6. Inconvenient locations or hours that preclude clients from accessing care
7. Lack of understanding, trust, and commitment on the part of health care providers

---

that nurses must take into account for culturally appropriate community-based care.

Assessment of Culturally Diverse Communities

A **cultural assessment** may be directed toward individual clients to assess their cultural needs (Leininger, 1991, 1995; see also Appendix A). In general, all successful cultural assessments have at their foundation extensive data to help them better understand and address the specific health needs and interests of their target populations. Individual cultural assessments are accomplished through the use of a systematic process. In community health nursing, the community is considered the client, and several models have been proposed to help nurses assess the community (Stanhope & Lancaster, 2006; Lowry & Martin, 2000), including the Andrews/Boyle Transcultural Nursing Assessment Guide for Individuals and Families in Appendix A. A community nursing assessment requires gathering relevant data, interpreting the database (including problem analysis and prioritization), and

identifying and implementing intervention activities for community health (Stanhope & Lancaster, 2006). Although the community nursing assessment focuses on a broader goal, such as improvement in the health status of a group of people, it is important to remember that it is often the characteristics of people that give every community its uniqueness. These common characteristics, which influence norms, values, religious practices, educational aspirations, and health and illness behaviors, are frequently determined by shared cultural experiences. Thus, adding the cultural component to a community nursing assessment strengthens the assessment base. Box 11-4 provides basic principles underlying all cultural assessments.

Nurses have become interested in using cultural data in nursing care. Leininger (1978, 1995) presented assessment domains within which to seek data to understand culture, and she has developed a tool to assess clients' cultural patterns by broadly looking at lifeways (Leininger, 1991). Inherent in most definitions of culture is the concept of shared cultural backgrounds or a way of life or a **worldview**. Thus, the concept of culture may be more easily applied to a community or group of persons than to an individual. An overview of selected cultural components is presented in Table 11-2. These components can be used to assess diverse cultural groups within a community. For example, using these components, a cultural assessment of the Navajo would provide the data detailed in Appendix B shown at the end of this text.

Community Nursing Interventions

Cultural Competence in Health Maintenance and Health Promotion

Leininger (1978, 1995) suggested that cultural groups have their own culturally defined ways of maintaining and promoting health. Pender suggested that "health promoting behaviors can be understood only by considering persons within their social, cultural, and environmental contexts" (1987, p. 16). Community nurses who have

BOX 11-4

Basic Principles of Cultural Assessment

1. **All cultures must be viewed in the context in which they have developed.** Cultural practices develop as a "logical" or understandable response to a particular human problem, and the setting as well as the problem must be considered. This is one reason why environmental and/or contextual data are so important.
2. **The underlying premises of the behavior must be examined.** For example, the Hispanic client's refusal to take a "hot" medication with a cold liquid is understandable if the nurse is aware that many Hispanic patients adhere to hot/cold theories of illness causation. There is often a range or spectrum of illness beliefs, with one end encompassing illnesses defined within the Western biomedical model and the other end firmly anchored within the individual culture (Huff, 1999). Obviously, the more widely disparate the differences between the biomedical model and the beliefs within the cultural group, the greater the potential for encountering resistance to biomedical interventions.
3. **The meaning and purpose of the behavior must be interpreted within the context of the specific culture.** An example would be the close relationship that is often seen in Hispanic cultures between mother and son; such an intense relationship might be viewed as abnormal in European American families.
4. **There is such a phenomenon as intracultural variation.** Not every member of a cultural group displays all the behaviors that we might associate with that group. For instance, not every Hispanic client will adhere to hot/cold theories of illness, and not every Hispanic mother will have a close personal relationship with her son. It is only by careful appraisal of the assessment data, and validation of the nurse's assessment with the client and family, that culturally competent care can be provided.

on health maintenance and promotion is considerable. Major cultural issues and considerations must be addressed before health maintenance and promotion programs are implemented for culturally diverse groups.

First, it is important to involve local community leaders or "elders" who are members of the cultural group being targeted to promote the acceptance of health promotion programs. Such a leader, for example, might be the pastor of an African American church in the rural south or a member of the tribal council for a Native American tribe. The nurse must also be sensitive to cultural differences in leadership styles. For example, the African American pastor may not speak in favor of the health education program from his or her pulpit but might choose instead to work through more informal networks. Numerous nurse researchers (Shambley-Ebron & Boyle, 2006; Abrums, 2004; and Boyle, Hodnicki, & Ferrell, 1999) found that African Americans tend to rely on spirituality and/or religious practices when they are ill. In addition to local community and religious leaders, it is important in the planning process to involve those who are most affected by the health-related problem. Those involved in planning and participating in the program's activities should likewise participate in its evaluation. Collaboration between the planner and the participants is often the key to success in community-based health programs (Kline, 1999).

Second, family members, churches, employers, and community work sites need to be involved in supporting a health promotion/education program by the use of networks that already exist. For example, a health education program about mammography and breast self-examination can be established at a work site that employs mostly women. A display could be set up in the cafeteria, dining room, or other accessible site. Women could view the educational material during breaks or after lunch.

Third, health messages are more readily accepted if they do not conflict with existing cultural beliefs. If the nurse plans to talk about prevention of teenage pregnancy to mothers and daughters at a local conservative church, he or

direct access to clients in the context of their daily lives should be especially aware of the importance of cultural knowledge in promoting and maintaining health because the promotion and maintenance of health occurs in the context of everyday lives rather than in the doctor's office or in a hospital. The range of cultural influences

TABLE 11-2 *Components of the Cultural Assessment*	
Cultural Component	**Description**
Family and kinship systems	Is the family nuclear, extended, or "blended"? Do family members live nearby? What are the communication patterns among family members? What is the role and status of individual family members? By age and gender?
Social life	What is the daily routine of the group? What are the important life cycle events such as birth, marriage, and death? How are the educational systems organized? What are the social problems experienced by the group? How does the social environment contribute to a sense of belonging? What are the group's social interaction patterns? What are its commonly prescribed nutritional practices?
Political systems	Which factors in the political system influence the way the group perceives its status vis-à-vis the dominant culture, e.g., laws, justice, and cultural heroes? How does the economic system influence control of resources such as land, water, housing, jobs, and opportunities?
Language and traditions	Are there differences in dialects or language spoken between health care professionals and the cultural group? How do major cultural traditions of history, art, drama, etc., influence the cultural identity of the group? What are the common language patterns in regard to verbal and nonverbal communication? How is the use of personal space related to communication?
Worldview, value orientations, and cultural norms	What are the major cultural values about the relationships of humans to nature and to one another? How can the groups' ethical beliefs be described? What are the norms and standards of behavior (authority, responsibility, dependability, and competition)? What are the cultural attitudes about time, work, and leisure?
Religion	What are the religious beliefs and practices of the group? How do they relate to health practices? What are the rituals and taboos surrounding major life events such as birth and death?
Health beliefs and practices	What are the group's attitudes and beliefs regarding health and illness? Does the cultural group seek care from indigenous health (or folk) practitioners? Who makes decisions about health care? Are there biologic variations that are important to the health of this group?

she could discuss these plans in advance with some of the mothers and the pastor and ask for ways to strengthen the church's support of abstinence programs. This is not the appropriate time to focus on contraception methods but to be sensitive to the group's religious values.

Fourth, language barriers and cultural differences are a very real problem in many larger U.S. cities. For example, in the U.S.–Mexico border areas, *promotoras* are used to disseminate messages in their own language and to help organize and present information that is culturally appropriate and understood by community members. The health care professional should not be afraid to ask for help and suggestions, and should make

it a point to find educational material such as brochures or videotapes in the appropriate language.

Last of all, sensitivity is essential to meeting health needs that exist within diverse cultural groups. For example, HIV/AIDS is spreading rapidly in some Hispanic and African American populations and is associated with intravenous drug use, violence, and the spread of crack cocaine use. In addition, the root causes of poverty and unemployment should be examined, and programs that improve overall economic status of culturally diverse communities should be developed. Culturally relevant treatment programs should be implemented. Many minority women who seek treatment programs for cocaine addiction encounter barriers that seem insurmountable. Treatment programs are not available in many areas, and child-care facilities are not provided—even in day-treatment programs. Thus, a young mother living in a rural area with children would not be able to find a treatment center that meets her needs. If she seeks admittance to a residential treatment program, she might have to agree to place her children in foster care. Evidence-Based Practice 11–2 discusses the culturally appropriate care for substance-dependent African American women.

Family Systems

Because the family is the basic social unit, it provides the context in which health promotion and maintenance are defined and carried out by family members within culturally diverse communities. The nurse can recognize and use the family's role in altering the health status of a family member and in supporting lifestyle changes. This requires an appreciation of the role of the family in diverse culture groups. African American families, for example, may demonstrate interchangeable roles for their male and female members, extended ties across generations, and strong social support systems, including the African American church, all of which can be tapped by a community health nurse to activate health and wellness in families (Abrums, 2004; Andrews, 2001).

Coping Behaviors

Culturally diverse clients often have distinct behaviors to cope with illness as well as to maintain and promote health. These behaviors may be traced to the health–illness paradigms that were discussed earlier in Chapter 4. Beliefs about hot and cold, yin and yang, harmony and balance may underlie actions to prevent disease and maintain health. Community nurses who understand their clients' cultural values and beliefs can assess their understanding of health and illness. These assessment data serve as the basis for planning health guidance and teaching strategies

that focus on incorporating cultural beliefs and practices in the nursing care plan. It seems likely that clients in the process of coping with illness and seeking help may involve a network of persons, ranging from family members and select laypersons to health care professionals.

Seeking social support is often seen as a means of coping. It is now evident that social support varies widely across people, cultural groups, and circumstances. Other studies of coping behaviors during an illness of a family member (Stewart, 1994; Picot, 1995) also show that interactions may differ remarkably at any one time during the illness, depending on intrapersonal, interpersonal, and environmental factors. Certainly, nurses working with multicultural populations will want to learn and understand how coping styles are used by individuals and family members as well as how these coping styles change over time.

Lifestyle Practices

Cultural influences have a significant impact on such health-promoting factors as diet, exercise, and stress management. Community health nurses should assess the implications of diet planning and teaching to clients and family members who adhere to culturally prescribed practices concerning foods. Some cultural groups believe that certain foods maintain or promote health. Some foods often are restricted during illness, just as there are "sick foods"—special dishes served to an ill person, such as the proverbial chicken soup. Cultural preferences determine the style of food preparation and consumption, the frequency of eating, the time of eating, and eating utensils. Milk is not always considered a suitable source of protein for Native Americans, Hispanics, Blacks, and some Asians because of their relatively high incidence of lactose intolerance.

Nurses who work with culturally different clients must evaluate patterns of daily living as well as culturally prescribed activities before they suggest forms of physical activity or exercise to clients. Exercise is often defined in terms of White middle-class values. Not everyone has

Evidence-Based Practice 11–2:

Cultural Care for Substance-Dependent African American Women

Substance abuse is in epidemic proportions in the United States and is currently defined as the nation's number-one public health problem. Caring for members of diverse cultural groups who abuse drugs and alcohol can be challenging. High rates of recidivism, relapse, and inadequate psychological support as well as lack of treatment facilities are among some of the issues in addressing substance dependence. In addition, health care providers have failed to address issues of culturally sensitive treatment strategies or gender issues. Clients from diverse cultural backgrounds have tended to be "treated" from a unicultural perspective, with limited approaches to fit the client's cultural background or needs.

This ethnonursing qualitative research study explored the meanings and expressions of care from 14 key and 18 general participants, all of whom were African American women. Four universal culture care themes were identified in the data.

1. Culture care for substance-dependent African American women meant taking time to listen and to understand them in a nonjudgmental manner, showing respect for and understanding of their traditional family, religious, spiritual, and cultural lifeways.
2. Culture care for African American women meant learning reciprocal support with other recovering women while forming alliances with adult females in developing recovery care networks.
3. Culture care was viewed as guidance and direction through suggestions by care providers.
4. Cultural care for African American women reflected concern for or about resolving past cultural pain experiences and ameliorating anger, guilt, fear, and shame.

Clinical Application

1. Understand and value that to be effective in providing culture care to African American women, health care providers must be knowledgeable about African Americans' religious, spiritual, philosophical, and cultural values and lifeways.
2. Recognize the influence of spirituality on health and incorporate spirituality in the provision of health care.
3. Assist African American women who are in treatment facilities to maintain family and kinship networks.
4. Spent time with African American women who are undergoing treatment for drug and alcohol abuse, to listen to and understand them and to show respect and concern for them.
5. Become knowledgeable about addictions and understand that recovery from substance abuse is a process.

Ehrmin, J. T. (2005). Dimensions of culture care for substance-dependent African American women. *Journal of Transcultural Nursing 16*(2), 117–125.

access to the tennis court at a local country club, and many individuals would not feel comfortable in such surroundings or in aerobics classes regardless of the setting. Some men might feel more comfortable playing basketball or hiking. Tribal dancing has become popular on some reservations for Native Americans. Helping clients plan physical activities that are culturally acceptable is only the first step in implementing a program of physical activity.

Another aspect of lifestyle that must be understood for the successful promotion of health and wellness is the manner in which culturally different clients manage stress. Stress management is learned from childhood through our parents, our social group, and our cultural group. Smoking and/or chewing tobacco, although not healthy habits, are often used to manage stress. Persons who choose to smoke greatly increase the risk of the development of heart disease and cancer. Debates currently rage about smoking in public places and the use of tobacco.

The use and abuse of alcoholic beverages are also related to lifestyle practices. Families coping with multiple stressors often feel overwhelmed by the challenges of everyday living, and individuals within families may develop dysfunctional ways of coping, such as alcohol abuse and domestic violence. Although many of these lifestyle practices are not associated with a group's culture per se, they are often found in groups whose members do not have appropriate options and/or alternatives and who are poor and unable to access other options. Evidence-Based Practice 11–3 discusses the problems and concerns of youth suicide in an American Indian tribe. Studies such as this one by Strickland, Walsh, and Cooper (2006) help us to understand the views and experiences of parents and elders in tribal communities about youth suicide, a particular concern for American Indian people.

Many cultural groups tend to express psychological distress through somatic symptoms, and some studies have found that women are at high risk for depression and somatic complaints. Indeed, for many immigrants and refugees, stress-related disorders such as posttraumatic stress disorder are relatively common. The presence of large numbers of families with altered family processes and unhealthy lifestyles within the community may create problems for all members of the larger community or society. The nurse who works in **community settings** will frequently encounter these families and is in an ideal position to act as their advocate, to refer them to appropriate care, and, in effect, to improve the health of the community at large.

The nurse may find that in some cultural groups, such as Mexican Americans, traditional healers, such as curanderas, can be helpful for persons with some emotional or psychologic disorders. In addition, health professionals such as physicians, dentists, and nurse practitioners may be more acceptable if they share the same ethnic heritage or at least speak the language of the client. In some aggregate ethnic settings, such as the Chinatown area in San Francisco, there are practitioners of traditional Chinese medicine as well as Western medicine, acupuncturists, neighborhood pharmacies, and herbalists, all of which are available to meet the diverse needs of that particular neighborhood.

Cultural Competence in Primary, Secondary, and Tertiary Preventive Programs

Nurses working in community settings use health-related concepts that are identified with the practice of community health nursing. Concepts such as "community as client" and "population-focused practice" were discussed briefly in the first sections of this chapter. Another important concept to community nurses is that of **levels of prevention**. Preventive care, consisting of primary, secondary, and tertiary activities, is directed toward high-risk groups or aggregates within a community setting. **Primary prevention** is composed of activities that prevent the occurrence of an illness, disease, or health risk. The preventive actions take place before the disease or illness occurs. **Secondary prevention** involves the early diagnosis and appropriate treatment of a condition or disease. **Tertiary prevention** focuses on reha-

Evidence-Based Practice 11–3:

Youth Suicide Prevention in a Pacific Northwest, American Indian Tribe

Suicide rates among American Indian youth in the United States are two to three times higher than the national average. Risk factors include abuse of alcohol, depression and hopelessness, family conflict and violence, and divorce and poverty. Community risks include discrimination, prejudice, and rapid change and instability. Researchers interviewed American Indian parents and elders to obtain their perspectives on community needs and to identify strengths within the community that might reduce suicide risk.

Parents and elders voiced concern about the vicious cycle of fractured families that contributes to difficulties in school and in obtaining employment, both of which perpetuate the further fracturing of families. Parents and elders worried about the loss of traditions and the effect of modern-day life on traditional family values and cultural practices. Cultural revitalization efforts were valued. Parents and elders believed that certain action would strengthen the community and reduce suicide risk. For example, youth mentoring programs, more cultural activities, support for economic development, and greater opportunities for youth recognition were identified.

Clinical Application

1. Accept and be sensitive to historical and contextual conditions under which stress, depression, and suicide ideation occur.
2. Use culturally relevant interventions as appropriate, such as story telling, demonstration, and role modeling.
3. Strengthen cultural values that enable youth to be strong and have hope for the future.
4. Recognize that the concept of family is remarkably different for American Indian people.
5. Direct community interventions to families, communities, and the larger systems in which social injustice and racial discrimination occur.

Strickland, C. J., Walsh, E., & Cooper, M. (2006). Healing fractured families: Parents' and elders' perspectives on the impact of colonization and youth suicide prevention in a Pacific Northwest American Indian Tribe. *Journal of Transcultural Nursing, 17,* 5–12.

bilitation and the prevention of recurrences or complications. The major aim of community-based preventive programs is to reduce the risk for the population at large rather than to prevent illnesses in specific individuals. As long as preventive actions are directed toward a given population rather than toward individuals, there is a chance of altering the general balance of forces so that even though not all will benefit, many will have a chance to avoid illness. This last section of this chapter discusses the use of cultural knowl-edge to plan community-nursing interventions for diverse cultural groups at the primary, secondary, and tertiary levels of prevention.

Primary Prevention: Prenatal Services in Mexican American Communities

OVERVIEW OF THE HEALTH CONCERN

For many years, public health agencies have tried to improve maternal and infant services to high-risk populations. In the 1980s, a special government report on minority health reported that only 58% of Mexican American mothers begin prenatal care in the first trimester, less than that of Blacks or non-Hispanic women (Heckler, 1985a). The neonatal mortality rate appeared good for Mexican American babies; still, by 1995, fewer Hispanic mothers began their prenatal care during the first trimester than did mothers of certain other ethnic origins (73.7% for Hispanic mothers versus 84.7% for White mothers and 82.1% for Asian and Pacific Islander mothers) (U.S. Department of Health and Human Services, Centers for Disease Control and Prevention [CDC], National Center for Health Statistics, 1995). Interestingly, even when Hispanic mothers seek prenatal care earlier in their pregnancy, the outcomes during pregnancy, labor, or the postpartum period are not improved (Goss, Lee, Koshar, Heilemann, & Stinson, 1997). The risk factors of pregnancy include age (both extremes), parity, and low socioeconomic status. In addition, numbers of children within the family (need for child care), transportation problems, and less assistance from a support system influence use of health services. Many women of Mexican American origin fall in these categories. Furthermore, an infant with health concerns often has negative and long-term consequences for the child and the mother as well as other family members. Obtaining early and regular prenatal care greatly enhances a young woman's chance of delivering a healthy, full-term baby. A program of primary prevention would focus on preventing infant mortality and other health problems in Mexican American mothers and their infants. Nursing care must be broadly focused, providing some specific services but also helping clients access other resources in the community.

Access to Care

There are various reasons why Mexican Americans might not seek care during pregnancy. Cost is often a factor, and in many areas of the country, Mexican Americans have tended to belong to poorer socioeconomic groups (Heckler, 1985a, 1985b). In 2005, the Pew Hispanic Center esti-

mated that nearly 11 million undocumented immigrants live in the United States, 6 million of whom are from Mexico (Passel, 2005). Undocumented immigrants face special problems with access to care: They lack health insurance, language, and knowledge regarding health services, and they fear their legal status.

The value of routine prenatal visits to a health care provider should be repeatedly emphasized, otherwise some Hispanic women may stop their regular visits because they are feeling well and are not accustomed to seeing a health care provider unless they are ill. The community health nurse can provide information about community resources and help clients access care early in pregnancy by referral to appropriate agencies. Nearly all states now provide programs that provide funds and services for low-income pregnant women. Although not a health program specifically, the Women, Infants, and Children (WIC) Program provides nutritious food and nutrition education to low-income pregnant and breast-feeding mothers, their infants, and their children under age 5 (U.S. Department of Agriculture, Food and Nutrition Service, 1999). The rate of low birth weight babies among infants born to women on WIC is 25% lower than for infants born to similarly situated women not on WIC. WIC is an example of one of the most popular, successful, and cost-effective public health programs (U.S. Department of Agriculture, Food and Nutrition Service, 1999; U.S. Department of Agriculture, Food and Nutrition Service, n.d.). Referring pregnant women to WIC services is a strong primary prevention intervention by community nurses.

Cultural Views About Modesty

Any prenatal program that serves Mexican American women may be underused unless consideration is given to some Mexican American women's modesty and reluctance to be examined by male health care providers. The use of female nurse practitioners and midwives is ideal for this population. In addition, some consideration should be given to incorporation of the traditional *parteras* (lay midwives) or *promotoras* (health workers) into the preventive educational services.

Language Barriers

It is absolutely essential in a prenatal program for a Mexican American population that the majority of health care professionals in the program be bilingual. If that is impossible, interpreters must be employed to facilitate the professional services. All prenatal classes should be offered in Spanish and English. This sometimes means that two classes must be offered concurrently; many Mexican American women speak predominantly either Spanish or English and would choose the class where they understand the language. The availability of health education material in Spanish is critical to reinforce teaching and anticipatory guidance. Videos may be more effective than brochures or other written material. In Berry's study (1999) of Mexican American women and prenatal care, the key informants who were bilingual spoke only Spanish within their homes because they did not want their children to forget their heritage. In some border communities such as Nogales, Arizona, the Hispanic population is high (93.6%), and most residents speak Spanish in their homes (Arizona Department of Health Services, Office of Health Systems Development, 2005).

Cultural Views of Motherhood and Pregnancy

Some evidence indicates that women of Mexican American culture may adhere to different value orientations and cultural views of motherhood and pregnancy than those found in mainstream American culture (Burk, Wieser, & Keegan, 1995). The Mexican American culture traditionally values motherhood, and young women are encouraged to prepare themselves for this role. Community health nurses, nurse practitioners, and professional midwives are in important positions to help pregnant women prepare for motherhood and its associated responsibilities. Understanding and reinforcing the approved cultural views of pregnancy will be helpful for clients because trust and mutual goal setting can develop more rapidly. All nursing interventions should incorporate family members, especially mothers and sisters, for support of the pregnant woman. Emphasizing the responsibility for the mother to be healthy for her baby's health and welfare is appropriate for this cultural group.

Traditional Pregnancy-Related Folk Beliefs of Mexican Americans

Many Mexican Americans adhere to traditional beliefs and practices related to pregnancy and childbirth. Additionally, children are greatly valued and are desired soon after marriage. As in many other cultures, Mexican Americans consider pregnancy, birth, and the immediate postpartum period as a time of great vulnerability for women and their newborns. Some traditional beliefs and practices related to pregnancy and childbirth are shown in Box 11–5. It is important

---

BOX 11-5

Selected Beliefs and Practices of Pregnancy and Childbirth in Traditional Mexican American Culture

- Avoid strong emotions such as anger and fear during pregnancy.
- Cool air is dangerous during pregnancy and should be avoided.
- Bathe often during pregnancy; be active so that the baby will not grow too big and hinder delivery.
- Eat a nutritious diet; "give in" to food cravings.
- Massage is helpful to place the baby in the right position for birth.
- Don't raise your arms above your head or sit with your legs crossed during pregnancy because these actions will cause knots in the umbilical cord.
- Moonlight should be avoided during pregnancy, especially during an eclipse, because it will cause a birth defect.
- After delivery, a 40-day period known as *la diet* or *la cuarentena* is observed. Certain activities and foods are restricted.
- Chamomile tea will relieve nausea and vomiting in pregnancy.
- Heartburn can be treated with baking soda.
- Laxatives and purges may be used to "clean" the intestinal tract.

for the culturally sensitive nurse to assess each client because each generation of childbearing women perceives pregnancy and birth differently (Nichols & Zwelling, 1997). In the Mexican American culture, it is important for the nurse to assess the views of members of the pregnant mother's support system, especially her mother, who belongs to an earlier generation and may adhere to more traditional values.

Mexican American Cultural Networks

Traditionally, the family is very important in Mexican American culture, and nursing care should be family focused. The most important social structural factor in the Mexican American culture is family and kinship ties. These ties often go beyond the family to a wide network of kin. Bauwens and Anderson (1992) observed that a Mexican American is expected to turn first to the family for help; if preventive services are to be effective, they must tap these kinds of cultural networks to ensure the support of community residents in preventive programs in their neighborhoods that involve family members, neighbors, or friends. Health care professionals face challenges such as language barriers, literacy levels, socioeconomic and educational levels, cultural backgrounds, and other subtle differences when they work with the varied Hispanic groups in the United States. It is also critically important to remember that there is tremendous diversity within Hispanic groups living in the United States.

USING CULTURAL COMPETENCE
AT THE PRIMARY LEVEL OF PREVENTION

The community health nurse should target for change certain high-risk behaviors during pregnancy, such as smoking, using drugs, consuming alcohol, and maintaining poor nutritional habits. Although there is no set rule of thumb, a Mexican American mother-to-be may respond to suggestions for change if she is convinced that her behavior will cause harm to her baby. Family and social support groups in Mexican American culture can also be helpful and supportive to expectant mothers wishing to make lifestyle changes. Some researchers have found that pregnant Latin women will attempt to stop smoking and will be successful with the help, support, and assistance of their families (Pletsch & Johnson, 1996).

Prenatal services should go beyond the birth of the baby to include information about breast-feeding and family-planning services. Traditionally, some health care professionals have assumed that family-planning services will not be accepted in a Mexican American population because of religious opposition and machismo—the need of the man to prove his manhood by having children or to believe in the biologic superiority of men. However, it may be that Mexican American men as well as women are interested in family planning and are concerned about the number of children they can support. This issue should be validated with individual clients and their spouses. During *la cuarentena*, the 40 days after the birth of the baby, women kin of the new mother often help with infant care, household tasks, and preparation of special foods for the mother (Berry, 1999). Many Hispanic families believe that chili and other spicy foods should be avoided during and immediately after pregnancy.

Strategies for promoting breast-feeding should be identified and encouraged. For example, educational levels, family experiences with breast-feeding, the husband's attitude, the need to return to work, and feelings of embarrassment are associated with infant-feeding choices among Mexican American women as well as other groups. These factors need to be explored with individual women to help them make the best choices for themselves and their babies. Traditionally, new Hispanic mothers may bind their abdomen as well as their baby's abdomen during the postpartum period. These customs should be supported by nurses who work with postpartum Mexican American women and their babies.

Secondary Levels of Prevention:
Type II Diabetes and Native Americans

OVERVIEW OF THE HEALTH CONCERN

Non–insulin-dependent diabetes (NIDD), or type II diabetes, is seen commonly among some

Native North Americans, and certain tribes have extremely high rates of the disease—154% higher than those for other groups in the United States (Hodge & Fredericks, 1999). By all accounts, the high rate of diabetes in Native North American groups is a leading health concern because diabetes is a leading cause of outpatient visits at Indian Health Service facilities. Further, Indian deaths resulting from renal failure alone were reported to be 290% higher than the national average in the United States (U.S. Department of Health and Human Services, 1993). Type II diabetes has become an epidemic and a national tragedy among many Native peoples.

The reasons for the epidemic of type II diabetes among some Native North Americans are not clear. It is believed that some Native North American tribes have an underlying genetic propensity for the disease that is triggered by changes in dietary practices, a sedentary lifestyle, and increasing obesity (Neel, 1962; West, 1978; Young, 1994). These factors have been complicated by social conditions such as poverty, as well as by problems of compliance or lack of adherence to medical regimens.

Because of the high rate of diabetes on some reservations, numerous secondary preventive services that focus on early diagnosis and treatment have been initiated. Many of them are modeled after programs that have been successful with White middle-class North Americans. Box 11-6 shows culturally related factors that could influence the success of secondary preventive programs for diabetes among some Native Americans. Readers are cautioned that validation of beliefs and practices should always take place

---

BOX 11-6

Beliefs and Practices Related to Diabetes Found in Some Native Americans

Nutritional Practices

- Diets are high in calories, carbohydrates, and fats.
- Sharing communal meals is a common and valued cultural practice.
- Some groups have a high incidence of obesity.
- Food preparation often adds fats and calories.
- Snack foods (potato chips, carbonated beverages, prepackaged pastries) are common.
- High intake of alcohol seriously compromises the treatment of diabetes.

Activity Levels/Fitness Practices

- Sedentary lifestyles have become common.
- Many reservations lack recreational facilities.
- Formal exercise activities are associated with the White man's culture and are not thought to be appropriate for Native Americans.

Beliefs and Values Related to Diabetes

- Ideal body image favors a heavier physique, and weight gain is considered normal; thinness is a cause for worry and concern.
- Concept of "control of one's body," i.e., weight, glucose levels, blood pressure, may conflict with values and norms of Native American culture. For example, Native American clients may be uncomfortable with comparison of individual performance against others or against the norms and standards of biomedical care.
- Many Native Americans are uncomfortable with discussing or exposing private body functions, such as providing urine samples or participating in blood testing in a public situation.
- Illness is a personal and unpleasant topic, and Native American clients may be uncomfortable when asked to talk about it.
- Diabetes is a "White man's disease"; Native Americans did not have diabetes until Whites came to this continent.
- The term "diabetic" may be offensive to some, and the label "diabetic clinic" may discourage clients from seeking health care services.
- White health professionals may be viewed with some suspicion and distrust, given the history of cultural contact between Whites and Native Americans.
- Because diabetes is so common in some tribal groups, there is a fatalism about the disease, especially if a family member already has diabetes.
- Beliefs and health practices surrounding diabetes may vary according to the Native American tribe.

with individual clients and families, and stereo-typing (thinking that all Native Americans are the same) should be avoided.

USING CULTURAL COMPETENCE AT THE SECONDARY LEVEL OF PREVENTION

Nursing interventions at the secondary level of prevention should focus on the implementation of healthful lifestyle changes that will ultimately decrease the complications of diabetes. Most of these are related to what health professionals call diet and exercise, but what is appropriate for Native North American culture is an emphasis on health and a healthy lifestyle.

Nurses should emphasize health and a healthy lifestyle rather than negative factors such as control of diabetes, prevention of complications, weight reduction, and exercise. The choice of words, as well as the emphasis, is important. For example, when teaching the client and family about diabetic diets, the nurse can substitute the word "nutrition" for "diet," thus removing the negative perceptions and leading to a nursing plan that emphasizes substitution rather than deprivation. Substituting fruits for candy bars and packaged pastries, whole grains for potato chips or doughnuts, and vegetables for sugared snacks will improve the client's nutritional status and lead to a healthier lifestyle. Special traditional foods, even fried bread, can be eaten on special occasions, and other types of bread can be substituted during regular meals.

Health education can be oriented toward individual clients and directed toward the family rather than provided in an impersonal clinic situation. Physical activities that are culturally congruent can be encouraged; again, the value of health and a healthy lifestyle should be stressed over exercise and weight reduction. Physical activities that are congruent with overall lifestyle and cultural context will be easier to incorporate into daily living situations.

Usually, the Native American family system is an extended family that includes several households of closely related kin. Family members become exceedingly important during times of crisis because they are a source of support, comfort, assistance, and strength. The importance of cultural ties with kin and other members of the reservation community always must be considered in planning for early diagnosis and treatment programs. It is in this context (family and community) that clients are encouraged and supported not only to seek care, but also to institute lifestyle changes that are congruent with cultural practices and that will enhance the health status of all members of the family and, ultimately, the tribal community.

The increasing rates of type II diabetes are of great concern to Native American communities. Introducing preventive health programs requires great sensitivity to cultural traditions and to the past experiences that native communities have had with health care and health research. Understanding the needs of community members is essential for the development of culturally appropriate programs, and each Native American community has its own cultural traditions and beliefs that make up the details of daily life. Understanding the needs of Native communities begins by asking them what they want and need from preventive programs rather than imposing ideas upon them. The best way to find out what matters to people is to get out into the community and talk to them. In Native American communities, it is wise to begin with respected and esteemed members of the tribal council.

Serious behavioral and social problems contribute to the high risk factors in American Indian groups. Suicide rates are rising, and deaths resulting from homicide, accidents, and injuries have resulted in increased American Indian mortality (Strickland, Walsh, & Cooper, 2006). In fact, suicide is the third leading cause of death among American Indian youth, ages 15–24 years (CDC, 2004). Evidence-Based Practice 11–3 shown earlier in this chapter offers both community- and family-based recommendations to reduce suicide risk. Newer threats to Indian health such as cancer, diabetes, nutritional diseases, and other illnesses caused by changing behaviors and environmental contaminants are on the rise. These problems contribute significantly to death and disease in Native communities (Hodge & Fredericks, 1999). Components of a Cultural Assessment for Traditional Navajo are shown in Appendix B at the end of this text. While specific to Navajo people, the components provide a framework that can be used to assess other Native communities.

Tertiary Levels of Prevention: Hypertension and African Americans

OVERVIEW OF THE HEALTH CONCERN

African Americans are a highly heterogeneous group and display considerable variation in health beliefs and behaviors. For the most part, this section will discuss a more traditional, rural African American culture, and the reader is advised to validate beliefs and behaviors with individual clients and communities.

Hypertension is a major risk factor for heart disease and stroke. Mean blood pressure levels are higher in Blacks than in European Americans, with a marked excess in Blacks. A decade ago, in a government study on minority health, Heckler stated, "Hypertensive Blacks were at least as likely as Whites of the same sex to be treated with antihypertensive medication and nearly as likely to have their blood pressure controlled" (1985a, p. 110). Heckler also noted that from 1968 to 1982, stroke mortality in Blacks declined 5%, and coronary heart disease also had decreased dramatically.

Control of hypertension has certainly been one factor responsible for this improvement. It is critical that efforts to treat hypertension in African American populations be continued. Unfortunately, appropriate care often has been complicated by discrimination, poverty, and limited access to care.

The goal of tertiary prevention is to reduce disability and prevent complications from developing. A major aim of nursing care in the implementation of tertiary activities is to help clients adjust to limitations in daily living, to increase their coping skills, to control symptoms, and in general to minimize the complications of disease by reducing the rate of residual damage in a given population. Cultural factors that should be considered in tertiary prevention programs for African Americans are shown in Box 11-7, Cultural Factors to Consider in Planning Tertiary Prevention for a Traditional African American Population.

USING CULTURAL COMPETENCE AT THE TERTIARY LEVEL OF PREVENTION

Community nurses have demonstrated competence in the management of community hypertension programs. Although these programs are vital to the early diagnosis and management of hypertension, they also include a component that focuses on helping clients manage a chronic disease—an aspect of tertiary prevention. The African American community should be involved in every aspect of community-based programs. The goals, objectives, and interventions of the services should reflect the expressed needs of the community target group. Hypertension programs should reflect the values, beliefs, and interests of the target community. Numerous studies have shown that African American churches are excellent sites for community-based clinics such as hypertension programs.

Poverty is often a problem in African American communities and, combined with the lasting effects of racism and discrimination, African Americans often experience severe economic deprivation. In 1998, 26.1% of all African Americans were living below the national poverty level. Forty percent of African American households are headed by females, often another contributing factor to families having insufficient socioeconomic resources (U.S. Census Bureau, 1998). Community health nurses are in the advantageous position of assessing clients and families in their own homes and neighborhoods. This provides an understanding of the daily life situation faced by clients that other health care professionals often lack. Community health nurses can bring this understanding to bear on helping clients with tertiary preventive activities.

BOX 11-7

Cultural Factors to Consider in Planning Tertiary Prevention for a Traditional African American Population

Language

African American communication concepts and patterns can be identified and used in community education programs.

Cultural Health Beliefs

Good health comes from good luck.
Health is related to harmony in nature.
Illnesses are classified as "natural" or "unnatural."
Illness may be God's punishment.
Maintenance of health is associated with "reading the signs," e.g., phase of the moon, seasons of the year, position of the planets.

Cultural Health Practices

The use of herbs, oils, powders, roots, and other home remedies may be common.

Cultural Healers

Older woman ("old lady") in the community who has a knowledge of herbs and healing.
Spiritualist who is called by God to heal disease or solve emotional or personal problems.
Voodoo priest/priestess who is a powerful cultural healer who uses voodoo, bone reading, etc., to heal or to bring about desired events.
Root doctor who uses roots, herbs, oils, candles, and ointments in healing rituals.

Time Orientation

May be present-time oriented, which makes preventive care more difficult to implement and maintain.

Nutritional Practices

Soul food takes its name from a feeling of kinship among Blacks and may be served at home, provided at church dinners, or served at home-style restaurants.
Diets may reflect traditional rural Southern foods such as greens, grits, corn bread, and chickpeas.

Economic Status

African Americans account for many persons in the lower socioeconomic strata in American society.

Educational Status

High aspirations for education, but socioeconomic status and other complex factors limit educational opportunities.

Family and Social Networks

Often strong extended family networks with a sense of obligation to relatives.

Self-concept

The importance of race has been a continual issue for the self-identity of African Americans.

Impact of Racism

Unfortunately, racism is still present, and a negative perception of the African American's skin color by health professionals will seriously interfere with efficacious health care.

Religion

African American churches have tremendous influence on the daily lives of their members because they serve as a source of spiritual and social support. (Boyle, Ferrell, Hodinicki, Muller, 1996).
The African American church acts as a caretaker for the cultural characteristics of Black culture (Abvums, 2004).

Biologic Variations

There is a high incidence of lactose intolerance and lactase deficiency; this has implications for diet planning if Black clients cannot tolerate milk or milk products.
There is a higher prevalence of hypertension among African Americans than among Europeans. Sickle cell anemia is more common among African Americans.

Adapted from Bloch, B. (1983). Nursing care of black patients. In M. S. Orque, B. Bloch, & L. S. Monroy (Eds.), *Ethnic nursing care: A multicultural approach* (pp. 81–113). St. Louis, MO: C. V. Mosby; and Andrews, M. M., & Bolin, L. (1993). The African American community. In J. M. Swanson & M. Albrecht (Eds.), *Community health nursing: Promoting the health of aggregates* (pp. 443–458). Philadelphia: W.B. Saunders.

Summary

Cultural concepts related to community health nursing practice were discussed. A framework for providing culturally sensitive nursing care was introduced to help nurses and other health professionals provide care to individuals and groups with diverse cultural backgrounds. These frameworks help nurses use cultural knowledge in assessing, planning, and implementing nursing care. This chapter explored the role of the family in transmitting beliefs and practices concerning health and illness. Cultural diversity within communities was addressed, and various subcultures, including refugees and immigrants, were discussed. A community case study of Afghan refugees was provided. Special concerns related to refugee populations were described. Cultural data about traditional Afghan culture were related, and examples of culturally competent care were provided.

Cultural concepts were explored as they relate to the community at large. A cultural assessment was described as an integral component of a community nursing assessment. Culturally competent nursing interventions for community health maintenance and health promotion were presented. Preventive care in the community is of particular importance to community health nursing. The use of cultural knowledge in primary, secondary, and tertiary levels of prevention was introduced. Examples of cultural diversity and levels of prevention were described to illustrate how cultural knowledge can be used in community health nursing practice.

REVIEW QUESTIONS

1. Describe four cultural concepts, and discuss how they can be used to provide transcultural nursing care to families and community aggregates.
2. Describe an example of how cultural factors influence the health of an aggregate group within the community. How do cultural factors influence illness levels in an aggregate group?
3. List the major cultural considerations in implementing preventive programs for culturally diverse groups. How can cultural considerations be used to identify barriers and facilitators for preventive programs?
4. Identify special health considerations in immigrant groups within the community.
5. Describe an approach to primary preventive health care for several cultural groups, e.g., Hispanics, African American, Amish, and Bosnian populations.
6. Describe secondary and tertiary programs targeting hypertension for elderly Chinese North Americans living in Chinatown in San Francisco.
7. Describe similarities and differences between folk and scientific health care systems. Give an example of each.

CRITICAL THINKING ACTIVITIES

1. Describe sociocultural factors and their impact on health care for a cultural group within your community. Evaluate the access to, availability of, and acceptability of various health care services. Is this cultural group at risk? Why?
2. Conduct a community cultural assessment of a group within your community. Critically analyze the cultural knowledge and/or information that should be considered when planning care for the group. Use the outline provided in Table 11–2 to identify and

collect cultural assessment data, i.e., family and kinship, social life, political systems, language, worldview, religious behaviors, health beliefs and practices, and health concerns. Compare and contrast the assessment of other groups in your community.

3. For a cultural group in your community, develop a program plan or intervention that has components of primary, secondary, and tertiary prevention.

4. Attend religious services at a church, temple, mosque, synagogue, or place of worship to learn about a religion different from your own. Assess how each church meets the unique needs of its congregation.

5. Identify alternative health care practitioners within your community. Which subcultures do they serve? Describe the kinds of care that they offer to residents.

REFERENCES

Abrums, M. (2004). Faith and feminism: How African American women from a storefront church resist oppression in healthcare. *Advances in Nursing Science, 27*(3), 187–201.

Akbar, S. H., & Burton, S. (2005). *Come back to Afghanistan: A California teenager's story.* New York City: Bloomsbury Publishing.

American Psychiatric Association. (1987). *Diagnostic and statistical manual of mental disorders* (3rd ed., rev.). Washington, DC: Author.

Anderson, E. T., & McFarlane, J. M. (2004). *Community as partner: Theory and practice in nursing* (4th ed.). Philadelphia: Lippincott Williams & Wilkins.

Andrew, M. M., & Bolin, L. (1993). The African American community. In J. M. Swanson & M. Albrecht (Eds.), *Community health nursing: Promoting the health of aggregates* (pp. 443–458). Philadelphia: W.B. Saunders.

Andrews, M. M. (2001). Cultural diversity and community health nursing. In M. A. Nies & M. McEwen (Eds.), *Community health nursing: Promoting the health of populations* (pp. 242–285). Philadelphia: W.B. Saunders Company.

Arizona Department of Health Services, Office of Health Systems Development. (2005). *Nogales Primary Care Area Statistical Profile.*

Aroian, K. J. (1993). Mental health risks and problems encountered by illegal immigrants. *Issues in Mental Health Nursing, 14,* 379–397.

Barth, F. (1987). Cultural wellsprings of resistance in Afghan Islam. In R. Klass (Ed.), *Afghanistan: The great game revisited* (pp. 187–202). Boston: Freedom House.

Bauwens, E., & Anderson, S. (1992). Social and cultural influences on health care. In M. Stanhope & J. Lancaster (Eds.), *Community health nursing: Process and health practice for promoting* (3rd ed., pp. 91–108). St. Louis, MO: C.V. Mosby.

Berry, A. B. (1999). Mexican American women's expressions of the meaning of culturally congruent prenatal care. *Journal of Transcultural Nursing, 10,* 203–212.

Bloch, B. (1983). Nursing care of Black patients. In M. S. Orque, B. Bloch, & L. A. Monrroy (Eds.), *Ethnic nursing care: A multicultural approach* (pp. 81–113). St. Louis, MO: C.V. Mosby.

Boyle, J. S., Ferrell, J., Hodnicki, D., & Muller, R. (1996). Going home: African American caregiving for adult children with human immunodeficiency virus disease. *Holistic Nursing Practice, 11,* 27–35.

Boyle, J. S., Hodnicki, D. R., & Ferrell, J. A. (1999). Patterns of resistance: African American mothers and adult children with HIV disease. *Scholarly Inquiry for Nursing Practice, 13,* 111–133.

Burk, M. E., Wieser, P. C., & Keegan, L. (1995). Cultural beliefs and health behaviors of pregnant Mexican American women: Implications for primary health care. *Advances in Nursing Science, 17*(4), 37–52.

CDC. (2004). *Suicide fact sheet.* Retrieved January 29, 2006, from http://www.cdc.gov/ncipe/factsheets/suifacts.htm

Clark, M. J. (2003). Care of the community or target group. In M. J. Clark (Ed.), *Nursing in the community* (4th ed., pp. 389–421). Stamford, CT: Appleton & Lange.

DeSantis, L. (1997). Building healthy communities with immigrants and refugees. *Journal of Transcultural Nursing, 9,* 20–31.

Ehrmin, J. T. (2005). Dimensions of culture care for substance-dependent African American women. *Journal of Transcultural Nursing, 16*(2) 117–125.

Flynn, B. C. (1997). Are we ready to collaborate for community based health services? *Public Health Nursing, 14*(3), 135–136.

Friedberg, R. M., & Hunt, J. (1995). The impact of immigrants on host country wages, employment and growth. *Journal of Economic Perspectives, 9*(2), 23–44.

Goodman, J. H. (2004). Coping with trauma and hardship among unaccompanied refugee youths from Sudan. *Qualitative Health Research, 14*(9), 1177–1196.

Goss, G. L., Lee, K., Koshar, J., Heilemann, M. S., & Stinson, J. (1997). More does not mean better; Prenatal visits and pregnancy outcome in the Hispanic population. *Public Health Nursing. 14,* 183–188.

Heckler, M. M. (1985a). *Report of the Secretary's Task Force on Black and Minority Health, Vol. I: Executive summary.* Washington, DC: U.S. Department of Health and Human Services.

Heckler, M. M. (1985b). *Report to the Secretary's Task Force on Black and Minority Health, Vol. 2: Crosscutting issues in minority health.* Washington, DC: U.S. Department of Health and Human Services.

Hodge, F. S., & Fredericks, L. (1999). American Indian and Alaska Native populations in the United States. In R. M.

Huff & M. V. Kline (Eds.), *Promoting health in multicultural populations* (pp. 269–289). Thousand Oaks, CA: Sage.

Huff, R. M. (1999). Cross-cultural concepts of health and disease. In R. M. Huff & M. V. Kline (Eds.), *Promoting health in multicultural populations* (pp. 23–40). Thousand Oaks, CA: Sage.

Huff, R. M., & Kline, M. V. (1999). *Promoting health in multicultural populations.* Thousand Oaks, CA: Sage.

Kirmayer, L. J. (1994). Suicide among Canadian Aboriginal peoples. *Transcultural Psychiatric Research Review, 31,* 3–58.

Kline, M. V. (1999). Planning health promotion and disease prevention programs in multicultural populations. In R. M. Huff & M. V. Kline (Eds.), *Promoting health in multicultural populations* (pp. 73–102). Thousand Oaks, CA: Sage.

Leininger, M. (1978). *Transcultural nursing: Concepts, theories and practices.* New York: John Wiley & Sons.

Leininger, M. (1991). Leininger's acculturation health care assessment tool for cultural patterns in traditional and nontraditional lifeways. *Journal of Transcultural Nursing, 2*(2), 40–42.

Leininger, M. (1995). *Transcultural nursing: Concepts, theories, research and practice.* New York: McGraw-Hill, Inc.

Lipson, J. (1991). Afghan refugee health: Some findings and suggestions. *Qualitative Health Research, 1,* 349–369.

Lipson, J. (1993). Afghan refugees in California: Mental health issues. *Issues in Mental Health Nursing, 14,* 411–423.

Lipson, J., & Meleis, A. (1983). Issues in health care of Middle Eastern patients. *Western Journal of Medicine, 139*(6), 854–861.

Lipson, J., & Miller, S. (1994). Changing roles of Afghan refugee women in the U.S. *Health Care for Women International, 15,* 171–180.

Lipson, J., & Omidian, P. (1992). Afghan refugees: Health issues in the United States. *Western Journal of Medicine, 157,* 271–275.

Lipson, J., & Omidian, P. (1997). Afghan refugee issues in the U.S. social environment. *Western Journal of Nursing Research, 19*(1), 110–126.

Lipson, J., Omidian, P., & Paul, S. (1995). Afghan health education project: A community survey. *Public Health Nursing, 12,* 143–150.

Lowry, L. W., & Martin, K. S. (2000). Organizing frameworks applied to community health nursing. In M. Stanhope & J. Lancaster (Eds.), *Community health nursing: Promoting health of aggregates, families and individuals* (5th ed., pp. 202–225). St. Louis, MO: C.V. Mosby.

McGeary, J. (2001, October 1). Afghanistan: The Taliban troubles. *Time,* 36–43.

Meleis, A. I. (1997). Immigrant transitions and health care: An action plan. *Nursing Outlook, 45,* 42.

Neel, J. V. (1962). Diabetes mellitus: A "thrifty" genotype rendered detrimental by progress. *American Journal of Human Genetics, 14,* 353–362.

Nichols, F. H., & Zwelling, E. (1997). *Maternal-newborn nursing: Theory and practice.* Philadelphia: W.B. Saunders Company.

Nies, M. A., & McEwen, M. (2007). *Community health nursing: Promoting the health of populations* (4th ed.). Philadelphia: W.B. Saunders Company.

NINR. (1995). *Community-based health care: Nursing strategies.* Bethesda, MD: U.S. Department of Health and Human Services.

NINR. (n.d.). *NINR's Strategic Plan on Reducing Health Disparities.* Retrieved December 8, 2006, from http://obssr.od.nih.gov/Content/Strategic_Planning/Health_Disparities/NINR.htm

Pender, N. J. (1987). Health and health promotion: Conceptual dilemmas. In M. E. Duffy & N. J. Pender (Eds.), *Proceedings of a wingspread conference: Conceptual issues in health promotion* (pp. 7–23). Indianapolis: Sigma Theta Tau International, Honor Society of Nursing.

Picot, S. J. (1995). Rewards, costs, and coping of African American caregivers. *Nursing Research, 44,* 147–152.

Pletsch, P. K., & Johnson, M. A. (1996). The cigarette smoking experiences of pregnant Latinas in the United States. *Health Care for Women International, 17,* 549–562.

Shambley-Ebron, D., & Boyle, J. S. (2006). Self-care and the cultural meaning of mothering in African American women with HIV/AIDS. *Western Journal of Nursing Research, 28*(1), 42–60.

Spector, R. E. (2003). *Cultural diversity in health and illness* (6th ed.). New York: Appleton-Century-Crofts.

Stanhope, M., & Lancaster, J. (2006). *Community health nursing: Promoting health of aggregates, families and individuals* (6th ed.). St. Louis, MO: C.V. Mosby.

Stewart, B. M. (1994). End-of-life family decision-making from disclosure of HIV through bereavement. *Scholarly Inquiry for Nursing Practice: An International Journal, 8,* 321–352.

Strickland, C. J., Walsh, E., & Cooper, M. (2006). Healing fractured families: Parents' and elders' perspectives on the impact of colonization and youth suicide prevention in a Pacific Northwest American Indian tribe. *Journal of Transcultural Nursing, 17,* 5–12.

United Nations Economic Commission for Europe, (n.d.). Retrieved December 8, 2006, from http://www.unece.org/stats/gender/glossary/r.html

U.S. Census Bureau. (1998). *Country of origin and year of entry into the U.S. of the foreign born, by citizenship status.* Available from http://www.bis.census.gov/cps/pub/1998/foreignborn.htm

U.S. Census Bureau News. (2004, March 18). *More diversity, slower growth: Census Bureau projects tripling of Hispanic and Asian Populations in 50 years; Non-Hispanic Whites may drop to half of total population.* Retrieved December 12, 2006, from http://www.census.gov/Press-Release/www/releases/archives/population/001720.html

U.S. Department of Agriculture, Food and Nutrition Service. (n.d.). *About WIC: How WIC helps.* Retrieved December 8, 2006, from http://www.fns.usda.gov/wic/aboutwic.howwichelps.htm

U.S. Department of Agriculture, Food and Nutrition Service. (1999).

U.S. Department of Health and Human Services. (1990). *Healthy people 2000. National Health Promotion and Disease Prevention Objectives.* Washington, DC: U.S. Government Printing Office.

U.S. Department of Health and Human Services. (1993). *Healthy people 2000 review.* Washington, DC: U.S. Government Printing Office.

U.S. Department of Health and Human Services. (2000). *Healthy people 2010. National health promotion and disease prevention objectives.* Retrieved July, 2002, from http:www.health.gov.healthypeople/document

U.S. Department of Health and Human Services, CDC, National Center for Health Statistics. (1995). *Health, United States, 1995*, (PHS No. 96-1232, p. 119). Washington, DC: U.S. Government Printing Office.

West, K. (1978). *Diabetes in American Indians: Advances in metabolic disorders*. New York: Academic Press.

Williams, C. A. (2006). Community-oriented nursing and community-based nursing, In M. Stanhope & J. Lancaster (Eds.), *Foundations of nursing in the community: Community oriented practice* (2nd ed., pp. 3–16). St. Louis, MO: Mosby, Inc.

Young, K. (1994). *The health of Native Americans*. New York: Oxford University Press.

Yount, S., McEwen, M., & Boyle, J. (in press). The United States–Mexico health care systems: Health care in the border region. *Journal of Transcultural Nursing*.

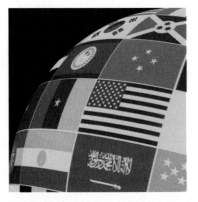

CHAPTER 12

Cultural Diversity in the Health Care Workforce

Margaret M. Andrews

LEARNING OBJECTIVES

1. Analyze past, present, and future trends in the racial and ethnic composition of the health care workforce.
2. Identify the cultural meaning of work and its influence on the corporate culture and organizational climate of health care organizations.
3. Critically examine the manner in which hatred, prejudice, racism, discrimination, and ethnoviolence manifest themselves in the health care workplace.
4. Critically analyze the cultural origins of conflict in the health care workforce.
5. Evaluate strategies for promoting effective cross-cultural communication and preventing conflict in the multicultural workplace.
6. Examine the process and content of cultural self-assessment for nurses and for health care organizations, institutions, and agencies.

The U.S. Department of Health and Human Services reports that in 2004, 81.8% of the RN population were estimated to be White (non-Hispanic), about 7.5% of RNs did not specify their racial/ethnic background, and 10.6% were in one or more of the identified racial and ethnic minority groups. In 2000, 12.3% of the RN population was estimated to be in one of the non-White racial/ethnic minority groups identified.

Of the nurses who indicated their racial/ethnic background in the 2004 survey, 88.4% (an estimated 2,380,639) were White, non-Hispanic; 4.6% or 122,495 were Black/African American, non-Hispanic; 3.3% or 89,976 were Asian or Pacific Islander, non-Hispanic; 1.8% or 48,009 were Hispanic; 0.4% or 9,453 were American Indian/Alaskan Native; and 1.5% were from two or more racial backgrounds (U.S. Department of Health and Human Services, Bureau of Health Professions, 2005). Refer to Figure 12–1.

Because of a change in definitions, comparisons of the racial/ethnic composition of the RN population to surveys prior to 2000 should be viewed carefully. In accordance with the Office of Management and Budget (OMB), the question regarding racial and ethnic background in the March 2000 survey was changed from the previous surveys. Nurses were asked to identify their ethnic background and then asked to identify all races that could best describe them. The information was aggregated to categories similar to those reported in previous years, with one additional grouping of non-Hispanics that reported being of mixed race (two or more races). In surveys prior to 2000, nurses had to choose from one of the racial/ethnic categories presented.

When both initial and post–registered nurse education are examined, Asian, Pacific Islander, and Black nurses are more likely than White and Hispanic nurses to have at least baccalaureate preparation. Somewhat similar findings prevail for graduate education among the racial and ethnic minorities, with 14.3% of Black registered nurses holding master's or doctor's degrees, compared with 13.3% of White nurses, 10.4% of Hispanic nurses, and 9.9% of Asian nurses (U.S. Department of Health and Human Services, Bureau of Health Professions, 2005).

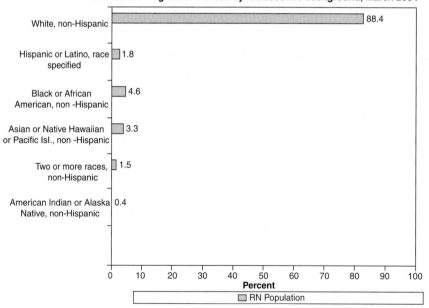

FIGURE 12-1. Distribution of registered nurses by racial/ethnic background, March 2004. (*Source*: U.S. Department of Health and Human Services, Bureau of Health Professions. [2004]. *The registered nurse population: Findings from the 2004 National Sample Survey of Registered Nurses*. Retrieved March 16, 2007, from http://bhpr.hrsa.gov/healthworkforce/rnsurvey04/2.htm)

The three most common employment settings for registered nurses in the United States are hospitals (56.2%), public or community health centers (14.9%), and ambulatory care (11.5%). More minority nurses than White nurses reported being currently employed in nursing (86.4% compared with 81%), and minority nurses were more likely to work full time than were their White counterparts (86% compared with 70%). Although fewer than 4% of licensed nurses in the United States are foreign educated, this percentage represents more than 101,000 nurses (U.S. Department of Health and Human Services, Bureau of Health Professions, 2005).

At 8.4%, the proportion of foreign-educated nurses working in Canada is almost double that in the United States (Canadian Institute for Health Information, 2005). Nevertheless, Canada continues to have less diversity in its nursing workforce than does the United States. For example, data from the 1996 Canadian Census indicate that only 10.7% of registered nurses employed in Canada identify themselves as members of a visible minority (Human Resources and Social Development Canada, 2001). There are also slightly fewer male nurses in Canada (5.6% of the registered nurse workforce) than in the United States (5.7% of the registered nurse workforce). However, as in the United States, the number of male registered nurses employed in Canada is on the rise (Canadian Institute for Health Information, 2005). In both Canada and the United States, there continues to be an increasingly diverse workforce.

The emerging U.S. and Canadian workforces are dramatically different from those in former times. In many health care settings there is diversity in race, ethnicity, religion, age, sexual orientation, and national origin. Recent strides in the women's movement have called attention to important gender differences and the manner in which changing societal roles of both men and women influence relationships in the **multicultural workplace**. See Evidence-Based Practice 12-1. The interrelationship between culture and the physical, mental, and emotional handicaps and disabilities of some health care workers must also be considered in the complex web called the **multicultural workforce.**

Women have historically constituted the majority of personnel in nursing and in many allied health disciplines. For the past 2 decades, women and members of racially and ethnically diverse groups have made significant inroads into health professions that were once overwhelmingly the province of White men. The largest gains for most culturally diverse groups, however, occurred during the mid- to late 1970s. Since that time, with the exception of Asians and Hispanics, **cultural diversity** in the health care fields has been relatively stable.

The Challenges and Opportunities of a Growing Multicultural Population and Health Care Workforce

A significant number of the U.S. and Canadian national health goals for the current decade and beyond involve specific objectives for improving the health status of members of the panethnic minority groups identified by both countries' federal governments, particularly those with low incomes. Meanwhile, culturally diverse cohorts of children, women of childbearing age, and the elderly are expected to grow, exacerbating the need for culturally competent providers of health care.

Since 1972 there has been an explosion in the numbers of people migrating to the United States and Canada, both with and without legal documentation. Overall, 12.4%, or 335.7 million people in the United States (U.S. Census Bureau, 2005b), and 18.4%, or 5.4 million people in Canada (Statistics Canada, 2001b), are foreign-born residents. The top 10 countries of origin for the foreign-born population in the United States are Mexico (30.7%), China (4.9%), Philippines (4.5%), India (4.0%), Vietnam (3.0%), El Salvador (2.8%), Korea (2.8%), Cuba (2.5%), Canada (2.3%), and the United Kingdom (1.9%) (U.S. Census Bureau, 2005b). In Canada, the largest number of immigrants (42%) comes from Europe. The remaining immigrants to Canada come mainly

Evidence-Based Practice 12–1:

Motivations and Experiences of Males in the Nursing Profession

This pilot study of the motivations and experiences of males in the nursing profession examines and critiques the available literature on males in nursing from both a historical and contemporary, present-day perspective and provides the foundation for a pilot study of 30 male nurses prior to professional registration and 30 male nurses after they have earned their professional registration. Preliminary data based on 42 male nurses who completed a mailed survey revealed the following themes: (1) inititial motivation for choosing nursing, including the influence of parents (particularly mothers); (2) lack of career advice for young men who might want to choose a career in nursing; (3) importance of altruism and caring in choosing a nursing career, with informants frequently reporting that they had experienced some form of a caring family situation prior to entering the profession; (4) age and cultural variations, e.g., attitude of Black males towards senior female colleagues, with some expressing concern at being "given orders by a woman"; (5) exclusion of males from certain specialties such as maternal–child nursing, and from certain gender-specific procedures; (6) high level of comfort caring for "older female patients," but discomfort caring for female patients who are about their same age; (7) preference of some male patients for the presence of male nurses, especially when shaving, bathing, or performing intimate procedures (e.g., catheterization); and (8) a need to convey their own sexuality and sexual orientation in subtle ways, e.g., confirming heterosexuality by referring to their wives or making negative remarks about homosexual male nurses.

Clinical Implications

Despite their historical significance to the nursing profession, the numbers of male nursing students and nurses have seldom exceeded 10% in the United States, Canada, or the United Kingdom. Findings from this preliminary pilot study confirm that some of the historic stereotypes about male nurses continue to exert a negative influence on young men as they make career choices. The major themes identified by the investigators need to be examined because they have implications for recruitment and retention strategies employed by schools of nursing and by employers of nurses. Limiting the clinical practice settings that are considered appropriate for males and excluding them from participating in specialties such as obstetric nursing or from performing certain procedures on female patients contributes to the perception by males that they are unwelcome in schools of nursing and in the nursing profession. Given the current shortage of nurses, the nursing profession collectively needs to explore how and where it markets itself to young men and the image of male nurses portrayed by the media.

Whittock, M., & Leonard, L. (2003). Stepping outside the stereotype. A pilot study of the motivations and experiences of males in the nursing profession. *Journal of Nursing Management, 11,* 242–249.

from Asia (37%), Central and South America (6%), the Caribbean and Bermuda (5%), and the United States (4%) (Statistics Canada, 2001b). Please note that although 2006 information

from Statistics Canada is in the process of being written, it is not currently available.

Because the health care workplace is a microcosm of the changing demographic patterns in society at large, the growing diversity among nurses and other members of the health care team frequently poses challenges and opportunities in the multicultural work setting (Case Studies 12–1 through 12–5).

When a Black patient was admitted to a small rural hospital with predominantly White staff and patients, nurses from one shift would include "Black male" in their report to the oncoming shift. When one of the few Black nurses began using "White male" or "White female" in her report, she was accused of "having an attitude" and "trying to instigate racial trouble."

CASE STUDY 12-2

When informed that a patient was requesting medication for pain, a Lutheran nurse of German heritage responded to a fellow nurse, "She's just a Jewish princess who complains about pain all the time." A Jewish laboratory technician overheard the remark and demanded to know what the nursing supervisor was going to do about the "blatant anti-Semitism" on the unit.

CASE STUDY 12-3

A slightly built Black male nurse asked to meet with the operating room nurse manager about a surgeon who had recently immigrated from Russia. The nurse complained, "Dr. Ivanovich keeps asking me why I became a nurse. He asks very personal questions about my sexual orientation and wants to know if I'm 'queer.' I consider this a hostile work environment and refuse to scrub for his surgical cases any more."

CASE STUDY 12-4

After receiving a report on a critically ill victim of a motor vehicle accident, Dr. Juan Valdez-Rodriguez, the physician on call, asked for the patient's name.

The reporting nurse said, "I don't know. Martinez, Hernandez, something like that. You'll recognize him when you see him—just another drunk Mexican who ran his pickup truck into a tree." Upon entering the examination room, the physician immediately recognized the victim as his cousin.

CASE STUDY 12-5

A nurse entered into a conversation with a Chinese American food service worker. Ms. Chin remarked that for the past 4 days she had been asked to be the interpreter for an elderly Chinese man on one of the units where she delivers food. "I don't want to offend the nurse manager who asked me to translate, but it is not right for a younger woman to speak for an older man. It is not our custom. Besides, my supervisor scolded me for being so slow to do my work. She thinks I have become lazy. Would you talk to the nurse manager for me?"

Transcultural Nursing Administration

According to Leininger, **transcultural nursing administration** refers to "a creative and knowledgeable process of assessing, planning, and making decisions and policies that will facilitate the provision of educational and clinical services that take into account the cultural caring values, beliefs, symbols, references, and lifeways of people of diverse and similar cultures for beneficial or satisfying outcomes" (1996, p. 30). Transcultural nursing administrative perspectives are essential for survival, growth, satisfaction, and achievement of goals in the multicultural workplace.

In the contemporary health care industry, nurse administrators necessarily focus their time and energy on issues such as cost–benefit outcomes, downsizing, territorial struggles with members of other disciplines, appropriate use of technology, and other important topics. With increasing frequency, nurse administrators are realizing the critical importance of transculturally based administrative practices that positively influence cost–benefit and quality outcomes.

With the increasing diversity among members of the health care workforce, nurses are challenged to develop and practice a new kind of administration known as transcultural nursing administration.

Cultural Perspectives on the Meaning of Work

The earliest recorded ideas about work refer to it as a curse, a punishment, or a necessary evil needed to sustain life. People of high status did not work, whereas slaves, indentured servants, and peasants worked. In contemporary society, the concept of work must be considered in its historical and cultural context. Cultural views about caring for the sick also must be considered because such care may be perceived as a divine calling for those with supernatural powers (some African tribes), a religious vocation (some ethnic Catholic groups), or an undignified occupation for lower-class workers (some Arab groups such as Kuwaitis and Saudi Arabians).

Cultural norms influence a staff member's consideration of group interest as opposed to individual interests in the multicultural workplace. Scholars have identified two major orientations embraced by people: individualism and collectivism. With **individualism**, importance is placed on individual inputs, rights, and rewards. Individualists emphasize values such as autonomy, competitiveness, achievement, and self-sufficiency. Most English-speaking and European countries have individualist cultures.

Collectivism entails the need to maintain group harmony above the partisan interests of subgroups and individuals. In collectivist cultures, values such as interpersonal harmony and group solidarity prevail. A staff member whose ethnic heritage is Asian or South American is likely to be influenced by collectivism. Amish and Mennonite groups also are considered collectivist cultures.

One of the most notable distinctions between people from individualist and collectivist cultures is the meaning of work. Individualists work to earn a living. People are expected to work; they need not enjoy it. Leisure or recreational activities frequently are pursued to alleviate the monotony of work. People from individualist cultures tend to dichotomize work and leisure. Individualist concepts of work reflect an orientation toward the future.

It also is useful to understand cultural differences about appropriate and desired behavior in the workplace. People from most individualist cultures are typically achievement oriented. Stereotypically, they want to do better, accomplish more, and take responsibility for their actions. They tend to develop personality traits such as assertiveness and competitiveness that facilitate these goals. In many collectivist cultures, however, qualities such as commitment to relationships, gentleness, cooperativeness, and indirectness are valued.

Some researchers have suggested that the motivational strategies of Japanese managers must appeal to the Japanese worker's sense of loyalty, commitment, and group orientation, whereas the motivation strategies of North American managers must appeal to the worker's sense of contract, rules, and individuality. Although some individuals have a combination of the two qualities, most staff members will display either an individualistic or a collectivistic orientation in the workplace. Nurses in leadership positions need to recognize the fundamental value system embraced by their staff members to understand why they behave as they do at work.

Corporate Cultures and Subcultures

Health care organizations are mini societies that have their own distinctive patterns of culture and subculture. One organization may have a high degree of cohesiveness, with staff working together like members of a single family toward the achievement of common goals. Another may be highly fragmented, divided into groups that think about the world in very different ways or that have different aspirations about what their organization should be. Just as individuals in a culture can have different personalities while sharing much in common, so can groups and organizations. This phenomenon is referred to as **corporate culture**. Corporate culture is a process of reality construction that allows staff to see and understand particular events, actions, objects, communications, or situations in distinctive ways. These patterns of understanding help people cope with the situations they encounter and provide a basis for making behavior sensible and meaningful.

Shared values, beliefs, meaning, and understanding are components of the corporate culture. The corporate culture is established and maintained through an ongoing, proactive process of reality construction. It is an active, living phenomenon through which staff members jointly create and re-create their workplace and world. One of the easiest ways to appreciate the nature of corporate culture and subculture is to observe the day-to-day functioning of the organization. Observe the patterns of interaction among individuals, the language that is used, the images and themes explored in conversation, and the various rituals of daily routine. Historical explanations for the ways things are done will emerge in discussions of the rationale for certain aspects of the culture.

The corporate culture metaphor is useful because it directs attention to the symbolic significance of almost every aspect of organizational life. Structures, hierarchies, rules, and organizational routines reveal underlying meanings that are crucial for understanding how organizations function. For example, meetings carry important aspects of organizational culture, which may convey a sense of conformity and order or of casual informality. The environment in which the meetings are held reflects the formality or informality of the organization.

Box 12–1 poses several questions that might be considered in the determination of the corporate culture of a health care organization, institution, or agency. The answers to the questions will provide a beginning understanding of the corporate culture of the organization.

BOX 12-1

Determining Corporate Culture

It is useful to pose the following questions when determining the corporate culture of an organization.
- Does the person presiding over the group stand or sit?
- Does the presider encourage discussion among group members or engage in a monologue?
- Are group members encouraged to express opinions freely, or is there pressure to silence those who express opposing points of view?
- How do group leaders and members dress?
- What message does the institutional dress code convey about the acceptance of cultural diversity?
- Do policies allow for cultural expressions in clothing, accessories, hair style, and related areas?
- Although most institutions require employees to wear identification badges or name tags, what flexibility does the individual have for self-expression and expression of cultural identity and affiliation?

Health care work environments are social settings that encompass many elements of a social system. It is useful to distinguish between the **organizational climate** of the work environment and the corporate culture. The organizational climate usually measures perceptions or feelings about the organization or work environment. The corporate or organizational culture, on the other hand, is what its members share—their beliefs, values, assumptions, rituals—often unconsciously. Culture provides the community, the sameness, and the consensus that makes those people unique and special.

Negative Attitudes and Behaviors in the Multicultural Workplace

Hatred, prejudice, bigotry, discrimination, racism, and violence represent negative attitudes or behaviors in the multicultural workplace, which must be considered. The formation of attitudes and strategies for changing these attitudes must also be considered.

Hatred

In some organizations, the use of racial, ethnic, sexual, and other derogatory remarks signals a disturbing underlying problem in the workplace. Why does hatred exist in the workplace? Although the reasons are complex and interconnected, some contributing factors include the early socialization of children to cultural and gender stereotypes, personal experiences (or lack of them) with people from diverse backgrounds, and exposure to negative societal attitudes.

According to Henderson (1994), **hatred** in the workplace is exacerbated during times of rapid immigration, periods of economic recession or depression, and high unemployment. Competition for sexual partners also is cited as a cause for hatred. Hatred can be the cause of tremendous hostility in the workplace. In some organizations, technology is used to transmit derogatory remarks electronically to individuals or targeted groups by e-mail or fax. Sites on the Internet that allow free expressions of hatred have proliferated. Those responsible justify their actions by citing either the Canadian Charter of Rights and Freedoms or the U.S. Constitution's First Amendment rights to freedom of expression.

Prejudice, Bigotry, and Discrimination

The term *prejudice* refers to inaccurate perceptions of others. Prejudice results in conclusions that are drawn without adequate knowledge or evidence. All people are prejudiced for or against other people. Prejudices in the community at large are acted out in the workplace. **Bigotry** connotes narrow-mindedness and an obstinate or blind attachment to a particular opinion or viewpoint. The bigot blames members of outgroups for various misfortunes. In their efforts to make expedient decisions, bigots react to concepts rather than to people.

Whereas prejudice and bigotry refer to attitudes, **discrimination** refers to behaviors and is defined as the act of setting one individual or group apart from another, thereby showing a difference or favoritism. Discriminatory behaviors, not attitudes, constitute the majority of intergroup problems. Although there are many laws against discriminatory behaviors, especially in the workplace, there are none against prejudice or bigotry (Henderson, 1994).

The nurse in Case Study 12–1 who points out in the report that the patient is Black may not have any conscious discriminatory intent. By departing from the usual practice of not mentioning race, however, she makes a statement that race is a variable that needs to be mentioned. In turn, this gives an opportunity for prejudices in the minds of the other nurses to surface. Keeping people of color exploitable is a foundation of racial inequality.

Contrary to popular writings, prejudices in the workplace are not limited to Black–White conflicts and confrontations. There is prejudice against various members of the workforce, including women, older workers, individuals with disabilities, foreign-born workers, and White workers.

In Case Study 12–2, the nurse's characterization of the patient experiencing pain as a "Jewish princess" is a transparently anti-Semitic remark. The ability to control the lives of people is a psychologic aspect of nursing that is often unconsciously manifested. The nurse in the case study may be exercising a certain degree of power over the patient, knowing that she is at the nurse's mercy for the relief of her pain. It also may reflect an underlying "scientific racism," i.e., that there are biologic differences between certain groups. The nurse may believe that there are different pain thresholds among persons of diverse backgrounds and that Jewish patients tend to have a relatively low tolerance for pain.

As discussed in Chapter 13 (Transcultural Aspects of Pain), the nurse's own ethnic background, religious affiliation, and personal experience with pain may contribute to her perceptions of the patient's need for pain relief. Although the nurse may be using "scientific racism" to rationalize her beliefs that a patient is requesting more pain relief than the average person, there is no excuse for the racist reference to her patient as a "Jewish princess." The nurse's racism adversely affects not only the patient, but also a fellow nurse and a laboratory technician. The racial slur is an example of an implicit cue passed on to others, in which the nurse perpetuates both prejudice against and stereotypes about Jewish people. The laboratory technician is likely to view the nurse, and perhaps by extension the entire multicultural workplace, as being hostile to Jews.

Prejudice is also based on sexual orientation, as illustrated in Case Study 12-3. The Black nurse expresses his concern with the hostile work environment created by the imposing Russian surgeon, who asks inappropriate questions about his sexual orientation. Because the offender is a recent immigrant, he may be unaware of cultural differences concerning appropriate topics for discussion in the workplace—though it is doubtful that his behavior would be widely accepted in a Russian operating room setting, either. Furthermore, the surgeon may have a limited English vocabulary and/or may be unaware of the negative connotation of the slang term "queer." These explanations for the surgeon's inappropriate behavior in the workplace do not excuse him; rather, they are offered as factors worthy of the nurse manager's consideration in an attempt to address the problem.

Racism

Racism implies that superior or inferior traits and behavior are determined by race. Racism connotes prejudice and discrimination. To understand racism in the workplace, distinctions need to be made among (1) institutional structures and personal behavior, and the relationship between the two; (2) the variation in both degree and form of expression of individual prejudice; and (3) the fact that racism is merely one form of a larger and more inclusive pattern of ethnocentrism that may be based on various factors, both racial and nonracial (Henderson, 1994; Williams & Rucker, 2000).

Racism is caused by a complex web of factors, including ignorance, apathy, poverty, historic patterns of discrimination against particular groups, and social stratification. In a classic work on racism, Brown (1973) posits that society "is racially divided and its whole organization...promotes racial distinctions" (p. 8). With this frame of reference, racial bias and discrimination have been built into most U.S. and Canadian institutions, and every citizen is a product of institutional racism. According to Henderson, "What is commonly called racism is part of the larger problem of ethnic identification, of power and powerlessness, and of the exploitation of the weak by the strong.... What most writers commonly call **race relations** should be properly understood in the larger context of **human relations**" (1994, p. 21) (emphasis added).

In the multicultural workplace, the expression of negative attitudes and behaviors by people toward others according to their identification as members of a particular group is of particular concern. The expression of these attitudes and behavioral patterns is learned as part of the cultural process. Negative group attitudes and destructive group conflicts are less likely to arise when employees treat each other as individuals and respond to each other on the basis of individual characteristics and behaviors (Williams & Rucker, 2000).

In Case Study 12-4, the nurse's remark "just another drunk Mexican" is an example of a stereotype that may have an element of truth in it but is nevertheless inaccurate. Although it is true that the majority of motor vehicle accidents are alcohol related, and that in this hospital a large proportion of those involved are Mexican Americans, it is untrue that all Mexican American men are alcoholics. By overgeneralizing in this way, the nurse fails to assess important information about the individual person and depersonalizes him through the stereotype. The nurse's apparent insensitivity to Dr. Valdez-Rodriguez's ethnic heritage is appalling. The pathos of the situation is further realized when the physician learns that the "just another drunk Mexican" accident victim is his cousin.

The career potential of staff from diverse backgrounds is frequently undermined by the relative lack of access to informal networks and mentors and by the expectation that these persons will assimilate into organizational cultures that are often intolerant of the cultures with which these staff members identify. These manifestations of discrimination can be expected to undermine the functioning of the health care organization. Paradoxically, the victims of mistreatment are often the perpetrators as well. The victim of mistreatment may, in turn, mistreat others. One explanation for this phenomenon is that people are likely to experience a form of internalized oppression as a result of low self-esteem.

Violence in the Workplace

Although not all hatred leads to violence, the number of reported attacks on gays and anti-Muslim and anti-Semitic incidents has increased significantly. **Ethnoviolence** is also increasing, not only in the United States and Canada, but worldwide. Blacks, Hispanics, homosexual men, Muslims, and Jews are the primary targets of hate crimes, many of which occur in the workplace. Although it is impossible to protect all employees and patients from violence in health care settings, reasonable steps must be taken to protect those believed to be at risk. Verbal threats and/or assaults by or against staff members should not be tolerated.

Health care administrators have a moral imperative to take reasonable steps in ensuring the physical safety of staff, patients/clients, and visitors. The institution's security officers and/or local police should be notified whenever violence is threatened. Some institutions require staff and visitors to pass through a metal detector when entering the premises, whereas others have posted security officers at entrances to ensure that only authorized persons are admitted. In extreme cases, it may be necessary to obtain a court order to prohibit an individual or group from the premises or to establish a safe perimeter so patients and staff may have safe access to the facility.

In recent years, attorneys representing health care institutions have sometimes found it necessary to obtain a court order to ensure a safe work environment during times of racial, ethnic, religious, and social discord. Unfortunately, some demonstrators with strong convictions have violated others' civil liberties and engaged in violent acts against those who disagreed with their point of view. The shooting of staff at clinics where abortions are performed is an extreme example of hatred that has resulted in violence. This violence is caused by a complex web of interconnected factors, including religious, moral, ethical, social, political, and cultural differences.

Formation of Attitudes

Attitudes are learned, not innate. Researchers have found that as children grow older they tend to forget that they were instructed in attitudes by their parents and significant other people. Around the age of 10, most children regard their attitudes toward people from different cultural backgrounds as being innate. Seldom do they recall being coached, resulting in **social amnesia**. When social amnesia develops, the individual tends to create elaborate rationalizations in an effort to account for learned attitudes toward certain groups of people in a society.

The superiority or inferiority of a group (versus an individual) is usually less obvious than an individual's behavior. Most staff members bring their cultural baggage to work with them, and their actions are molded and shaped by peer pressure. The values, behaviors, and customs of those in the outgroup are labeled as "strange" or "unusual." As children, many staff learned to reject people who were culturally different and to view differences as being synonymous with inferiority. In the insightful words of Carl Jung:

> We still attribute to the other fellow all the evil and inferior qualities that we do not like to recognize in ourselves, and therefore have to criticize and attack him, when all that has happened is that an inferior soul has emigrated from one person to another. The world is still full of *betes noirs* and scapegoats, just as it formerly teemed with witches and werewolves (1968, p. 65).

Changing Attitudes

Although some argue that the focus should be on behavior change rather than **attitude change**, others maintain that hatred, prejudice, bigotry, racism, discrimination, and ethnoviolence begin with an individual's attitudes toward certain groups. Staff members' attitudes can be changed in several ways, but they require commitment by all levels of management within an organization. They also require a certain degree of openness and receptivity by the individual.

Efforts to change staff members' attitudes about people from culturally diverse groups should center on communication. Several approaches have been used by organizations. The first, called the **formal attitude change approach**, is based on learning theories: on the assumption that people are rational, information-processing beings who can be motivated to listen to a message, hear its content, and incorporate what they have learned when it is advantageous to do so. There is an actual or expected reward for embracing diversity.

The second, known as the **group dynamics approach**, assumes that staff members are social beings who need culturally diverse coworkers as they adjust to environmental changes. The amount of change depends on people's attitudes toward diversity, their attention to the message and to the communicator, their understanding of the message, and their acceptance of the message. Acceptance of diversity is likely to be enhanced by activities that provide tangible rewards for staff. It is seldom enough for top management to urge staff members to embrace diversity as a moral imperative.

Cultural Values in the Multicultural Workplace

Cultural values frequently lie at the root of cross-cultural differences in the multicultural workplace. Values form the core of a culture. Time orientation, family obligations, communication patterns (including etiquette, space/distance, touch), interpersonal relationships (including long-standing historic rivalries), gender/sexual orientation, education, socioeconomic status, moral/religious beliefs, hygiene, clothing, meaning of work, and personal traits exert influences on individuals within the multicultural health care setting.

What is the importance of learning about the values of people from diverse cultural groups? Values exert a powerful influence on how each person behaves, reacts, and feels. In the multicultural workplace, values affect people's lives in four major ways. Values underlie *perceived needs, what is defined as a problem, how conflict is resolved,* and *expectations of behavior.* When cultural values of individual staff members conflict with the organizational values or those held by coworkers, challenges, misunderstandings, and difficulties in the workplace become inevitable. You must use these inevitable conflicts as opportunities to foster cross-cultural understanding among staff members from diverse backgrounds and to enhance cross-cultural communication.

Cultural Perspectives on Conflict

The term *conflict* is derived from Latin roots (*confligere,* "to strike against") and refers to actions that range from intellectual disagreement to physical violence. Frequently, the action that precipitates the conflict is based on different cultural perceptions of the situation. According to some social scientists, when participants in a conflict are from the same culture, they are more likely to perceive the situation in the same way and to organize their perceptions in similar ways.

By examining proverbs used by members of various cultural groups, it is possible to better understand differences in the way conflict is viewed. Table 12–1 summarizes selected proverbs that relate to conflict and its resolution. The dominant culture's proverbs emphasize that people should behave assertively and deal with conflict through direct confrontation. Other cultures—particularly collectivist groups—may promote avoidance of confrontation and emphasize harmony (e.g., Native North Americans,

TABLE 12-1 *Cross-Cultural Perspectives on Proverbs and Conflict*

Proverb	Value
Dominant Culture	
The squeaky wheel gets the grease.	Aggressiveness
	Direct confrontation
Tell it like it is.	Direct confrontation
	Honesty even if it hurts the other
Take the bull by the horns.	Direct confrontation
Shoot first, ask questions later.	Aggressiveness
	Direct confrontation
	Protection of individual rights (versus good of the group)
Might makes right.	Aggressiveness
	Dominance
Japanese	
The nail that sticks out gets hammered.	Not calling attention to oneself
	Going along with the group
	Harmony and balance
Senegalese	
Misunderstandings do not exist; only the failure to communicate does.	Strive to understand the other's point of view
	Harmony and balance is normal state, not conflict and confrontation
Zen	
He who knows does not speak, and he who speaks does not know.	Listen to the other's side during conflict
	Silence
Arab	
The hand of Allah is with the group.	Primacy of group good (versus individual)
Haste comes from the devil.	Patience
	Conflict resolution takes time

Alaskan Natives, Amish, and Asians). The culture-based choices that lead people in these opposite directions are a major source of conflict in the workplace.

Many people from individualist cultures view conflict as a healthy, natural, and inevitable component of all relationships. People from many collectivist cultures, on the other hand, have learned to internalize conflict and to value harmonious relationships above winning arguments and "being right." To many people of Native North American and Asian descent, conflict is not healthy, desirable, or constructive. In the Arab world, mediation is critical in resolving disputes, and confrontation seldom works. Mediation allows for saving face and is rooted in the realization that all conflicts do not have simple solutions.

The assertive, confrontational, direct style of communicating is characteristic of people from individualistic cultures, whereas the cooperative, conciliatory style is a more collectivist or Eastern mode of managing conflict. When attempting to influence others during a disagreement, for example, nurses from China, Japan, and other collectivist cultures may use covert conflict prevention strategies to minimize interpersonal conflicts. Nurses from individualistic cultures are more likely to rely on the overt confrontation of ideas and argumentation by reason.

In Case Study 12–5, the Chinese food service worker demonstrates the cultural value for harmonious relationships, indirect communication, and nonconfrontational resolution of conflict. The nurse manager has inadvertently placed Mrs. Chin in an awkward position by violating Chinese norms concerning gender and age. In traditional Chinese culture, it is inappropriate for a younger person to speak for an older one and for a female to speak for a male. Serving as an interpreter for the elderly Chinese man has been uncomfortable for both Mrs. Chin and the patient. Mrs. Chin's value for harmonious relationships in the workplace prevents her from speaking directly to the nurse manager and food service supervisor about the problem. By involving the staff nurse as an intermediary with the nurse manager, she is attempting to convey her dissatisfaction with the situation in a nonconfrontational, indirect, and polite manner. She also attempts to avoid appearing like a complaining, disgruntled employee who is unwilling to cooperate with other workers. For these reasons,

she is reluctant to bring the problem to her food service supervisor's attention. She believes that she must please those in authority, foster harmonious relationships, and avoid direct confrontation if she is to be a valuable employee of the hospital.

Cultural Origins of Conflict

Let's examine some cultural values and the manner in which they may result in conflict in the multicultural workplace. The origins of cultural conflict result from influences on the organization and on individuals. As indicated in Figure 12-2 , political, economic, technologic, and legal factors influence the corporate culture and the organizational climate of both organizations and their employees. For organizations owned and operated by religious groups, religious influences must be considered. For example, in a hospital owned and operated by a Roman Catholic religious order, abortions, tubal ligations, and other gynecologic procedures may be prohibited. Factors such as educational background, socioeconomic status, culture, moral and religious beliefs,

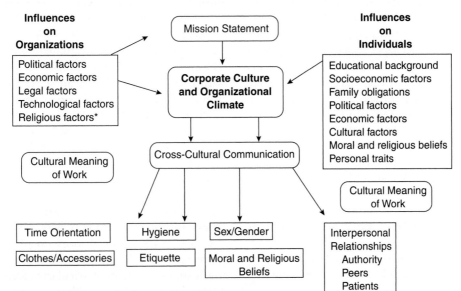

* For organizations owned and operated by religious groups.

FIGURE 12-2. Origins of conflict in the multicultural health care setting.

and personal traits of employees must also be considered when determining the cultural origins of conflict. Staff members contribute to the perception that values are in conflict. Although there are many conflicting values that underlie problems, the following areas will be explored in the remainder of this chapter: cultural perspectives on family obligations, personal hygiene, cross-cultural communication (including etiquette and touch), clothing and accessories, time orientation, interpersonal relationships (including historic rivalries between groups), gender/sexual orientation, and moral and religious beliefs (including dietary practices).

Cultural Perspectives on Family Obligations

Although family is important in all cultures, the constellation (e.g., nuclear, single-parent, extended, same-sex), emotional closeness among members, social and economic commitments among members, and other factors vary cross-culturally. Both staff nurses and those in administrative positions frequently report difficulty with requests from nurses of diverse cultural backgrounds that pertain to **family obligations**.

Some nurses from different cultures have been labeled as uncommitted to their work and/or disinterested in their nursing careers because family is a higher priority than job or career. The so-called *appliance nurse* has long been recognized among members of the dominant culture as well. Given that it is highly unlikely (and undesirable) that the nurse manager will be successful at changing fundamental family-related values, the most useful approach is to focus on the problematic behavior. For example, if excessive absenteeism is the undesirable behavior, the nurse manager should arrange for a face-to-face meeting in which the problematic behavior is discussed. In addition, the use of peer pressure by coworkers also can be helpful in changing the undesirable behavior as fellow workers communicate to the individual why his or her behavior is troublesome. It is generally useful to identify the reason(s) for the excessive absenteeism and to explore culturally appropriate strategies for resolving the problem, such as

use of the natural social support that is culturally expected of extended family members. The solution is seldom simple, as the following case analysis illustrates.

Independence from the family, for example, is highly valued by many from the dominant cultural groups in the United States and Canada, but it ranks very low in the hierarchy of people from most Middle Eastern and Asian cultures. In the latter groups, the family is highly valued, and the individual's lifelong duties toward the family are explicit. Thus, absence from work for family-related reasons may be considered legitimate and important by workers from some cultures but may be perceived as an unnecessary inconvenience to the supervisor. For example, a Mexican American staff member may submit a last-minute request for vacation time to visit with a distant cousin who has unexpectedly arrived in town after traveling a great distance. The Mexican American staff member thinks, "What a great opportunity to develop a stronger relationship with a distant member of my mother's family. How nice that cousin Juan has traveled so far to see me. I've been thinking about making a trip to Mexico next year, so perhaps I can stay with Juan during my visit. Surely my nurse manager understands how important family relationships are to Mexican Americans and will be able to rearrange the unit schedule to accommodate my request." The nurse manager may think, "What's wrong with these Mexican American staff? Don't they want to work? This vacation request means that I'll have to redo the schedule for the entire unit. If I permitted everyone to submit last-minute vacation requests, I'd go crazy. What's the big deal about a distant cousin coming to visit, anyway?"

Ideas about the importance of anticipating and controlling the future vary significantly from culture to culture. Whereas some staff members place a high priority on planning for retirement, accumulating sick days, and purchasing insurance, others, particularly recent immigrants with family obligations in their homelands, may be more concerned with current obligations and living in the present. Similarly, some workers in high-risk jobs will participate actively in preventive immunization programs aimed at hepatitis and influenza, whereas others bewilder managers by saying, "What will be, will be. I can't spend time worrying about something that may or may not happen in the future."

Cultural Perspectives on Personal Hygiene

Another value that influences behavior is found in the proverb "cleanliness is next to godliness." This proverb highlights the value for cleanliness, including an obsession with eliminating or minimizing natural bodily odors—as evidenced by the plethora of deodorants, douches, body lotions, mouthwashes, and the like with hundreds of different fragrances. Members of the dominant culture sometimes have difficulty with staff members from other cultures who are not unduly bothered by body odors and see no reason to mask nature's original smells. In some cases, the staff member may come from a country in which water is scarce and bathing is restricted. Other staff members may be following religious or cultural practices that prohibit bathing during certain phases of the menstrual cycle, after the delivery of a baby, and at other times. Nurse managers and other supervisors frequently find the sensitive topic of **hygiene** difficult to discuss with staff from diverse cultural backgrounds.

Cross-Cultural Communication

Underlying the majority of conflicts in the multicultural health care setting are issues related to effective **cross-cultural communication**, both verbal and nonverbal. Even when one is dealing with staff members from the same cultural background, it requires administrative skill to decide whether to speak with someone face to face, send an electronic or paper memorandum, contact the person by telephone, or opt not to communicate about a particular matter at all. The nurse must exercise considerable judgment when making decisions about effective methods for communicating with staff members and patients from diverse cultural backgrounds, considering a sense of timing, tone and pitch of voice, choice of location for face-to-face interactions, and related

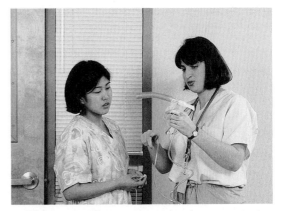

FIGURE 12-3. Effective cross-cultural communication among staff is necessary to ensure optimal patient care. (Copyright B. Proud)

matters (Figure 12-3). Communication difficulties caused by differences in language and accent become compounded on the telephone. It is sometimes necessary to counsel recent immigrants from non–English-speaking countries to refrain from giving or receiving medical orders by telephone until their English language skills have developed (Nixon & Bull, 2006; Samovar, Porter, & McDaniel, 2006).

In the United States, approximately 52 million people age 5 or older, or 19% of the total U.S. population, speak languages other than English. In rank order, the most frequently spoken languages are Spanish (62%), Chinese (4%), French (3%), Tagalog (3%), Vietnamese (2%), German (2%), and Korean (2%) (U.S. Census Bureau, 2005a). In Canada, 66% of the total population speak English most often, and 21% speak French most often. In rank order, the most frequently spoken languages in Canada other than English and French include Chinese (2.3%), Punjabi (1.4%), Italian (6%), Spanish (5%), Portuguese (4%), Arabic (0.4%), and German (0.4%) (Statistics Canada, 2001a). It is estimated that the United States will continue to attract about two-thirds of the world's immigration and that 85% of the immigrants will come from Central and South America. Immigration rates to Canada are also predicted to remain proportionally high, with

BOX 12-2

Strategies to Promote Effective Cross-Cultural Communication in the Multicultural Workplace

- Pronounce names correctly. When in doubt, ask the person for the correct pronunciation.
- Use proper titles of respect: "Doctor," "Reverend," "Mister." Be sure to ask for the person's permission to use his or her first name, or wait until you are given permission to do so.
- Be aware of gender sensitivities. If uncertain about the marital status of a woman or her preferred title, it is best to refer to her as Ms. (pronounced mizz) initially, then ask how she prefers to be called at the first opportunity.
- Be aware of subtle linguistic messages that may convey bias or inequality, for example, referring to a white man as Mister while addressing a Black female by her first name.
- Refrain from Anglicizing or shortening a person's given name without his or her permission. For example, calling a Russian American "Mike" instead of Mikhael, or shortening the Italian American Maria Rosaria to Maria. The same principle applies to the last name, or surname.
- Call people by their proper names. Avoid slang such as "girl," "boy," "honey," "dear," "guy," "fella," "babe," "chief," "mama," "sweetheart," or similar terms. When in doubt, ask people if they are offended by the use of a particular term.
- Refrain from using slang, pejorative, or derogatory terms when referring to persons from ethnic, racial, or religious groups, and convey to all staff that this is a work environment in which there is zero tolerance for the use of such language. Violators should be counseled immediately.
- Identify people by race, color, gender, and ethnic origin only when necessary and appropriate.
- Avoid using words and phrases that may be offensive to others. For example, "culturally deprived" or "culturally disadvantaged" imply inferiority, and "non-White" implies that White is the normative standard.
- Avoid cliches and platitudes such as "Some of my best friends are Mexicans" or "I went to school with Blacks."
- Use language in communications that includes *all* staff rather than excludes some of them.
- Do not expect a staff member to know all the other employees of his or her background or to speak for them. They share ethnicity, not necessarily the same experiences, friendships, or beliefs.
- Communications describing staff should pertain to their job skills, not their color, age, race, sex, or national origin.
- Refrain from telling stories or jokes demeaning to certain ethnic, racial, age, or religious groups. Also avoid those pertaining to gender-related issues or persons with physical or mental disabilities. Convey to all staff that there will be zero tolerance for this inappropriate behavior. Violators should be counseled immediately.
- Avoid remarks that suggest to staff from diverse backgrounds that they should consider themselves fortunate to be in the organization. Do not compare their employment opportunities and conditions with those people in their country of origin.
- Remember that communication problems multiply in telephone communications because important nonverbal cues are lost and accents may be difficult to interpret.
- Provide staff with opportunities to explore diversity issues in their workplace, and constructively resolve differences.

approximately 250,000 immigrants being admitted each year. Box 12–2 suggests strategies for promoting effective cross-cultural communication in the multicultural workplace.

CULTURAL PERSPECTIVES ON TOUCH

Differences in behavioral norms in the multicultural workforce are often inaccurately perceived. Typically, people from Asian cultures are not as overtly demonstrative of affection as are Whites or Blacks. Generally they refrain from public embraces, kissing, and loud talking or laughter. Affection is expressed in a more reserved manner. Whites and Blacks may be perceived as boisterous, loud, ill mannered, or rude by comparison. In some cases, staff members from different cultures may send messages through their use of touch that are not intended. Special attention to male–female relationships is warranted in the multicultural workplace. In general, it is best to refrain from touching staff members of either sex unless necessary for the accomplishment of a job-related task, such as the provision of safe patient care. For nurses who tend to be more tactile, it is important to consciously refrain from placing one's hand on another's arm or shoulder, as frequently happens during ordinary conversation. For a further discussion of this topic, see Chapter 2.

CULTURAL PERSPECTIVES ON ETIQUETTE

Values frequently underlie cultural expectations of behavior, including matters of **etiquette**, the conventional code of good manners that governs behavior. For example, some people from Hispanic, Middle Eastern, and African cultures expect the nurse manger to engage in social conversation and to establish personal and social rapport before giving assignments or orders for the day's work. In developing interpersonal relationships, a high value is placed on getting to know about a person's family, personal concerns, and interests before discussing job-related business. The nurse manager's reluctance to engage in self-disclosure about personal matters may leave the impression that he or she is uncaring and is not interested in the staff member. These behaviors by the manager are not conducive to building productive, harmonious relationships and may be misunderstood by staff members from diverse backgrounds. Similarly, some cultures value formal greetings at the start of the day or whenever the first encounter of the day occurs—a practice found even among close family members. For example, it is important to say, "Good morning, Mr. Okoro. There has been a change in your patient's insulin orders," rather than immediately "getting to the point" without recognizing by name the person to whom you are speaking.

Cultural Perspectives on Clothing and Accessories

Most health care institutions have a **dress code** or policy statement about clothing and accessories worn by staff in various parts of the facility (e.g., delivery room, operating room, specialty units). It is important to review these documents periodically from a cultural perspective. For example, modification of the dress code may be necessary to accommodate Hindu women dressed in saris, Sikh men who wear turbans, Amish and Mennonite women who wear bonnets and men who wear straw or black felt hats, Muslim women and Roman Catholic nuns who cover their heads with veils, and Arab men who wear kaffiyehs. Special consideration may need to be given to some Blacks and others who wear jewelry and other accessories in their hair, particularly when the hair is braided.

Cultural Perspectives on Time Orientation

In some cases, cultural differences in **time orientation** create difficulty in the workplace. This may manifest itself when staff members from diverse cultures are tardy, take excessive time for breaks, and fail to complete assignments within the expected time frame. These differences may be interrelated with the cultural meaning of work, religious practices, and cross-cultural communication issues. It is important to be explicit in the job-related expectations about punctuality, the schedule for breaks, and time allotted for assignments.

If a staff member develops a pattern of tardiness, the reason(s) should be explored. Although a uniform standard of punctuality needs to be applied to all staff members, it may be useful to listen to the staff member's explanation and ask what he or she thinks will rectify the problem. The reasons for problems with punctuality may range from child care to car repair needs. Solutions may include the mobilization of cultural resources, such as using extended family members to look after dependents, or networking with coworkers who might be able to recommend a reliable auto mechanic. It is important to listen attentively without rendering judgment or dictating solutions with which the person has not agreed.

It is sometimes useful to divide an assignment into subtasks with specific time lines for each activity. If the staff member has difficulty completing the assignment within the allotted time, it is important to follow up with a discussion of the reasons why there were problems. This follow-up discussion should be conducted in a positive, proactive manner and viewed as an opportunity to promote cross-cultural communication, not as a punitive or disciplinary measure.

Cultural Perspectives on Interpersonal Relationships

AUTHORITY FIGURES, PEERS, SUBORDINATES, AND PATIENTS

As indicated in Figure 12-4 , there are cultural differences in interpersonal relationships involving authority figures, peers, subordinates, and patients. To examine, these cultural differences, consider the following example. Dr. Kelly, an Irish American physician, gave an order for vital signs to Kim Li, a Chinese American nurse. The nurse perceived the order as unnecessary (but not harmful) to the patient, i.e., she thought the physician was requesting vital signs more frequently than was warranted by the patient's condition. Nurse Li refrained from questioning the physician or negotiating with him out of respect for his position of authority and the value she placed on maintaining harmony in the relationship. Nurse Li said nothing and carried out the physician's order.

At the change of shift, the charge nurse became angry because she concurred with the assessment that Dr. Kelly had ordered vital signs too frequently and thought that Nurse Li should have confronted the physician about the order.

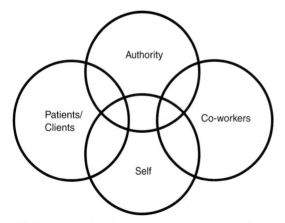

FIGURE 12-4. Cultural perspectives on interpersonal relationships.

Nurse Li intentionally chose to avoid questioning Dr. Kelly's order because she perceived him as an authority figure and wanted to foster harmony and balance. In her cultural value system, causing conflict through direct confrontation would be perceived negatively. She would have experienced lowered self-esteem and "loss of face" if she had been responsible for causing disharmony in the nurse–physician relationship. The charge nurse, on the other hand, perceived the physician as a colleague whose respect would be earned by assertive, direct communication with him.

LONG-STANDING HISTORIC RIVALRIES

The U.S. and Canadian media are replete with news, documentaries, human-interest stories, and related programs pertaining to nations with long-standing historic rivalries. Within nations there might be intergroup conflict such as the rivalries and civil war involving the Sunni and Shia Islamic groups in Iraq. At any given moment, there are numerous armed conflicts between two or more nations or between factions within nations. On occasion, the multicultural workplace becomes a battleground, where long-standing historic rivalries and more recent geopolitical differences are reenacted in the form of interpersonal conflict between two or more staff members. After ruling out other potential sources of conflict, it may be worth examining the ethnic heritage and national origins of staff members for possible reasons. For example, the nurse manager may observe a pattern of strained relationships between an Israeli physician and Palestinian physicians, nurses, laboratory technicians, physical therapists, and other health care providers. Similar observations may be made concerning staff members from countries known to be rivals, such as North and South Korea, Russia and Afghanistan, Iran and Iraq, India and Pakistan, and so forth.

Cues that may signal underlying historic rivalries include (1) the expression of high levels of emotional energy when a staff member is interacting with a person from a rival group and the topic does not seem to warrant it; (2) sudden, uncharacteristic behavior changes when the staff member is in the presence of a person from the rival group, e.g., an ordinarily cordial staff member unexpectedly becomes acrimonious for no apparent reason; (3) the repeated expression of strong opinions about historical, political, and current events involving rival nations or factions; and (4) inappropriate attempts to persuade others to adopt the staff member's partisan views about the rivalry.

Cultural Perspectives on Gender and Sexual Orientation

Women have historically constituted the majority of personnel in nursing and in many allied health disciplines. Currently, women constitute 94.3% of the nursing profession in the United States (U.S. Department of Health and Human Services, Bureau of Health Professions, 2005) and 94.4% of the nursing profession in Canada (Canadian Institue for Health Information, 2005). Although Chapter 2 provides information about gender and sexual orientation, a few remarks about issues in the multicultural workplace will be made here. The complex interrelationship between gender and culture has been studied extensively. In the health care setting, nurses of both genders may face the biases and preconceptions of physicians, fellow nurses, and other health care providers. The issue is further complicated by cultural beliefs about relationships with authority figures and cross-national perspectives on the status of various health care disciplines. For example, in many less developed nations, nursing is a low-status occupation. In some oil-rich Arab countries (e.g., Saudi Arabia, Kuwait), care for the sick is carried out by health care providers who are hired from abroad for the purpose of caring for the bodily needs of the sick—an activity that is considered unacceptable in its cultural context.

Men in nursing and other health care disciplines dominated by women continue to struggle as minority members of their professions. In the multicultural health care workplace, both men and women face the gender biases that exist in society. These issues frequently emerge in verbal

and nonverbal communication and in interpersonal relationships. Our language also betrays covert gender biases and preconceptions. For example, the expression "male nurse" is sometimes used, but seldom does one hear about the "female nurse" because that term is considered redundant and unnecessary. An extensive analysis of workplace issues concerning gay, lesbian, bisexual, and transgendered staff members is beyond the scope of this text, but these types of diversity must be considered in the multicultural workplace.

Cultural Perspectives on Moral and Religious Beliefs

In some circumstances, **moral and religious beliefs** may underlie conflicts in the multicultural workplace. Consider the following dilemmas:

- A nurse who believes that it is morally wrong to drink alcohol refuses to carry out a physician's order for the therapeutic administration of alcohol as a sedative–hypnotic or to administer medicines with an alcohol base (e.g., cough syrup).
- A nurse who believes that humankind should not unleash the power of nuclear energy refuses to care for cancer patients undergoing irradiation.
- A Roman Catholic nurse working in the operating room refuses to scrub for abortions, tubal ligations, vasectomies, and similar procedures because of religious prohibitions.
- A Jehovah's Witness nurse refuses to hang blood or counsel patients concerning blood or blood products.
- A Seventh-Day Adventist nurse who cites biblical reasons for following a vegetarian diet is unwilling to conduct patient education involving diets that contain meat.
- Muslim and Jewish staff members express concern that the hospital cafeteria fails to serve foods that meet their religious requirements.

These moral and religious issues reflect the diversity that characterizes staff members in the health care workplace. The challenge is to balance the health care needs and rights of patients with the moral and religious beliefs of health care providers. In some instances, it may be impossible to provide the services demanded by the organization's mission statement if all nurses refuse to engage in a particular activity. There may be legal implications for refusing to provide patients with certain services, e.g., those related to reproductive health. In the clinical world, the options available to accommodate the diverse moral and religious beliefs of staff members frequently depend on the size of the organization, the moral and religious proclivities of workers, the attitudes and beliefs of managers, the organizational climate, fiscal constraints, and other factors. The challenge faced by nurse managers is to balance the conflicting moral and religious beliefs of diverse groups with the achievement of organizational goals. This must be accomplished in a manner that is respectful of the moral and religious beliefs of staff members.

Conflicting Role Expectations: Staff Educated Abroad

Many graduates of foreign nursing programs are currently practicing as registered nurses in the United States and Canada. The majority of these nurses practicing in the United States were educated in the Philippines (50.2%); a markedly increased number have come from Asia and the British Commonwealth countries, the United Kingdom (8.4%), Ireland (1.5%), and Australia, New Zealand, and Canada (20.2%) in recent years. Smaller numbers of nurses have come from Nigeria (2.3%), India (1.3%), Jamaica (1.1%), Israel (1%), and South Korea (1%) (U.S. Department of Health and Human Services, Bureau of Health Professions, 2005). In Canada, the majority of foreign-educated nurses come from the Philippines (30.5%), the United Kingdom (18.9%), the United States (6.5%), and India (5%). (Canadian Institute for Health Information, 2005). Similar trends prevail for foreign-educated physicians, laboratory technicians, and other health care providers in the United States and Canada.

Role is defined as the set of expectations and behaviors associated with a specific position. Considerable research has been conducted on the patient sick role and on the roles of nurses, physicians, and other health care providers. Furthermore, it is suggested that persons entering the United States or Canada from a similar culture (e.g., Australia, England, Ireland) with English as the primary language may experience a lesser degree of culture shock than someone from a more diverse culture. For example, it is suggested that staff members from Australia or the United Kingdom will experience less difficulty with cultural adjustment to the United States or Canada than will persons from the Near and Middle East, Asia, or Africa, where language, religion, dress, and many other components of culture may be markedly different. Although social scientists speculate that people from similar cultures are more readily able to relate to one another, health care providers must be able to transcend cultural differences and to recognize that there are differences in role expectations.

Discrepancies in role expectations tend to create intrapersonal and interpersonal conflict. For example, nurses in Taiwan, the Philippines, and many African nations expect the families of patients to participate significantly in caregiving during the patient's hospitalization. Family members, who may be encouraged to remain with the patient around the clock, provide all aspects of personal hygiene often sleeping on the floor or in uncomfortable lounge chairs.

In many countries, nurses have considerably expanded roles, and their scope of practice is correspondingly broader. For example, in Nigeria it is clearly stated by the Board of Nursing and Midwifery that nurses diagnose and treat common illnesses such as malaria, typhoid, cholera, tetanus, and similar maladies. To graduate from a nursing program in the Philippines, nursing students must deliver a minimum of 25 babies unassisted and also assist at major and minor surgical procedures. In Haiti, nurses routinely start intravenous lines, perform episiotomies, and repair lacerations. In the mastery of technical skills, recent graduates of many foreign nursing programs have logged a considerable number of hours of clinical experience, often as apprentices mentored by experienced nurses who serve as their clinical faculty.

Some British and Irish nurses perceive U.S. and Canadian nurses as "junior physicians," second-guessing and anticipating therapy. Many perceive that in Great Britain and Ireland, nurses have greater freedom in ordering nursing modalities without a physician's orders. For example, decubitus ulcer care, ambulation, dressings, and nutritional therapy are all nurse-initiated activities based on nursing assessment. British and Irish nurses also expect that the nursing role includes activities that are defined by U.S. and Canadian nurses as nonnursing activities. For example, in many British hospitals, nurses are expected to clean patients' units after discharge and prepare them for the next admission.

In many nations, nurse midwives are primarily responsible for obstetric care. In some ways, the United States and Canada are anomalous with so much emphasis on the medically dominated specialty of obstetric medicine. Viewing childbirth as a medical problem, rather than a normal physiologic process, reveals an underlying philosophic difference between the U.S. and Canadian health care delivery systems and those in other nations. Some nurses who have been educated abroad are both nurses and midwives; thus, the transition to the medically dominated U.S. and Canadian models may leave them feeling underutilized and confused about the roles of the obstetrician and the maternal–child nurse or nurse midwife.

Because of the shortage of qualified health care providers in many less developed countries, there usually are fewer interdisciplinary differences about the nature and scope of practice for various health care disciplines. There are also various categories of licensed and unlicensed health care providers who contribute to the overall health and well-being of people in countries around the world. For example, there are feldshers in the former Soviet Union, barefoot doctors in China, and herbalists in nearly every nation.

Cultural Assessment in the Multicultural Workplace

Cultural self-assessment in the multicultural workplace focuses on (1) staff members and their beliefs about multiculturalism in the workplace (**individual cultural self-assessment**) or (2) the entire or particular unit or division of a health care organization, institution, or agency (**organizational cultural self-assessment**).

Individual Cultural Self-Assessment

As indicated in Chapter 1, it is important for nurses to be aware of their own ethnocentric tendencies. This is best accomplished when individuals review their cultural attitudes, values, beliefs, and practices. Figure 12–5 shows the importance of cultural values in the workplace, and Table 12–2 contains the individual cultural assessment instrument, which is one instrument used for gathering cultural data about staff members and their beliefs about multiculturalism in the workplace. By gathering responses to the individual cultural assessment instrument, nurse managers can identify staff perceptions about diversity issues and determine what management strategies might be useful. A culturally diverse workforce should be a strength in meeting the needs of culturally diverse patients and should be viewed as an asset. Nurse managers,

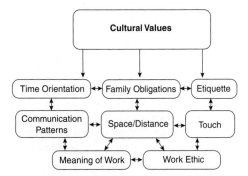

FIGURE 12-5. Influence of cultural values in the multicultural workplace.

TABLE 12-2 *Individual Cultural Assessment Instrument*

	Strongly Agree	Agree	No Opinion	Disagree	Strongly Disagree
1. Open acknowledgment and/or general discussion of cultural diversity occurs in my work environment.	1	2	3	4	5
3. Multicultural education or awareness programs are emphasized in my work environment.	1	2	3	4	5
5. I have personally experienced communication or interaction difficulties with a manager because of my ethnic, cultural, gender, or racial values.	1	2	3	4	5
7. Coworkers in my work environment tend to "hang out" during lunch or breaks with workers from the same cultural background.	1	2	3	4	5
9. Members of my own culture are participants on existing work committees or task forces that help set direction for the work environment.	1	2	3	4	5
11. In my work environment, I have access to work-related growth and development opportunities like my coworkers.	1	2	3	4	5
13. In my work environment, coworkers communicate verbally and/or through body language in ways that demean my culture or race.	1	2	3	4	5
15. All workers in my work environment are held to the same standards of job performance regardless of gender, race, or cultural background.	1	2	3	4	5
17. Staff in my work environment are more successful if they share the same cultural values and ancestry as the manager.	1	2	3	4	5
19. When bicultural or multicultural conflict occurs in my work area, cultural, gender, and racial influences are openly discussed as part of the conflict resolution steps.	1	2	3	4	5
2. It is important that openness and general discussion of cultural diversity take place in my work setting.	1	2	3	4	5
4. Multicultural education and awareness program emphasis is important in my work environment.	1	2	3	4	5
6. It is important that various cultural values are understood and respected by all managers working in a multicultural environment.	1	2	3	4	5
8. It is important for management to facilitate work and to plan culturally mixed social activity for the workers and my work environment.	1	2	3	4	5
10. It is important for management to ensure that the cultures of all workers in my work environment are represented on work committees.	1	2	3	4	5
12. It is important for managers to recognize and encourage growth opportunities equally for all workers.	1	2	3	4	5

(Continued on following page)

TABLE 12-2 *Individual Cultural Assessment Instrument (continued)*

	Strongly Agree	Agree	No Opinion	Disagree	Strongly Disagree
14. It is important for managers to work with staff to increase sensitivity to cultural values and perceptions that will help to reduce or eliminate racial and cultural barriers.	1	2	3	4	5
16. It is important for managers to have systems to identify and analyze which employees receive promotions and growth experiences, and to consider biases that influence performance standards so that they are achievable for all groups of staff.	1	2	3	4	5
18. It is important for the administration to recognize, reward, and value the managers who successfully promote, manage, and retain a harmonious multicultural work force.	1	2	3	4	5
20. It is important for managers to facilitate, promote, and participate in open dialogue about cultural influences and diverse perceptions that occur because of differences in ethnicity or gender.	1	2	3	4	5

Modified and used with permission. From Davis, P. D. (1995). Enhancing multicultural harmony. Nursing Management 26(7), 32D-32E © Springhouse Corporation.

however, need to release the cultural talents of this workforce.

Cultural Self-Assessment of Health Care Organizations, Institutions, and Agencies

Before engaging in a cultural self-assessment of a health care organization, institution, or agency, it is necessary to consider both content and process. Box 12–3 illustrates recommended content in a sample instrument. The instrument may be used to assess an entire organization, such as a hospital; a long-term care facility; a home health agency; or another institution, organization, or agency, or it may be modified for the assessment of a particular unit or division. For example, staff in the operating room, specialty units, home health care division, ambulatory care area, and so forth may perceive a need to engage in an organizational self-assessment because of changing demographics in popu-

lations served or concerns with quality of care for diverse patients. Figure 12–6 provides a schematic representation of the cultural self-assessment of a health care organization, institution, or agency.

The Process of Cultural Self-Assessment by Organizations, Institutions, and Agencies

Although the manner in which the cultural self-assessment is carried out will vary for each institution, organization, or agency and for different units or divisions within it, the process remains fundamentally the same. After identifying key staff members to lead the institutional cultural self-assessment process, the leaders should communicate the purpose of the cultural self-assessment to those who will be participating in it. It is important to involve grassroots members of the staff and to solicit input from the patient population served through interviews, focus groups, written surveys, or other methods. The process of cultural self-assessment by organiza-

BOX 12-3

Cultural Assessment of an Organization, Institution, or Agency

Demographics/Descriptive Data

- What types of cultural diversity are represented by clients, families, visitors, and others significant to the clients? Indicate approximate numbers and percentages according to the conventional system already used for reporting census data.
- What types of cultural diversity are represented? What types of diversity are present among patients, physicians, nurses, x-ray technicians, and other staff? Indicate approximate numbers and percentages by department/discipline.
- How is the organization, institution, or agency structured? Who is in charge? How do you assess the administrators in terms of support for cultural diversity and interventions to foster multiculturalism?
- How many key leaders/decision makers within the organization, institution, or agency come from culturally diverse backgrounds?
- What languages are spoken by patients, family members/significant others, and staff?

Assessment of Strengths

- What are the cultural strengths or positive characteristics and qualities?
- What institutional resources (fiscal, human) are available to support multiculturalism?
- What goals and needs related to cultural diversity already have been expressed?
- What successes in making services accessible and culturally appropriate have occurred to date? Highlight goals, programs, and activities that have been successful.
- What positive comments have been given by clients and significant others from culturally diverse backgrounds about their experiences with the organization, institution, or agency?

Assessment of Community Resources

- What efforts are made to use multicultural community-based resources (e.g., anthropology and foreign languages faculty and students from area colleges and universities, community organizations for ethnic or religious groups, and similar resources)?
- To what extent are leaders from racial, ethnic, and religious communities involved with the institution (e.g., invited to serve on boards and advisory committees)?

- To what extent is there political and economic support for multicultural programs and projects?

Assessment of Weakness/ Areas for Continued Growth

- What are the cultural weaknesses, limitations, and areas for continued growth?
- What could be done to better promote multiculturalism?

Assessment from the Perspective of Clients and Families

- How do clients (and families/significant others) evaluate the multicultural aspects of the organization, institution, or agency? Do quality assurance data indicate that clients from various cultural backgrounds are satisfied/dissatisfied with care? Be specific.
- How adequate is the system for translation and interpretation? What materials are available in the client's primary language (in written and other forms such as audiocassettes, videotapes, computer programs)? *Note:* the literacy level of clients must be assessed.
- Are educational programs available in the languages spoken by clients?
- Are cultural and religious calendars used in determining scheduling for preadmission testing, procedures, educational programs, follow-up visits, or other appointments?
- Are cultural considerations given to the acceptability of certain medical and surgical procedures (e.g., amputations, blood transfusions, disposal of body parts, and handling various types of human tissue)?
- Are cultural considerations a factor in administering medicines? How familiar are nurses, physicians, and pharmacists with current research in ethnopharmacology?
- If a client dies, what cultural considerations are given during postmortem care? How are cultural needs associated with dying addressed with the family and others significant to the deceased? Does the roster of religious representatives available to nursing staff include traditional spiritual healers such as shamans and medicine men/women as well as rabbis, priests, elders, and others?

(Continued on following page)

BOX 12-3 (continued)

Cultural Assessment of an Organization, Institution, or Agency

Assessment from an Institutional Perspective

- To what extent do the philosophy and mission statement support, foster, and promote multiculturalism and respect for cultural diversity? Is there congruence between philosophy/mission statement and reality? How is this evident?
- To what extent is there administrative support for multiculturalism? In what ways is support present or absent? Provide evidence to support this.
- Are data being gathered to provide documentation concerning multicultural issues? Are there missing data? Are data disseminated to appropriate decision makers and leaders within the institution? How are these data used?
- Are opportunities for continuing professional education and development in topics pertaining to multiculturalism provided for nurses and other staff?
- Are there racial, ethnic, religious, or other tensions? If so, try to objectively and nonjudgmentally assess their origins and nature in as much detail as possible.
- Are adequate resources being allocated for the purpose of promoting a harmonious multicultural health care environment? If not, indicate areas in which additional resources are needed.
- What multicultural library resources and audiovisual and computer software are available for use by nurses and other staff?

- What efforts are made to recruit and retain nurses and other staff from racially, ethnically, and religiously diverse backgrounds? What other types of diversity (e.g., sexual orientation) are fostered or discouraged?
- How would you describe the cultural climate of the institution? Are ethnic/racial/religious jokes prevalent? Are negative remarks or comments about certain cultural groups permitted? Who is doing the talking and who is listening to negative comments/jokes?
- Are human resources initiatives pertaining to advertising, hiring, promotion, and performance evaluations free from discrimination?
- Are cultural and religious considerations reflected in staff scheduling policies for nursing and other departments?
- Are policies and procedures appropriate from a multicultural perspective? What process is used for reviewing them for cultural appropriateness and relevance?

Assessment of Need and Readiness for Change

- Is there a need for change? If so, indicate who, what, when, where, why, and how.
- Who is in favor of change? Who is against it?
- What are the anticipated obstacles to change?
- What financial and human resources would be necessary to bring about the recommended changes?

---

tions, institutions, and agencies involves collecting demographic and descriptive data, identifying strengths and limitations, assessing the need and readiness for change, identifying community resources, evaluating the effectiveness of changes, and implementing any necessary revisions.

DEMOGRAPHIC AND DESCRIPTIVE DATA

As with any assessment, begin by gathering demographic and descriptive data. It is highly likely that some of these data have already been collected and stored centrally. If reports containing the necessary data are available, the group should review and discuss them as part of the cultural assessment process. Data such as types and numbers of diverse patients and staff members should be determined. There should be an assessment of the predominant languages spoken and of the effectiveness of the system being used for translation and interpretation.

STRENGTHS AND LIMITATIONS

After the data have been gathered, a team of key leaders should convene to critically review and analyze them. Because this will be an active working group, membership should be limited to approximately 12 people. If the group is larger, consideration should be given to division into smaller subgroups. The purpose of the review is

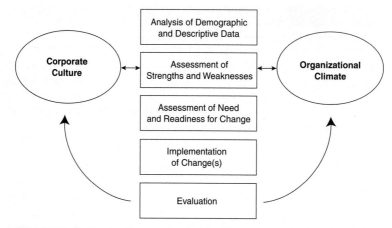

FIGURE 12-6. Cultural self-assessment of health care organization, institution, or agency.

to assess the strengths, limitations, and areas for continued growth in terms of promoting a harmonious multicultural environment for patients and staff members of diverse backgrounds. It is important to identify strengths and limitations from both an **emic** (insider) and an **etic** (outsider) perspective (i.e., from the viewpoint of health care providers [insiders] and patients, those significant to them, and visitors [outsiders]). For example, although the staff may believe the system is structured adequately to meet the needs of linguistically diverse persons, it would be important to compare that perception with the patients' point of view. From their perspective, examine the ways in which cultural aspects are part of the care provided. From the institutional perspective, critically examine the infrastructure for philosophic, fiscal, and human resources that reflect a commitment—or lack of one—to promoting harmony in the multicultural workplace. Throughout the process, comparative analyses are made between input from staff members and that from patients to identify strengths and limitations.

NEED AND READINESS FOR CHANGE

Once the strengths and limitations have been identified, there should be an assessment of the need and readiness for change. If changes are needed, it is important to identify why, who, what, when, where, and how. Identify the fiscal and human resources that will be needed to bring about the recommended change(s).

Be sure to anticipate staff **resistance to change**. Determine who is likely to favor and oppose the proposed change, anticipate obstacles to it, and develop contingency plans. Different people will see different meanings in activities by organizations to become more culturally diverse. Members of the federal minority groups may see job opportunities, whereas White men may complain of reverse discrimination. Depending on the nature of the recommendation and the corporate culture of the organization, an action plan should accompany the recommendation, i.e., specifically what does the group believe ought to be done? Although most staff members will support the change, it is insufficient for nurse managers and supervisors to say, "A new law has been passed mandating diversity" or "Hospital policy requires diversity." Resistance can be expected to increase to the degree that staff members influenced by the changes have pressure on them to change, and it will decrease to the degree they are actively involved in planning diversity activities. Resistance can be expected if the changes are made on personal grounds rather than as requirements, sanctions, or policies. Finally, resistance can be expected if the organizational culture is ignored. There are informal as well as formal norms within every organization. An effective change will neither ignore old customs nor abruptly create new ones. As with most change, timing is important.

COMMUNITY RESOURCES

In developing an action plan for change, be sure to assess the community resources available to assist with goal achievement. For example, it may be possible to invite leaders from ethnic communities to provide staff in-service programs aimed at increasing understanding of the health care needs of persons from diverse backgrounds. A second example might be to involve foreign-language faculty and students from area colleges and universities to assist with translation for linguistically diverse patients and clients. A final example might be to invite clergy to discuss health-related religious beliefs and practices (Parsons & Reiss, 1999). If organizational resources are limited, it may be possible to identify community-based resources that are available at low cost.

EVALUATION OF THE EFFECTIVENESS OF CHANGES AND IMPLEMENTATION OF REVISIONS

After implementation of the recommended changes, an evaluation of their effectiveness should be conducted, and revisions should be made as needed. In recognition of the rapid pace of change in contemporary health care, the process of institutional cultural self-assessment should be repeated at periodic intervals. Mateo and Smith (2001) note that although significant fiscal and human resources are expended by organizations in diversity initiatives, there is a need to be more diligent in monitoring and evaluating outcomes. They recommend the development of a grid that articulates goals, diversity initiatives, and outcome measures.

Promoting Harmony in the Multicultural Workplace

After conducting a cultural assessment of the health care organization, institution, or agency, the nurse will have data about the strengths and weaknesses; fiscal, human, and community resources; areas in which to pursue change; and readiness of the staff to engage in change.

As indicated in Box 12–4, there are **facilitators** and **barriers** to promoting harmony in the multicultural workplace. Facilitators include identification of the cultural values of the organization, institution, or agency; clear articulation of the mission statement and policies about diversity; zero tolerance for discrimination; effective cross-cultural communication; skill with conflict resolution involving diversity; and commitment to multiculturalism at all levels of management. The barriers that must be overcome include hatred, prejudice, bigotry, racism, discrimination, and ethnoviolence. Negative behaviors aimed at employees, patients, their families, others significant to them, and other visitors, based on race, ethnicity, religion, gender, sexual orientation, national origin, class, or handicap/ disability should not be tolerated. All employees should be apprised that there will be zero toler-

---

BOX 12-4

Promoting Harmony in the Multicultural Workplace

Facilitators

Identification of cultural values of the organization, institution, or agency

Mission statement and policies about diversity

Zero tolerance for discrimination

Effective cross-cultural communication

Skill with conflict resolution involving diversity

Commitment to multiculturalism at all levels of management

Barriers

Hatred

Prejudice

Bigotry

Racism

Discrimination

   (Negative attitudes or behaviors based on race, ethnicity, religion, gender, sexual orientation, national origin, class, handicap/disability)

ance for those who engage in negative behaviors, and management staff at all levels should be given the authority to impose sanctions when violations occur.

Summary

Given the demographic composition of contemporary U.S. and Canadian societies, nurses will continue to find both challenges and opportunities as they practice nursing in multicultural health care settings. Microcosms of society at large, health care organizations, institutions, and agencies will consist of staff members from increasingly diverse backgrounds. It is important to remember that culture influences the manner in which people perceive, identify, define, and solve problems in the workplace. Among the complex and interrelated factors that must be considered when workplace diversity is addressed are cultural perspectives on values, the meaning of work, interpersonal relationships, cross-cultural communication patterns (including etiquette, touch, space/distance), gender and sexual orientation, moral and religious beliefs, hygiene, and clothing. Characteristics of the staff member such as individual preferences, biases and prejudices for and against certain groups, educational background, and previous experiences living and working in culturally diverse settings also must be considered.

Understanding cultural differences in the workplace and developing skill in conflict resolution will continue to be needed in transcultural nursing administration in the new millennium. The successful transcultural nurse administrator will behave respectfully toward others from diverse backgrounds and will implement policies that promote cultural understanding, knowledge, and skill in the workplace. Nurses in leadership and management positions will apply the principles of transcultural nursing to the multicultural workplace, just as they have done in the past to provide culturally competent and congruent care for patients.

REVIEW QUESTIONS

1. Compare and contrast the concepts of hatred, prejudice, racism, discrimination, and ethnoviolence. Critically examine the manner in which they may manifest themselves in the health care workplace.
2. What is meant by transcultural nursing administration? How is transcultural nursing administration useful for nurses who hold leadership positions in multicultural health care settings?
3. How do the cultural meanings of work embraced by staff from diverse cultures influence the corporate culture and organizational climate of contemporary health care institutions, organizations, and agencies?
4. Identify strategies to promote effective cross-cultural communication in the multicultural workplace.
5. Critically analyze the cultural origins of conflict that may arise in the health care workplace.
6. Review the process and content of cultural self-assessment by organizations, institutions, and agencies. What aspects of the change process must be considered during engagement in cultural self-assessment?
7. Identify facilitators and barriers to promoting harmony in the multicultural workplace.

CRITICAL THINKING ACTIVITIES

1. Using the guidelines in Box 12–3, conduct a cultural assessment of a health care organization, institution, or agency. Alternatively, you may use the guidelines to gather assessment data on a unit or department within a larger facility.

2. Ask at least 10 nurses working at a health care organization, institution, or agency (hospital, long-term care facility, prison, home health care agency, or related facility) if they would be willing to respond to the items found in the instrument in Table 12–2, Individual Cultural Assessment Instrument. Average the numeric responses for each of the 20 items to identify trends. Write a 1-page summary of your findings that includes a critical analysis of the results. What do the responses tell you about the organizational climate and corporate culture that prevail within the health care facility?

3. Reflect on your personal experience with hatred, prejudice, bigotry, racism, discrimination, and/or ethnoviolence. Were you the victim or the perpetrator? How did you feel during the incident(s)? Discuss your responses with another member of the class, preferably someone from a different cultural background from your own.

4. From a cultural perspective, critically examine the dress code or policy statement about clothing and accessories that are permitted for staff at a health care organization, agency, or institution. How effectively does the code or policy address the widespread diversity that characterizes our contemporary health care workforce? Identify the strengths and limitations of the dress code or policy statement. What modifications or changes would you recommend to accommodate the attire worn by staff from diverse cultures?

5. Choose two of the five case studies presented at the beginning of the chapter, and analyze them from the perspective of a nurse manager. For the purpose of analysis, assume the role of nurse manager, and critically examine approaches you might use to change the negative attitudes and behaviors of those mentioned in the case studies.

REFERENCES

Brown, I. C. (1973). *Understanding race relations.* Englewood Cliffs, NJ: Prentice-Hall.

Canadian Institute for Health Information. (2005). *Workforce trends of regulated nurses in Canada, 2005* [Data file]. Available from http://secure.cihi.ca/cihiweb/dispPage.jsp?cw_page=statistics_results_topic_nurses_e&cw_topic=Health%20Human%20Resources&cw_subtopic=Nurses. Retrieved December 29, 2006.

Henderson, G. (1994). *Cultural diversity in the workplace.* Westport, CT: Praeger.

Human Resources and Social Development Canada. (2001). *Canadian citizen workforce population showing representation by employment equity occupational groups and unit groups (2001 NOC) for women, aboriginal peoples and visible minorities* (Table 14) [Data file]. Employment Equity Data Report. Retrieved December 29, 2006, from http://www.hrsdc.gc.ca/en/lp/lo/lswe/we/ee_tools/data/tables/annual/2001/Table14.pdf

Jung, C. A. (1968). In G. Adler, *The Collected Works of Carl Jung* (Vol. 10). Princeton, NJ: University Press.

Kalbach, M. A., & Kalbach, W. E. (2000). *Perspectives on ethnicity in Canada.* Toronto: Harcourt Canada.

Leininger, M. M. (1996). Founder's focus. Transcultural nursing administration: An imperative worldwide. *Journal of Transcultural Nursing, 8*(1), 28–33.

Mateo, M. A., & Smith, S. P. (2001). Workforce diversity: Challenges and strategies. *Journal of Multicultural Nursing & Health, 7*(2), 8–12.

Nixon, Y., & Bull, P. (2006). Cultural communication styles and accuracy in cross-cultural perception: A British and Japanese study. *Journal of Intercultural Communication, 12.* Available from http://www.immi.se/intercultural/

Parsons, L. C., & Reiss, P. L. (1999). Promoting collaborative practice with culturally diverse populations. *Seminars for Nurse Managers, 7*(1), 160–165.

Samovar, L. A., Porter, R. E., & McDaniel, E. R. (2006) *Intercultural communication: A reader.* Belmont, CA: Thomson/Wadsworth.

Statistics Canada. (2001a). *Detailed language spoken at home, frequency of language spoken at home and sex for population, for Canada, provinces, territories, census population areas and census agglomerations, 2001 Census.* Retrieved January 28, 2007, from http://www12.statcan.ca/english/census01/products/standard/themes/RetrieveProductTable.cfm?Temporal=2001&PID=55536&APATH=3&GID=431515&METH=1&PTYPE=55440&THEME=41&FOCUS=0&AID=0&PLACENAME=0&PROVINCE=0&SEARCH=0&GC=0&GK=0&VID=0&VNAMEE=&VNAMEF=&FL=0&RL=0&FREE=0

Statistics Canada. (2001b). *Immigrant status and place of birth of respondent, sex and age groups for population, for Canada, provinces, territories, census metropolitan areas, 2001 Census.* Retrieved January 27, 2007, from http://www12.statcan.ca/english/census01/Products/standard/themes/DataProducts.cfm?S=1&T=43&ALEVEL=2&FREE=1

U.S. Census Bureau. (1995). Employed civilians by occupation, sex, race, and Hispanic origin: 1995. In Section 13: Labor Force Employment and Earnings, *Current Population Reports.* Washington, DC: U.S. Government Printing Office.

U.S. Census Bureau. (2005a). *Language spoken at home by ability to speak English for the population 5 years and over* (Table C16001) [Data file]. 2005 American Community Survey. Retrieved January 27, 2007, from http://factfinder.census.gov/servlet/DTTable?_bm=y&-state=dt&-ds_name=ACS_2005_EST_G00_&-CONTEXT=dt&-mt_name=ACS_2005_EST_G2000_C16001&-redoLog=true&-_caller=geoselect&-geo_id=01000US&-geo_id=NBSP&-format=&-_lang=en

U.S. Census Bureau. (2005b). *Place of birth for the foreign-born population* (Table C05006) [Data file]. 2005 American Community Survey. Retrieved January 27, 2007, from http://factfinder.census.gov/servlet/DTTable?_bm=y&-geo_id=01000US&-ds_name=ACS_2005_EST_G00_&-_lang=en&-redoLog=false&-mt_name=ACS_2005_EST_G2000_C05006&-format=&-CONTEXT=dt

U.S. Department of Health and Human Services, Bureau of Health Professions. (2001). *The registered nurse population: National sample survey of registered nurses.* Washington, DC: U.S. Government Printing Office.

U.S. Department of Health and Human Services, Bureau of Health Professions. (2005). *Preliminary Findings: 2004 National Sample Survey of Registered Nurses.* Retrieved from http://bhpr.hrsa.gov/healthworkforce/reports/rnpopulation/preliminaryfindings.htm

Williams, D. R., & Rucker, T. D. (2000). Understanding and addressing racial disparities in health care. *Minority Health, 2*(1), 30–39.

PART FOUR

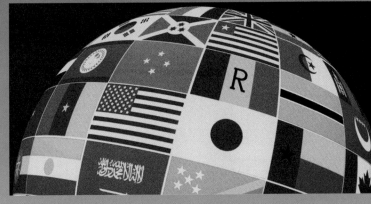

CONTEMPORARY CHALLENGES IN TRANSCULTURAL NURSING

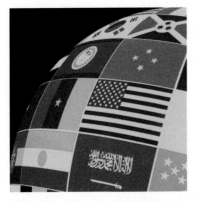

CHAPTER 13

Transcultural Aspects of Pain

Patti Ludwig-Beymer

Pain, a universally recognized phenomenon, is an important area of consideration in nursing practice. While the capacity to treat pain has never been greater, pain is undertreated (Bonham, 2001). In a nationally representative sample of African American, Hispanic, and White subjects, approximately one-third in each group reported "frequent or persistent pain" for 3 months or longer during the previous year. White subjects reported experiencing longer pain with less intensity; significantly fewer Hispanic subjects reported visiting a physician for pain; and African American subjects were more likely to have used prescription medication for pain (Portenoy, Ugarte, Fuller, & Haas, 2004).

Pain is a frequent and compelling reason for seeking health care and is a common result of many diagnostic, surgical, and treatment procedures. Chronic pain is now considered to be the most frequent cause of disability in the United States and in other industrialized nations. Chronic pain has often been mismanaged and has resulted in decreased quality of life, medical expense, lost work hours, and lawsuits. The elderly are at special risk for pain. One study found that 51% of nursing home residents reported pain every day (Ferrell & Ferrell, 1990), and other studies have reported that approximately 70% of elderly people living in the community experience some degree of pain regularly (Crook, Rideout, & Brown, 1984; Roy & Thomas, 1986; Sorkin, Rudy, Hanlon, Turk, & Steig, 1990). Acute pain is also common. For example, a large number of patients with breast cancer experience postsurgical pain at the site of incision. Research suggests that Latinas and African Americans are more likely to report this pain (Eversley et al., 2005). Even in acute care settings, pain may not be adequately treated, and the ethnicity of patients affects pain management (Todd, Samaroo, & Hoffman, 1993). Data from numerous studies suggest that White males receive more interventions than women and minorities. In degenerative spinal disorders, for example, surgery recommendations were more common in White males than in Asian, Black, or Hispanic males or any females (Taylor et al., 2005). Similarly, racial differences in the use of joint replacement cannot be explained by pain resulting from osteoarthritis (Ang, Ibrahim, Burant & Kwoh, 2003). In addition, there is considerable variation in the use of epidurals to manage pain in the laboring patient (see Evidence-Based Practice 13-1)

The management of pain is particularly important in nursing because nurses often encounter people either experiencing or anticipating pain. Of equal importance, pain management has traditionally been a nursing responsibility. Thus, nurses are in an ideal position to assess pain and to take action to alleviate it. Many nurses, however, may not be sufficiently prepared to care for patients in pain. Inadequacies in pain management may result from lack of knowledge about pain management and disease processes. Ferrell, Virani, Grant, Vallerand, and McCaffery (2000) surveyed 50 textbooks used in nursing education and found that pain constituted only 0.5% of the total text content. Pharmacologic management of pain was identified as a particular weakness.

Pain is a private experience and is influenced by a variety of factors, as summarized in Table 13-1. Culture has long been recognized in nursing practice and research as a factor that influences a person's expression of and reaction to pain. Expectations about pain and its manifestations and management are embedded in a cultural context. The definition of pain, like that of health or illness, is culturally influenced. Zborowski (1952, 1969) has made perhaps the greatest contribution to our understanding of cultural responses to pain and the subjective nature of the pain experience (see Evidence-Based Practice 13-2).

Definition of Pain

Definitions of pain are quite diverse, partly because of the complex nature of pain and partly because of the many different existing perspectives on pain. The term *pain* is derived from the Greek word for penalty, which helps to explain the long association between pain and punishment in Judeo-Christian thought. The medical profession has dominated our understanding of pain since the late 1800s. Consequently, pain has come to be defined as a sensation associated with real or potential tissue damage involving chemical disturbances along neurologic pathways. In the United States, the national guidelines on acute pain management define pain as an unpleasant sensory and emotional experience arising from actual or potential tissue damage or described in terms of such damage (U.S. Department of Health and Human Services, 1992).

However, pain is much more variable and modifiable than has previously been believed. Variations within and among people and cultures have been identified. Pain measurements

Evidence-Based Practice 13–1:

Use of Epidurals for Pain Management

The impact of race/ethnicity and insurance coverage as determinants of epidural use for childbirth pain management was analyzed from a large national database. While race was not a significant risk factor for not receiving an epidural, ethnicity was strongly associated with nonuse of epidurals. Hispanic women were twice as likely as non-Hispanic women not to have an epidural. In addition, women who reported publicly funded insurance (Medicaid) were almost twice as likely not to receive an epidural procedure when compared to women with private or no insurance. The decision for epidural use may come from the mothers' cultural expectations and/or physicians' choice related to clinical or economic reasons.

Clinical Application

This study suggests major differences in the management of labor pain. The ethnic differences may reflect patient preference or provider reluctance to discuss the epidural option with Hispanic women. The strong link with type of insurance is a troubling indicator of disparity in access to health care resources.

Atherton, M. J., Feeg, V. D., & El-Adham, A. F. (2004). Race, ethnicity, and insurance as determinants of epidural use: Analysis of a national sample survey. *Nursing Economics, 22*(1), 6–13.

are summarized in Table 13-2. These measurements include **sensation threshold, pain threshold, pain tolerance,** and **encouraged pain tolerance.** Stimuli that would produce intolerable pain in one person may be embraced by another. For example, in some cultures, initiation rites and other rituals involve procedures generally associated with severe pain, but the participants reportedly feel little or no pain (Melzack & Wall, 1983).

Pain perception, then, cannot be defined simply in terms of particular kinds of stimuli. Rather, pain is a highly personal experience, depending on cultural learning, the meaning of the situation, and other factors unique to the individual. Pain is subjective, occurring whenever the experiencing person says it does. The meaning of painful stimuli for individuals, the way individuals define their situation, and the impact of previous personal experiences all help determine the experience of pain (McCaffery & Pasero, 1999).

Culturally Competent Nursing Care for Clients in Pain

Six helpful strategies for dealing with the client in pain are identifying **personal attitudes,** creating an effective **nurse–client relationship,** establishing **nurse competence,** assessing pain, managing pain, and clarifying responsibility. Transcultural concepts are integrated into these strategies. When these strategies are not used, culturally insensitive care may result.

Identifying Personal Attitudes

Nurses bring their own attitudes about pain to each client interaction. Some research suggests that nurses, as part of a **nursing subculture,** have been socialized to have certain pain expectations, as summarized in Table 13-3. Nurses must understand and confront their own personal beliefs about pain and suffering. It is helpful for

TABLE 13-1 *Factors That Affect Expressions of Pain*

Factor	Explanation
Family	Experiences and attitudes of one's family affect response to painful situation.
Cultural group	Patterned attitudes toward pain behavior exist in every culture, and appropriate and inappropriate expressions of pain are thus culturally prescribed.
	Cultural responses to pain can be divided into two categories: stoic and emotive. Patients who are stoic are less likely to express their pain, whereas emotive patients are more likely to verbalize the expressions of pain.
Emotional factors	Perceived significance of pain affects response to pain.
Gender	Studies suggest that women tend to express distress and strain related to pain more openly and more often than men (Kleinman, 1988; Lawlis, Achterberg, Kenner, & Kopetz, 1984; Encandela, 1993).
Spirituality and religious heritage	Studies suggest that spiritually focused or strongly religious people find meaning and expression for their pain through religious doctrines (Kotarba, 1983; Ohnuki-Tierney, 1984, Encandela, 1993).
Age	Specific biological and psychosocial factors influence elderly people's perceptions and experience of pain. Elderly people may believe that pain is a normal part of aging and should be tolerated, staff are too busy to hear complaints of their pain, and telling nurses about pain may result in further testing and expenses. The elderly may also be resigned to pain, ambivalent about the benefits of pain relief, and reluctant to express pain. (For further information, see Melding, 1991; Herr & Mobily, 1991; Hofland, 1992; Witte, 1989; and Yates, Dewar, & Fentiman, 1995.)

individual nurses to identify how they view, express, and manage their own pain. Nurses must also identify their beliefs about clients' expression of pain. For example, is a nurse truly nonjudgmental, or does the nurse prefer the patient to express pain stoically? The learner activities at the end of this chapter will assist nurses in this process. Identifying personal cultural beliefs is the first step in recognizing how these beliefs may interfere with truly therapeutic nurse–client relationships.

Creating an Effective Nurse–Client Relationship

The issue of power and powerlessness always colors the relationship between the person in pain and the health care provider. Because pain is a wholly subjective experience that cannot be proved or verified, people in pain are at the mercy of the health care provider to whom they chose to disclose information about their pain. The health care provider may decide to believe or disbelieve the person's account of pain, ignore it completely, or intentionally or inadvertently make it worse.

Thus, in nursing practice, it is important to establish an effective and supportive nurse–client relationship. The quality of the relationship may be as important as the pain-relieving skills or techniques used. The nurse should strive to create a relationship with the client that is characterized by genuineness, empathy, warmth, and respect. These caring behaviors constitute the essence of transcultural nursing. A positive relationship incorporates respect for the client and avoidance of stereotyping.

Respect Clients as Individuals

Nurses must respect clients as unique individuals and recognize that culture is an important aspect

Evidence-Based Practice 13–2:
Zborowski's Classic Study of Pain

An anthropologist, Zborowski studied 103 patients on a Veterans Administration hospital medical-surgical unit using a variety of qualitative methods, including questionnaires, unstructured interviews, and direct observations. Data were collected from four cultural groups: Irish Americans, Italian Americans, Jewish Americans, and "Old Americans" (defined as third-generation Americans).

Zborowski compared pain interpretation, significance of pain, and other specific aspects of the pain experience, such as intensity, duration, and quality, across the four cultural groups. He found that Irish Americans had difficulty describing and talking about pain, showed little emotion with pain, deemphasized the pain, and withdrew socially when experiencing pain. Italian Americans were expressive in their pain and preferred the company of others when in pain. They tended to request immediate pain relief by any means possible and were generally happy when the pain was relieved. Like the Italian Americans, the Jewish Americans preferred company while in pain, sought relief from pain, and freely expressed their pain through crying, moaning, and complaining. However, the Jewish American men were skeptical and suspicious of the pain and were concerned about the implications of the pain. The "Old Americans" were precise in defining pain, displayed little emotion, and preferred to withdraw socially when in pain.

Clinical Application

Zborowski maintained that cultural traditions dictate whether to expect and tolerate pain in certain situations as well as how to behave during a painful experience. In addition, cultural groups expect individuals to conform to these culturally prescribed rules and norms. Despite some methodologic flaws, Zborowski's research remains the classic study of cross-cultural pain responses.

Zborowski, M. (1952). Cultural components in response to pain. *Journal of Social Issues, 8,* 16–30, and Zborowski, M. (1969). *People in pain.* San Francisco: Jossey-Bass.

of that individuality. For example, nurses must recognize that clients hold a variety of beliefs about pain. In addition to recognizing the existence of different perspectives on pain, nurses must acknowledge that clients are entitled to their own belief systems.

Respect the Client's Response to Pain

Although personal values and cultural expectations differ, nurses must accept the rights of clients to respond to pain in the way they deem appropriate. Clients should never be made to feel ashamed of their responses to pain, even if the responses are not congruent with what nurses consider typical. Nurses need to remember that **pain expressions** vary widely and that no expression of pain is inherently good or bad.

The nurse who is aware of cultural differences and understands clients in terms of cultural backgrounds will respond effectively and appropriately to their needs. Such a nurse will not be disturbed by the emotional expressiveness of a client whose culture expects and encourages open expression of pain. Similarly, the sensitive nurse will not mistake the stoic attitude of a client from another culture for lack of pain.

TABLE 13-2 *Measurement of Pain*

Type of Pain	Definition	Impact of Culture
Sensation threshold	Lowest stimulus that results in tingling or warmth	Research suggests that most people, regardless of cultural background, have a uniform sensation threshold
Pain threshold	Point at which the individual reports that a stimulus is painful	Cultural background appears to have some effect on this measure of pain
Pain tolerance	Point at which the individual withdraws or asks to have the stimuli stopped	Cultural background appears to have a strong effect on pain tolerance levels
Encouraged pain tolerance	Amount of painful stimuli an individual accepts when encouraged to tolerate increasingly higher levels of stimulation	Cultural differences have been documented

TABLE 13-3 *The Nursing Subculture: Expectations About Pain*

Expectations	Description
Silent suffering	Social customs and practices in society at large, particularly in health care, have been dominated by White Anglo-Saxon Protestants. Regardless of their ethnic backgrounds, most nurses have been somewhat influenced by these dominant values and beliefs. The majority of nurses in the United States and Canada are White, middle-class women who have been socialized to believe that self-control is better than open displays of strong feelings. Nurses may be socialized to place a high value on self-control in response to pain. (For further information, see Benoliel & Crowley, 1974; Acheson, 1988; and Howell, Butler, Vincent, Watt-Watson, & Stearns, 2000).
Ability to describe pain	Nurses expect people to be objective about the very subjective experience of pain. In clinical practice, nurses may expect a person experiencing pain to report it and give a detailed description of it but to display few emotional responses to the pain.
Pain inferences	Individuals who are in frequent contact with people in pain may become insensitive to pain. Nurses may deny or downplay the pain they observe in others. Research suggests that the ethnic background of both the client and the nurses is an important determinant for inference of suffering caused by both physical and psychological distress. One study asked nurses from 13 countries to infer physical and psychologic pain for clients described in brief case studies. Nurses from these cultures differed markedly. Korean nurses inferred the highest level of psychologic distress, followed by Puerto Rican and Ugandan nurses. Nepalese, Taiwanese, and Belgian nurses inferred the least amount of psychological distress. Korean nurses also inferred the greatest amount of physical pain, followed by Japanese and Indian nurses. Nurses from Belgium, the United States, and England inferred the least amount of physical pain. (For further information, see Baer, Davitz, & Lieb, 1970; Davitz & Davitz, 1975,

Never Stereotype a Person on the Basis of Culture

Culture should never be used as a basis on which to stereotype an individual. Intragroup differences in pain perception and expression have been well documented in pain research (Wolff & Langley, 1977). When providing care, the nurse should take into account many aspects of the experience, including the pain itself, the client's culture, the psychologic aspects of the situation, and additional needs of the client. Expressions of pain vary widely within each culture, and nurses must anticipate and accept these variations.

Establishing Nurse Competence

Nurses must demonstrate and establish their competence for clients. The manner in which nurses present themselves and their care may greatly influence their reception. For example, research indicates that the status of the person who suggests that a treatment will be effective influences the extent to which individuals believe the suggestion (Neufeld, 1970). Clients should feel comfortable with both the technical and interpersonal skills of nurses. An important aspect of establishing credibility relates to the nurse's ability to provide culturally competent care.

Part of establishing interpersonal competence involves being available to the client who is experiencing pain. This may entail staying with the client, providing privacy to the client, or using ordinary touch as an adjunct to pain relief. Research findings indicate that nurses often provide "instrumental touch," such as dressing changes and technology-related touch. However, "caring touch" is essential for comforting clients, generating warmth, decreasing anxiety, diminishing pain, and creating a bond (Figure 13–1).

In addition, nurses should not assume that they are the only people available to clients in pain. Involvement of family members in the nursing care may be helpful. Friends, volunteers, and other health care providers may also provide care and help relieve pain. The ideal caregiver is at least partially determined by culture. For example, a member of a particular culture may prefer

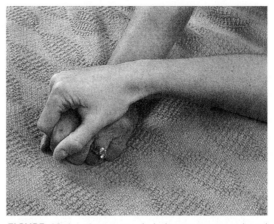

FIGURE 13-1. Caring touch helps to create a bond between client and nurse and provides comfort to the client. A reassuring handclasp uses touch to express concern and interest. (© Copyright B. Proud)

a caregiver of the same gender. These restrictions should be respected and honored as much as possible.

Assessing Pain

According to Leininger (1991), the emic, or insider perspective, presents a true knowledge base for providing culturally congruent care. Perception is a crucial component of pain assessment and forms the basis of subsequent decisions about pain management. Nurses obtain the most useful results when they approach **pain assessment** not as a task but as an important interaction with the client. Self-report is the single most reliable indicator of the existence and intensity of pain (National Institutes of Health, 1987). In practice, however, nurses tend to use other, less reliable measures for assessing pain. For example, McCaffery, Ferrell, and Pasero (2000) found that five of the six top factors identified by nurses as useful in assessing the patient's degree of suffering were influenced by the patient's culture. These factors include facial expression, position and movement, vocalization, request for relief, and verbalization. The danger in using these measures alone is that nurses may overlook clients who do not show the expected signs of distress. Neither vital signs nor behavior can substitute for self-report of pain.

When people in pain realize that others do not believe the existence of their pain, they experience stress and increased pain intensity. Nurses need to try to understand how the client is experiencing pain and convey that understanding to the client. Because the word *pain* has so many different meanings and refers to such a variety of sensations, clarifying clients' experience of pain will be helpful for both nurses and clients. Assessing pain in the elderly presents additional challenges. Despite these challenges, however, the nurse is responsible for knowing the person's pain history and established coping mechanisms.

The assessment of pain has three major objectives. First, it allows the nurse to understand what the client is experiencing. Second, it evaluates the effect that the experience of pain is having on the client. Third, it sometimes allows for a determination of the physical cause of the pain. The first two objectives are described in the next section. The third objective falls primarily within the domain of medicine rather than nursing and is therefore not addressed.

Understanding the Experience

To understand what the client is experiencing, the nurse seeks information about the location, duration, intensity, and type of sensation. The main task is to facilitate communication about what is being experienced. Cultural sensitivity (as described in Chapter 2) must always be a component of pain assessment. A variety of pain assessment tools have been developed and are briefly summarized in Table 13–4. Although the tools have different formats, they are meant to assess the same type of information. However, the usefulness of basic pain assessment tools across cultures is not sufficient to ensure high quality of care for clients with different cultural backgrounds (McCaffery & Pasero, 1999).

Tan, Jensen, Thornby, & Anderson (2005) compared Black and White patients and found that Black patients reported lower perceived control over pain, more external pain-coping strategies, and a stronger belief that others should be solicitous when they experience pain. In addition, Black patients reported higher levels of depression and disability, even when controlling for pain severity.

The nurse must remember that pain expressions will vary among clients and even with the same client in different situations. For example, stress resulting from fear of cancer may result in an increased expression of pain. Clients experiencing chronic pain may display less intense nonverbal behavior relative to their pain than do clients experiencing acute pain. The absence of nonverbal pain behaviors such as grimacing and squinting, however, does not signify the absence of pain. Variations must also be acknowledged within cultures.

Evaluating the Effect

Often the most difficult aspect of pain assessment is evaluating the effect of the experience on the client. At the most fundamental level, the nurse must avoid dictating to clients what effect the pain "should" be having on them. Instead, the meaning of the experience should come from the clients. An assessment of actual responses to pain should include gathering data on what a particular behavior means to each client.

A baseline understanding of the client and his or her response to pain is essential. The nurse needs to assess the type of interventions desired by the client. For example, does the client want traditional interventions, nurturing behaviors, psychologic support, physical interventions, or a combination of these interventions? The role of the family or social support network in providing these interventions should also be assessed. Children should be asked about their preferred coping strategies for managing pain. Parental preferences must also be acknowledged (see Evidence Based Practice 13–3).

Managing the Pain

Undertreatment of pain has been identified as a problem for many years. The Agency for Health Care Policy and Research issued guidelines

TABLE 13-4 *Pain Assessment Tools*

Tool	Description
The Visual Analog Scale (VAS)	This is a vertical or horizontal line with the words *no pain* on one end and *pain as bad as it can be* on the other end (Scott & Huskisson, 1976). Cultures that read from top to bottom or right to left will understand the vertical presentation, while those who read from left to right will be comfortable with the horizontal display.
Numerical Rating Scale	This scale asks individuals to rate their pain on a scale of 0–5 or 0–10. The numerical rating scale correlates well with the visual analog scale (Ohnhaus & Adler, 1975; Cork, Isaac, Elsharydah, Zavisca, & Alexander, 2004), and the 0–10 scale is more precise than the 0–5 scale (Carpenter & Brockopp, 1995). The scale is widely used in clinical practice and can be easily administered to critically ill patients. It is available in Chinese, English, French, German, Greek, Hawaiian, Hebrew, Italian, Japanese, Korean, Pakistan, Polish, Russian, Samoan, Spanish, Tagalog, Tongan, and Vietnamese (McCaffery & Pasero, 1999). The scale may not be reliable when used with cognitively impaired individuals (Kaasalainen & Crook, 2003).
Face Rating Scales	A number of face rating scales have been developed. The Wong-Baker Faces Pain Rating Scale is available in Chinese, English, French, Italian, Portuguese, Romanian, Spanish, and Vietnamese. It has been used in children age 3 and older (Wong & Baker, 1988). Another helpful tool for assessing pain in children is the Oucher Scale (Villarruel & Denyes, 1991). It allows children in pain to compare their pain intensity with pictures of children in pain. It is available in Caucasian, African American, and Hispanic versions (Beyer & Kuott, 1998).
The Brief Pain Inventory (BPI) tool	The Brief Pain Inventory (BPI) tool takes about 15 minutes to complete and is helpful when behavioral expressions for pain vary. It has been found to be reliable and valid in the United States (Cleeland, 1982; Zelman, Gore, Dukes, Tai & Brandenburg, 2005), Singapore (Cleeland & Ryan, 1994), France, the Philippines, and China (Cleeland et al., 1996).
The Adolescent Pediatric Assessment Tool	The Adolescent Pediatric Assessment Tool which takes about 20 minutes to complete, is a multidimensional self-reported pain assessment tool that includes a body outline, a word graphic rating scale, and a qualitative descriptive word list of 67 words representing sensory, affective, evaluative, and temporal dimensions of pain. It has been used effectively to assess complex pain such as sickle cell disease in children and adolescents (Crandell & Savedra, 2005).

related to acute pain management in "recognition of the widespread inadequacy of pain management" (U.S. Department of Health and Human Services, 1992). Several studies (Cohen, 1980; Teske, Daut, & Cleeland, 1983; Rankin & Snider, 1984) suggest that nurses' perception of pain does not coincide with the patients', which results in increased suffering for patients. In addition, Dudley and Holm (1984) found that nurses tended to infer a greater degree of psychologic distress than physical distress from pain. This may lead to inappropriate interventions, such as psychologic support without other pain interventions.

Evidence-Based Practice 13–3:

Parental Preferences for Involvement in Painful Procedures

Clinicians sometimes make assumptions about parental preferences to remain present during their child's painful procedures. Jones, Qazi, & Young (2005) examined ethnic differences in parents' desire to remain present for venipuncture, laceration repair, lumbar puncture, fracture reduction, and critical resuscitation. Overall, White, Black and Hispanic parents (both English and Spanish speaking) wished to remain with their child. The only statistically significant differences were that English-speaking Hispanic parents were less likely to wish to remain during critical resuscitation and more likely to want physicians to decide whether they should be present, while Black parents were less likely to want physicians to decide whether they should be present. Parents generally preferred to actively participate through coaching and soothing rather than simply observing.

Clinical Application

Parents should be offered the option of remaining with their child during painful procedures, and their preferences should be respected.

Jones, M., Qazi, M., & Young, K. D. (2005). Ethnic differences in parent preference to be present for painful medical procedures. *Pediatrics, 116*(2, Pt. 1, Suppl.) e191–197.

The administration of analgesia may differ by cultural group, and medications may be withheld from less vocal clients. For example, Streltzer and Wade (1981) studied postcholecystectomy pain in Whites, Hawaiians, and Asians. They found that nurses limited the amount of analgesia given to all groups and gave significantly fewer analgesics to Japanese, Filipino, and Chinese patients, who were least vocal about pain in the study.

Thus, it is important for nurses to take several active roles in pain management. First, the nurse must base his or her interventions on pain assessment rather than personal beliefs. Second, the nurse must intervene and obtain medical orders for analgesia when the patient requires it.

Clarifying Responsibilities

Responsibilities in pain relief should always be clarified with clients so that they know what they can do to achieve relief. For example, a member of a particular cultural group may consider it inappropriate to report having pain. The client may need permission to request pain relief. A simple statement such as, "please tell me when your pain returns" may be all that is needed. This will allow the client to feel in control of the situation and involved in pain management. In addition, the nurse should assess how the client ordinarily copes with pain. This will identify some potentially effective therapeutic techniques, which are outlined later in this chapter. Above all, the nurse must be open to alternative forms of treatment.

Nurse–client collaboration is essential in pain management. Too often, nurses approach a situation as if they had all the answers. Clearly, this attitude is not helpful. Instead, the client should be involved in actively setting goals. The client should not be left alone to manage the situation. Similarly, the health team should not manage the client's condition without his or her input. Instead, health professionals and clients should work together to meet the challenge of pain. It is clearly the health professional's responsibility to elicit and evaluate cultural knowledge that can be used in pain management.

Clinical Application

Several case studies are presented in this section to illustrate principles of pain management, using a transcultural-nursing framework. It is important to emphasize the great variation that exists within cultures. Differences exist among individuals in any culture in terms of the perception and expression of pain. Nurses should avoid stereotyping patients or assuming that an individual will respond to pain in a certain way based only on his or her culture.

Culturally Competent Nursing Care of a Black Adolescent with Sickle Cell Crisis

In this section, culturally insensitive and culturally competent nursing actions are presented for a client with sickle cell crisis. Additionally, detailed information on the specific physiology of **sickle cell pain** is presented. Case Study 13-1A highlights culturally insensitive nursing actions.

CASE STUDY 13-1A

Jamil Jones is a 13-year-old Black male with sickle cell disease. He has arrived in the emergency department writhing and screaming in pain. His grandmother is crying and shouting, "Why can't you help him? He's hurting!"

Jamil is well known in the emergency department; this is his second visit this month. In a very insensitive manner, health care providers sometimes refer to these patients as "frequent flyers," meaning that they frequently receive care in the emergency department. Staff members are frustrated with his frequent visits, and they express concern that he is addicted to the pain medication. They also believe that the discharge education they provide is ignored, contributing to frequent crises.

In report, one nurse states: "Jamil's back. Same pain. Is he making it up? Why doesn't he do what we tell him to? He wouldn't have all these problems. He's failing school; he stays home all the time and just lies around. We'll get him stabilized and send him home with a prescription for pain medication. He'll probably sell the pain meds on the street. Might even be taking some street drugs. Who knows? No wonder he ends up back here so often."

Case Analysis

This interchange demonstrates a lack of understanding of two important aspects of care: sickle cell disease (SCD) and the cultural dynamics in play during family and professional interactions. It also portrays cultural stereotyping on the part of the nurse. Let's examine each of the nurse's statements.

SICKLE CELL PAIN

SCD is an autosomal recessive inherited condition that occurs primarily in the African American population; the sickle mutation is located on chromosome 11. SCD is the most common genetic disorder of the blood (Edwards et al., 2005). The life expectancy of a person with SCD has increased from 14 years in 1973 to 50 years in 2003 (Claster & Vichinsky, 2003). One in 12 African Americans in the United States carries the trait for SCD (Jakubik, 2000). An estimated 50,000 Americans have the disease, and approximately 2.5 million people carry the sickle cell trait (Beyer, Platt, Kinney, & Treadwell, 1999). The disease is characterized by a defective hemoglobin molecule that causes red blood cells to become sickle (crescent) shaped when partially or totally deoxygenated. This causes hemolysis and vaso-occlusion, with impaired circulation, inadequate oxygenation, pain, and tissue infarction. The disease is recurrent and unpredictable, causing physiologic and psychologic distress. The pain, triggered when misshapen blood cells create capillary blockages, is episodic and severe. In fact, the degree of pain has been compared to the pain of a myocardial infarction, although individuals with myocardial infarction typically receive more aggressive and immediate attention to prevent further infarction. The nurse needs to recognize and acknowledge that the pain associated with SCD is real, rather than minimizing it.

A basic understanding of the pathophysiology of vaso-occlusion is important for proper nursing care. Pain in SCD is complex, requiring continuous adjustment of comfort measures, especially analgesics. Nursing care must incorporate multisystem assessments and interventions that are developmentally appropriate. Pain control, hydration, establishment of trust, and support of individual and family coping are needed to improve recovery and reduce long-term complications.

Pain is a common and important problem for children with SCD, but it has been undertreated and understudied. According to one study, most children are still in pain during crisis despite receiving nalbuphine by intravenous infusion drip (Beyer, 2000). Another study found that 43% of children aged 4 to 18 reported intense pain levels during vaso-occlusive episodes; older children reported higher levels of pain than did younger children. The most frequently used pain management tools were acetaminophen with codeine, fluids, and ibuprofen. Self-care behaviors used by the children included the application of heat, sleeping, reading, and exercising. These interventions helped children to remain in their normal environment and experience some control over their disease (Conner-Warren, 1996).

Living with vaso-occlusive episodes is physically and psychosocially stressful for adolescents. They experience feelings of helplessness as a result of their interrupted lives and their feelings of being discounted by some individuals during a vaso-occlusive event. The unpredictable pain episodes can be incapacitating and may affect the way children view themselves, relate to others, set goals, and approach activities and situations (Jacob, 2001). Common emotional responses may include anger, hostility, depression, disenfranchisement, death anxiety, and fatalism (Strickland, Jackson, Gilead, McGuire, & Quarles, 2001).

McLeod-Fletcher (1996) found that adolescents with SCD who believed they could control and decrease vaso-occlusive episodes used cognitive and behavioral coping strategies that were associated with positive adjustment. Adolescents engaged in a variety of behaviors to control the vaso-occlusive event. This allowed them to decrease the impact of the event, maintain a positive outlook for the future, and make a difficult situation tolerable. Psychologic approaches are commonly used in an attempt to improve coping ability in patients with SCD, but the outcomes have not been carefully studied or researched.

The lack of an established patient–care provider relationship in an emergency department may increase the incidence of patient stereotyping and may result in the failure to properly treat pain (Bonham, 2001). Interestingly, patients who are treated at centers that see primarily Black or Hispanic patients and patients treated at university centers may receive inadequate analgesia compared to patients who received care in other settings. Inadequate prescribing of analgesics may result from many factors, such as concern for potential drug abuse, financial resources, and difficulty in assessing pain because of differences in language and cultural backgrounds (Cleeland, Gonin, Baez, Loehrer, & Pandya, 1997). Physicians and nurses bring preconceived notions about the patient's need for pain medication. These perceptions are often tied to race/ethnicity rather than illness. Care providers are often unaware of their behavior (Dimsdale, 2000). As a result of the treatment they receive, patients and families may feel distrustful, humiliated, intimidated, demoralized, frustrated, angry, and abused. The relationship between provider and patient may become adversarial. The lack of cultural understanding and socioeconomic differences between provider and patient may contribute to the problems.

SCHOOL ABSENCES AND DRUG ABUSE

Studies suggest that school absences are frequent in children with SCD and that standardized academic achievement is approximately one standard deviation below the normative mean for the broader population, with class grades below a C average (Eaton, Haye, Armstrong, Pegelow, & Thomas, 1995). The nurse should be aware of this issue and should not minimize the situation. Also, though drug abuse is a serious problem, there is no reason to suspect drug abuse in every African American male patient who arrives in the emergency department. This represents racial profiling: a severe type of stereotyping.

ADDICTION TO PAIN MEDICATIONS

It is important for patients, families, and clinicians to understand the differences among tolerance, dependence, and addiction. Tolerance and dependence are involuntary and predictable physiologic changes that develop with the repeated administration of narcotics. Tolerance occurs when larger doses are needed to obtain the same effect. Dependence exists if withdrawal symptoms occur when a narcotic is stopped abruptly. Addiction refers to marked psychologic and physiologic dependence on a substance, beyond voluntary control.

While a growing body of literature suggests that only a small percentage of patients without a prior substance abuse history become addicted to opioids appropriately prescribed for analgesia, many health professionals are concerned about contributing to substance abuse problems in patients. This fear is termed "opioidophobia" (Resnick & Rehm, 2001). Emergency department physicians tend to overestimate addiction rates for individuals with SCD (Shapiro, Benjamin, Payne, & Heidrich, 1997). Waldrop and Mandy (1995) found that 8% of staff physicians, 17% of residents, and 13% of nurses in an emergency department estimated that patients with SCD experiencing pain were opioid dependent. This is far in excess of estimates made regarding other populations of patients and may reflect stereotyping and prejudice. It could lead to the inappropriate withholding of pain medication from patients with SCD. In addition, when they believe that health care professionals view them as drug dependent, SCD patients respond with anger and hostility (Strickland, Jackson, Gilead, McGuire, & Quarles, 2001).

Delivering Culturally Competent Care

Although the emergency department staff cannot address all the issues outlined in the case study in an ongoing way, they can and should provide culturally competent care by acknowledging the pain, providing appropriate pain medication, assessing the usual coping strategies, providing assistance in using the pain strategies, and establishing trust.

ACKNOWLEDGING PAIN

Staff members must acknowledge that Jamil is an adolescent in pain. One way to acknowledge this is to rapidly triage the patient into the "very urgent" category (Newcombe, 2002). In addition, treatment of pain in SCD requires a comprehensive team strategy (Claster & Vichinsky, 2003). The use of an acute pain consultant may prove beneficial.

There is no denying that the vaso-occlusion in SCD is extremely painful. It has been estimated that 90% of hospital admissions among patients with SCD are for the treatment of acute pain (Ballas, 1998). The unpredictability of painful episodes adds to patients' discomfort. Rather than minimizing the experience, staff members must recognize the pain and encourage dialogue about it. Staff members must assess the location, duration, intensity, and type of pain.

Considering pain assessment tools, one study found that African-American children preferred the Wong-Baker Faces Pain Rating Scale over the African-American Oucher Scale (Luffy & Grove, 2003). In addition, Jamil may find the Oucher Scale to be too childish, and he should therefore be encouraged to quantify his pain using numbers or words. This will help build a trusting relationship between Jamil and the nursing staff. It will also help family members know that their loved one is believed and is receiving competent care.

ASSESSING USUAL COPING STRATEGIES

In addition to assessing the pain, it is essential for the nurse to assess how Jamil typically copes with his pain. Because he is an adolescent, Jamil needs a sense of control or mastery over the experience. Coping strategies allow some measure of control. When the nurse asks Jamil how he has handled pain in the past, she helps him identify his own strengths and coping mechanisms.

APPROPRIATE PAIN MEDICATION

Rapid, accurate assessment of the patient's condition and prompt delivery of pain relief are essential. The American Pain Society recognizes that the undertreatment of pain in SCD is common (Jacob, 2001). Patients also believe that nurses and physicians do not always respond appropriately to an adolescent's need for pain relief (Lauderdale, 2003). Pain management should be aggressive to relieve pain and allow patients to achieve maximal function (Preboth, 2000). Long used in pain control, meperidine is no longer the drug of choice for managing acute pain (McDermot, 2003; D'Arcy, 2004). Some emergency departments have developed pain management protocols for patients with sickle cell crisis, using morphine or hydromorphone rather than meperidine (Blank et al., 2005). Use of protocols has resulted in increased patient satisfaction and cost savings (Perlman, Myers-Phariss, & Rhodes, 2004). Initiating patient-controlled analgesia in a pediatric emergency department has been shown to decrease time to treatment and was preferred by patients (Meltzer-Lange, Walsh-Kelly, Lea, Hillery, & Scott, 2004).

Pain medication should be based on Jamil's analgesic history and should be titrated in response to qualitative and quantitative pain assessment. Patients with SCD have experienced considerable pain and may be more tolerant to pain medications than the general population (Hammer, Geier, Aksoy, & Reynolds, 2003). However, low analgesic use may lead to poor outcomes such as little relief and reduced functional status (Jacob, 2001). Under no circumstances should the staff belittle or minimize Jamil's pain.

When responding to clinical vignettes, emergency department physicians developed similar treatment plans for pain management regardless of the race or ethnicity mentioned in the vignette (Tamayo-Sarver et al., 2003). However, a large survey of emergency departments found that opioids are less likely to be prescribed for Blacks than for Whites, particularly for migraines and back pain. Differences were not significant for Whites and Hispanics (Tamayo-Sarver, Hinze,

Cydulka, & Baker, 2003). Compounding the situation, some individuals discount pain as a major stressor for adolescents with SCD during the vaso-occlusive event (McLeod-Fletcher, 1996). Jamil needs information on what he is receiving for pain and what he can expect from the medication.

PROVIDING ASSISTANCE IN USING COPING STRATEGIES

Although medications are important during the vaso-occlusive crisis, they do not constitute the only strategy that nurses should use for pain management. Jamil needs to be encouraged to use existing coping strategies and develop additional ones. His family and friends should also be involved. In addition, the nurse might select other strategies that have been found to be helpful by others with SCD. For example, when the pain is under control, Jamil could be encouraged to find out more about SCD and to share what he has learned with his care providers, who can confirm his understanding and acknowledge his mastery of information. Often, this will help mitigate the helplessness that is commonly felt by adolescents with SCD.

Research on coping mechanisms is mixed, with some studies suggesting little variation by race or ethnicity and others suggesting potentially important ethnic influences on pain coping. Prayer, however, is more often reported as coping mechanisms for African Americans and Hispanics (Edwards, Moric, Husteldt, Buvanendran, & Ivankovish, 2005; Hastie, Riley, & Fillingim, 2004; Ang, Ibrahim, Burant, Siminoff, & Kwoh, 2002); prayer, hoping, and diverting attention are used together as a coping technique more often with Blacks than with Whites (Jordan, Lumley, & Leisen, 1998), and religion is a major source of coping for those with SCD (Strickland, Jackson, Gilead, McGuire, & Quarles, 2001; Harrison et al., 2005). Interestingly, this holds true in Muslim as well as Christian patients. Voigtman (2002) found that religious precepts derived from Islamic teaching support tolerance for pain and suffering, as well as seeking a cure. A plan of care that includes appropriate pain management, staff training, patient education, and diversional resources has been found to improve lengths of stay, cost per case, and patient satisfaction (Jamison & Brown, 2002).

In addition, Jamil could be encouraged to keep a daily pain diary as this provides a simple and cost-effective means of collecting data (Gil et al., 2000; Dampier, Ely, Brodecki, & O'Neal, 2002) and enhances patients' ability to communicate about and cope with their disease (Maikler, Broome, Bailey, & Lea, 2001). There is little evidence for the use of psychological treatments, such as relaxation and cognitive behavioral therapy, in patients with SCD (Eccleston, Yorke, Morley, Williams & Mastroyannopoulou, 2004; Anie & Green, 2005). However, a keeping positive mood (Gil et al., 2004) and decreasing negative thoughts during vaso-occlusive crisis (Hayes & Fletcher, 2000) may serve to offset the consequences of pain.

ESTABLISHING TRUST

The actions just described will help to establish a relationship of trust between Jamil, his grandmother, and the nursing staff. However, it is important to realize that trust will not develop immediately. Dorsey, Phillips, and Williams (2001) found that patients with SCD reported lower satisfaction with nurses' caring behaviors than did patients with other medical conditions. In addition, many members of the African American community are somewhat distrustful of health care providers and indeed of many organizations, institutions, and officials. Some of this distrust harkens back to atrocities committed in the name of research, such as the Tuskegee study that allowed African American men with syphilis to remain untreated for years. Some of the distrust is related to society at large. Shared group historical experiences and individual experiences with prejudice, discrimination, and racial profiling affect every interaction with institutions and individuals. Often, predominately White health care professionals are not aware of the degree of distrust. An understanding of the shared history of African Americans is helpful to health care providers. The nurse interacting with Jamil and

his family needs to be aware of this dimension and must make every effort to be open, welcoming, and honest.

FOLLOW-UP REFERRAL

Obviously, the emergency department staff can address only a small part of Jamil's care. Across the nation, emergency departments are inundated with patients, and they exist to provide acute care to very ill patients. However, the emergency department must be viewed as part of a continuum of care. Most likely, Jamil will be admitted to the hospital and then will be discharged to his home. Jamil cannot be allowed to fall between the cracks in our health care system. Instead, the hospital needs to be sure Jamil has appropriate follow-up care after discharge. This may include both medical and psychosocial follow-up care.

Case Revisited

Let's take another look at the case of Jamil Jones. Case Study 13–1B highlights culturally competent nursing care.

CASE STUDY 13-1B

Jamil Jones is a 13-year-old Black male with sickle cell disease. He has arrived in the emergency department writhing and screaming in pain. His grandmother is crying and shouting, "Why can't you help him? He's hurting!"

Jamil is well known in the emergency department; this is his second visit this month. Staff members are frustrated by his frequent visits. Chris Brown, the nurse assigned to Jamil's care, understands that previous discharge planning has been unsuccessful. She wonders what she can do differently to help Jamil and his family.

Chris Brown begins by going immediately to Jamil's bedside. "I know you're in pain, Jamil," she says. "The doctor is ordering you something to manage your pain. The medicine you had last time seemed to work well. How does that sound to you?"

Jamil responds, "Yes—but hurry, please. It's worse than last time."

The nurse nods and turns to Jamil's grandmother. "I'll go get the medicine right away. In the meantime, Jamil might like to listen to some of his favorite music. Remember how that helped him last time? How does that sound, Jamil?"

Jamil states, "No, no, I don't want that. I want to talk to mom. Does she know I'm here?"

Jamil's grandmother is happy to be of help. She tells Jamil she will call his mother, who is at work, and let her know her son is in the emergency department. The nurse leaves to get the pain medication. When she returns, she finds Jamil talking to his mother on the telephone, with his grandmother at his side.

In report, one nurse states: "Jamil's back—can you believe it? Same pain. Is he making it up? Why doesn't he do what we tell him to? He wouldn't have all these problems. He's failing school; he stays home all the time and just lies around. We'll get him stabilized and send him home with a prescription for pain medication. He'll probably sell the pain meds on the street. Might even be taking some street drugs. Who knows? No wonder he ends up back here so often."

Chris Brown speaks up: "You know, sickle cell disease is very complicated. I don't understand it all, but I think we might be missing something with Jamil and with other patients who come to us. What do you think about scheduling some staff education on it? And for Jamil, I'd really like social services to see him. We need to make sure he sees his doctor after he goes home, and he gets the follow-up he needs."

Culturally Competent Nursing Care of a Hospitalized Lebanese American Patient in Pain

This section presents the case of a hospitalized Lebanese American patient in pain to illustrate additional principles of pain management using a transcultural nursing framework (Case Study 13-2).

CASE STUDY 13-2

Mrs. Abdullah is a 45-year-old woman admitted to the hospital with multiple injuries after an automobile accident. Mrs. Abdullah was born in Lebanon, moved to the United States in her early 20s, and is a U.S. citizen. She speaks English fluently.

Ms. Smith, the nurse assigned to provide care to Mrs. Abdullah, arrives in the room to perform her admission assessment. Mrs. Abdullah lies quietly in the bed, providing monosyllabic responses to Ms. Smith's questions and failing to make eye contact. Ms. Smith knows that Mrs. Abdullah received strong pain medication in the emergency department, and she hopes that Mrs. Abdullah will rest after her trauma. When questioned, Mrs. Abdullah neither confirms nor denies pain, but she does moan and cry as soon as the nurse leaves the room. A few hours later, Mrs. Abdullah's husband and sister arrive to visit. Ms. Smith is surprised when she is confronted in the hall by Mr. Abdullah, who shouts: "How can you let my wife lie there without giving her something for pain? What kind of inhumane place is this?"

Let's examine what has occurred in this encounter. The nurse has assumed that Mrs. Abdullah will tell her when her pain returns. However, Reizian and Meleis (1986) suggest that Arab Americans have a present-time orientation to pain similar to that described in Italian Americans by Zborowski (1952, 1969). As such, Arab Americans tend to focus on the immediacy of the pain. Pain is viewed as unpleasant—to be avoided or controlled at all costs. Pain responses are private and are reserved for immediate family members, and families often oversee and make decisions about the care.

When responses are shared with family members but not with health care professionals, conflicts may arise. In this situation, Mrs. Abdullah has discussed her pain with her family but not with her nurse. To provide culturally competent care, Ms. Smith needs to take the following actions:

- Assess pain level at frequent intervals
- Ask the client to describe how she usually copes with pain
- Clarify with the client and family how pain will be reported and managed
- Provide interventions as appropriate to the situation

- Discuss with family members their role in assisting Mrs. Abdullah
- Recognize that Mrs. Abdullah may always feel most comfortable discussing her pain with her family

Making the family a part of care is an excellent way to assist patient and family and enhance the quality of care. In addition, the nurse should be aware that Arab Americans often use metaphors and analogies to describe their pain. The nurse can encourage this type of communication. Last, the nurse should be aware that different pain episodes result in different responses. Some pain, such as labor pain, induces loud moans, groans, and screams. These responses are part of the coping strategies for pain. The nurse should provide privacy as required.

Culturally Competent Nursing Care of a German-American Man with Cancer Pain

This final scenario of a German-American man with cancer pain further illustrates the principles of pain management through culturally competent nursing actions (Case Study 13–3).

CASE STUDY 13-3

Mr. Schwartz is an 82-year-old man of German-American descent who received a diagnosis of stomach cancer 2 years ago. He has multiple physical problems, including postherpetic neuralgia and acute pain that remained after the herpes zoster ("shingles") that occurred 10 years ago. Mr. Schwartz underwent a partial gastrectomy when the cancer was diagnosed and received chemotherapy for 18 months. He has been losing weight despite the high-calorie meals and frequent snacks prepared for him by his wife.

Mr. Schwartz has decided that he wants no further medical interventions for his cancer. With the support of his family and his physician, Mr. Schwartz has enrolled in a hospice program, with care provided by his wife and family in his home. Mrs. Berry, the hospice nurse, finds Mr. Schwartz

to be cooperative and pleasant. He makes jokes with hospice staff and answers their questions in a jovial way. When asked about pain, he changes the subject, although he winces when touched, grits his teeth, and disengages when pain is discussed. Mrs. Schwartz tells the nurses that she knows when her husband is in pain because he snaps at her.

Mrs. Berry is a gentle, compassionate, and knowledgeable nurse. She understands that Mr. Schwartz is a private individual and doesn't wish to discuss his pain. She tells him that she understands and respects his feelings and that her job is to make him as comfortable as possible. She discusses the situation with the doctor and obtains an order for a strong pain medication. She talks with Mr. and Mrs. Schwartz about the intended effects of the medication and also alerts them to the side effects of the medicine. She helps them determine the best timing for the medicine.

After several doses, Mr. Schwartz confesses, "This is the first time I haven't had pain in 10 years." He dies 3 months after beginning hospice, at peace and in no pain.

This case demonstrates the positive impact of a culturally competent nurse. The nurse collected data about the pain experience from a variety of sources, including the patient and family members. In addition, the nurse understood the pathophysiology of both stomach cancer and postherpetic neuralgia. She intervened on the part of the patient, obtained the necessary order, educated the patient and family members on what to expect, and involved them in decision making about Mr. Schwartz's care.

Unfortunately, there is still a tendency to undermedicate for pain, even within hospice programs. This tendency exists both in the United States and in other countries. Studies show that 75% to 90% of cancer pain in terminally ill patients is well controlled when the World Health Organization approach is used: Mean medication doses are as high as 30 mg of morphine every 4 hours. However, appropriate doses are often not used.

The barriers to effective palliative care appear to be similar worldwide (Rhymes, 1996). A German-language study of cancer pain treatment (cited in Rhymes, 1996) found that only 322 of 16,630 cancer patients received strong opiates, adjuvant therapy was rarely used, and treatment for breakthrough pain was rarely given. Health care professionals may be concerned about addiction and respiratory depression or may think that morphine is a drug only for those actively dying. Similar beliefs exist among patients and family members. For example, a study in Poland (cited in Rhymes, 1996) identified common lay myths, including the belief that morphine is to be given only in the very last stages of disease, it will cause addiction, and if it is used too early, there will be nothing stronger to use for pain relief.

Complementary and Alternative Practices for Pain

Many practices have been used for centuries in the management of pain. However, the predominant biomedical system has adapted very few of these techniques, resulting in the growth of complementary and alternative medicine (CAM). Research indicates that alternative therapies were used by 42% of persons in both the United States and Canada in 1997 (Eisenberg et al., 2000; National Council for Reliable Health Information, 1998). Nearly 48% of Hispanic and Vietnamese elderly report using CAM over the past year, with most not informing their physicians of the use. Pain was the most common indicator for use of CAM in Hispanics (Najm, Reinsch, Hoehler, & Tobis, 2003). Adolescents are also using CAM therapies. In a cross-sectional survey of Midwest urban adolescents, 68.1% reported using one or more CAM therapies. Most commonly, adolescents used CAM for alleviation of physical pain. However, very few adolescents disclosed their use to health care providers (Braun, Bearinger, Halcon, & Pettingell, 2005).

Patients are turning to CAM for several reasons, which include the following:

- Frustration with conventional medicine
- Increasing evidence of the influence of lifestyle, nutrition, and emotions on disease
- Expectations of wellness rather than just the absence of symptoms
- Desire to take less medication and decrease health costs
- Increasing awareness of other cultures and their practices

Physicians and nurses are being encouraged to consider CAM therapies as they manage care (Novey, 2000; Ang-Lee, Moss, & Yuan, 2001). In addition, 25% of the hospitals in major metropolitan areas offer some CAM medicine ("Alternative Therapies Come," 2001). Many of these hospitals use relaxation, hypnosis, acupuncture, and acupressure to help patients reduce their need for pain medication.

This section is not designed to prepare the nurse to deliver the alternative practices described. Instead, it is meant to sensitize the nurse to the many options available to clients. In addition, the nurse and the client may choose together to use some of the techniques summarized in Table 13-5, including **relaxation techniques**, **transcendental meditation**, **autogenic training**, **hypnosis**, **yoga**, **distraction**, **imagery**, **cutaneous stimulation**, **herbal remedies** (Figure 13-2), **religious rituals**, **biofeedback**, **acupuncture** (Figure 13-3), and **acupressure**.

In CAM therapies, the connection between mind, body, and spirit is emphasized. The culturally competent nurse must talk with patients about their use of CAM therapies. To begin dialogue, the nurse might simply ask what the patient is doing to reduce pain or improve health. As the patient identifies the use of CAM therapies, the nurse can explore areas such as these:

- The safety and effectiveness of the therapy
- The experience of the practitioner
- The cost of therapy (most patients must pay for CAM therapies themselves because they are typically not covered by insurance)
- The benefits and risks of therapy
- Other activities, therapies, or medications to be avoided during the CAM therapy

TABLE 13-5 *Complementary and Alternative Methods of Pain Control*

Acupressure	Acupressure involves a deep-pressure massage of the appropriate acupoints. Shiatsu is the most widely known form of acupressure, used in Japan for more than 1,000 years to treat pain and illness and maintain general health. (For more information, see Novey, 2000.)
Acupuncture	Acupuncture, practiced for at least 3,000 years, is a method of preventing, diagnosing, and treating pain and disease by the skilled insertion of special needles into the body at designated locations and at various depths and angles. According to Chinese thought, life energy, or ch'i, constantly flows and energizes humans through a pattern known as meridians. Ch'i may be intercepted at various acupoints throughout the body. Acupuncture has been used as an alternative to other forms of analgesia for many minor surgical procedures in China. It has also been used in the treatment of pain in a variety of other countries. There are no simple explanations for the mechanisms that underlie the analgesia-producing effects of acupuncture. However, research has documented the release of endorphins into the vascular system during acupuncture, contributing to pain relief (Novey, 2000).
Alexander Technique	This is based on the belief that tension restricts movement and tightens the body. An Alexander Technique teacher works to restore freedom of movement and enhance body awareness by applying subtle adjustments in posture and alignment (Novey, 2000).
Aromatherapy	Aromatherapy may take a variety of forms, including aesthetic (aromas used for pleasure), holistic (aromatherapy used for general stress), environmental (aromas used to manipulate mood), and clinical (essential oils used for specific measurable outcomes). Aromatherapy has been used in pain management to enhance strong analgesics. The specific essential oils used are based on the type of pain (see Novey, 2000).
Autogenic training	This emphasizes passive attention to the body. The training, which was first recognized within the biomedical model in 1910, incorporates elements of hypnotism, spiritualism, and various yogic disciplines. (See Luthe and Schultz, 1970, for specific meditative exercises.)
Benson's relaxation response	Relaxation is achieved through six basic steps: Sit quietly, close eyes, deeply relax all muscles, breathe through nose, continue for 20 minutes, and allow relaxation to occur at its own pace. (For further information, see Benson, 1976.)
Biofeedback	Biofeedback techniques use instrumentation to provide a client with information about changes in bodily functions of which the person is usually unaware. Clients are taught to manipulate and control their degree of relaxation and tension by way of biofeedback training using electroencephalography (EEG) or electromyogram (EMG) muscle potential.
Craniosacral therapy	This manual procedure is used to remedy distortions in the structure and function of the brain, spinal cord, skull, and sacrum. It is used to treat chronic pain and migraine headaches (see Novey, 2000).
Cutaneous stimulation	This reduces the intensity of pain or makes the pain more bearable. Types of cutaneous stimulation for pain relief include massage/pressure, vibration, heat or cold application, topical application, and transcutaneous electrical nerve stimulation (TENS). Stimulation need not be applied directly to the painful site to be effective (McCaffery, 1990).

(Continued on following page)

TABLE 13-5 *Complementary and Alternative Methods of Pain Control (continued)*

Distraction	Distraction from pain is a kind of sensory shielding in which one is protected from the pain sensation by focusing on and increasing the clarity of sensations unrelated to the pain. Research suggests that distraction techniques, like pain, may be a cultural phenomenon. Clinical and research findings suggest that distraction may be a potent method of pain relief, usually by increasing the client's tolerance for pain by placing pain at the periphery of awareness. Distraction techniques include watching television, listening to music, reading, telling jokes, walking, playing with pets, crocheting, doing housework, interacting with children, animal-assisted therapy, and getting out of the house. Distraction appears to place the pain at the periphery of awareness. (For further information, see McCaffery, 1990; Miller, Hickman, & Lemasters, 1992; Zadinsky & Boyle, 1996; and Kaplan & Ludwig-Beymer, 2005.)
Herbal remedies	Herbal treatments have been used in many cultures for centuries. Although adherence to herbalism diminished in the West, interest is currently increasing, as exemplified by the popularity of herbal teas. Many of the herbs used have a physiologic effect and must be understood by the health care professional. (For additional details, see Novey, 2000.)
Hypnosis	This technique was introduced into Western medical practice in the 18th century by Franz Anton Mesmer. A hypnotic state may be induced either by a hypnotist or by the client (autohypnosis). Hypnosis is based on the power of suggestion and the process of focusing attention. It has been used as an adjunct to other pain-relieving therapies and has been found to be helpful in dentistry, surgery, and childbirth as well as malignancies.
Imagery	Imagery techniques for physical healing date back hundreds of years. Guided imagery involves using one's imagination to develop sensory images that decrease the intensity of pain or that become a nonpainful or pleasant substitute for pain. During guided imagery the client is alert, concentrating intensely and imagining sensory images. Research suggests that pleasant imagery can effectively reduce the perception of postsurgical pain. Music therapy is being used with increased frequency to augment imagery and other relaxation techniques. (For further information, see McCaffery & Pasero, 1999; and Novey 2000.)
Progressive relaxation	Originated by Jacobson (1964), this is probably the most widely used relaxation technique today. The method teaches the client to concentrate on various gross muscle groups in the body by first tensing and then relaxing each group.
Reiki Therapy	"Reiki" is a Japanese word meaning *life energy*. In this therapy, a Reiki master or Reiki practitioner uses hands to effect healing. (See Reiki Infocenter, n.d.)
Relaxation techniques	Many relaxation techniques result in physiologic changes that reduce the damaging effects of stress and promote a sense of physical, mental, and spiritual well-being. All these techniques result in an altered state of consciousness and produce a decrease in sympathetic nervous system activity. Each technique requires a calm and quiet environment, a comfortable position, a mental device or image, and a willingness to let relaxation happen.

(Continued on following page)

TABLE 13-5 *Complementary and Alternative Methods of Pain Control* (continued)

Religious rituals	Clients should be encouraged to use their religious practices as they desire to help in pain management. Privacy should be provided as needed. Prayer, chanting, songs, amulets, and charms should be respected and incorporated into the care provided. Christianity has included the notion of healing through divine intervention since its inception. Roman Catholic clients in pain may wish to pray the rosary or attend mass. Clients of many Christian denominations may actively seek healing through prayer and other rituals. Jewish clients experiencing pain may ask to speak to a rabbi. In other faith traditions, a shaman may conduct a religious ritual for the purpose of healing or pain relief. In this context, the illness or pain is viewed as a disorder of the total person, involving all parts of the individual as well as relationships to others. Working with client, family members, and others, the shaman focuses on strengthening or stimulating the client's own natural healing powers.
Trager	Practitioners move the client's trunk and limbs in a gently rhythmic way. These noninvasive movements help to release physical and mental patterns, allowing the recipient to experience new sensations of freedom and lightness (see Novey, 2000).
Transcendental meditation	This type of meditation is taught individually, involves the use of a specific mantra during the meditation, and was originally developed by the Maharishi Mahesh Yogi, an Indian scholar and teacher.
Yoga	Yoga techniques have been used within the Hindu culture for thousands of years. Yoga involves the practice of both physical exercise (hatha yoga) and meditation (raja yoga). The correct performance of yoga results in deep relaxation without drowsiness or sleep.

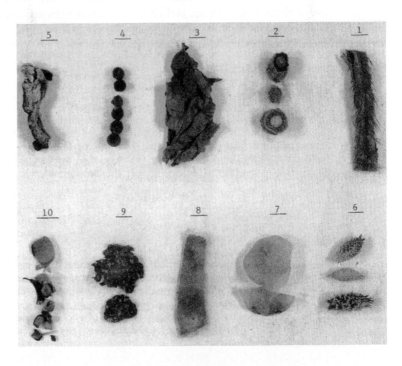

FIGURE 13-2. Pictured here are some of the herbs used in complementary and alternative methods of pain control. The client brews the herbs into a tea then drinks it on an empty stomach. (Reprinted by permission of William Arnold, MD, Advocate Medical Group and Advocate Lutheran General Hospital, Park Ridge, IL)

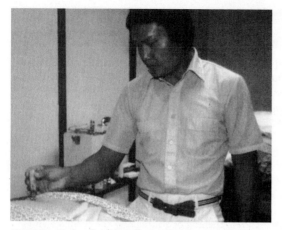

FIGURE 13-3. Traditionally a Chinese practice, acupuncture has gained acceptance in the United States and Canada. Research reveals that the procedure produces an analgesic effect because it causes the release of enkephalin, a naturally occurring endorphin that has opiate-like effects. The practitioner shown here is using moxibustion (heat) to enhance the therapeutic effects of acupuncture.

As seen in this brief overview, several alternative practices may be used to assist clients in the management of pain. Some practices involve only the nurse and the client. Other techniques involve different types of healers, family members, and significant others. Nurses who are familiar with these techniques will feel more comfortable suggesting, observing, participating in, or performing a variety of healing practices.

Summary

Pain has been experienced throughout the ages. Sophisticated pharmacologic interventions do not necessarily relieve pain, which people define, express, cope with, and manage in a variety of ways. Culture is a major influence in this process. Culture helps determine the innermost feelings of the individual. According to Mead, the behavior of an individual may be understood only in terms of the behavior of the whole social group of which he or she is a member (Mead, 1934). To examine the phenomenon of pain in its entirety, a model of pain is needed. This model incorporates physical, psychologic, social, and cultural factors, which interact and define the pain experience for individuals.

Nurses practicing in the United States and Canada come in contact with people from a variety of cultural backgrounds. In addition, nurses encounter clients experiencing pain in virtually every clinical setting. Recognizing cultural differences in beliefs about pain and suffering, and cultural views about appropriate responses to pain, can prevent misunderstanding and lead to the delivery of culturally competent care.

REVIEW QUESTIONS

1. How is pain defined?
2. How does the expression of pain vary by culture? By gender? By type of pain?
3. How does the nursing subculture view pain? What are nurses' typical expectations for expressions of pain by others?
4. What tools may appropriately be used for assessing pain?
5. How might the nurse demonstrate his or her competence to clients and families?
6. What alternative practices might be used by clients experiencing pain? How might nurses support these practices?

CRITICAL THINKING ACTIVITIES

1. Think about the last time you experienced pain. Describe it. How intense was the pain? What do you think caused the pain? Did you want others to know about it? How did you respond to the pain? Did you want to be alone or with other people? What treatments did you use for the pain? Did you worry about the pain?

2. Ask five of your friends or relatives what treatments they use when they have a headache. Be sure to ask about folk remedies and who taught them to use a particular treatment. Identify similarities and differences compared with the treatments you use.

3. Think about one of the clients in pain for whom you have provided care. How did that client respond to pain? How did you help the client? How would you modify your practice based on what you have learned in this chapter?

4. Identify three times when you have encouraged (or have seen others encourage) a client to accept more pain. What words were used? How were family members involved? What was the ultimate outcome? Did you realize you were applying principles of encouraging tolerance to pain?

5. Select several clients with different cultural backgrounds. Assess their pain, using several different tools. Which tools are most helpful? Are your clients able to use numbers to describe their pain? Can they draw pictures or use colors to describe their pain? What words do they use to describe their pain?

REFERENCES

Acheson, E. S. (1988). *Nurses' inferences of pain and the decision to intervene for culturally different patients.* Unpublished doctoral dissertation, University of Texas at Austin.

Alternative therapies come to America's hospitals. (2001, August). *Vitality Notes, 3.*

Ang, D. C., Ibrahim, S. A., Burant, C. J., & Kwoh, C. K. (2003). Is there a difference in the perception of symptoms between African Americans and whites with osteoarthritis? *Journal of Rheumatology, 30*(6), 1305–1310.

Ang, D. C., Ibrahim, S. A., Burant, C. J., Siminoff, L. A., & Kwoh, C. K. (2002). Ethnic differences in the perception of prayer and consideration of joint arthroplasty. *Medical Care, 40*(6), 471–476.

Ang-Lee, M. K., Moss, J., and Yuan, C. S. (2001). Herbal medicines and perioperative care. *Journal of the American Medical Association, 286*(2), 208–216.

Anie, K. A., & Green, J. (2002). Psychological therapies for sickle cell disease and pain (Art. No.: CD001916, DOI: 10.1002/14651858.CD001916). *Cochrane Database of Systematic Reviews 2002, 2.* Retrieved in 2005 from The Cochrane Library at http://www.mrw.interscience.wiley.com/cochrane/clsysrev/articles/CD001916/frame.html

Atherton, M. J., Feeg, V. D., & El-Adham, A. F. (2004). Race, ethnicity, and insurance as determinants of epidural use: Analysis of a national sample survey. *Nursing Economic$, 22*(1), 6–13.

Baer, E., Davitz, L. J., & Lieb, R. (1970). Inferences of physical pain and psychological distress in relation to verbal and nonverbal patient communication. *Nursing Research, 19,* 388.

Ballas, S. K. (1998). *Sickle cell pain: Progress in pain research and management* (Vol. 11, pp. 51–89). Seattle: IASP Press.

Benoliel, J. Q., & Crowley, D. M. (1974). *The patient in pain: New concepts.* New York: American Cancer Society.

Benson, H. (1976). *The relaxation response.* New York: Avon Books.

Beyer, J. E. (2000). Judging the effectiveness of analgesia for children and adolescents during vaso-occlusive events of sickle cell disease. *Journal of Pain and Symptom Management, 19*(1), 63–72.

Beyer, J. E., & Kuott, C. B. (1998). Construct validity estimation for the African-American and Hispanic versions of the Oucher Scale. *Journal of Pediatric Nursing, 13*(1), 20–31.

Beyer, J., Platt, A. F., Kinney, T. R., & Treadwell, M. (1999). Practice guidelines for the assessment of children with sickle cell pain. *Journal of the Society of Pediatric Nurses, 4*(2), 61–73.

Blank, F. S. J., Li, H., Henneman, P. L., Smithline, H. A., Santoro, J. S., Provost, et al. (2005). A descriptive study of heavy emergency department users at an academic emergency department reveals heavy ED users have better access to acre than average users. *Journal of Emergency Nursing, 31*(2), 139–144.

Bonham, V. L. (2001). Race, ethnicity, and pain treatment: Striving to understand the causes and solutions to the disparities in pain treatment. *Journal of Law, Medicine & Ethics, 29*(1), 52–68.

Brau, C. A., Bearinger, L. H., Halcon, L. L., & Pettingell, S. L. (2005). Adolescent use of complementary therapies. *Journal of Adolescent Health, 37*(1), JAH Online Exclusives, 76.e1–9.

Carpenter, J., & Brockopp, D. (1995). Comparison of patents' ratings and examination of nurses' responses to pain intensity rating. *Cancer Nursing, 18,* 292–298.

Claster, S., & Vichinsky, E. P. (2003). Managing sickle cell disease. *British Medical Journal, 327*(7424), 1151–1155.

Cleeland, C. S. (1982). *Brief pain inventory.* Houston, TX: The Pain Research Group.

Cleeland, C. S., Gonin, R., Baez, L., Loehrer, P., & Pandya, K. J. (1997). Pain and treatment in minority patients with cancer. *Annals of Internal Medicine, 127,* 813–816.

Cleeland, C. S., Nakamura, Y., Mendoza, T. R., Edwards. K. R., Douglas, J., & Serlin, R. C. (1996). Dimensions of the impact of cancer in a four country sample: New information from a multidimensional scaling. *Pain, 67,* 267–273.

Cleeland, C. S., & Ryan, H. (1994). Pain assessment: Global use of the Brief Pain Inventory. *Annals of Academy of Medicine, 23,* 129–138.

Cohen, F. L. (1980). Postsurgical pain relief: Patients' status and nurses' medication choices. *Pain, 9*(1), 265–274.

Conner-Warren, R. L. (1996). Pain intensity and home pain management of children with sickle dell disease. *Issues in Comprehensive Pediatric Nursing, 19,* 183–195.

Cork, R. C., Isaac, I., Elsharydah, A., Zavisca, F., & Alexander, L. (2004). A comparison of the Verbal Rating Scale and the Visual Analog Scale for pain assessment. *Internet Journal of Anesthesiology, 8*(1), 1–3.

Crandell, M., & Savedra, M. (2005). Multidimensional assessment using the adolescent pediatric pain tool: A case report. *Journal for Specialists in Pediatric Nursing, 10*(3), 115–113.

Crook, J., Rideout, E., & Brown, G. (1984). The prevalence of pain complaints in a general population. *Pain, 18,* 299–314.

Dampier, C., Ely, B., Brodecki, D., & O'Neal, P. (2002). Characteristics of pain managed at home in children and adolescents with sickle cell disease by using diary self-reports. *Journal of Pain, 3*(6), 461–470.

D'Arcy, Y. (2004). Managing sickle-cell crisis. *Nursing 2004, 34*(1), 24–25.

Davitz, L. J., & Davitz, J. R. (1975). How do nurses feel when patients suffer? *American Journal of Nursing, 75,* 1505.

Davitz, J. R., & Davitz, L. J. (1981). *Influences of patients' pain and psychological distress.* New York: Springer-Verlag.

Davitz, L. J., Sameshima, Y., & Davitz, J. (1976). Suffering as viewed in six different cultures. *American Journal of Nursing, 76,* 1296.

Dimsdale, J. E. (2000). Stalked by the past: The influence of ethnicity on health. *Psychosomatic Medicine, 62,* 161–170.

Dorsey, C., Phillips, K. D., & Williams, C. (2001). Adult sickle cell patients' perceptions of nurses' caring behaviors. *ABNF Journal, 12*(5), 95–100.

Dudley, S. R., & Holm, K. (1984). Assessment of the pain experience in relation to selected nurse characteristics. *Pain, 18*(2), 179–186.

Eaton, M. L., Haye, J. S., Armstrong, F. D., Pegelow, C. H., & Thomas, M. (1995). Hospitalizations for painful episodes:

Association with school absenteeism and academic performance in children and adolescents with sickle cell anemia. *Issues in Comprehensive Pediatrics, 18*(1), 1–9.

Eccleston, C., Yorke, L., Morley, S., Williams, A. C. de C., & Mastroyannopoulou, K. (2003). Psychological therapies or the management of chronic and recurrent pain in hildren and adolescents (Art. No.: CD003968. DOI: 10.1002/14651858.CD003968). *Cochrane Database of Systematic Reviews 2003, 1.* Retrieved in 2004 from The Cochrane Library at http://www.mrw.interscience.wiley.com/cochrane/clsysrev/articles/CD003968/frame.html

Edwards, C. L., Scales, M. T., Loughlin, C., Bennett, G. G., Harris-Peterson, C., De Castro, L. M., et al. (2005). A brief review of the pathophysiology, associated pain, and psychosocial issues in sickle cell disease. *International Journal of Behavioral Medicine, 12*(3), 171–179.

Edwards, R. R., Moric, M., Husteldt, B., Buvanendran, A., & Ivankovich, O. (2005). Ethnic similarities and differences in the chronic pain experience: A comparison of African American, Hispanic and white patients. *Pain Medicine, 6*(1), 88–98.

Eisenberg, D. M., Davis, R. B., Ettner, S. L., Appel, S., Wilkey, S., Van Rompay, M., et al. (2000). Trends in alternative medicine use in the United States, 1990–1997: Results of a follow-up national survey. *Journal of the American Medical Association, 283*(7), 884.

Encandela, J. A. (1993). Social science and the study of pain since Zborowski: A need for a new agenda. *Social Science Medicine, 36*(6), 783–791.

Eversley, R., Esrin, D., Dibble, S., Wardlaw, L., Pedrosa, M. & Favila-Penney, W. (2005). Post-treatment symptoms among ethnic minority breast cancer survivors. *Oncology Nursing Forum, 322,* 250–256.

Ferrell, B., Virani, R., Grant, M., Vallerand, A., & McCaffery, M. (2000). Analysis of pain content in nursing textbooks. *Journal of Pain and Symptom Management, 19*(2), 216–228.

Ferrell, B. R., & Ferrell, B. A. (1990). Easing the pain. *Geriatric Nursing, 11,* 175–178.

Gil, K. M., Carson, J. W., Porter, L. S., Scipio, C., Bediako, S. M., & Orringer, E. (2004). Daily mood and stress predict pain, health care use, and work activity in African-American adults with sickle-cell disease. *Health Psychology, 23*(3), 267–274.

Gil, K. M., Porter, L., Ready, J., Workman, E., Sedway, J., & Anthony, K. K. (2000). Pain in children and adolescents with sickle cell disease: An analysis of daily pain diaries. *Children's Health Care, 29*(4), 225–241.

Hammer, M., Geier, K. A., Aksoy, S., & Reynolds, H. M. (2003). Perioperative care for patients with sickle cell who are undergoing total hip replacement as treatment for osteonecrosis. *Orthopaedic Nursing, 22*(6), 384–397.

Harrison, M. O., Edwards, C. L., Koenig, H. G., Bosworth, H. B., Decastro, L., & Wood, M. (2005). Religiosity/spirituality and pain in patients with sickle cell disease. *Journal of Nervous and Mental Disease, 193*(4), 250–257.

Hastie, B. A., Riley, J. L., & Fillingim, R. B. (2004). Ethnic differences in pain coping: Factor structure of the Coping Strategies Questionnaire and Coping Strategies Questionnaire—Revised. *Journal of Pain, 5*(6), 304–316.

Hayes, J. S., & Fletcher, C. (2000). Appraisal and coping with vaso-occlusive crisis in adolescents with sickle cell disease. *Pediatric Nursing, 26*(3), 319–324.

Herr, K. A., & Mobily, P. R. (1991). Complexities of pain assessment in the elderly: Clinical considerations. *Journal of Gerontological Nursing, 17,* 12–19, 44–45.

Hofland, S. L. (1992). Elder beliefs: Blocks to pain management. *Journal of Gerontological Nursing, 18,* 19–24, 39–40.

Howell, D., Butler, L., Vincent, L., Watt-Watson, J., & Stearns, N. (2000). Influencing nurses' knowledge, attitudes, and practice in cancer pain management. *Cancer Nursing, 23*(1), 55–63.

Jacob, E. (2001). *Pain in children with sickle cell anemia.* Unpublished doctoral dissertation, University of California, San Francisco.

Jacob, E. (2001). Pain management in sickle cell disease. *Pain Management Nursing, 2*(4), 121–131.

Jacob, E. (2001). The pain experience of patients with sickle cell disease. *Pain Management Nursing, 2*(3), 74–83.

Jacobson, E. (1964). *Self-operations control: A manual of tension control.* Chicago: National Foundation for Progressive Relaxation.

Jakubik, L. D. (2000). Care of the child with sickle cell disease: Acute complications. *Pediatric Nursing, 26*(4), 373–380.

Jamison, C., & Brown, H. N. (2002). A special treatment program for patients with sickle cell crisis. *Nursing Economic$, 20*(3), 126–132.

Jones, M., Qazi, M., & Young, K. D. (2005). Ethnic differences in parent preference to be present for painful medical procedures. *Pediatrics, 116*(2, Pt 1, Suppl.), e191–197.

Jordan, M. S., Lumley, M. A., & Leisen, J. C. C. (1998). The relationships of cognitive coping and pain control beliefs to pain and adjustment among African-American and Caucasian women with rheumatoid arthritis. *Arthritis Care and Research, 11*(2), 80–88.

Kaasalainen, S., & Crook, J. (2003). A comparison of pain-assessment tools for use with elderly long-term-care residents. *Canadian Journal of Nursing Research, 35*(4), 59–71.

Kaplan, P., & Ludwig-Beymer, P. (2005). *The impact of animal assisted therapy (AAT) on the use of pain medications after a surgical procedure in an acute care hospital.* Paper presented at the Second Annual Nursing Science Fair: Evidence Based Practice. Naperville, IL: Edward Hospital and Health Services.

Kleinman, A. (1988). *The illness narratives.* New York: Basic Books.

Kotarba, J. (1983). *Chronic pain: Its social dimension.* Beverly Hills, CA: Sage.

Lauderdale, G. (2003). *The lived experience of African American adolescents with sickle cell disease.* Unpublished doctoral dissertation, University of Virginia, Charlottesville.

Lawlis, G. G., Achterberg, J., Kenner, L., & Kopetz, K. (1984). Ethnic and sex differences in response to clinical and induced pain in chronic spinal pain patients. *Spine, 9,* 751–754.

Leininger, M. M. (1991). *Cultural care diversity and universality: A theory of nursing.* New York: National League for Nursing.

Luffy, R., & Grove, S. K. (2003). Examining the validity, reliability, and preference of three pediatric pain measurement tools in African-American children. *Pediatric Nursing, 29*(1), 54–59.

Luthe, W., & Schultz, J. H. (1970). *Autogenic therapy: Medical applications.* New York: Grune & Stratton.

Maikler, V. E., Broome, M. E., Bailey, P., & Lea, G. (2001). Childrens' and adolescents' use of diaries for sickle cell pain. *Journal for Specialists in Pediatric Nursing, 6*(4), 161–169.

McCaffery, M. (1990). Nursing approaches to nonpharmacological pain control. *International Journal of Nursing Studies, 27*(1), 1–5.

McCaffery, M., & Pasero, C. (1999). *Pain: A clinical manual for nursing practice* (2nd ed.). St. Louis, MO: Mosby.

McCaffery, M., Ferrell, B. R., & Pasero, C. (2000). Nurses' personal opinions about patients' pain and their effect on recorded assessments and titration of opioid doses. *Pain Management Nursing, 1*(3), 79–87.

McDermot, P. A. (2003). Recognizing normeperidine toxicity. *Nursing2003, 33*(3). 24.

McLeod-Fletcher, C. (1996). *Appraisal and coping with vaso-occlusive crisis in adolescents with sickle cell disease.* Unpublished doctoral dissertation, University of Miami, Florida.

Mead, G. (1934). *Mind, self and society.* Chicago: University of Chicago Press.

Melding, P. S. (1991). Is there such a thing as geriatric pain? *Pain, 46,* 119–121.

Melzack, R., & Wall, P. D. (1983). *The challenge of pain.* New York: Basic Books.

Melzer-Lange, M. D., Walsh-Kelly, C. M., Lea, G., Hillery, C. A., & Scott, J. P. (2004). Patient-controlled analgesia for sickle cell pain crisis in a pediatric emergency department. *Pediatric Emergency Care, 20*(1), 2–4.

Miller, A. C., Hickman, L. C., & Lemasters, G. K. (1992). A distraction technique for control of burn pain. *Journal of Burn Care and Rehabilitation, 13*(5), 576–580.

Najm, W., Reinsch, S., Hoehler, F. & Tobis, J. (2002). Use of complementary and alternative medicine among the ethnic elderly. *Alternative Therapies in Health and Medicine, 9*(3), 50–57.

National Council for Reliable Health Information. (1998, January/February). Canadians increase use of alternative medicine. *NCAHF Newsletter, 21*(1), 1. Retrieved January 10, 2002, from Health Source: Nursing/Academic Edition database http://www.ncahf.ovg/nl/1998/index.html

National Institutes of Health (1987). The integrated approach to the management of pain. *Journal of Pain and Symptom Management, 2,* 35–44.

Newcombe, P. (2002). Pathophysiology of sickle cell disease crisis. *Emergency Nurse, 9*(9), 19–22.

Novey, D. W. (2000). *Clinician's complete reference to complementary and alternative medicine.* St. Louis; Mosby.

Ohnhaus, E. E., & Adler, R. (1975). Methodological problems in the measurement of pain: A comparison between the Verbal Rating Scale and the Visual Analogue Scale. *Pain, 1*(4), 379–384.

Perlman, K. M., Myers-Phariss, S., & Rhodes, J. C. (2004). A shift from demerol (meperidine) to dilaudid (hydromorphone) improves pain control and decreases admissions to patients in sickle cell crisis. *Journal of Emergency Nursing, 30*(5), 439–446.

Portenoy, R. K., Ugarte, C., Fuller, I., & Haas, G. (2004). Population-based survey of pain in the United States: Differences among white, African American and Hispanic subjects. *Journal of Pain, 5*(6), 317–328.

Preboth, M. (2000). Management of pain in sickle cell disease. *American Family Physician, 61*(5), 1544–1546.

Reiki Infocenter. (n.d.). Accessed December 28, 2005, at www.holistic-online.com/Reiki/hol_Reiki_home.htm

Reizian, A., & Meleis, A. I. (1986). Arab-Americans' perceptions of and responses to pain. *Critical Care Nurse, 6*(6), 30–37.

Resnik, D., & Rehm, M. (2001). Pain and sickle cell anemia. *Hastings Center Report, 31*(3).

Rhymes, J. A. (1996). Barriers to effective palliative care of terminal patients. *Clinics in Geriatric Medicine, 12*(2), 407–416.

Roy, R., & Thomas, M. (1986). A survey of chronic pain in an elderly population. *Canadian Family Physician, 32,* 513–516.

Scott, J., & Huskisson, E. C. (1976). Graphic representation of pain. *Pain, 2*(2), 175–184.

Shapiro, B. S., Benjamin, L. J., Payne, R., & Heidrich, G. (1997). Sickle cell–related pain: Perceptions of medical practitioners. *Journal of Pain and Symptom Management, 14*(3), 168–174.

Sorkin, B. A., Rudy, T. E., Hanlon, R. B., Turk, D. C., & Steig, R. L. (1990). Chronic pain in older and younger patients: Differences are less important than similarities. *Journal of Gerontology, 45,* 64–68.

Streltzer, J., & Wade, T. C. (1981). The influence of cultural group on the undertreatment of postoperative pain. *Psychosomatic Medicine, 43*(5), 397–403.

Strickland, O. L., Jackson, G., Gilead, M., McGuire, D. B., & Quarles, S. (2001). Use of focus groups for pain and quality of life assessment in adults with sickle cell disease. *Journal of Black Nurses' Association, 12*(2), 36–43.

Tamayo-Sarver, J. H., Dawson, N. V., Hinze, S. W., Cydulka, R. K., Wigton, R. S., & Albert, J. M., et al. (2003). The effect of race/ethnicity and desirable social characteristics on physicians' decisions to prescribe opioid analgesics. *Academic Emergency Medicine, 10*(11), 1239–1248.

Tamayo-Sarver, J. H., Hinze, S. W., Cydulka, R. K., & Baker, D. W. (2003). Racial and ethnic disparities in emergency department analgesic prescription. *American Journal of Public Health, 93*(12), 2067–2073.

Tan, G., Jensen, M. P., Thornby, J., & Anderson, K. O. (2005). Ethnicity, control appraisal, coping, and adjustment to chronic pain among black and white Americans (2005). *Pain Medicine, 6*(1), 18–28.

Taylor, B. A., Casas-Ganem, J., Vaccaro, A. R., Hilibrand, A. S., Hanscom, B. S., & Albert, T. J. (2005). Differences in the work-up and treatment of conditions associated with low back pain by patient gender and ethnic background. *Spine, 30*(3), 359–364.

Teske, K., Daut, R. L., & Cleeland, C. S. (1983). Relationship between nurses' observation and patients' self-reports of pain. *Pain, 16,* 289–296.

Todd, K. H., Samaroo, N., & Hoffman, J. R. (1993). Ethnicity as a risk factor for inadequate emergency department analgesia. *Journal of the American Medical Association, 269*(12), 1537–1539.

U.S. Department of Health and Human Services. (February, 1992). *Acute pain management: Operative or medical procedures and trauma.* Rockville, MD: Agency for Health Care Policy and Research, Public Health Service, U.S. Department of Health and Human Services.

Villarruel, A., & Denyes, M. (1991). Pain assessment in children: Theoretical and empirical validity. *Advances in Nursing Science, 14,* 32–41.

Voigtman, J. L. (2002). *Learning to suffer: Pain response in a community of Saudi Arab children with sickle cell disease.* Unpublished doctoral dissertation, University of Arizona, Tucson.

Waldrop, R. D., & Mandy, C. (1995). Health professional perceptions of opioid dependence among patients with pain. *American Journal of Emergency Medicine, 13*(5), 529–531.

Witte, M. (1989). Pain control. *Journal of Gerontological Nursing, 15,* 32–37, 40–41.

Wolff, B. B., & Langley, S. (1977). *Cultural factors and the response to pain. Culture, disease, and healing.* New York: Macmillan.

Wong, D. & Baker, C. (1988). Pain in children: Comparison of assessment scales. *Pediatric Nursing, 14,* 9–17.

Yates, P., Dewar, A., & Fentiman, B. (1995). Pain: The view of elderly people living in long-term residential care settings. *Journal of Advanced Nursing, 21,* 667–674.

Zadinsky, J. K., & Boyle, J. S. (1996). Experiences of women with chronic pelvic pain. *Health Care for Women International, 17,* 223–232.

Zborowski, M. (1952). Cultural components in response to pain. *Journal of Social Issues, 8,* 16–30.

Zborowski, M. (1969). *People in pain.* San Francisco: Jossey-Bass.

Zelman, D. C., Gore, M., Dukes, E., Tai, K. S., & Brandenburg, N. (2005). Validation of a modified version of the Brief Pain Inventory for painful diabetic neuropathy. *Journal of Vascular Nursing, 23*(3), 97–104.

C H A P T E R

14

Religion, Culture, and Nursing

Margaret M. Andrews

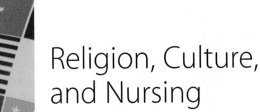

LEARNING OBJECTIVES

1. Explore the meaning of spirituality and religion in the lives of clients across the life span.
2. Identify the components of a spiritual needs assessment for clients from diverse cultural backgrounds.
3. Examine the ways in which spiritual and religious beliefs can be incorporated into the nursing care of clients from diverse cultures.
4. Discuss cultural considerations in the nursing care of dying or bereaved clients and families.
5. Describe the health-related beliefs and practices of selected religious groups in North America.

As an integral component of culture, religious beliefs may influence a client's explanation of the cause(s) of illness, perception of its severity, and choice of healer(s). In times of crisis, such as serious illness and impending death, religion may be a source of consolation for the client and family and may influence the course of action believed to be appropriate.

The first half of this chapter discusses dimensions of religion, religion and spiritual nursing care, religious trends in the United States and Canada, and contributions of religious groups to the health care delivery system. The second half highlights the health-related beliefs and practices of selected religions, which are presented in alphabetic order.

Dimensions of Religion

Religion is complex and multifaceted in both form and function. Religious faith and the institutions derived from that faith become a central focus in meeting the human needs of those who believe. "Not a single faith fails to address the issues of illness and wellness, of disease and healing, of caring and curing. Stated more positively, most faiths were born as, at least in part, efforts to heal" (Marty, 1990, p. 14; Scherer, 1996; Woods & Ironson, 1999). Consequently, the influence of religion on health-related matters requires a few preliminary remarks.

Religious Factors Influencing Human Behavior

First, it is necessary to identify specific religious factors that may influence human behavior. No single religious factor operates in isolation but rather exists in combination with other religious factors. Faulkner and DeJong (1966) have proposed **five major dimensions of religion:** experiential, ritualistic, ideologic, intellectual, and consequential.

Experiential Dimension

The experiential dimension recognizes that all religions have expectations of members and that the religious person will at some point in life achieve direct knowledge of ultimate reality or will experience religious emotion. Every religion recognizes this subjective religious experience as a sign of religiosity.

Ritualistic Dimension

The ritualistic dimension pertains to religious practices expected of the followers and may include worship, prayer, participation in sacraments, and fasting.

Ideologic Dimension

The ideologic dimension refers to the set of beliefs to which its followers must adhere in order to call themselves members. Commitment to the group or movement as a social process results, and members experience a sense of belonging or affiliation.

Intellectual Dimension

The intellectual dimension refers to specific sets of beliefs or explanations or to the cognitive structuring of meaning. Members are expected to be informed about the basic tenets of the religion and to be familiar with sacred writings or scriptures. The intellectual and the ideologic are closely related because acceptance of a dimension presupposes knowledge of it.

Consequential Dimension

The consequential dimension refers to religiously defined standards of conduct and to prescriptions that specify what followers' attitudes and behaviors should be as a consequence of their religion. The consequential dimension governs people's relationships with others.

Religious Dimensions in Relation to Health and Illness

Obviously, each religious dimension has a different significance when related to matters of health and illness. Different religious cultures may emphasize one of the five dimensions to the relative exclusion of the others. Similarly, individuals may develop their own priorities related to the dimension of religion. This affects the nurse providing care to clients with different religious beliefs in several ways. First, it is the nurse's role to determine from the client, or from significant others, the dimension or combinations of dimensions that are important so that the client and nurse can have mutual goals and priorities.

Second, it is important to determine what a given member of a specific religious affiliation believes to be important. The only way to do this is to ask either the client or, if the client is unable to communicate this information personally, a close family member.

Third, the nurse's information must be accurate. Making assumptions about clients' religious belief systems on the basis of their cultural, or even religious, affiliation is imprudent and may lead to erroneous inferences. The following case example illustrates the importance of verifying assumptions with the client.

Observing that a patient was wearing a Star of David on a chain around his neck and had been accompanied by a rabbi upon admission, a nurse inquired whether he would like to order a kosher diet. The patient replied, "Oh, no. I'm a Christian. My father is a rabbi, and I know it would upset him to find out that I have converted. Even though I'm 40 years old, I hide it from him. This has been going on for 15 years now."

The key point in this anecdote is that the nurse validated an assumption with the patient before acting. Furthermore, not all Jewish persons follow a kosher diet or wear a Star of David.

Fourth, even when individuals identify with a particular religion, they may accept the "official" beliefs and practices in varying degrees. It is not the nurse's role to judge the religious virtues of clients but rather to understand those aspects related to religion that are important to the client and family members. When religious beliefs are translated into practice, they may be manipulated by individuals in certain situations to serve particular ends; that is, traditional beliefs and practices are altered. Thus, it is possible for a Jewish person to eat pork or for a Catholic to take contraceptives to prevent pregnancy.

Although some find it necessary to label such occurrences as exceptional or accidental, such a point of view tends to ignore the fact that change can and does occur within individuals and within groups. Homogeneity among members of any religion cannot be assumed. Perhaps the individual once embraced the beliefs and practices of the religion but has since changed his or her views, or perhaps the individual never accepted the religious beliefs completely in the first place. It is important for the nurse to be open to variations in religious beliefs and practices and to allow for the possibility of change. Individual choices frequently arise from new situations, changing values and mores and exposure to new ideas and beliefs. Few people live in total social isolation, surrounded by only those with similar religious backgrounds.

Fifth, ideal norms of conduct and actual behavior are not necessarily the same. The nurse is frequently faced with the challenge of understanding and helping clients cope with conflicting norms. Sometimes conflicting norms are manifested by guilt or by efforts to minimize or rationalize inconsistencies.

Sometimes norms are vaguely formulated and filled with discrepancies that allow for a variety of interpretations. In religions having a lay organization and structure, moral decision making may be left to the individual without the assistance of members of a church hierarchy. In religions having a clerical hierarchy, moral positions may be more clearly formulated and articulated for members. Individuals retain their right to choose regardless of official church-related guidelines, suggestions, or even religious laws; however, the individual who chooses to violate the norms may experience the consequences of that violation, including social ostracism, public removal from membership rolls, or other forms of censure.

Religion and Spiritual Nursing Care

For many years, nursing has emphasized a holistic approach to care in which the needs of the total person are recognized. Most nursing textbooks emphasize the physical and psychosocial needs of clients rather than ways to address spiritual needs. Little has been written about guidelines for providing spiritual care to culturally diverse clients. Because the nurse provides holistic health care, addressing spiritual needs becomes essential.

Religious concerns evolve from and respond to the mysteries of life and death, good and evil, and pain and suffering. Although the religions of the world offer various interpretations of these phenomena, most people seek a personal understanding and interpretation at some time in their lives. Ultimately, this personal search becomes a pursuit to discover God or some unifying truth that will give meaning, purpose, and integrity to existence (Ebersole & Hess, 2003).

Before spiritual care for culturally diverse clients is discussed, an important distinction needs to be made between religion and spirituality. **Religion** refers to an organized system of beliefs concerning the cause, nature, and purpose of the universe, especially belief in or the worship of God or gods. **Spirituality** is born out of each person's unique life experience and his or her personal effort to find purpose and meaning in life.

The goal of **spiritual nursing care** is to assist clients in integrating their own religious beliefs about God or a unifying truth into the ultimate reality that gives meaning to their lives in relationship to the health crisis that has precipitated the need for nursing care. Spiritual nursing care promotes clients' physical and emotional health as well as their **spiritual health**. When providing care, the nurse must remember that the goal of spiritual intervention is not, and should not be, to impose his or her religious beliefs and convictions on the client (White, 2007).

Although spiritual needs are recognized by many nurses, spiritual care is often neglected. Among the reasons why nurses fail to provide spiritual care are the following: (1) they view religious and spiritual needs as a private matter concerning only an individual and his or her creator; (2) they are uncomfortable about their own religious beliefs or deny having spiritual needs; (3) they lack knowledge about spirituality and the religious beliefs of others; (4) they mistake spiritual needs for psychosocial needs; and (5) they view meeting the spiritual needs of clients as a family or pastoral responsibility, not a nursing responsibility.

Spiritual intervention is as appropriate as any other form of nursing intervention and recognizes that the balance of physical, psychosocial, and spiritual is essential to overall good health. Nursing is an intimate profession, and nurses routinely inquire without hesitation about very personal matters such as hygiene and sexual habits. The spiritual realm also requires a personal, intimate type of nursing intervention.

In the United States and Canada, efforts to integrate spiritual care and nursing have been underway for several decades. For example, in 1971 at the White House Conference on Aging, the spiritual dimension of care was defined as those aspects of individuals pertaining to their inner resources, especially their ultimate concern, the basic value around which all other values are focused, the central philosophy of life that guides their conduct and the supernatural and nonmaterial dimensions of human nature. The spiritual dimension encompasses the person's need to find satisfactory answers to questions about the meaning of life, illness, or death (Ebersole & Hess, 2003; Moberg, 1971).

In 1978, the Third National Conference on the Classification of Nursing Diagnoses recognized the importance of spirituality by including **"spiritual concerns," "spiritual distress,"** and **"spiritual despair"** in the list of approved diagnoses. Because of practical difficulties, these three categories were combined at the 1980 National Conference into one category, spiritual distress, which is defined as disruption in the life principle that pervades a person's entire being and that integrates and transcends the person's biologic and psychosocial nature. Moberg (1981) acknowledges the multidimensional nature of spiritual concerns and defines them as the human need to deal with sociocultural deprivations, anxieties and fears, death and dying, personality integration, self-image, personal dignity, social alienation, and philosophy of life.

Cultural Assessment of Religious and Spiritual Issues

As discussed in Chapter 3, cultural assessment includes assessment of the relationship between religious and spiritual issues as they relate to the health care status of the client. In the integration of health care and religious/spiritual beliefs, the focus of nursing intervention is to help the client maintain his or her own beliefs in the face of the health crisis and to use those beliefs to strengthen individual coping patterns. If the religious beliefs are contributing to the overall health problem (e.g., guilt, remorse, expectations), you can conduct a **spiritual assessment**. To be therapeutic, begin by asking questions that clarify the problem, and nonjudgmentally support the client's problem solving.

Summarized in Box 14–1 are guidelines for assessing spiritual needs in clients from diverse cultural backgrounds (Figure 14–1).

Spiritual Nursing Care for Ill Children and Their Families

Religion is especially important to clients during periods of crisis. In a broad sense, any hospitalization or serious illness can be viewed as stressful and therefore has the potential to develop into a crisis. You may find that religion plays an especially significant role when a child is seriously ill and in circumstances that include dying, death, or bereavement.

Illness during childhood may be an especially difficult clinical situation. Children as well as adults have spiritual needs that vary according to their developmental level and the religious climate in the family. Parental perceptions about the illness of their child may be partially influenced by religious beliefs. For example, some parents may believe that a transgression against a religious law has caused a congenital anomaly in their offspring. Other parents may delay seeking medical care because they believe that prayer should be tried first.

The nurse should be respectful of parents' preferences regarding the care of their child. When parental beliefs or practices threaten the child's well-being and health (from your perspective), you are obligated to discuss the matter with the parents. It may be possible to reach a compromise in which parental beliefs are respected and necessary care is provided. On rare occasions, it may become a legal matter. Religion may be a source of consolation and support to parents, especially those facing the unanswerable questions associated with life-threatening illness in their children.

Spiritual Nursing Care for the Dying or Bereaved Client and Family

"All Americans do not mourn alike. Mourning is cultural behavior and we live in a multicultural society. But the way we are raised dictates patterns we regard as proper or natural. Just as we celebrate holidays or marriages differently, we also mourn differently. The mourning customs of others may seem unusual when compared to your tradition, but like yours, they help people cope with death" (Adams, 1994).

Nurses inevitably focus on restoring health or on fostering environments in which the client returns to a previous state of health or adapts to physical, psychological, or emotional changes. However, one aspect of care that is often avoided or ignored, though every bit as crucial to clients and their families, is death and the accompanying dying and grieving processes.

Death is indeed a universal experience, but one that is highly individual and personal. Although each person must ultimately face death alone, rarely does one person's death fail to affect others. There are many rituals, serving many purposes, which people use to help them cope with death. These rituals are often determined by cultural and religious orientation. Situational factors, competing demands, and individual differences are also important in determining the dying, bereavement, and grieving behaviors that are considered socially acceptable.

The role of the nurse in dealing with dying clients and their families varies according to the needs and preferences of both the nurse and client, as well as the clinical setting in which the interaction occurs. By understanding some of the

---

BOX 14-1

Assessing Spiritual Needs in Culturally Diverse Clients

Environment

- Does the client have religious objects, such as a Bible, prayer book, devotional literature, religious medals, rosary or other type of beads, photographs of historic religious persons or contemporary church leaders (e.g., Pope, church president), paintings of religious events or persons, religious sculptures, crucifixes, objects of religious significance at entrances to rooms (e.g., holy water founts, a mezuzah, or small parchment scroll inscribed with an excerpt from the Bible), candles of religious significance (e.g., Paschal candle, menorah), shrine, or other?
- Does the client wear clothing that has religious significance (e.g., head covering, undergarment, uniform)?
- Are get-well greeting cards religious in nature or from a representative of the client's church?
- Does the client receive flowers or bulletins from his or her church?

Behavior

- Does the client appear to pray at certain times of the day or before meals?

- Does the client make special dietary requests (e.g., kosher diet, vegetarian diet, or diet free from caffeine, pork, shellfish, or other specific food items)?
- Does the client read religious magazines or books?

Verbalization

- Does the client mention God (Allah, Buddha, Yahweh), prayer, faith, church, or religious topics?
- Does the client ask for a visit by a clergy member or other religious representative?
- Does the client express anxiety or fear about pain, suffering, or death?

Interpersonal Relationships

- Who visits? How does the client respond to visitors?
- Does a priest, rabbi, minister, elder, or other church representative visit?
- How does the client relate to the nursing staff? To his or her roommate(s)?
- Does the client prefer to interact with others or to remain alone?

Spiritual Care: The Nurse's Role, 3d Ed., by Judith Allen Shelly and Sharon Fish. © 1998 by InterVarsity Press, Christian Fellowship of the USA. Used by permission of InterVarsity Press, P.O. Box 1400, Downers Grove, IL 60515.

---

cultural and religious variations related to death, dying, and bereavement, the nurse can individualize the care given to clients and their families.

Nurses are often with the client through various stages of the dying process and at the actual moment of death, particularly when death occurs in a hospital, nursing home, extended care facility, or hospice. The nurse often determines when and whom to call as the impending death draws near. Knowing the religious, cultural, and familial heritage of a particular client as well as his or her devotion to the associated traditions and practices may help the nurse determine whom to call when the need arises.

Religious Beliefs Associated with Dying

Universally, people want to die with dignity. Historically this was not a problem when individuals died at home in the presence of their friends and families. Now, when more and more people are dying in institutions (hospitals, nursing homes, and extended care facilities), ensuring dignity throughout the dying process is more complex. Once death is seen as a problem for professional management, the hospital displaces the home, and specialists with different kinds and degrees of expertise take over for the family.

The way in which people commemorate death tells us much about their attitude and philosophy of life and death. Although it is beyond the scope of this book to explore the philosophic and psychological aspects of death in detail, some points will be made that relate to nursing care.

Preparation of the Body

A nurse may or may not actually participate in the rituals associated with death. When people

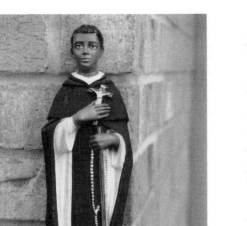

FIGURE 14-1. This statue commemorates the Roman Catholic Saint Martin De Porres. Born in Peru during the 16th century to a Spanish father and a Black mother, Martin De Porres studied medicine, which he later, as a member of the Dominican Order, put to use in helping the poor. Some Catholics honor him as the patron saint of African Americans. When assessing the needs of clients from diverse backgrounds, nurses can observe for the presence of religious objects in the client's home or yard.

die in the United States and Canada, they are usually transported to a mortuary, where the preparation for burial occurs.

In many cultural groups, preparation of the body has traditionally been very important. Whereas members of many cultural groups have now adopted the practice of letting the mortician prepare the body, there are some, particularly new immigrants, who want to retain their native and/or religious customs. For example, for certain Asian immigrants it is customary for family and friends of the same sex to wash and prepare the body for burial or cremation. In other situations, the family or religious representatives may go to the funeral home to prepare the body for burial by dressing the person in special religious clothing.

If a person dies in an institution, it is common for the nursing staff to "prepare" the body according to standard procedure. Depending on the ethnoreligious practices of the family, this may be objectionable—the family members may view this washing as an infringement on a special task that belongs to them alone. If the family is present, you should ask family members about their preference. If ritual washings will eventually take place at the mortuary, you may carry out the routine procedures and reassure the family that the mortician will comply with their requests, if that has in fact been verified.

North American **funeral** customs have been the topic of lively discussion. The initial preparation of the body has been described in the following way:

"After delivery to the undertaker, the corpse is in short order sprayed, sliced, pierced, pickled, trussed, trimmed, creamed, waxed, painted, rouged and neatly dressed...transformed from a common corpse into a beautiful memory picture. This process is known in the trades as embalming and restorative art, and is so universally employed in the U.S. and Canada that the funeral director does it routinely without consulting the corpse's family. He regards as eccentric those few who are hardy enough to suggest it might be dispensed with. Yet no law requires it, no religious doctrine commends it, nor is it dictated by considerations of health, sanitation or even personal daintiness. In no part of the world but in North America is it widely used. The purpose of embalming is to make the corpse presentable for viewing in a suitably costly container, and here too the funeral director routinely without first consulting the family prepares the body for public display" (Kalish & Reynolds, 1981, p. 65).

This extensive preparation and attempt to make the body look "alive," "just as he used to" or "just as if she were asleep," may reflect the fact that Anglo North Americans have come into contact with death and dying less than have other cultural groups. Anglo North Americans constitute a culture-bound ethnic group, and the avoidance of death may reflect cultural and religious differences. For example, if a patient has died and a family member does not want to see the body until the mortician has "fixed it up," this request needs to be respected, regardless of your personal beliefs.

Funeral Practices

By their very nature, people are social beings who need to develop social attachments. When these social attachments are broken by death, people need to bring closure to the relationships. The funeral is an appropriate and socially acceptable time for the expression of sorrow and grief. Although there are some mores that dictate acceptable behaviors associated with the expression of grief, such as crying and sobbing, the wake and funeral are generally viewed as times when members of the living social network can observe and comfort the grieving survivors in their mourning and say a last good-bye to the dead person. It is important to keep in mind that even the terms used for the wake and the funeral may vary according to religious and cultural beliefs. What is called a *wake* in many North American religions may be called a *viewing* or *calling hours* by others.

Customs for disposal of the body after death vary widely. Muslims have specific rituals for washing, dressing, and positioning the body. In traditional Judaism, cosmetic restoration is discouraged, as is any attempt to hasten or retard decomposition by artificial means. As part of their lifelong preparation for death, Amish women sew white burial garments for themselves and for their family members (Wenger, 1991). For the viewing and burial, faithful Mormons are dressed in white temple garments. Burial clothes and other religious or cultural symbols may be important items for the funeral ritual. If such items are present, you should ensure that they are taken by the family or sent to the funeral home.

Believing that the spirit or ghost of the deceased person is contaminated, some Navajos are afraid to touch the body after death. In preparation for burial, the body is dressed in fine apparel, adorned with expensive jewelry and money, and wrapped in new blankets. After death, some Navajos believe that the structure in which the person died must be burned. There are specific members of the culture whose role is to prepare the body and who must be ritually cleansed after contact with the dead.

Funeral arrangements vary from short, simple rituals to long, elaborate displays. Among the Amish, family members, neighbors, and friends are relied on for a short, quiet ceremony. Many Jewish families use unadorned coffins and stress simplicity in burial services. Some Jews fly the body to Jerusalem for burial in ground considered to be holy. Regardless of economic considerations, some groups believe in lavish and costly funerals.

Attitudes Toward Death

TABOOS

In some cultures, people believe that particular omens, such as the appearance of an owl or a message in a dream, warn of approaching death. Breaking a taboo may be believed to cause death, and the nurse may be seen as the responsible agent! The literature contains numerous reports of incidents in which nurses have removed objects of religious and spiritual significance that are believed to have healing powers from clients and patients of all ages—rosaries from the cribs of infants, necklaces worn by elderly Native Americans, and so forth. In some cases, the intention of the nurse was benevolent, as when the nurse indicated that the item was removed to be kept in a safe place with other valuables.

Voodoo beliefs and practices are known to exist in North America. Incidents of sudden death or minor injuries after hexing have been attributed to the power of suggestion and to total social isolation, which have been thought to trigger fatal physiologic responses and sensitization of the autonomic nervous system.

AWARENESS OF DYING

Whether individuals should be made aware of their impending death has been debated extensively by physicians, nurses, and others. In the Kalish and Reynolds (1981) study, 71% of Anglos, 60% of African Americans, 49% of Japanese Americans, and 37% of Mexican Americans favored telling clients that they were dying (Stolley & Koenig, 1997). Each cultural group believed that the physician was the most appropriate person to communicate the information, whereas a family member was the second most appropriate choice. However, individual preferences should be respected. In some cultures, not telling the dying individual of his or her impending death is a way for that person to be allowed to "save face."

Unexpected Death, Violent Death, and Suicide

Acceptance of sudden, violent death is difficult for family members in most societies. For example, suicide is strictly forbidden under Islamic law. In the Filipino culture, suicide brings shame to the individual and to the entire family. Many Christian religions prohibit suicide and may impose sanctions even after death for the "sin." For example, a Roman Catholic who commits suicide may be denied burial in blessed ground or in a Catholic cemetery. In some religions, a church funeral is not permitted for a suicide victim, requiring the family to make alternative arrangements. This imposition of religious law can further add to the grief of surviving family members and friends.

The Northern Cheyenne believe that suicide, or any death resulting from a violent accident, disturbs the individual's spiritual balance. This disharmony is termed *bad death* and is believed to render the spirit earthbound in its wanderings, thus preventing it from entering the spirit world. A **good death** among the Tohono O'odham comes at the end of a full life, when a person is prepared for death. A bad death, by contrast, occurs unexpectedly and violently, leaving the victim without a chance to settle affairs or to say good-bye.

"A 'bad death' is 'bad' because evil caused it, which leaves the soul of the dead unrestful, unfulfilled, and desirous of returning to the living out of a longing for what has been taken away. The soul returns to the living, although not out of malevolence, to visit loved ones. It is on these visits that the dead can bring a form of *ka: cim mumkidag* (staying-Indian-sickness) to the

living—hence their dangerousness" (Kozak, 1991, p. 214).

In addition to exploring Tohono O'odham (Papago) categories of death, Kozak looks at the larger causes of the increase in violent deaths, arguing "that shifting mortality trends indicate shifts in other aspects of society" (Kozak, 1991, p. 211). Increased deaths are tied to declining economic conditions on the reservation, where jobs have disappeared.

"...the O'odham's economic transition has meant either migrating away from family and friends to find work or remaining on the reservation at home usually to confront extreme unemployment and welfare dependency. Neither option is considered satisfactory or desirable. The social and psychologic side effects of these economic transformations are highlighted, in an inverse relationship in alcohol and drug abuse, violence, and a general increase in dependency" (Kozak, 1991, p. 213).

The categories of "good" and "bad" deaths among the Tohono O'odham have implications for research on excess deaths. Accidents, homicide, and suicide produce bad deaths; in Tohono O'odham eyes, these are deaths that should not occur, deaths that should be avoided if possible. "Bad" deaths are excess deaths. If the medical community's concern is with eliminating excess deaths, it must also be concerned with the larger cultural, social, and economic context in which these deaths occur. Other causes of death, while still important, may affect a people to a much lesser degree. Diabetes mellitus, for example, most often affects people of more advanced years and, because of its slow progress, allows them to prepare for death. This is still an excess death by Western medical standards, but it is not a "bad" death (Hickey & Hall, 1993; Huttlinger, Krefting, Drevdahl, Tree, Bacca, & Benally, 1992).

Death memorials provide a place for the dead to go without bringing harm to the living and a place for the living to go to help the dead to a proper afterlife. Among the Tohono O'odham, there has been a notable increase in violent deaths, particularly for young males, since 1955. Motor vehicle accidents caused the majority of these violent deaths, Tohono O'odham people marked them with roadside death memorials or shrines. Suicides and homicides are also sometimes commemorated with death memorials.

Deaths resulting from nonviolent but untimely causes can be equally difficult for the patient, family, and friends. Cancers and chronic diseases may give the patient and family time to "prepare" for the death, but the death still occurs and must receive attention.

Holism

Buddhism has a holistic approach to death. To the Buddhist way of thinking, illness is inevitable and is a consequence of events and actions taken, not necessarily in this life but also in previous lives. The Buddhist believes in the cause and effect of events in this life as well as in previous lives. There is an acceptance of death, which means that the choice has been made to anticipate the grief and accept the inevitability of death. This does not mean resignation or the denial of conventional medicine. It does mean moving peacefully from the presence of loving family and friends into the next existence.

The Death of a Child

Although a great deal has been written about children's conceptions of death, cross-cultural studies have not yet been reported. Children develop a concept of death through innate cognitive development, which has significant cultural variations, and through acquired notions conveyed by the family, which vary according to the family's cultural beliefs. Thus, it is unsafe to assume that all children, regardless of family culture, will develop parallel concepts of and reactions to death.

Most children's initial experiences with death occur with the loss of a pet rather than a person. Because of reduced childhood mortality and delayed adult mortality, Western children are much less exposed to death in family than they used to be, and they tend to be sheltered from the experience. The current lack of direct exposure of children to death is both a class phenomenon and a cultural phenomenon.

In many societies of the Western world, children are considered precious, valued, and vulnerable; they are protected and are often the first to be saved in emergencies. In less developed societies, by contrast, parents are less likely to see most of their children grow into adulthood because of a very high infant mortality rate. As a result, a child's life may be viewed as less valued and precious than an adult's, but it is still viewed as valuable to the parents and other loved ones. Regardless of the sociocultural situation, each society has a special view of the significance of children and their death as it affects the bereaved family.

Bereavement, Grief, and Mourning

Bereavement is a sociologic term indicating the status and role of the survivors of a death. **Grief** is an affective response to a loss, whereas **mourning** is the culturally patterned behavioral response to a death. What differs between races and cultural groups is not so much the feelings of grief but their forms of expression or mourning.

Different family systems may alleviate or intensify the pain experienced by bereaved persons. In the typical nuclear Anglo North American family, the death of a member leaves a great void because the same few individuals fill most of the roles. By contrast, cultural groups in which several generations and extended family members commonly reside within a household may find that the acute trauma of bereavement is softened by the fact that the familial role of the deceased is easily filled by other relatives. It should be noted, however, that the loss is experienced and mourned irrespective of the person's cultural background.

Although nurses frequently encourage clients and their families to express their grief openly, many people are reluctant to do so in the institutional setting. The nurse often sees family members when they are still in shock over the death and are responding to the situation as a crisis rather than expressing their grief. Three-fourths of Blacks, Japanese, and Anglos stated that they would try hard to maintain control of their emotions in public, whereas less than two-thirds of Mexican Americans were concerned with the public expression of grief. When asked about crying, either publicly or privately, 88% of Mexican American, 71% of Japanese, 70% of Anglos, and 60% of Blacks indicated that this was acceptable, particularly in private (Kalish & Reynolds, 1981).

When asked who would be sought for comfort and support in a time of bereavement, these groups most frequently named a family member or a member of the clergy. In an institutional setting, a nurse who has been with the patient and family throughout the dying process may be surprised at the time of death when the grieving persons turn to other family, and the nurse is "left out."

Although the experience of grief is a universal phenomenon, a nurse should recognize that the expression of grief is strongly influenced by cultural factors. For example, mourning may vary according to the lines of emotional attachment. In matrilineal societies, a woman may be expected to grieve for male members of her maternal family, such as fathers and brothers, but not for her spouse.

It is not uncommon for a surviving spouse to have a serious illness within a year or two after the death. Although the exact reasons for this are unknown, the stress of losing a spouse seems to render the surviving partner more vulnerable to illness. Caring for a person who is seriously ill but who is also mourning a recent death requires added sensitivity by the nurse to the patient's emotional needs.

Some mourning rituals are highly structured and lengthy, whereas others are relatively simple and short. In the Jewish tradition, there are five successive stages of mourning, which extend for a year and include practices that influence virtually every aspect of life.

Summary of Beliefs Related to Death and Dying

Contemporary bereavement practices of various cultural and religious groups demonstrate the wide range of expressions of bereavement. Each group reflects practices that best meet its members' needs. Once you understand this, you can better appreciate their role in promoting a culturally appropriate grieving process and realize that hindering or interfering with practices that

the client and family find meaningful can disrupt the grieving process. Bereaved people can experience physical and psychological symptoms, and they may succumb to serious physical illnesses, leading even to death. Although bereavement is regarded as a universal stressor, the magnitude of the stress and its meaning to the individual vary significantly cross-culturally. For example, one Western misconception is that it is more stressful to mourn the death of a child than the death of an older or more distant relative. Yet, cross-cultural studies show that emotional attachments to relatives vary significantly and are not based on Western concepts of kinship (Duffy, 2006).

Although traditional funeral and postfuneral rituals have benefited both bereaved persons and their social groups in their original settings, the influence of the contemporary Western urban setting is unknown. It is likely that in North America, most individuals have assimilated U.S. and Canadian practices in varying degrees. You should obtain information from individual clients in a caring manner, explaining that you wish to provide culturally appropriate nursing care.

Religious Trends in the United States and Canada

The United States and Canada are cosmopolitan nations to which all of the major and many of the minor faiths of Europe and other parts of the globe have been transplanted. Religious identification among people from different racial and ethnic groups is important because religion and culture are interwoven. In a recent survey, 64% of Latino and 50% of Black congregations in the United States regard their churches as a means of preserving their cultural heritage, whereas fewer than one-third of White congregations link their religious denomination with the preservation of cultural heritage (Pew Forum, 2007). During the past 25 years, there has been an unusually large group of immigrants from Asia and Latin America. The changing composition of the Asian population has resulted in a proportional decrease in Christians with a corresponding proportional rise in those professing Asian religions (e.g., Buddhism, Hinduism, Islam). These immigration patterns have resulted in significant shifts. For example, there are three times as many Hindus in the United States today as there were in 1990. Most of the Latin American immigrants, on the other hand, are Roman Catholic, although the numbers are not large enough to make a significant statistical shift overall (U.S. Census Bureau, 2000).

With such a complex mosaic of religions, no one has succeeded in enumerating all the denominations. Table 14–1 details the statistical breakdown of major religious affiliations of the United States and Canada (Figure 14–2). Selected religious groups and their respective memberships numbers in the United States and Canada are identified in Table 14–2.

As discussed, a wide range of beliefs frequently exists within religions—a factor that adds complexity. Some religions have a designated spokesperson or leader who articulates, interprets, and applies theological tenets to daily life experiences, including those of health and illness. These leaders include Jewish rabbis, Catholic priests, and Lutheran ministers. Some churches rely more heavily on individual conscience, whereas others entrust decisions to a group of

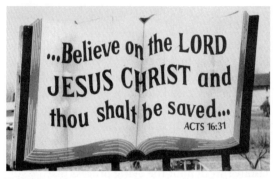

FIGURE 14-2. Approximately 77% of North Americans report religious affiliation with a Christian church. Of the 52% affiliated with Protestant groups in the United States, Baptists account for 29%; Methodists, 13%; Lutherans, 8%; Presbyterians, 3.6%; and Episcopalians, 2.5%. Catholics make up 24%. Those belonging to non-Christian religions total 6% to 7% of the population, whereas those reporting no religious affiliation account for 13% to 17%.

individuals or to a single person vested with ultimate authority within their church.

Although it is impossible to address the health-related beliefs and practices of any religion adequately, this chapter offers a brief overview of some groups. Some of the world's religions fall into major branches or divisions, such as Vaishnavite and Shaivite Hinduism; Theravada and Mahayana Buddhism; Orthodox, Reform, and Conservative Judaism; Roman

TABLE 14-1 *Major Religious Affiliations of U.S. and Canada (%)*

	USA	Canada	World
Christianity	76.5	77.1	32.9
Atheism, Agnosticism, no affiliation	13.2	17	12.5
Judaism	1.4	1.1	0.2
Islam	0.5	2.0	19.9
Buddhism	0.5	1	6
Hinduism	0.4	0.9	14
Major Christian Faith Groups			
Roman Catholic	245	50.8	32.3
Protestant	52	35	9.2
Eastern Orthodox	2.0	1.4	

Source: www.religioustolerance.org, accessed on March 18, 2007.

TABLE 14-2 *Membership for Selected Religious Bodies in the United States and Canada*

Religious Body (year reported)	Membership
African Methodist Episcopal Church (2006)	2,500,000
African Methodist Episcopal Zion Church (2006)	1,432,795
American Baptist Churches in the USA (2006)	1,424,840
Assemblies of God (2006)	2,779,095
Baptist Bible Fellowship International (2006)	1,200,000
Buddhist (1990)	780,000
Christian Churches and Churches of Christ (2006)	1,071,615
Church of God in Christ (2006)	5,499,875
Church of Jesus Christ of Latter-Day Saints (2006)	5,999,177
Churches of Christ (2006)	1,500,000
Episcopal Church (2006)	2,284,233
Evangelical Lutheran Church of America (2006)	4,930,429
Greek Orthodox Diocese America (2006)	1,500,000
Hindu (1990)	227,000
Islam (2002)	6,000,000 to 7,000,000
Jehovah's Witnesses (1999)	1,029,902
Jewish (1998)	7,320,000
Lutheran Church–Missouri Synod (2006)	2,463,747
Muslim/Islamic (1990)	3,600,000
National Baptist Convention of America, Inc. (2006)	3,500,000
National Baptist Convention, USA, Inc. (2006)	5,000,000
National Missionary Baptist Convention, USA, Inc. (2006)	2,500,000
Orthodox Church in America (2006)	1,064,000
Pentecostal Assemblies of the World, Inc. (2006)	1,500,000
Presbyterian Church (USA) (2006)	3,189,573
Progressive National Baptist Convention, Inc. (2006)	2,500,000
Roman Catholic Church (2006)	67,820,833
Southern Baptist Convention (2006)	16,267,494
United Church of Christ (2006)	1,265,786
United Methodist Church (2006)	8,186,254

Yearbook of American and Canadian Churches, 2006

Catholic, Orthodox, and Protestant Christianity, and Sunnite and Shi'ite Islam. There also are subdivisions into what are often called denominations, sects, or schools of thought and practice.

Contributions of Religious Groups to the Health Care Delivery System

In the United States and Canada, many denominations own and operate health care institutions and make significant fiscal contributions that help control health care costs. For example, the Roman Catholic Church, the largest single denomination in the United States, is also a major stakeholder in the health care field. According to the *Catholic Almanac* (2000), the nation's nearly 600 Catholic hospitals treat 17.2 million patients annually and account for approximately 10% of all hospital beds. In addition, the Catholic Church is responsible for treating 84,723, 272 patients at its 573 hospitals and 6,054,544 individuals at its 392 other health-related centers. Moreover, under direct Catholic auspices, there are 79 nonresidential schools for the handicapped; 14 facilities for the deaf and hearing impaired; 4 centers for the blind and visually impaired; 517 facilities for the aged; 72 facilities for abused, abandoned, neglected, and emotionally disturbed children; 116 centers for those with developmental disabilities; 2 residences for the orthopedically and physically handicapped; 8 cancer hospitals; and 11 substance abuse centers (U.S. Conference of Catholic Bishops, 2007).

Catholic Charities USA, an umbrella agency that oversees nonhospital work, reports that its agencies serve more than 10 million people each year, often functioning as a centralized referral source for clients ultimately treated in non-Catholic agencies (*Catholic Almanac*, 2000).

Similarly, there are many Jewish hospitals, day-care centers, extended care facilities, and organizations to meet the health care needs of Jewish and non-Jewish persons in need. For example, the National Jewish Center for Immunology and Respiratory Medicine is a research and treatment center for respiratory, immunologic, allergic, and infectious diseases, whereas the Council for Jewish Elderly provides a full range of social and health care services for seniors, including adult day care, care/case management, counseling, transportation, and advocacy.

Many other denominations, including the Lutheran, Mennonite, Methodist, Muslim, and Seventh-Day Adventist groups, own and operate hospitals and health care organizations similar to those described previously.

In Canada, hospital care, outpatient care, extended care, and medical services have been publicly funded and administered since the Medical Care Act of 1966. However, before the Medical Care Act and into the present, religious organizations have made important contributions to the health and well-being of Canadians at individual, community, and societal levels. For example, countless church-run agencies, charities, and facilities offer care and social support to individuals and families coping with such conditions as chronic illness, disability, poverty, and homelessness. At the national level, church-run organizations, such as the Catholic Health Asso-

ciation of Canada, are committed to addressing social justice issues that affect the health system and offer leadership through research and policy development regarding health care ethics, spiritual and religious care, and social justice.

Amish

The term *Amish* refers to members of several ethnoreligious groups who choose to live separately from the modern world through manner of dress, language, family life, and selective use of technology. There are four major orders or affiliating groups of Amish: (1) *Old Order Amish*, the largest group, whose name is often used synonymously with "the Amish"; (2) the ultraconservative *Swartzentruber* and *Andy Weaver Amish*, both more conservative than the Old Order Amish in their restrictive use of technology and shunning of members who have dropped out or committed serious violations of the faith; (3) the less conservative *New Order Amish*, which emerged in the 1960s with more liberal views of technology but with an emphasis on high moral standards in restricting alcohol and tobacco use and in courtship practices; and (4) the *Liberal Beachy Amish*.

The total population of Amish is estimated at 160,000, spread throughout more than 220 settlements in 21 states and one Canadian province (about 1/20th of 1% of the total populations of the United States and Canada). In 1900, there were approximately 5,000 Amish, representing the number who immigrated to the United States during the 18th and 19th centuries. During the 20th century, however, the population grew as the Amish became less frequent targets for conversion and growing numbers of children (80% to 85%) chose, as adults, to be baptized Amish. As a result, the population grew to 85,000 by 1979 and has nearly doubled that number today. More than half are younger than age 18 (Donnermeyer, 1997).

General Beliefs and Religious Practices

The imperative to remain separate is the common theme of the nearly 500-year history of the

Amish and is based on the following scripture passages:

"Be not conformed to this world, but be ye transformed by the renewing of your mind"

(Romans 12:2)

"Be ye not unequally yoked together with unbelievers; for what fellowship hath righteousness with unrighteousness? and what communion hath light with darkness?"

(II Corinthians 6:14)

The Amish are direct descendants of a branch of Anabaptists (which means "to be rebaptized") that emerged during the Protestant Reformation and resided in Switzerland, the Netherlands, Austria, France, and Germany. Anabaptists stressed adult baptism, separation from and nonassimilation with the dominant culture, conformity in dress and appearance, marriage to others within the group, nonproselytization, nonparticipation in military service, and a disciplined lifestyle with an emphasis on simple living. These basic tenets remain today.

A former Catholic priest from the Netherlands named Menno Simmons (1496–1561) wrote down the beliefs and practices of the Anabaptists, who became known as **Mennonites**. In 1693, under the leadership of a church elder named Jacob Ammann (1656–1730), a more conservative group broke away and formed the group currently known as the Amish.

Core Characteristics

According to Donnermeyer (1997), there are **five core characteristics of the Amish**.

SUBCULTURE

First, the Amish are a subculture: a group with beliefs, values, and behaviors that are distinct from the greater culture of which the group is a part. The Amish maintain their separateness and distinctiveness from United States and Canadian societies in a variety of ways. Geographically, the Amish live close together in areas referred to as settlements and rely primarily on the horse and buggy for transportation.

The Amish continue to practice their faith in the tradition of Anabaptism, which includes small church districts of a few dozen families led by a bishop, church services that rotate from house to house of each family (no church building), the practice of adult baptism, communion twice a year, and shunning. Church leaders are chosen through a process of nomination and drawing by lot, and they serve for life. All but a few Amish marry, extended family remains important, and divorce is rare. The Amish dress in distinctive clothing (plain colors and mostly without buttons and zippers). They speak a form of German among themselves known as Pennsylvania Dutch or High German, and they sometimes refer to non-Amish as the "English."

ORDUNG

The second core feature of the Amish is the *ordung*, which is used for passing on religious values and way of life from one generation to the next. Parts of the *ordung* are based on specific biblical passages, but much of it consists of rules for living the Amish way.

MEIDUNG/SHUNNING

The third characteristic of the Amish is *meidung*, the practice of shunning members who have violated the *ordung*. After all members of the church district have discussed the case and agreed to impose *meidung*, the individual is separated from the rest of his or her community. It is the church's method of enforcing the *ordung*. *Meidung* is an important way of maintaining both a sense of community among Amish and a sense of separation from the rest of the world. Sanctions for violations against important values, beliefs, and behaviors that define distinctiveness from the majority culture enable the Amish to retain their religious and cultural identity. In most cases, when *meidung* is applied, it is for a limited time. *Meidung* applies only to Amish adults who have been baptized, not to their unbaptized children. Children of Amish who choose not to be baptized often become members of neighboring Mennonite congregations and maintain contact with their Amish relatives.

With less serious violations of the *ordung*, a member is visited privately by the deacon and a minister, and the matter is resolved quietly. For more serious offenses, the punishment is carried out publicly during a church service. A few offenses, such as adultery and divorce, are automatically conditions of excommunication. By displaying deep sorrow and repentance for an offense, excommunicated members can be allowed back, but this is not easily accomplished.

SELECTIVE USE OF TECHNOLOGY

The fourth core characteristic is the selective use of technology. The Amish selectively use many modern technologies, but only if they do not threaten their ability to maintain a community of believers. Technologically, the Amish restrict the use of electricity in their homes and farms, and they limit their use of telephones. Although they ride in automobiles, trains, and airplanes, they do not operate them. Tractors for farm field-work might reduce the opportunity for sons and daughters to help parents with farm chores, and the farm would become larger, reducing the number available for future generations. Thus, technology is not inherently bad, but when its consequences result in destruction of family and community life, it is avoided (Figure 14–3).

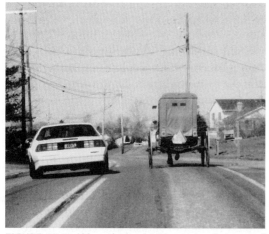

FIGURE 14-3. Although the Amish restrict their use of technology for reasons that are, in part, health related, they ironically find themselves at a high risk for accidents that frequently result from the careless use of technologic developments by non-Amish neighbors.

GELASSENHEIT

The fifth and final core characteristic of the Amish is *gelassenheit*. This term means "submission," or yielding to a higher authority, and it represents a general guide for behavior among Amish members. *Gelassenheit* represents the high value that the Amish place on maintaining a sense of community, which is accomplished by not drawing too much attention to one's self. Amish cite *gelassenheit* as the reason they avoid having their photographs taken and prohibit mirrors in their homes.

Holy Days and Sacraments

Amish hold church services every other Sunday on a rotating basis in the homes or barns of church district members. The church services last several hours with hymns, scriptures, and services in High German or Pennsylvania Dutch. The family hosting the services is expected to provide a meal for all in attendance. Christmas celebrations include family dinners and exchanges of gifts. Weddings last all day and include eating and singing. An important part of Amish life is informal visiting. Families often visit one another without advance notice, and it is common for unexpected visitors to stay for a meal. Amish observe adult baptism and communion twice a year.

Social Activities (Dating, Dancing)

The Amish strive for high standards of conduct in both their private and public lives. This includes chastity before marriage and humility in dress, language, and behavior. The function of dating is to afford individuals an opportunity to become acquainted with each other's character. Couples contemplating marriage may engage in a practice called bundling, in which they lie together in bed, fully clothed, without having sexual contact.

Substance Use

Alcoholic beverages and drugs are forbidden unless prescribed by a physician. Tobacco use is prohibited.

Health Care Practices

Illness is seen as the inability to perform daily chores; physical and mental illness are equally accepted. Health care practices within the Amish culture are varied and include folk, herbal, and homeopathic medicine and Western biomedicine. Unlike the use of episodic biomedicine, however, preventive medicine may be seen as against God's will. The use of the Western biomedical health care system is largely episodic and crisis oriented. If Western biomedicine fails, there is no hesitancy in visiting an herb doctor, pow-wow doctor (a practitioner of a folk healing art, known as *brauche*, in which touch is used to heal), or a chiropractor. Folk, professional, and alternative care are often used simultaneously. Cost, access, transportation, and advice from family and friends are the major factors that influence healing choices (Wenger, 1990).

Medical and Surgical Interventions

The use of narcotic drugs is prohibited. There are no restrictions against the use of blood, blood products, or vaccines if advised by health care providers.

Practices Related to Reproduction

The Amish believe that the fundamental purpose of marriage is the procreation of children, and couples are encouraged to have large families. Children are economic assets to the family because they assist their parents with housework, farm chores, gardening, and family business. Women are expected to have children until menopause. If situations arise that justify sterilization (e.g., removal of cancerous reproductive organs), those called upon to make the decisions would rely on the best medical advice available and the council of the church leaders. Although the Amish family structure is patriarchal, the grandmother is often a key decision maker concerning reproductive and other health-related issues.

Abortion is inconsistent with Amish values and beliefs. Artificial insemination, genetics, eugenics, and stem cell research are also inconsistent with Amish values and beliefs.

Religious Support System for the Sick

VISITORS

Individual members of local and surrounding communities assist and support one another in time of need. From cradle to grave, each person knows that he or she will be cared for by those in the community. **Friendscraft** is a unique three-generational extended family support network inherent in the Amish community that provides informal support, emotional and financial assistance, and advice. The extended family consists of aunts, uncles, cousins, and grandparents, who usually live only a few miles away and can be counted on to assist in times of illness.

TITLE OF RELIGIOUS REPRESENTATIVE

The Amish do not use religious titles. There are approximately 1,100 Amish church districts in the United States and Canada, each representing about 20 to 35 families, and a minimal hierarchy of church leaders (a bishop, deacon, and two ministers). The bishop is the spiritual head; the deacon assists the bishop and is responsible for donations to help members with medical bills and other expenses; and the ministers help the bishop with preaching at church services and providing spiritual direction for the church district and its members. Although bishops meet periodically, there is no church hierarchy above the level of the church district. Because the Amish are surrounded by American and Canadian societies, which continuously exert strong economic and cultural pressures that are incompatible with Amish values, the Amish represent a subculture that is among the most "self-consciously engineered of all societies" (Donnermeyer, 1997, p. 9).

CHURCH ORGANIZATIONS TO ASSIST THE SICK

Individual members of local church districts look after the needs of the sick person and his or her family.

Practices Related to Death and Dying

Prolongation of life (right to die) and euthanasia are personal matters that may be discussed with the bishop, ministers, and/or family members.

Autopsy is acceptable in the case of medical necessity or legal requirement but is seldom performed on the Amish. Although there is no specific prohibition, the Amish usually prefer to bury the intact body and generally do not donate body parts for medical research. Bodies are buried in small cemeteries in Amish communities on private property.

Addendum: Meeting Health Expenses

The Amish beliefs in self-sufficiency, separation from the world, and mutual aid have resulted in their rejection of formal assistance that comes from outside the Amish community. For example, the Amish obtained exemption for self-employed workers from Social Security, including Medicare, in 1965 on religious grounds and received exemption for all Amish workers from these programs in 1988. Amish seldom purchase commercial health insurance; instead, they have traditionally relied on personal savings and various methods of mutual assistance within the immediate and larger Amish community to meet their medical expenses. It is expected that each family has planned for future health care needs (e.g., childbirth and minor illness), but it is recognized that catastrophic illnesses resulting in extensive medical expenses do sometimes occur. In these instances, the Amish community provides assistance, usually through participation in one of the Amish Hospital Aid plans.

As indicated in Evidence-Based Practice 14–1, changing occupational patterns among the Amish have resulted in shifting views toward commercial health insurance. According to Donnermeyer (1997), in Holmes County, Ohio, only 32.9% of Amish breadwinners earn their living as farmers: 24.5% are active farmers, 4% are retired farmers, and 3.4% hold dual occupations (both farm and nonfarm). Similar trends have been reported among other Amish settlements, where 30% to 80% of adult men work in nonfarm wage labor jobs in construction, factories, and home-based shops (e.g., cabinetmaking, harness making, blacksmithing, and so forth). The underlying reasons for the change are attributed

to two factors: population growth and difficulty finding sufficient farmland for the growing numbers of Amish.

Baha'i International Community

The Baha'i Faith is an independent world religion. It has members in approximately 340 countries and localities and represents 1,900 ethnic groups and tribes. North American membership is 161,366, and worldwide membership is 7,666,000.

General Beliefs and Religious Practices

The writings that guide the life of the **Baha'i International Community** comprise numerous works by Baha'u'llah, prophet–founder of the Baha'i Faith. Central teachings are the oneness of God, the oneness of religion, and the oneness of humanity. Baha'u'llah proclaimed that religious truth is not absolute but relative, that Divine Revelation is a continuous and progressive process, that all the great religions of the world are divine in origin, and that their missions represent successive stages in the spiritual evolution of human society.

For Baha'is, the basic purpose of human life is to know and worship God and to carry forward an ever-advancing civilization. To achieve these goals, they strive to fulfill certain principles:

1. Fostering of good character and the development of spiritual qualities, such as honesty, trustworthiness, compassion, and justice.
2. Eradication of prejudices of race, creed, class, nationality, and gender.
3. Elimination of all forms of superstitions that hamper human progress, and achievement of a balance between the material and spiritual aspects of life. An unfettered search for truth and belief in the essential harmony of science and religion are two aspects of this principle.

Evidence-Based Practice 14–1:

Old Order Amish and Commercial Health Insurance

Although Old Order Amish families have in the past been prohibited from using commercial health insurance on religious grounds, the increasing cost of hospitalization, combined with changing occupational patterns by the Amish, has resulted in a change in health care use patterns. The data for the study were obtained through observation of participants and informal open-ended interviews with Old Order Amish families residing in Geauga County, Ohio. The findings indicate that there is an increasing tendency for Old Order Amish families in this county to use health insurance provided by non-Amish employers. The pattern is associated with increased use of biomedical health services, which is related to the availability of extensive health services and facilities in neighboring Cleveland.

Clinical Application

The Old Order Amish is a dynamic group that has managed to survive at least partially because they have selectively incorporated new components into their cultural system. One important change over the past few generations involves the transition from an agrarian way of life to one based on wage labor and the accompanying increased use of employer-provided commercial health insurance. The researchers also noted that an additional cost for Amish seeking biomedical health care is transportation—a sum that may equal or exceed that paid to the health care provider. Perhaps the most important consideration for nurses is to understand that Old Order Amish society is dynamic and that there is greater heterogeneity between and within congregations than might be expected from the outward manifestations of conformity in dress and selective use of technology.

Greksa, L. P., & Korbin, J. E. (1997). Influence of changing occupational patterns on the use of commercial health insurance by the Old Order Amish. *Journal of Multicultural Nursing & Health, 3*(2), 13–18.

4. Development of the unique talents and abilities of every individual through the pursuit of knowledge and the acquisition of skills for the practice of a trade or profession.
5. Full participation of both sexes in all aspects of community life, including the elective, administrative, and decision-making processes, along with equality of opportunities, rights, and privileges of men and women.
6. Fostering of the principle of universal compulsory education.

Baha'is may not be members of any political party, but they may accept nonpartisan government posts and appointments. They are enjoined to obey the government in their respective countries and, without political affiliation, may vote in general elections and participate in the civic life of their communities.

The Baha'i administrative order has neither priesthood nor ritual; it relies on a pattern of local, national, and international governance created by Baha'u'llah. Institutions and programs are supported exclusively by voluntary contributions from members.

The Baha'i International Community has consultative status with the United Nations Economic and Social Council and with the United Nations Children's Fund. It is also affiliated with the United Nations Environment Program and with the United Nations Office of Public Information.

The World Center of the Baha'i Faith is in Israel, established in the two cities of Haifa and 'Akka. The Universal House of Justice, the supreme elected council, administers the affairs of the Baha'i world community in Haifa.

Holy Days and Sacraments

Extending from sunset to sunset are Baha'i holy days, feast days, and days of fasting. These holy days are not contraindications to medical care or surgery.

Although the Baha'i Faith does not have sacraments in the same sense that Christian churches do, it does have practices that have similar meanings to members. These practices include the recitation of obligatory prayers and participation in the observance of holy days and the Nineteen-Day Fast, which is mandatory for all Baha'is between the ages of 15 and 70 years. Exceptions are made for illness, travel away from home, and pregnancy. **Fasting** occurs from sunrise to sunset for an entire Baha'i month, which consists of 19 days.

Social Activities (Dating, Dancing)

Baha'is strive for high standards of conduct in both their private and public lives; this includes chastity before marriage; moderation in dress, language, and amusements; and complete freedom from prejudice in their dealings with peoples of different races, classes, creeds, and orders.

The Baha'i Faith forbids monastic celibacy, noting that marriage is fundamental to the growth and continuation of civilization. The function of dating is to afford individuals an opportunity to become acquainted with each other's character. Those contemplating marriage are encouraged to engage in some form of work and service together—a practice intended to promote assessment of their own maturity and readiness for marriage as well as to improve their knowledge of the character and values of the prospective marriage partner.

Substance Use

Alcoholic beverages and drugs are forbidden unless prescribed by a physician. Tobacco use is strongly discouraged.

Health Care Practices

With an attitude of harmony between religion and science, Baha'is are encouraged to seek out competent medical care, to follow the advice of those in whom they have confidence, and to pray.

Medical and Surgical Interventions

The use of narcotic drugs is prohibited except by prescription. There are no restrictions against the use of blood, blood products, or vaccines if health care providers advise them. Amputations, organ transplants, biopsies, and circumcision are also permitted if advised by health care providers.

Practices Related to Reproduction

BIRTH CONTROL

Baha'is believe that the fundamental purpose of marriage is the procreation of children. Individuals are encouraged to exercise their discretion in choosing a method of family planning. Baha'u'llah taught that to beget children is the highest physical fruit of man's existence. The Baha'i teachings imply that birth control constitutes a real danger to the foundations of social life; it is against the spirit of Baha'i law, which defines the primary purpose of marriage to be the rearing of children and their spiritual training. It is left to each husband and wife to decide how many children they will have. Baha'i teachings state that the soul appears at conception. Therefore, it is improper to use a method that produces an abortion after conception has taken place (e.g., intrauterine device). Methods that result in permanent sterility are not permissible under normal circumstances. If situations arise that justify sterilization (e.g., removal of cancerous reproductive organs), those called upon to make the decision would rely on the best medical advice available and their own consciences.

AMNIOCENTESIS

Amniocentesis is permitted if advised by health care providers.

ABORTION

Members are discouraged from using methods of contraception that produce abortion after conception has taken place (e.g., intrauterine device). A surgical operation for the purpose of preventing the birth of an unwanted child is strictly forbidden.

Baha'i teachings state that the human soul comes into being at conception. Abortion and surgical operations for the purpose of preventing the birth of unwanted children are forbidden unless circumstances justify such actions on medical grounds. In this case, the decision is left to the consciences of those concerned, who must carefully weigh the medical advice they receive in the light of the general guidance given in the Baha'i writings.

ARTIFICIAL INSEMINATION

Although there are no specific Baha'i writings on artificial insemination, Baha'is are guided by the understanding that marriage is the proper spiritual and physical context in which the bearing of children must occur. Couples who are unable to bear children are not excluded from marriage because marriage has other purposes besides the bearing of children. The adoption of children is encouraged.

EUGENICS AND GENETICS

The Baha'is view scientific advancement as a noble and praiseworthy endeavor of humankind. Baha'i writings do not specifically address these two branches of science.

Religious Support System for the Sick

Individual members of local and surrounding communities assist and support one another in time of need. Religious titles are not used. Individual members of local communities look after the needs of the sick.

Practices Related to Death and Dying

Because human life is the vehicle for the development of the soul, Baha'is believe that life is unique and precious. The destruction of a human life at any stage, from conception to natural death, is rarely permissible. The question of when natural death has occurred is considered in the light of current medical science and legal rulings on the matter.

Autopsy is acceptable in the case of medical necessity or legal requirement. Baha'is are permitted to donate their bodies for medical research and for restorative purposes. Local burial laws are followed. Unless required by state law, Baha'i law states that the body is not to be embalmed. Cremation is forbidden. The place of burial must be within 1 hour's travel from the place of death. This regulation is always carried out in consultation with the family, and exceptions are possible.

Buddhist Churches of America

Buddhism is a general term that indicates a belief in Buddha and encompasses many individual churches. In 1999, there were approximately 780,000 Buddhists in North America, and the worldwide membership was greater than 500 million.

The Buddhist Churches of America is the largest Buddhist organization in mainland United States. This group belongs to the largest subsect of Jodo Shinshu Buddhism (Shin Buddhism), Honpa Hongwanji, which is the largest traditional sect of Buddhism in Japan. The Jodo Shinshu sect was started by Shinran (1173–1263) in Japan; its headquarters are in Kyoto, Japan. The group of churches in Hawaii is a different organization of Shin Buddhism, called Honpa Hongwanji Mission of Hawaii. There are numerous Buddhist sects in the United States and Canada, including Indian, Sri Lankan, Vietnamese, Thai, Chinese, Japanese, Tibetan, and so on.

Gautama Buddha founded Buddhism in the 6th century BC in northern India. In the 3rd century BC, Buddhism became the state religion of

India and spread from there to most of the other Eastern nations. The term *Buddha* means "enlightened one."

At the beginning of the Christian era, Buddhism split into two main groups: Hinayana, or southern Buddhism, and Mahayana, or northern Buddhism. Hinayana retained more of the original teachings of Buddha and survived in Sri Lanka (formerly Ceylon) and southern Asia. Mahayana, a more social and polytheistic Buddhism, is strong in the Himalayas, Tibet, Mongolia, China, Korea, and Japan.

General Beliefs and Religious Practices

Buddha's original teachings included the **Four Noble Truths** and the **Noble Eightfold Way**, the philosophies of which affect Buddhist responses to health and illness. The Four Noble Truths expound on suffering and constitute the foundation of Buddhism. The truths consist of (1) the truth of suffering, (2) the truth of the origin of suffering, (3) the truth that suffering can be destroyed, and (4) the way that leads to the cessation of pain.

The Noble Eightfold Way gives the rule of practical Buddhism, which consists of (1) right views, (2) right intention, (3) right speech, (4) right action, (5) right livelihood, (6) right effort, (7) right mindfulness, and (8) right concentration. **Nirvana**, a state of greater inner freedom and spontaneity, is the goal of all existence. When one achieves Nirvana, the mind has supreme tranquility, purity, and stability (Hinnell, 1984).

Although the ultimate goals of Buddhism are clear, the means of obtaining those goals are not religiously prescribed. Buddhism is not a dogmatic religion, nor does it dictate any specific practices. Individual differences are expected, acknowledged, and respected. Each individual is responsible for finding his or her own answers through awareness of the total situation.

Holy Days

"The major Buddhist holy day is Saga Dawa (or Vesak) which is the observance of Sakyamuni

Buddha's birth, enlightenment and parinirvana. This holiday falls during the months of May or June. It is based on a lunar calendar, and therefore the actual date varies from year to year." (University of Virginia Health System, 2006a) (Figure 14-4). Although there is no religious restriction for therapy on those days, they can be highly emotional, and a Buddhist patient should be consulted about his or her desires for medical or surgical intervention. Some Buddhists may fast for all or part of this day.

Sacraments

Buddhism does not have any sacraments. A ritual that symbolizes one's entry into the Buddhist faith is the expression of faith in the Three Treasures (Buddha, Dharma, and Sangha).

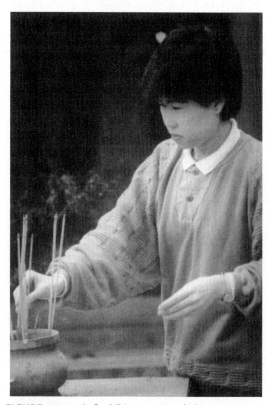

FIGURE 14-4. A Buddhist woman lights incense in remembrance of deceased ancestors.

Diet

Moderation in diet is encouraged. Specific dietary practices are usually interconnected with ethnic practices. Some branches of Buddhism have strict dietary regulations while others do not. It is important to inquire about the patient's preferences.

Health Care Practices

Buddhists do not believe in healing through a faith or through faith itself. However, Buddhists do believe that spiritual peace and liberation from anxiety by adherence to and achievement of awakening to Buddha's wisdom can be important factors in promoting healing and recovery.

Medical and Surgical Interventions

There are no restrictions in Buddhism for nutritional therapies, medications, vaccines, and other therapeutic interventions. Buddha's teaching on the Middle Path may apply here; he taught that extremes should be avoided. What may be medicine to one may be poison to another, so generalizations are to be avoided. Medications should be used in accordance with the nature of the illness and the capacity of the individual. Whatever will contribute to the attainment of Enlightenment is encouraged. Treatments such as amputations, organ transplants, biopsies, and other procedures that may prolong life and allow the individual to attain Enlightenment are encouraged.

Practices Related to Reproduction

The immediate emphasis is on the person living now and the attainment of Enlightenment. If practicing birth control or having an amniocentesis or sterility test will help the individual attain Enlightenment, it is acceptable.

Buddhism does not condone the taking of a life. The first of Buddha's Five Precepts is abstention from taking lives. Life in all forms is to be respected. Existence by itself often contradicts this principle (e.g., drugs that kill bacteria are given to spare a patient's life). With this in mind, it is the conditions and circumstances surrounding the patient that determine whether abortion, therapeutic or on demand, may be undertaken.

Religious Support System for the Sick

Buddhist priests often offer support to the ill client. Support of the sick is more of an individual practice in keeping with the philosophy of Buddhism.

Practices Related to Death and Dying

If there is hope for recovery and continuation of the pursuit of Enlightenment, all available means of support are encouraged. If life cannot be prolonged so that the person can continue to search for Enlightenment, conditions might permit euthanasia. If the donation of a body part will help another continue the quest for Enlightenment, it might be an act of mercy and is encouraged. The body is considered but a shell; therefore, autopsy and disposal of the body are matters of individual practice rather than of religious prescription. Burial usually consists of a brief graveside service after a funeral at the temple. Cremations are common (Chapman, 1991).

Religious Objects

Prayer beads and images of Sakyamuni Buddha and other Buddhist deities may be utilized for specific prayer or meditation practices.

Addendum

The headquarters of the Buddhist Churches of America are at 1710 Octavia Street, San Francisco, California 94109 (Telephone: [415] 776-5600). Additional material is available at the Buddhist Bookstore of the Buddhist Churches of America Headquarters. Information on Buddhism and temple locations in Canada can be found at http://buddhismcanada.com/

Catholicism (according to the Roman Rite)

With a North American membership of approximately 97 million (2006) and a worldwide membership of more than 1 billion, some 32 rites exist within **Catholicism**. Of these, the Roman Rite is the major body.

General Beliefs and Religious Practices

The Roman Catholic Church traces its beginnings to about 30 AD, when Jesus Christ is believed to have founded the church. Catholic teachings, based on the Bible, are found in declarations of church councils and popes and in short statements of faith called creeds. The oldest and most authoritative of these creeds are the Apostle's Creed and the Nicene Creed, the latter being recited during the central act of worship, called the Eucharistic Liturgy, or Mass. The creeds summarize Catholic beliefs concerning the Trinity and creation, sin and salvation, the nature of the church, and life after death.

Holy Days

Catholics are expected to observe all Sundays (including Easter Sunday) as holy days. Sunday or holy day worship services may be conducted any time from 4 p.m. on Saturday until Sunday evening. Other days are set aside for special liturgical observance are Christmas (December 25th); Solemnity of Mary, Mother of God (January 1st); Ascension Thursday (the Lord's bodily ascension into Heaven, observed 40 days after Easter), Feast of the Assumption (August 15th), All Saints Day (November 1st), and the Feast of the Immaculate Conception (December 8th).

Sacraments

The Roman Catholic Church recognizes seven sacraments: Baptism, Reconciliation (formerly Penance or Confession), Holy Communion or the **Eucharist** (Figure 14–5), Confirmation, Matrimony, Holy Orders, and Anointing of the Sick (formerly Extreme Unction).

Religious Objects

Rosaries, prayer books, and holy cards are often present and are of great comfort to the patient and his or her family. They should be left in place and within reach of the patient whenever possible (University of Virginia Health System, 2006e).

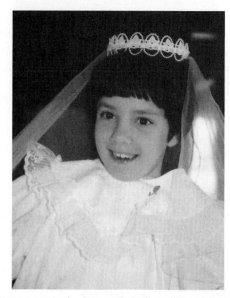

FIGURE 14-5. In the Roman Catholic tradition, when children reach the age of reason (about 7 years), they continue the ongoing initiation into their religion by making their First Communion. In addition to the religious ritual, there are sometimes cultural traditions surrounding this event, many of which involve a family celebration after the religious services have concluded.

Diet (Foods and Beverages)

The goods of the world have been given for use and benefit. The primary obligation people have toward foods and beverages is to use them in moderation and in such a way that they are not injurious to health. Fasting in moderation is recommended as a valued discipline. There are a few days of the year when Catholics have an obligation to fast, which means to abstain from meat and meat products. Catholics fast and abstain on Ash Wednesday and Good Friday, and abstinence is required on all of the Fridays of Lent. The sick are never bound by this prescription of the law. Healthy persons between the ages of 18 and 62 are encouraged to engage in fasting and abstinence as described.

Social Activities (Dating, Dancing)

The major principle is that Sunday is a day of rest; therefore, only unnecessary servile work is prohibited. The seven holy days are also considered days of rest, although many persons must engage in routine work-related activities on some of these days.

Substance Use

Alcohol and tobacco are not evil per se. They are to be used in moderation and not in a way that would be injurious to one's health or that of another party. The misuse of any substance is not only harmful to the body, but also sinful.

Health Care Practices

In time of illness, the basic rite is the **Sacrament of the Sick**, which includes anointing of the sick, communion if possible, and a blessing by a priest. Prayers are frequently offered for the sick person and for members of the family. The Eucharistic wafer (a small unleavened wafer made of flour and water) is often given to the sick as the food of healing and health. Other family members may participate if they wish to do so.

Medical and Surgical Interventions

As long as the benefits outweigh the risk to the individuals, judicious use of medications is permissible and morally acceptable. A major concern is the risk of mutilation. The Church has traditionally cited the **principle of totality**, which states that medications are allowed as long as they are used for the good of the whole person. Blood, blood products, and amputations are acceptable if consistent with the principle of totality. Biopsies and circumcision are also permissible.

The transplantation of organs from living donors is morally permissible when the anticipated benefit to the recipient is proportionate to the harm done to the donor, provided that the loss of such an organ does not deprive the donor of life itself or of the functional integrity of his or her body.

Practices Related to Reproduction

Birth Control

The basic principle is that the conjugal act should be one that is love giving and potentially life giving. Only natural means of contraception, such as abstinence, the temperature method, and the ovulation method are acceptable. Ordinarily, artificial aids and procedures for permanent sterilization are forbidden. Birth control (anovulants) may be used therapeutically to assist in regulating the menstrual cycle.

Amniocentesis

The procedure in and of itself is not objectionable. However, it is morally objectionable if the findings of the amniocentesis are used to lead the couple to decide on termination of the pregnancy or if the procedure injures the fetus.

Abortion

Direct abortion is always morally wrong. Indirect abortion may be morally justified by some circumstances (e.g., treatment of a cancerous uterus in a pregnant woman). Abortion on demand is prohibited. The Roman Catholic Church teaches the sanctity of all human life, even of the unborn, from the time of conception.

Sterility Tests and Artificial Insemination

The use of sterility tests for the purpose of promoting conception, not misusing sexuality, is permitted. Although artificial insemination has been debated heavily, traditionally it has been looked on as illicit, even between husband and wife.

Eugenics, Genetics, and Stem Cell Research

Research in the fields of eugenics and genetics is objectionable. This violates the moral right of the individual to be free from experimentation and also interferes with God's right as master of life and human beings' stewardship of their lives. Some genetic investigations to help determine genetic diseases may be used, depending on their ends and means. There is support for research using adult stem cells but opposition for the use of embryonic stem cells.

Religious Support System for the Sick

Visitors

Although a priest, deacon, or lay minister usually visits a sick person alone, the family or other significant people may be invited to join in prayer.

In fact, that is most desirable since they too need support.

The priest, deacon, or lay minister will usually bring the necessary supplies for administration of the Eucharist or administration of the Sacrament of the Sick (in the case of a priest). The nursing staff can facilitate these rites by ensuring an atmosphere of prayer and quiet and by having a glass of water on hand (in case the patient is unable to swallow the small wafer-like host). Consecrated wine can be made available but is usually not given in the hospital or home. The nurse may wish to join in the prayer. Candles may be used if the patient is not receiving oxygen. The priest, deacon, or lay minister will usually appreciate any information pertaining to the patient's ability to swallow. Any other information the nurse believes may help the priest or deacon respond to the patient with more care and effectiveness would be appreciated.

Catholic laypersons of either sex may visit hospitalized or homebound elderly or sick persons. Although they may not administer the Sacrament of the Sick or the Sacrament of Reconciliation, they may bring Holy Communion (the Eucharist).

TITLE OF RELIGIOUS REPRESENTATIVE

The titles of religious representatives include Father (priest), Mr. or Deacon (deacon), Sister (Catholic woman who has taken religious vows), and Brother (Catholic man who has taken religious vows).

ENVIRONMENT DURING VISIT BY RELIGIOUS REPRESENTATIVE

Privacy is most conducive to prayer and to the administration of the sacraments. In emergencies, such as cardiac or respiratory arrest, medical personnel will need to be present. The priest will use an abbreviated form of the rite and will not interfere with the activities of the health care team.

CHURCH ORGANIZATIONS TO ASSIST THE SICK

Most major cities have outreach programs for the sick, handicapped, and elderly. More serious needs are usually handled by Catholic Charities and other agencies in the community or on the local parish level. Organizations such as the St. Vincent DePaul Society may provide material support for the poor and needy as well as some counseling services, depending on the location. In the United States, the Catholic Church owns and operates hospitals, extended care facilities, orphanages, maternity homes, hospices, and other health care facilities. Although the majority of tertiary care facilities in Canada are publicly owned, many such institutions are strongly influenced by the leadership of the Catholic Church and its members. It is usually best to consult the pastor or chaplain in specific cases for local resources.

Practices Related to Death and Dying

PROLONGATION OF LIFE (RIGHT TO DIE)

Members are obligated to take ordinary means of preserving life (e.g., intravenous medication) but are not obligated to take extraordinary means. What constitutes extraordinary means may vary with biomedical and technologic advances and with the availability of these advances to the average citizen. Other factors that must be considered include the degree of pain associated with the procedure, the potential outcome, the condition of the patient, economic factors, and the patient's or family's preferences.

EUTHANASIA

Direct action to end the life of patients is not permitted. Extraordinary means may be withheld, allowing the patient to die of natural causes.

AUTOPSY AND DONATION OF BODY

Autopsy and donation of body are permissible as long as the corpse is shown proper respect and there is sufficient reason for doing the autopsy. The principle of totality suggests that this is justifiable, contributing to the betterment of the person who does the giving.

DISPOSAL OF BODY AND BURIAL

Ordinarily, bodies are buried. Cremation is acceptable in certain circumstances, such as to avoid spreading a contagious disease. Because life is considered sacred, the body should be treated with respect. Any disposal of the body should be done in a respectful and honorable way.

Christian Science (Church of Christ, Scientist)

Christian Science accepts physical and moral healing as a natural part of the Christian experience. Members believe that God acts through universal, immutable, spiritual law. They hold that genuine spiritual or Christian healing through prayer differs radically from the use of suggestion, willpower, and all forms of psychotherapy, which are based on the use of the human mind as a curative agent. In emphasizing the practical importance of a fuller understanding of Jesus' works and teachings, Christian Science believes healing to be a natural result of drawing closer to God in one's thinking and living. The church does not keep membership data; there are 3,000 congregations worldwide.

General Beliefs and Religious Practices

Holy Days

Besides the usual weekly day of worship (Sunday), other traditional Christian holidays are observed on an individual basis. Worldwide, Wednesday evenings are observed as times for members to gather for testimony meetings.

Sacraments

Although sacraments in a strictly spiritual sense have deep meaning for Christian Scientists, there are no outward observances or ceremonies. Baptism and Holy Communion are not outward observances but deeply meaningful inner experiences. Baptism is the daily purification and spiritualization of thought, and communion is finding one's conscious unity with God through prayer (Christian Science Publishing Society, 1994).

Social Activities (Dating, Dancing) and Substance Use

Members are encouraged to be honest, truthful, and moral in their behavior. Although every effort is made to preserve marriages, divorce is recognized. The Christian Science Sunday School teaches young people how to make their religion practical in daily life as related to school studies, social life, sports, and family relationships. Members abstain from alcohol and tobacco; some abstain from tea and coffee.

Health Care Practices

Viewed as a by-product of drawing closer to God, healing is considered proof of God's care and one element in the full salvation at which Christianity aims. Christian Science teaches that faith must rest not on blind belief but on an understanding of the present perfection of God's spiritual creation. This is one of the crucial differences between Christian Science and **faith healing** (Christian Science Publishing Society, 1994).

The practice of Christian Science healing starts from the biblical basis that God created the universe and human beings "and made them perfect." Christian Science holds that human imperfection, including physical illness and sin, reflects a fundamental misunderstanding of creation and is therefore subject to healing through prayer and spiritual regeneration.

An individual who is seeking healing may turn to Christian Science practitioners, members of the denomination who devote their full time to the healing ministry in the broadest sense. In cases requiring continued care, nurses grounded in the Christian Science faith provide care in facilities accredited by the mother church, the First Church of Christ, Scientist, in Boston, Massachusetts. Individuals may also receive such care in their own homes. Christian Science nurses are trained to perform the practical duties a patient may need while also providing an atmosphere of warmth and love that supports the healing process. No medication is given, and physical application is limited to the normal measures associated with hygiene. *The Christian Science Journal*, a monthly publication, contains a directory of qualified Christian Science practitioners and nurses throughout the world.

Before they can be recognized and advertised in *The Christian Science Journal*, practitioners must have instruction from an authorized teacher of Christian Science and provide substantial evidence of their experience in healing. There are some 4,000 Christian Science practitioners throughout the world. Practitioners who speak other languages may also be listed in appropriate editions of *The Herald of Christian Science*, which is published in 12 languages.

The denomination has no clergy. Practitioners are thus lay members of the Church of Christ, Scientist, and do not conduct public worship services or rituals. Their ministry is not an office within the church structure but is carried out on an individual basis with those who seek their help through prayer. Both members and nonmembers are welcome to contact practitioners by telephone, by letter, or in person for help or for information.

Christian Science practitioners are supported not by the church but by payments from their patients. Their ministry is not restricted to local congregations but extends worldwide. Many insurance companies include coverage of payments to practitioners and Christian Science nursing facilities in their policies. In spite of such superficial resemblances to the health care professions, the work of Christian Science practitioners involves a deeply religious vocation, not simply alternative health care. Practitioners do not use medical or psychologic techniques.

The term *healing* applies to the entire spectrum of human fears, grief, wants, and sin, as well as to physical ills. Practitioners are called upon to give Christian Science treatment not only in cases of physical disease and emotional disturbance but also in family and financial difficulties, business problems, questions of employment, schooling problems, theological confusion, and so forth. The purpose of prayer, or Christian Science treatment, is to deal with these interrelated and complex problems of establishing God's law of harmony in every aspect of life. When healings are accomplished through perception and living of spiritual truth, they are effective and permanent. Physical healing is often the manifestation of a moral and spiritual change (Christian Science Publishing Society, 1978, 1994).

Ordinarily, a Christian Science practitioner and a physician are not employed in the same case, because the two approaches to healing differ so radically. During childbirth, however, an obstetrician or qualified midwife is involved. Because bone setting may be accomplished without medication, a physician is also employed for repair of fractures if the patient requests this medical intervention. In cases of contagious or infectious disease, Christian Scientists observe the legal requirements for reporting and quarantining affected individuals. The denomination recognizes public health concerns and has a long history of responsible cooperation with public health officials.

Christian Scientists are not arbitrarily opposed to doctors. They are always free to make their own decisions regarding treatment in any given situation. They generally choose to rely on spiritual healing because they have seen its effectiveness in the experience of their own families and fellow church members—experience that goes back more than 100 years and in many families for three or four generations. Where medical treatment for minor children is required by law, Christian Scientists strictly adhere to the requirement. At the same time, they maintain that their substantial healing record needs to be seriously considered in determining the rights of Christian Scientists to rely on spiritual healing for themselves and their children. They do not ignore or neglect disease, but they seek to heal it by the means they believe to be most efficacious.

Medical and Surgical Procedures

Christian Scientists ordinarily do not use medications. Immunizations and vaccines are acceptable only when required by law. Ordinarily, members do not use blood or blood components. A Christian Scientist who has lost a limb might seek to have it replaced with a prosthesis. Christian Scientists are unlikely to seek transplants and are unlikely to act as donors. Christian Scientists do not normally seek biopsies or any sort of physical examination. Circumcision is considered an individual matter.

Practices Related to Reproduction

Matters of family planning (i.e., birth control) are left to individual judgment. Because abortion involves medication and surgical intervention, it is normally considered incompatible with Christian Science. Artificial insemination is unusual among Christian Scientists, and they are opposed to programs in the field of eugenics and genetics.

Religious Support System for the Sick

As discussed previously, Christian Scientists have their own nurses and practitioners. No special religious titles are used. Although each branch church elects two Readers for Sunday and Wednesday services, Christian Scientists are a church of laymen and laywomen. Organizations to assist the sick include Benevolent Homes, staffed by Christian Science nurses, and visiting home nurse services.

Practices Related to Death and Dying

A Christian Science family is unlikely to seek medical means to prolong life indefinitely. Family members pray earnestly for the recovery of a person as long as the person remains alive.

Euthanasia is contrary to the teachings of Christian Science. Most Christian Scientists believe that they can make their particular contribution to the health of society and of their loved ones in ways other than donation of the body. Disposal of the body is left to the individual family to decide. The individual family decides the form of burial and burial service.

Addendum

A wide variety of books and journals are published by the Christian Science Publishing Society in Boston, Massachusetts. Most major cities have Christian Science Reading Rooms, which carry these publications and which are staffed by church members, who are available to provide additional information.

The Church of Jesus Christ of Latter-Day Saints (Mormonism)

The Church of Jesus Christ of Latter-Day Saints, commonly known as **Mormonism**, is a Christian religion established in the United States in the early 1800s. North American membership in 2006 was approximately 6 million, and the worldwide membership was approximately 12 million.

General Beliefs and Religious Practices

Holy Days/Special Days

Sunday is the day observed as the Sabbath in the United States. In other parts of the world the Sabbath may be observed on a different day; in Israel, for example, members observe the Sabbath on Saturday.

Sacraments

Sacraments are commonly called **ordinances**.

ORDINANCES OF SALVATION

1. Baptism at the age of accountability (8 years or after); never performed in infancy or at death; always by immersion
2. Confirmation at the time of baptism to receive the gift of the Holy Ghost
3. Partaking of the sacrament of the Lord's Supper at weekly Sunday sacrament meetings
4. Endowments*
5. Celestial Marriage*
6. Vicarious ordinances*

*These ordinances occur in temples. Temples are sacred places of worship that are accessible only to observant Mormons, who are "worthy" to enter them as seemed by their local religious leaders.

Ordinances of Comfort, Consolation, and Encouragement

1. Blessing of babies
2. Blessing of the sick
3. Consecration of oil for use in blessing of the sick
4. Patriarchal blessings
5. Dedication of graves

After being deemed worthy to go to a temple, a member of the Church of Jesus Christ of Latter-Day Saints will wear a special type of underclothing, called a **garment**. In a health care setting, the garment may be removed to facilitate care. As soon as the individual is well, he or she is likely to want to wear the garment again. An elderly person may not wish to part with the garment in the hospital. The garment has special significance to the person, symbolizing covenants or promises the person has made to God.

Diet

Members of this church have a strict dietary code called the **Word of Wisdom.** This code prohibits all alcoholic beverages (including beer and wine), hot drinks (i.e., tea and coffee, although not herbal tea), tobacco in any form, and any illegal or recreational drugs.

Fasting to a member means no food or drink (including water), usually for 24 hours. Fasting is required once a month on the designated fast Sunday. Pregnant women, the very young, the very old, and the ill are not required to fast. The purpose of fasting is to bring oneself closer to God by controlling physical needs. The person is expected to donate the price of what has not been eaten to the church to be used to care for the poor.

Social Activities (Dating, Dancing)

The Church of Jesus Christ of Latter Day Saints has a wide variety of activities for its youth and encourages group activities until young people are at least 16. Young men are highly encouraged to perform missions for the church for 2 years at their own expense, beginning at the age of 19 years. Women may go on missions when they are

21, but marriage is more strongly emphasized for them.

Substance Use

Alcohol, caffeinated beverages (such as tea, coffee, and soda), and tobacco are forbidden. In recent years, "recreational drugs" and nonmedically indicated sedatives and narcotics have also been considered forbidden substances.

Health Care Practices

The members of the Church of Jesus Christ of Latter-Day Saints believe that the power of God can be exercised on their behalf to bring about healing at a time of illness. The ritual of blessing the sick consists of one member (Elder) of the priesthood (male) anointing the ill person with oil and a second Elder "sealing the anointing with a prayer and a blessing." Commonly, both Elders place their hands on the individual's head. Faith in Jesus Christ and in the power of the priesthood to heal, requisite to the healing use of priesthood, does not preclude medical intervention but is seen as an adjunct to it. Mormons believe that medical intervention is one of God's ways of using humans in the healing process.

Medical and Surgical Procedures

There is no restriction on the use of medications or vaccines. It is not uncommon to find many members using herbal folk remedies, and it is wise to explore in detail what an individual may already have done or taken. There is no restriction on the use of blood or blood components.

Surgical intervention is a matter of individual decision in cases of amputations, transplants, and organ donations (of both donor and recipient). Biopsies and resultant surgical procedures are also a matter of individual choice. The circumcision of infants is viewed as a medical health promotion measure and is not a religious ritual.

Practices Related to Reproduction

Birth Control

According to church doctrine, one of the major purposes of life is procreation; therefore, any form of prevention of the birth of children is contrary to church teachings. Exceptions to this policy include ill health of the mother or father and genetic defects that could be passed on to offspring.

AMNIOCENTESIS

Amniocentesis is a matter of individual choice. However, even if the fetus is found to be deformed, abortion is not an option unless the mother's life is in danger.

ABORTION

Abortion is forbidden in all cases except when the mother's life is in danger. Even in these circumstances, abortion is looked upon favorably only if the local priesthood authorities, after fasting and prayer, receive divine confirmation that the abortion is acceptable.

In the event of pregnancy resulting from rape, the church position is that the child should be born and put up for adoption if necessary, rather than be aborted. The final decision rests with the mother. No official church sanction is used if she chooses to abort the child. Abortion on demand is strictly forbidden.

STERILITY/FERTILITY TESTING AND ARTIFICIAL INSEMINATION

Because bearing children is so important, all measures that can be taken to promote having children are acceptable. Artificial insemination is acceptable if the semen is from the husband.

RELIGIOUS OBJECTS

Copies of scriptures are often found at the bedside of members of this church. Reading these scriptures often brings comfort during times of illness. Scriptures sacred to members of the Church of Jesus Christ of Latter-Day Saints include the Bible (Old and New Testament), the Book of Mormon, Doctrine and Covenants, and Pearl of Great Price.

Religious Support System for the Sick

VISITORS

The Church of Jesus Christ of Latter-Day Saints has a highly organized network, and many church representatives are likely to visit a hospitalized member, including the bishop and two counselors (leaders of the local congregation), home teachers (two men assigned to visit the family each month), and visiting teachers (two women assigned to visit the female head of household each month). Friends within the local congregation can also be expected to visit.

TITLE OF RELIGIOUS REPRESENTATIVE

Various titles are used for members of this church's hierarchy. The term *Elder* is generally acceptable regardless of a man's position, and the term *Sister* is acceptable for women.

ENVIRONMENT NEEDED FOR HEALTH-RELATED RITUALS

To perform a blessing of the sick, the Elders performing the blessing need privacy and, if possible, quiet. They generally bring a vial of consecrated oil with which to anoint the person. If they plan to perform a Sacrament of the Lord's Supper, they usually bring what they need with them. Bread and water are used for this ordinance.

CHURCH ORGANIZATIONS TO ASSIST THE SICK

The Relief Society is the organization for helping members. It is organized by the women of the church, who work closely with priesthood leaders to determine the general needs of members, including use of the church-run welfare organization. Church members who are in need may receive local help, such as child care when parents are ill or hospitalized and money for medical expenses.

Practices Related to Death and Dying

Whenever possible, medical science and faith healing are used to reverse conditions that threaten life. When death is inevitable, the effort is to promote a peaceful and dignified death. Members of this church firmly believe that life continues beyond death and that the dead are reunited with loved ones; therefore, the belief is that death is another step in eternal progression (Green, 1992a, 1992b).

Euthanasia is not acceptable because members hold the belief that life and death are in the hands of God, and humans must not interfere in any way. Autopsy is permitted with the consent of the next of kin and within local laws. Organ donation is permitted; it is an individual decision. Cremation is discouraged but not forbidden; burial is customary. A local priesthood member dedicates the graves.

Hinduism

The **Hindu** religion may be the oldest religion in the world. There are more than 1.4 billion Hindus worldwide, with a North American following of approximately 1.3 million members.

General Beliefs and Religious Practices

No common creed or doctrine binds Hindus together. There is complete freedom of belief. One may be monotheistic, polytheistic, or atheistic; however the basis of Hindu belief is the unity of everything. The major distinguishing characteristic is the social caste system.

The religion of Hinduism is founded on sacred, written scripture called the **Vedas**. **Brahman** is the principle and source of the universe and the center from which all things proceed and to which all things return. **Reincarnation** is a central belief in Hinduism. The law of **karma** determines life. According to karma, rebirth is dependent on moral behavior in a previous stage of existence. Life on earth is transient and a burden. The goal of existence is liberation from the cycle of rebirth and redeath and entrance into what in Buddhism is called nirvana (a state of extinction of passion).

The practice of Hinduism consists of roles and ceremonies performed within the framework of the **caste system**. These rituals focus on the main socioreligious events of birth, marriage, and death. Hindu temples are dwelling places for deities to which people bring offerings. There are numerous places for religious pilgrimage.

Holy Days (based on a lunar calendar)
1. Purnima (day of full moon)
2. Janamastami (birthday of Lord Krishna)
3. Ramnavmi (birthday of Rama)
4. Shivratri (birth of Lord **Shiva**)
5. Navaratri (nine holy days occurring twice a year; in about April and October)
6. Dussehra
7. Diwali
8. Holi

Diet, Social Activities (Dating, Dancing), and Substance Use

The eating of meat is forbidden because it involves harming a living creature. Social activities are strictly limited by the caste system. Substance use is not restricted.

Health Care Practices

Some Hindus believe in faith healing; others believe illness is God's way of punishing people for their sins.

Medical and Surgical Procedures

The use of medications, blood, and blood components is acceptable. Persons who lose a limb are not outcasts from society. Loss of a limb is considered to be caused by "sins of a previous life." Organ transplantations are acceptable for both donors and recipients.

Practices Related to Reproduction

All types of birth control are acceptable. Amniocentesis is acceptable, although not often available. No Hindu policy exists on abortion, either therapeutic or on demand. Artificial insemination is not restricted, but it is not often practiced because of lack of availability.

Noting the exact time of a baby's birth is very important because it is used to determine the baby's horoscope. Males are not circumcised. Breast-feeding is expected. The infant is traditionally given a name on the 10th day following the birth, although in American hospitals the child is sometimes named at birth.

Religious Objects

A small picture of a deity may be found at the bedside. Prayer is often accompanied by the use of "mala beads" (prayer beads) and a "mantram" (a sound representing an aspect of the divine). Facing North or East during prayer is preferable but not required (University of Virginia Health System, 2006b).

Religious Support System for the Sick

Religious representatives use the title of priest. Church organizations to assist the sick do not exist; family and friends within the caste provide help.

Practices Related to Death and Dying

No religious customs or restrictions exist related to the prolongation of life. Life is seen as a perpetual cycle, and death is considered as just one more step toward nirvana. Euthanasia is not practiced. Autopsy is acceptable. The donation of body or parts is also acceptable.

Cremation is the most common form of body disposal. Ashes are collected and disposed of in holy rivers. The fetus or newborn is sometimes buried.

Islam

Islam is a monotheistic religion founded between 610 and 632 AD by the prophet Muhammad. Derived from an Arabic word meaning "submission," Islam literally translated means "submission to the will of God." A follower of Islam is called **Moslem** or **Muslim**, which means "one who submits." The current North American membership is approximately 6–7 million, and the worldwide membership ranges between 2–3 billion (Nimer, 2002).

Muhammad, revered as the prophet of **Allah** (God), is seen as succeeding and completing both Judaism and Christianity. Good deeds will be rewarded at the last Judgment, whereas evil deeds will be punished in hell.

General Beliefs and Religious Practices

Pillars of Faith

Islam has five essential practices, or **Pillars of Faith**. These are (1) the profession of faith (Sha-

hada), which requires bearing witness to one true God and acknowledging Muhammad as his messenger; (2) ritual prayer five times daily at dawn, noon, afternoon, sunset, and night, facing Mecca, Saudi Arabia, Islam's holiest city (salat); (3) almsgiving (zakat) to the needy, reflecting the Koran's admonition to share what one has with those less fortunate, including widows, orphans, homeless persons, and the poor; (4) fasting from dawn until sunset throughout Ramadan, during the ninth month of the Islamic lunar calendar; and (5) making a pilgrimage to Mecca at least once during one's lifetime (Hajj).

Sources of Faith

The sources of the Islamic faith are the **Qur'an (Koran)**, which is regarded as the uncreated and eternal Word of God, and **Hadith** (tradition), regarded as sayings and deeds of the prophet Muhammad. All Muslims recognize the existence of the Sharia and the five categories into which it divides human conduct: required, encouraged, permissible, discouraged, and prohibited.

Sects of Islam

Various sects of Islam have developed. When Muhammad died, a dispute arose over the leadership of the Muslim community. One faction, the *Sunni*, derived from the Arabic word for "tradition," felt that the caliph, or successor of Muhammad, should be chosen as Arab chiefs customarily are: by election. Therefore, they supported the succession of the first four (the "rightly guided") caliphs who had been Muhammad's companions. The other group maintained that Muhammad chose his cousin and son-in-law, Ali, as his spiritual and secular heir and that succession should be through his bloodline. In 680 AD, one of Ali's sons, Hussein, led a band of rebels against the ruling caliph. In the course of the battle Hussein was killed, and with his death began the *Shi'a*, sometimes called the *Shi'ite* movement, whose name comes from the word meaning "partisans of Ali." The Shi'a and the Sunni are the two major branches of Muslims; the Sunni constitute about 85% of the total. The

Sunni are found in Lebanon, the West Bank, Jordan, and throughout Africa, whereas the Shi'a are in Iran, Iraq, Yemen, Afghanistan, and Pakistan. The Shi'a and the Sunni also have different rituals, practices, and structural and political orientations.

Holidays, Special Observances, and Sacraments

Days of observance in Islam are not "holy" days but days of celebration or observance. The Muslims follow a lunar calendar, so the days of observance change yearly.

Each Muslim observance has its own significance. They are listed here in the same order in which they occur in the Muslim lunar calendar, and their standard Arabic names are used. However, the Arabic spellings for the names of the holidays may vary, or local names may be used.

Muharram 1 Rasal-Sana (or New Year): The first day of the first month, celebrated much the same as the first day of the year is celebrated throughout the world.

Muharram 10 Ashura (the 10th of the first month): A religious holiday through which pious Muslims may fast from dawn to sunset. For Shi'ite Muslims, this is a special day of sorrow, commemorating the assassination of the prophet's grandson, Hussein.

Rabi'i 12 Maulid al-Nabi: The birthday of the prophet Muhammad. In some regions this holiday goes on for many days; it is a time of festivities and exchanging of gifts.

Rajab 27 Lailat al-Isra wa al Miraj (literally, "The Night of the Journey and Ascent"): Commemorates Muhammad's night journey from Mecca to the al-Aqsa mosque in Jerusalem and his ascent to heaven and return on the same night.

Sh'ban 14: This is the 14th night of the 8th month of Sh'ban. It is widely celebrated by pious Muslims and is sometimes called the Night of Repentance. It is treated in many parts of the Muslim world as a New Year's celebration.

Ramadan (the 9th month of the Muslim year): This entire month is devoted to meditation and spiritual purification through self-discipline. It is a period of abstinence from eating, drinking, smoking, and sexual relations. The fast is an obligation practiced by Muslims throughout the world unless they are old, infirm, traveling, or pregnant. The fast is from sunup to sundown, at which time a meal (*Iftar*) is taken.

Ramadan 27 Lailat al-Qadir (next to the last night of the fasting month): This is simply called the Night of Power and Greatness, and it is by custom a very special holy time. It commemorates the time when revelation was first given to Muhammad.

Shawwal 1 "Id ad-Fitr": This is called the Lesser Feast because it begins immediately after the month-long Ramadan feast. It is perhaps Islam's most joyous festival, marking as it does the end of the month of abstinence and the cleansing of the believer. It usually lasts for 2 or 3 days. Families and friends visit one another's homes, new clothes and presents are exchanged, and sweet pastries are a favorite treat.

Dhu al-Hijjah 1–10: Muslims, if they are able, are obliged to undertake a pilgrimage to Mecca at least once in their lifetime. This journey, called the Hajj, is performed during the last month of the Muslim calendar, Dhu al-Hijjah.

Dhu al-Hijjah 10: All Muslims, whether they are on the pilgrimage or at home, participate in the feast of the sacrifice, Id al-Adha, which marks the end of the Hajj on the 10th of Dhu al-Hijjah. The feast is the Feast of the Sacrifice, called the Greater Feast, and is observed by the slaughtering of animals and distribution of the meat. In some places this is done individually. The meat is shared equally among the family and the poor. Sometimes the slaughtering takes place in public areas, and the meat is then distributed.

Sacraments are not observed.

Diet and Substance Use

Eating pork and drinking alcoholic or other intoxicating beverages are strictly prohibited. In all cases, moderation in one's life is expected. Some Muslims consume meat that has been ritually slaughtered by the process called **halal**, which means "the lawful or that which is permitted by Allah."

Fasting during the month of Ramadan is one of the pillars of Islam. Children (boys: 7 years old, girls: 9 years old) and adults are required to fast. Pregnant women, nursing mothers, the elderly, and anyone whose physical condition is so fragile that a physician recommends not fasting are exempt from fasting but are expected to fast later in the year or to feed a poor person to make up for the unfasted Ramadan days.

Religious Objects

A prayer rug and the Koran are often present with a Muslim patient and should not be handled or touched by anyone who is ritually unclean. Nothing should be placed on top of these items. Some Muslims may wear an amulet, which is a black string or a silver or gold chain, on which sections of the Koran are attached. If worn by the patient it should not be removed and should remain dry (University of Virginia Health System, 2006c).

Health Care Practices

Muslim women typically prefer to have female physicians and health care providers, while men prefer male physicians and health care providers. Faith healing is not acceptable unless the psychological health and morale of the patient are deteriorating. At that time, faith healing may be used to supplement the physician's efforts.

Medical and Surgical Procedures

There are no restrictions on medications. Even items normally forbidden (e.g., pork derivatives) are permitted if prescribed as medicine. The use of blood and blood components is not restricted. Amputations are not restricted. Organ transplantations are acceptable for both donor and recipient. Biopsies are acceptable. No age limit is fixed, but circumcision is practiced on boys at an early

age. For adult converts, it is not obligatory, although it is sometimes practiced.

Practices Related to Reproduction

BIRTH CONTROL

All types of birth control are generally acceptable in accordance with the law of "what is harmful to the body is prohibited." The family physician's advice on method of contraception is required. The husband and wife should agree on the method.

AMNIOCENTESIS

Amniocentesis is available in many Islamic countries. "Progressive" doctors and expectant parents use amniocentesis only to determine the status of the fetus, not the sex of the child; this is left in the hands of God.

ABORTION

No official policy on abortion, either therapeutic or on demand, exists. There is a strong religious objection to abortion, which is based on Muhammad's condemnation of the ancient Arabian practice of burying unwanted newborn girls alive.

ARTIFICIAL INSEMINATION, EUGENICS, AND GENETICS

Artificial insemination is permitted only if from the husband to his own wife. No official policy exists on practices in the fields of eugenics and genetics. Different Islamic schools of thought accept differing opinions.

Religious Support System for the Sick

In Islam, care of the physical body is not regarded highly. In many wealthy, oil-rich Middle Eastern nations, expatriates are hired to staff hospitals and provide for health care. Even in the United States, care of the sick does not resemble the Catholic corporal work of mercy or the Jewish mitzvah. Islamic clerics, called imams, may provide guidance that could be helpful for emotional and psychological disorders. Formal, organized support systems to assist the sick do not exist; family and friends provide emotional and financial support.

Practices Related to Death and Dying

The right to die is not recognized in Islam. Any attempt to shorten one's life or terminate it (suicide or otherwise) is prohibited. Euthanasia is thus not acceptable. Autopsy is permitted only for medical and legal purposes. The donation of body parts or body is acceptable, without restrictions.

Burial of the dead, including fetuses, is compulsory. It is important in Islam to follow prescribed burial procedures. Under conditions that cause fragmentation of the body, sections of the burial ritual may be omitted. The burial procedure consists of five steps:

1. Ghasl El Mayyet: Rinsing and washing of the dead body according to Muslim tradition. Muslim women cleanse a woman's body; Muslim men cleanse a man's body.
2. Muslin: After being washed three times, the body is wrapped in three pieces of clean white cloth. The Muslim word for "coffin" is the same as that for "muslin."
3. Salat El Mayyet: Special prayers for the dead are required.
4. The body should be processed and buried as soon as possible. The body should always be buried so that the head faces toward Mecca.
5. Burial of a fetus: Before a gestational age of 130 days, a fetus is treated like any other discarded tissue. After 130 days, the fetus is considered a fully developed human being and must be treated as such.

Jehovah's Witnesses

North American membership of the **Jehovah's Witnesses** is 1,029,902; worldwide membership is approximately 6,035,564.

General Beliefs and Religious Practices

Many North Americans have at one time or another encountered ministers of the **Watch Tower Bible and Tract Society**, known as Jehovah's Witnesses. The name Jehovah's Witnesses (the name that members prefer) is derived from the Hebrew name for God (**Jehovah**) according to the King James Bible. Thus, Jehovah's Witnesses is a descriptive name, indicating that members profess to bear witness concerning Jehovah, his Godship, and his purposes. Every Bible student devotes approximately 10 hours or more each month to proselytizing activities.

Holy Days and Sacraments

Although Witnesses do not celebrate Christmas, Easter, or other traditional Christian holy days, a special observance of the Lord's Supper is held. Witnesses and others may attend this important meeting, but only those numbered among the 144,000 chosen members (Revelation 7:4) may partake of the bread and wine as a symbol of the death of Christ and the dedication to God. This memorial of Christ's death should take place on the day corresponding to Nisa 14 of the Jewish calendar, which occurs sometime in March or April. These elite members will be raised with spiritual bodies (without flesh, bones, or blood) and will assist Christ in ruling the universe. Others who benefit from Christ's ransom will be resurrected with healthy, perfected physical bodies (bodies of flesh, bones, and blood) and will inhabit this earth after the world has been restored to a paradisiacal state. Sacraments are not observed.

Social Activities (Dating, Dancing) and Substance Use

Youth are encouraged to socialize with members of their own religious background. Members abstain from the use of tobacco and hold that drunkenness is a serious sin. Alcohol used in moderation, however, is acceptable.

Health Care Practices

The practice of faith healing is forbidden. However, it is believed that reading the scriptures can comfort the individual and lead to mental and spiritual healing.

Medical and Surgical Procedures

MEDICATIONS

To the extent that they are necessary, medications are acceptable.

BLOOD AND BLOOD PRODUCTS

Blood in any form and agents in which blood is an ingredient are not acceptable. Blood volume expanders are acceptable if they are not derivatives of blood. Mechanical devices for circulating the blood are acceptable as long as they are not primed with blood initially. In some cases, children have been made wards of the court so they could receive blood when a medical condition mandating blood transfusion was life threatening. This can threaten the standing of the child in the community and must be approached with great care.

The determination of Jehovah's Witnesses to abstain from blood is based on scriptural references and precedents in the history of Christianity. Courts of justice have often upheld the principle that each individual has a right to bodily integrity, yet some physicians and hospital administrators have turned to the courts for legal authorization to force blood to be used as a medical treatment for an individual whose religious convictions prohibit the use of blood (Sugarman, Churchill, Moore, & Waugh, 1991).

SURGICAL PROCEDURES

Although surgical procedures are not in and of themselves opposed, the administration of blood during surgery is strictly prohibited (Smith, 1986). There is no church rule pertaining to the loss of limbs or the amputation of body parts. If they are a violation of the principle of bodily mutilation, transplants are forbidden. However, this is usually an individual decision. Blood may not be used in this or any surgical procedure. Biopsies are acceptable. Circumcision is an individual decision.

Practices Related to Reproduction

Sterilization is prohibited because it is viewed as a form of bodily mutilation. Other forms of birth control are left to the individual. Amniocentesis is acceptable. Both therapeutic and on-demand abortions are forbidden. Sterility testing is an individual decision. Artificial insemination is forbidden both for donors and for recipients. Jehovah's Witnesses do not condone any activities in the areas of eugenics and genetics; they are considered to interfere with nature and therefore are unacceptable.

Religious Support System for the Sick

Individual members of congregation, including elders, visit the ill. Visitors pray with the sick person and read scriptures. Because members do not smoke, it is preferred that patients be placed in rooms where no smoking is allowed. If a man, the religious representative is referred to as "Mr." or "Elder"; if the religious representative is female, she is called "Ms." or "Mrs." Religious titles are not generally used. Individuals and members of the congregation look after the needs of the sick.

Practices Related to Death and Dying

The right to die or the use of extraordinary methods to prolong life is a matter of individual conscience. Euthanasia is forbidden. An autopsy is acceptable only if it is required by law. No parts are to be removed from the body. The human spirit and the body are never separated. The donation of a body is forbidden. Disposal of the body is a matter of individual preference. Burial practices are determined by local custom. Cremation is permitted if the individual chooses it.

Addendum

Jehovah's Witnesses are opposed to saluting the flag, serving in the armed forces, voting in civil elections, and holding public office. These prohibitions are related to belief in a theocracy that is in harmony with their understanding of New Testament Christianity. Governed by a body of individuals, members united with the theocracy are to dissociate themselves from all activities of the political state and give full allegiance to "Jehovah's organization." This practice is related to the belief that Jesus Christ is King and Priest and that there is no need to hold citizenship in more than one kingdom. Members also refrain from gambling.

A pamphlet entitled *Jehovah's Witnesses and the Question of Blood* may be obtained free of charge from the World Headquarters for the Jehovah's Witnesses at 117 Adams Street, Brooklyn, NY, 11201.

Judaism

Judaism is an Old Testament religion that dates back to the time of the prophet Abraham. Worldwide, there are approximately 18 million Jews. Membership includes approximately 7 million members in the United States and 371,000 members in Canada.

General Beliefs and Religious Practices

Judaism is a monotheistic religion. Jewish life historically has been based on interpretation of the laws of God as contained in the **Torah** and explained in the **Talmud** and in oral tradition. Ancient Jewish law prescribed most of the daily actions of the people. Diet, clothing, activities, occupation, and ceremonial activities throughout the life cycle were all part of Jewish daily life.

Today there are at least three schools of theological thought and social practice in Judaism. The three main divisions include Orthodox, Conservative, and Reform. There is also a fundamentalist sect, called Hasidism. Hasidic Jews cluster in metropolitan areas and live and work only within their Jewish communities.

Any person born of a Jewish mother or anyone converted to Judaism is considered a Jew. All Jews are united by the core theme of Judaism, which is expressed in the **Shema**, a prayer that professes a single God.

Holy Days

The Sabbath is the holiest of all holy days. The Sabbath begins each Friday, 18 minutes before sunset and ends on Saturday, 42 minutes after sunset, or when three stars can be seen in the sky with the naked eye.

Other Holy Days are as follows:

1. Rosh Hashanah (Jewish New Year)
2. Yom Kippur (Day of Atonement, a fast day)
3. Sukkot (Feast of Tabernacles)
4. Shmini Atzeret (8th Day of Assembly)
5. Simchat Torah
6. Chanukah (Festival of Lights, or Rededication of the Temple in Jerusalem)
7. Asara B'Tevet (Fast of the 10th of Tevet)*
8. Fast of Esther
9. Purim
10. Passover
11. Shavuot (Festival of the Giving of the Torah)
12. Fast of the 17th of Tammuz
13. Fast of the 9th of Av (Commemoration of the Destruction of the Temple)

Holy days are very special to practicing Jews. If a condition is not life threatening, medical and surgical procedures should not be performed on the Sabbath or on holy days. Preservation of life is of greatest priority and is the major criterion for determining activity on holy days and the Sabbath. If a Jewish patient is hesitant to receive urgent and necessary treatment because of religious restrictions, a rabbi should be consulted.

Sacraments/Rituals

Brit milah, the covenant of circumcision, is performed on all Jewish male children on the 8th day after birth (Figure 14–6). Although circumcision is a surgical procedure, for Jews it is a fundamental religious obligation. Circumcision is usually performed by a **mohel**, a pious Jew with special training, or by the child's father. Because the severing of the foreskin constitutes the essence of the ritual, the practice of having a non-Jewish or nonobservant physician perform the circumcision in the presence of a rabbi or other person who pronounces the blessing is not acceptable according to Jewish law. Circumcision

---

*Not observed by liberal or Reform Jews.

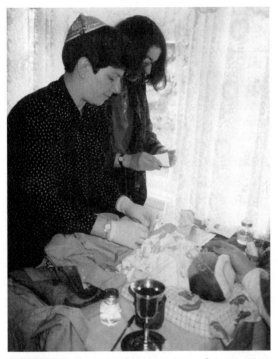

FIGURE 14-6. The *brit milah*, or covenant of circumcision, is being performed in the home of this 8-day-old Jewish infant by two mohels, one of whom is a Jewish pediatrician.

may be delayed if medically contraindicated. For example, if the child has hypospadias, a congenital defect of the urethral wall for which surgical repair usually occurs at age 3 years and requires the use of the foreskin in reconstructive plastic surgery, the circumcision may be delayed. At times, Jewish law requires postponement of circumcision, though contemporary medical science recognizes no potential threat to the health of the baby (e.g., for physiologic jaundice). As soon as the jaundice disappears, the brit milah may be performed. In Reform and Conservative traditions, girls mark the 8th day of life with a dedication ceremony in which prayers and blessings are invoked on her behalf.

The bar mitzvah (meaning "son of the commandment") is a confirmation ceremony for boys at age 13 that has been preceded by extensive religious study, including mastery of key Torah passages in Hebrew. In Reform and Conservative traditions, the bas (or bat) mitzvah (meaning "daughter of the commandment") is the equivalent ceremony for girls.

Diet

The dietary laws of Judaism are very strict; the degree to which they are observed varies according to the individual. Strictly observant Jews never eat pork, never eat predatory fowl, and never mix milk dishes and meat dishes. Only fish with fins and scales are permissible; shellfish and other water creatures are prohibited.

The word **kosher** comes from the Hebrew word *kashrut* that means "proper" All animals must be ritually slaughtered to be kosher. This means that the animal is to be killed by a specially qualified person, quickly, with the least possible pain. More colloquially, many people think that "kosher" refers to a type of food. If a patient asks for kosher food, it is important to determine what he or she means.

Religious Objects

On the Sabbath and on holidays it is customary to light two candles in candleholders. Many Jewish men and some women wear *kipot* or *yarmulkes* (small head coverings) and *tallith* prayer shawls when praying. A *siddur* or prayer book may also be present (University of Virginia Health System, 2006d).

Social Activities (Dating, Dancing)

Like all ethnic groups, Jews tend toward endogamy. Social activities that might lead to marriage outside the faith are discouraged. However, it is recognized that a significant number of individuals in Jewish society will seek partners outside of the Jewish faith. When this occurs, every effort is made to bring the non-Jewish partner into Judaism and to keep the Jewish partner a member and part of Jewish society.

Substance Use

The guideline is moderation. Wine is a part of religious observance and used as such. Drunkenness is not a sign of a good Jew. Historically, Jews well connected with their faith have had a low incidence of alcoholism.

Health Care Practices

Medical care from a physician in the case of illness is expected according to Jewish law. There are many prayers for the sick in Jewish liturgy. Such prayers and hope for recovery are encouraged.

Medical and Surgical Procedures

There are no restrictions when medications are used as part of a therapeutic process. There is a prohibition in Judaism against ingesting blood (e.g., blood sausage, raw meat). However, this does not apply to receiving blood transfusions. Beliefs and practices related to body mutilation (e.g., organ transplantation, amputations) vary widely among Jews. Individual beliefs should be explored with the client before any procedure that involves body mutilation.

Practices Related to Reproduction

BIRTH CONTROL

It is said in the Torah that Jews should be fruitful and multiply; therefore, it is a *mitzvah* (a good deed) to have at least two children. Since the Holocaust of World War II, it has been increasingly acceptable to have more children to replace those that were lost. It is permissible to practice birth control in traditional and liberal homes (Forsythe, 1991).

In the past, contraception was limited to the woman; vasectomy was prohibited. Currently, Judaism permits contraception by either partner, although Hasidic and Orthodox Jews rarely use vasectomy.

ABORTION

Although therapeutic abortion is always permitted if the health of the mother is jeopardized, traditional Judaism regards the killing of an unborn child to be a serious moral offense, whereas liberal Judaism permits it with strong moral admonitions (i.e., it is not to be used as a means of birth control). The fetus, although not imbued with the full sanctity of life, is a potential human being and is acknowledged as such.

STERILITY TESTING AND ARTIFICIAL INSEMINATION

Sterility testing is permissible when the goal is to enable the couple to have children. Artificial insemination is permitted under certain circumstances. A rabbi should be consulted in each individual case.

EUGENICS AND GENETICS

Jews have an understandable aversion to genetic engineering because of the experimentation carried on during the Nazi era. At the same time, eugenic practices are permitted under a limited range of circumstances. The Jewish belief in the sanctity of life is a guiding factor in rabbinical counseling.

Religious Support System for the Sick

VISITORS

The most likely visitors will be family and friends from the synagogue. To visit the sick is a mitzvah of service (an obligation, a responsibility, and a blessing). There are often many Jewish social service agencies to help those in need. The Jewish Federation and Jewish Community Service are two large organizations that provide services to fulfill a variety of needs.

TITLE OF RELIGIOUS REPRESENTATIVE

The formal religious representative from a synagogue is the rabbi. A visit from the rabbi may be spent talking, or the rabbi may pray with the person alone or in a *minyan*, a group of 10 adults, 13 years or older. If the patient is male and strictly observant, he may wish to have a prayer shawl (*tallith*), a cap (*kippah*), and *tefillin* (special symbols tied onto the arms and forehead). If the patient's own materials are not at the hospital, it may be necessary to ask that they be brought. Prayers are often chanted. If possible, privacy should be provided.

Practices Related to Death and Dying

PROLONGATION OF LIFE (RIGHT TO DIE)

A person has the right to die with dignity. If a physician sees that death is inevitable, no new therapeutic measures that would artificially extend life need to be initiated. It is important to know the precise time of death for the purpose of honoring the deceased after the first year has passed.

EUTHANASIA

Euthanasia is prohibited under any circumstances. It is regarded as murder. However, in the administration of palliative medications that carry the calculated risk of overdose, the amelioration of pain is paramount.

AUTOPSY

Any unjustified alteration in a corpse is considered a desecration of the dead, to be avoided in normal circumstances. When postmortem examinations are justified, they must be limited to essential organs or systems. Needle biopsy is preferred. All body parts must be returned for burial. Jewish family members may ask to consult with a rabbinical authority before signing an autopsy consent form.

DONATION OF BODY PARTS

This is a complex matter according to Jewish law. If it seems necessary, consultation with a rabbi should be encouraged (Weiss, 1988).

BURIAL

The body is ritually washed at a funeral home after death, if possible by members of the Chevra Kadisha (Ritual Burial Society). The body is then clothed in a simple white burial shroud. Embalming, a process wherein the blood of the deceased is replaced by an embalming fluid, and cosmetic treatment of the body are forbidden. Public viewing of the body is considered a humiliation of the dead. Relatives are forbidden to touch or embrace the deceased, except when involved in preparation for interment. The exact time of burial is significant for sitting shiva, the mourning period. After death in an institution, a nurse may wash the body for transport to the funeral home. Ritual washing then occurs later. Human remains, including a fetus at any stage of gestation, are to be buried as soon as possible. Cremation is not in keeping with Jewish law.

Addendum

Additional information can be obtained from Synagogue Council of America, 432 Park Avenue South, New York, NY 10016, phone: (212) 686-8670; or the Canadian Jewish Congress, 100 Sparks Street Suite 650, Ottawa, Ontario, K1P 5B7, phone: (613) 233-8703, fax: (613) 233-8748, or e-mail: canadianjewishcongress@cjc.ca

Mennonite Church

Membership in the Mennonite Church is 122,545 in the United States, 207,970 in Canada, and 1,250,000 worldwide.

Mennonites take their name from Menno Simons, an Anabaptist bishop who united a fragmented group of Anabaptists in the early 1500s. Simons had been a Catholic priest in Holland but left the church over theological differences after his brother was killed as an Anabaptist. The word "Anabaptist" comes from the doctrine that baptism to be valid must be upon confessed faith.

General Beliefs and Religious Practices

Mennonites believe that each person is responsible before God to make decisions based on his or her understanding of the Bible. For this reason, there are minimal official statements or regulations. Even when these are to be found, e.g., the Mennonite Confession of Faith, they are perceived by members as guidelines rather than proclamations to supplant individual responsibility. It should also be noted that the Mennonite faith encompasses a wide spectrum of cultural circumstances, which are more responsible for variations among individual Mennonites than is the basic theology, which is relatively uniform. It is therefore necessary to ascertain individual preferences and to work with patients on a one-to-one basis rather than stereotyping according to religious affiliation.

Holy Days and Sacraments

Mennonites observe the religious days of the traditional Christian churches. Observance places no restrictions on health-related procedures on these days. Mennonites observe Baptism and Holy Communion as official church sacraments. Patients will request sacraments as necessary. Neither sacrament is believed necessary for salvation.

Social Activities (Dating, Dancing)

No restrictions are placed on social activities.

Health Care Practices

Healing is believed to be a part of God's work in the human body through whatever means he chooses to use, whether medical science or healing that comes in answer to specific prayer. There is no religious ritual to be applied unless the patient asks for one in whatever way is personally meaningful. Sometimes anointing of oil is practiced.

Medical and Surgical Procedures

No specific guidelines or restrictions exist for the administration of medications, blood and blood components, or surgical procedures.

Practices Related to Reproduction

BIRTH CONTROL

All types of contraception are acceptable. The choice is left to the individual.

ABORTION

Therapeutic abortions are acceptable. Mennonites generally believe that on-demand abortion must be decided according to the specifics of individual cases. The church has chosen to avoid making a ruling that must be followed unquestionably. The individual must follow her own conscience and learn to live with the consequences. Some parts of the Mennonite Church have adopted statements opposing abortion on demand.

ARTIFICIAL INSEMINATION

The church does not have regulations regarding artificial insemination. The individual conscience and point of view of the patient need to be respected. Usually, artificial insemination is sought only if husband and wife are donor and recipient, respectively.

EUGENICS AND GENETICS

The church accepts scientific endeavor as a valid activity that needs to respect all of God's creation. The concerns of eugenics and genetics in its future potential have not been fully confronted. Mennonites believe that God and human beings work together in caring for and improving the world.

Practices Related to Death and Dying

The church does not believe that life must be continued at all cost. Health care professionals should decide whether to take heroic measures on the basis of the patient's individual circumstances and the emotional condition of the family. When life has lost its purpose and meaning beyond hope of meaningful recovery, most Mennonites feel that relatives should not be censured for allowing life-sustaining measures to be withheld.

Euthanasia as the termination of life by an overt act of the physician is not condoned. Autopsy and the donation of the body are acceptable, without restrictions. Procedures for disposal of body and burial follow local customs and legal requirements.

Native North American Churches

Differentiating Native North American health care practices from their religious and cultural beliefs is much more difficult than with the other religions presented in this chapter. Native North Americans represent 2 million people and more than 300 tribal units within North America. Each group has individual beliefs and practices, yet they maintain a similar nonprescriptive attitude toward health care.

There is in the United States and Canada today a specific religion called the **Native American Church** or **Peyote Religion**. Encompassing members of many tribes, its focus is on the revival of Native North American culture, beliefs, and spirituality.

When trying to support a Native American in physical or psychological crisis, the nurse needs to remember several seemingly unrelated facts. First, the non-Westernized Native North American belief about disease is not necessarily based on symptoms. Disease may be attributed to intrusive objects, soul loss, spirit intrusion, breach of taboo, or sorcery. Disease may also be attributed to natural or supernatural causes (Vogel, 1970). Second, the Native North American may embrace an organized, usually Christian, religion and still be a member of a particular Native North American tribe. Native North Americans also balance "modern theories of disease" with long-standing tribal beliefs or customs. Therefore, during illness and particularly hospitalization, Native North Americans may ask to see a priest or minister as well as a tribal "medicine man" or *curandero*. Visits from these persons will likely be spiritually supportive, although the form of the support may vary greatly.

The spiritual basis for much of Native North American belief and action is symbolized by the number four. This number, which pervades much North American Indian thought, is seen in the extended hand, which means life, unity, equality, and eternity. The clasped hand symbolizes unity, the spiritual law that binds the universe.

It is this unity on which decisions should be made. Questions about abortion, the use of drugs, giving and receiving blood, the right to life, euthanasia, and so on do not have dogmatic "yes" or "no" answers; rather, answers are based on the situation and the ultimate unity or disunity that a decision would produce.

To the Native North American, everything is cyclical. Communication is the key to learning and understanding; understanding brings peace of mind; peace of mind leads to happiness; and happiness is communicating. Other guidelines also function in groups of four (Steiger, 1975).

The four guidelines toward self-development are

1. Am I happy with what I am doing?
2. What am I doing to add to the confusion?
3. What am I doing to bring about peace and contentment?
4. How will I be remembered when I am gone, in absence and in death?

The four requirements of good health are

1. Food
2. Sleep
3. Cleanliness
4. Good thoughts

The four divisions of nature are

1. Spirit
2. Mind
3. Body
4. Life

The four divisions of goals are

1. Faith
2. Love
3. Work
4. Pleasure

The four ages of development are the

1. Learning age
2. Age of adoption
3. Age of improvement
4. Age of wisdom

The four expressions of sharing are

1. Making others feel you care
2. Expressing interest
3. Expressing friendship
4. Expressing belonging

Unity, the great spiritual law, also can be expressed in four parts:

1. Going into the silence in spirit, mind, and body
2. The union through which all spirituality flows
3. A goal toward communicating with all things in nature
4. Recognized through sense, emotions, and impressions

In concert with the belief in the interconnectedness of all things, natural remedies in the form of herbal medicine are often used. (It is interesting to note that Native North American folk medicine and herbal remedies provided the forerunners of many of today's pharmaceutical remedies.) Herbal treatments are still used today and may be requested by Native North American patients in a Western medical setting.

A nurse caring for a Native North American client should be careful to obtain a careful and complete history, including a list of whatever native remedies have been tried. The patient may not know the names of herbs used in treatment, and the tribal medicine man or woman may need to be consulted.

Respecting the concept that religion, medicine, and healing are inseparable to the Native North American, one must be sensitive to the fact that asking for the names of native medicines or descriptions of healing practices tried in an attempt to cure the person before his or her entrance into the Western medical system is not just simply obtaining a history, but also entering into the realm of what might be not only private, but also very sacred. The nurse must use care and sensitivity and show deep respect for the information received.

Protestantism

In its broadest meaning, **Protestantism** denotes the whole movement within Christianity that originated in the 16th century with Martin Luther and the Protestant Reformation. Historically and traditionally, the chief characteristics of Protestantism are the acceptance of the Bible as the only source of infallible revealed truth, the belief in the universal priesthood of believers, and the doctrine that Christians are justified in their relationship to God by faith alone, not by good works or dispensations of the church.

It is difficult to accurately categorize Protestant churches and impossible to mention them all because there are more than 30,000 denominations. Protestantism is basically non-Roman Western Christianity, and it can be divided into four major forms: Lutheran, Anglican, Reformed, and free (or independent) church (Johnson, Kurian & Barett, 2001).

Lutheranism

The oldest and second-largest Protestant religion, Lutheranism, began in 1517 with Martin Luther's split from the Roman Catholic Church. Lutherans emphasize theological doctrine and spirituality. Many North American Lutherans are of German or Scandinavian heritage.

Anglicanism

Anglicanism is represented by the established Church of England and similar churches. Unlike most other Protestant churches, they have an episcopal system of government in which each church or parish is served by a priest, who is supervised by a bishop. A bishop supervises a group of churches called a diocese. A bishop, in turn, is responsible to a council of bishops. Anglican churches allow their clergy to marry. The Methodist church was established by followers of John Wesley, an 18th-century Anglican who sought to bring reform to the Church of England. Wesley's movement spread to the United States and Canada in the 18th century.

Reformed Denominations

The Reformed denominations include Presbyterianism and are based on the teachings of John Calvin and his followers. These churches are distinguished from Lutheranism and Anglicanism, which maintain symbolic and sacramental traditions that originated before the Protestant Reformation.

Free or Independent Churches

Free or independent churches, including the Baptists, Congregationalists, Adventists, and

Churches of Christ exercise congregational government. Each local denomination is an independent autonomous unit, and there is no official doctrine.

With 27 million members, the Baptist church makes up more than 10% of the population of the United States. Black and White Baptist church denominations exist separately. The largely White Southern Baptist Convention has about 12 million members, whereas 9 million Blacks (30% of all Blacks in the United States) are members of the National Baptist Conventions.

Health Care Practices

Given the wide diversity that exists within Protestant denominations, it is beyond the scope of this text to identify health-related beliefs and practices for each group. Selected Protestant denominations (e.g., Seventh-Day Adventists, Jehovah's Witnesses) have been identified separately because they have significant health-related practices. For further information about specific Protestant churches, you are encouraged to visit www.adherents.com or the official Web pages of the various groups for a synopsis of their beliefs.

Seventh-Day Adventists

North American membership of **Seventh-Day Adventists** is approaching 1,000,000; worldwide membership now exceeds 10.65 million.

Doctrinally, Seventh-Day Adventists are heirs of the interfaith Millerite movement of the late 1840s, although the movement officially adopted the name Seventh-Day Adventist in 1863. Between 1831 and 1844, William Miller, a Baptist preacher and former army captain in the War of 1812, launched the "great second advent awakening," which eventually spread throughout most of the Christian world. At first, the work was largely confined to North America, but it quickly spread to Switzerland, Africa, Italy, Egypt, and many other nations.

General Beliefs and Religious Practices

Seventh-Day Adventists accept the Bible as their only creed and hold certain fundamental beliefs to be the teaching of the Holy Scriptures. The official statements by the General Conference of the Seventh-Day Adventists concerning the scriptures, the Trinity, creation, nature of man, the great controversy (Christ versus Satan), life, death, resurrection, and other topics may be found at www.adventist.org

Holy Days

The seventh day (Saturday) is observed as the Sabbath, from Friday at sundown to Saturday at sundown. The Sabbath is the day that God blessed and sanctified. It is a sacred day of worship and rest. Saturday worship services are held, as are weekly evening prayer meetings (usually midweek).

Sacraments/Rituals

There are three church ordinances: (1) baptism by immersion, (2) the Ordinance of Humility, and (3) the Lord's Supper or Communion. There are no rituals at the time of birth. There is no requirement for a final sacrament at death. If requested by an individual or family member, the dying person might be anointed with oil.

Diet

Seventh-Day Adventists believe that because the body is the temple of God, it is appropriate to abstain from any food or beverage that could prove harmful to the body. Because the first human diet consisted of fruits and grains, the Church encourages a vegetarian diet. Nevertheless, some members prefer to eat meat and poultry. Based on a passage in Leviticus 11:3, nonvegetarian members refrain from eating foods derived from any animal having a cloven hoof that chews its cud (e.g., meat derived from pigs, rabbits, or similar animals). Although fish with fins and scales are acceptable (e.g., salmon), shellfish are prohibited. Consumption of some birds is prohibited, but common poultry such as chicken and turkey are acceptable. Fermented beverages are prohibited. Fasting is practiced, but only when members of a specific church elect to do so. Practiced in degrees, fasting may involve abstention from food or liquids. Fasting is not encouraged if it is likely to have adverse effects on the individual.

Social Activities (Dating, Dancing) and Substance Use

Dancing is not encouraged as a form of recreation or social activity. Members are encouraged to date other members or persons holding similar beliefs and values. Members should abstain from the use of fermented beverages and tobacco products.

Health Care Practices

The church believes in divine healing and practices anointing with oil and prayer, in addition to accepting healing brought about by medical intervention. Since 1865, the church has maintained chaplains and physicians as inseparable in its institutions.

Medical and Surgical Procedures

Adventists operate one of the world's largest religiously operated health systems, including a medical school. **The Health Ministries** include 166 hospitals and sanitariums, 117 nursing homes and retirement centers, 371 clinics and dispensaries, 30 orphanages and children's homes, and 12 airplanes and medical launches. Physical medicine and rehabilitation are emphasized and recommended, along with therapeutic diets. There are no restrictions on the use of vaccines. Similarly, there are no restrictions on the use of blood and blood products, amputations, organ transplants, donation of organs, biopsies, and circumcisions.

Practices Related to Reproduction

The use of birth control is an individual decision; the church prohibits cohabitation except between husband and wife. There are no restrictions on amniocentesis. Therapeutic abortion is acceptable if the mother's life is in danger and in cases of rape and incest. On-demand abortion is unacceptable because Adventists believe in the sanctity of life. Artificial insemination between husband and wife is acceptable. Although the church views practices in the fields of eugenics and genetics as an individual decision, it upholds the principle of responsibility in dealing with children.

Religious Support System for the Sick

At the request of the sick person or the family, the pastor and elders of the church will come together to pray and anoint the sick person with oil. The religious representative is referred to as Doctor, Pastor, or Elder. There is a worldwide Seventh-Day Adventist health system, which includes hospitals and clinics.

Practices Related to Death and Dying

Although there is no official position, the church has traditionally followed the medical ethics of prolonging life and euthanasia. Autopsy and the donation of the entire body or parts are acceptable. No directives or recommendations exist regarding disposal of the body. No specific directives concerning burial exist; this is an individual decision.

Addendum

The Seventh-Day Adventist church is opposed to the use of hypnotism in the practice of medicine or under any other circumstance.

Unitarian Universalist Church

Worldwide, **Unitarian Universalist** membership is 800,000, with a North American membership of 221,760.

General Beliefs and Religious Practices

Unitarianism was officially organized in 1774 in England. This organization occurred after a long history of debate and dissension regarding the nature of God, particularly regarding the Trinitarian concept, which existed in various forms in the Catholic and Protestant religions. The Unitarian Universalist Association is the modern institutional embodiment of two separate denominations that grew out of movements and faith traditions extending back to the Christian Reformation era (14th to 16th century). Universalist convictions include the belief that all creation will ultimately be drawn back to its divine source and that no person or thing would be ultimately and forever excluded. The Unitarian conviction is reflected in the belief that God is ultimately and absolutely one.

Holy Days and Sacraments

No religious holy days are celebrated. Members come from various cultural and religious backgrounds and observe special days according to their own heritage and desire.

Normal milestones of life (birth, marriage, death) may be celebrated religiously. Although it is uncommon, puberty and divorce may include religious observances.

Unitarian Universalism does not believe in a need for sacraments. Baptism of infants and occasionally of adults is sometimes performed as a symbolic act of dedication. The Lord's Supper is administered in some congregations.

Diet and Substance Use

No restrictions on diet exist. Substances should be used according to reason.

Health Care Practices

Faith healing is considered largely superstitious and wishful thinking. Members believe in use of the empirical method, reason, and science to facilitate healing.

Medical and Surgical Procedures

The use of medications is not restricted. The use of blood and blood products is similarly not restricted. Amputations, organ transplants, and biopsies are not restricted. Circumcision is viewed as a health practice, not a religious one.

Practices Related to Reproduction

Unitarian Universalists strongly favor all types of birth control as a human right. Both therapeutic and on-demand abortion are acceptable. Members strongly favor the right of the mother to decide. Amniocentesis is not restricted and is encouraged if medical evaluation deems it necessary. Sterility testing is acceptable; in fact, more research is encouraged. Both donation and receipt of artificial insemination are acceptable and strongly favored as a human right.

Practices Related to Death and Dying

Members favor the right to die with dignity. Personhood is sacred, not the spark of life. Members tend to favor nonaction, including withdrawal of technical aids when death is imminent or when the patient has made a written request in advance. Autopsy is recommended. The donation of the body is acceptable, and donation to a medical school for study occurs frequently. Cremation is most common. Burial of a fetus is rare. A memorial service in the church or at home without the body present is customary.

Summary

Religious and cultural beliefs are interwoven and influence a client's understanding of illness and health care practices. In times of serious illness and death, religion may be a source of consolation for the client. Five dimensions of religion influence human behavior, including health-related practices. The goal of spiritual nursing care is to assist clients in integrating their own religious beliefs about God or a unifying truth into the ultimate reality that gives meaning to their lives in relationship to the health care crisis that has precipitated the need for nursing care. For the nurse providing spiritual nursing care, issues related to death and dying are of particular importance. Health-related beliefs and practices of select religions are important to understand, especially considering the diverse religious groups in the United States and Canada. Evidence-Based Practice 14–2 provides information regarding other research done on this topic, and Box 14–2 summarizes some of the religious and nonreligious holidays covered in this chapter.

Evidence-Based Practice Box 14-2:

Spirituality, Religion, Culture, and Health

Considerable scientific research has analyzed the potential connection among spiritual and religious practices, culture, and health. A metasynthesis of findings involving more than 7,000 participants in 25 research studies pertaining to spirituality, religion, intercessory prayer, culture, and health revealed the following:

- Regular participation in spiritual or religious practices lowers the overall mortality rate of the population by 12% to 46% per year (in 11 studies).
- Mortality for African Americans who participate in religious services at least weekly decreases by 10% for women and 17% for men (in one study).
- For the elderly, regular attendance at religious services improves physical health and psychological well-being (in two studies).
- People with high levels of religious beliefs or spirituality have lower levels of cortisol, cholesterol, and cardiac arrhythmias in response to stress (in three studies).
- Positive thinking that is associated with spirituality and religion produces nearly a 30% drop in perception of pain (in one study).
- Religious experience such as meditation lowers blood pressure (in 14 studies).
- Spirituality is connected to immune and endocrine functioning (in three studies).
- Spirituality and religion are associated with a slower progression of Alzheimer's disease (in two studies).
- People who pray before surgery have better surgical outcomes and report feeling less anxious before and after surgery, indicated one study. (Another study found the opposite outcome, i.e., more complications after surgery.)
- Women who attend weekly religious services are more successful in cigarette smoking cessation (in three studies).
- Men and women who attend weekly religious services are more successful in adhering to a cardiac rehabilitation program after being diagnosed with coronary artery disease (in one study).
- Intercessory prayer increases the success of women undergoing in vitro fertilization, (in one study).
- Faster recovery from depression, anxiety, and bereavement was reported for Christian, Muslim, and Buddhist patients (in one study).
- Some people undergoing surgery may not wish to know that others are offering prayers on their behalf (in one study).
- Hispanic men with HIV did not report religion as being helpful in coping with their disease (in one study).

(Continued on following page)

Evidence-Based Practice Box 14-2: *(continued)*

Spirituality, Religion, Culture, and Health

Clinical Application

While some of the studies have methodological limitations and most are epidemiological investigations, this growing body of research supports nurses' encouragement of patients who find daily or weekly prayer and other religious or spiritual practices to be meaningful. The best clinical practices demonstrated by nurses would include the following:

- Taking a spiritual and religious history on each patient
- Asking, "Do spiritual or religious beliefs or practices provide comfort or cause distress?"
- Encouraging patients to engage in spiritual and religious practices that they find satisfying and meaningful without imposing their own beliefs or practices on others
- Refraining from implying that religion is good or bad, only that it can provide comfort or cause stress
- Recognizing that, in times of physical or emotional stress such as hospitalization, people who do not regularly participate in spiritual or religious practices might turn to these practices for comfort, support, and hope
- Respecting that spiritual and religious practices can influence the patient's coping by providing
  - An optimistic worldview
  - A hopeful perspective on life, even in the face of serious or terminal diagnoses
  - A sense of empowerment and control

Butler, S. M., Koenig. H. G., Puchalski, C., Cohen, C., & Sloan, R. (2003). *Is prayer good for your health? A critique of the scientific research.* Heritage Lecture #816. Accessed on March 18, 2007, at www.heritage.org/Research/Religion

Dupre, M. E., Franzese, A. T., & Parrado, E. A. (2006). Religious attendance and mortality: Implications for the Black-White mortality crossover. *Demography, 43*(1), 141–164.

Gordon, S. (2006). *Spirituality can soothe body and soul.* Accessed on March 18, 2007, at www.healthfinder.gov.

Lyvers, M., Barling, N., & Harding-Cook, J. (2006). Effect of belief in "psychic healing" on self-reported pain in chronic pain sufferers. *Journal of Psychosomatic Research, 60*(1), 59–61.

Musick, M. A., House, J., & Williams, D. (2004). Attendance at religious services and mortality in a national sample. *Journal of Health & Social Behavior, 45,* 198–213.

Roberts, L., Ahmed, I., & Hall, S. (2007). *Cochrane Database of Systematic Reviews, 1,* pp. 1–2. Accessed on March 18, 2007, at www.cochrane/clsysrev/articles/CD000368.html

---

BOX 14-2

Religious and Nonreligious Holidays in the United States and Canada

This calendar is a guide to religious and nonreligious holidays that are celebrated in the United States and Canada. The list is not exhaustive but is given to encourage the reader to be aware of the many holidays and festivals that are reflective of the great mixture of religious and ethnic groups in North America.

A = African American	H = Hindu	O = Eastern Orthodox Christian
B = Buddhist	I = Islam	P = Protestant
Ba = Baha'i	J = Jewish	RC = Roman Catholic
C = Christian (general)	Ja = Jain	S = Sikh
Ci = Civic holiday	M = Mormon	

January

1 New Year's Day Ci
1 Feast of St. Basil O
6 Epiphany C
7 Nativity of Jesus Christ O
3rd Monday Martin Luther King, Jr. Birthday
    Observance Ci

February

Black History Month (U.S.)
8 Scout Day Ci
14 Valentine's Day Ci
Mid-month President's Day (U.S.) Ci
Other holidays that often fall in February according to the lunar calendar
Chinese New Year B
Ramadan (30 days) I
Nehan-e (Death of Buddha) B
Vasant Panchami (Advent of Spring) H, Ja
Ash Wednesday RC, P
Purim J

March

Women's History Month (U.S.) Ci
17 St. Patrick's Day C
25 Annunciation C
Other holidays that often occur in March according to the lunar calendar
Eastern Orthodox Lent begins O
Higan-e (First Day of Spring) B
Naw-Ruz (Baha'i and Iranian New Year)
Palm Sunday RC, P
First Day of Passover (8 days) J
Holi (Spring Festival) H, Ja
Maundy Thursday RC, P
Good Friday RC, P
Easter C, RC, P, M
Mahavir Jayanti (Birth of Mahavir) Ja

April

16 Yom Ha'atzmaut (Israel Independence Day) J
Holidays that often occur in April according to the lunar calendar
Hanamatsuri (Birth of Buddha) B
Yom Hashoah (Holocaust Remembrance Day) J, Ci
Baisakhi (Brotherhood) S
Huguenot Day P
Ramavani (Birth of Rama) H
Palm Sunday O
Holy Friday O
Easter O

May

5 Cinco de Mayo Ci
23 Victoria Day (Canada)
30 Memorial Day Ci
Holidays that often occur in May according to the lunar calendar
Shavuot J
Idul-Adha (Day of Sacrifice) I
Ascension Day RC, P
Pentecost RC, P

June

12 Anne Frank Day Ci
14 Flag Day (U.S.) Ci
24 Nativity of St. John the Baptist RC, P, O
Holidays that often occur in June according to the lunar calendar
Ratha-yatra H
Ascension Day O
Muharam (I)
Pentecost O
Islamic New Year I
Hindu New Year H

(Continued on following page)

BOX 14-2 (continued)

Religious and Nonreligious Holidays in the United States and Canada

July

1 Canada Day (Canada) Ci
4 Independence Day (U.S.) Ci
24 Pioneer Day M
Holidays that often occur in July according to the lunar calendar
Obon-e B

August

6 Transfiguration C
15 Feast of the Blessed Virgin Mary RC, O

September

1st Monday Labor Day (U.S.) Ci
15 National Hispanic Heritage Month (30 days) Ci
17 Citizenship (U.S. Constitution) Ci
19 San Gennaro Day RC
25 Native American Day Ci
Holidays that often occur in September according to the lunar calendar
Higan-e (First Day of Fall) B
Rosh Hashanah (Jewish New Year: 2 days) J

October

12 Columbus Day (U.S.) Ci
Thanksgiving Day (Canada) Ci
24 United Nations Day Ci
31 Reformation Day P
31 Halloween RC, P, Ci
Holidays that often occur in October according to the lunar calendar

Dusserah (Good over Evil) H, JA
Yom Kippur (Atonement) J
Sukkot (Tabernacles) J
Shemini 'Azeret (end of Sukkot) J
Diwali, or Dipavali (Festival of Lights) H, Ja

November

1 All Saints Day RC, P
11 Veterans Day Ci
25 Religious Liberty Day Ci
1st Tuesday Election Day (U.S.) Ci
4th Thursday Thanksgiving Day (U.S.) Ci
Holidays that often occur in November according to the lunar calendar
Baha'u'llah Birthday Ba
Guru Nanak Birthday S

December

6 St. Nicholas Day C
8 Feast of the Immaculate Conception RC
10 Human Rights Day Ci
12 Festival of Our Lady of Guadalupe (Mexico-Hispanic) RC
25 Christmas C, RC, P, M, Ci
Holidays that often occur in December according to the lunar calendar
Bodhi Day (Enlightenment) B
Hanukkah (Jewish Festival of Lights: 8 days) J
Kwanzaa (7 days) A

REVIEW QUESTIONS

1. When assessing the spiritual needs of clients from diverse cultural backgrounds, what key components should you consider?
2. In providing nursing care for the dying or bereaved client and family, what cultural considerations should the nurse include in the plan?
3. Compare and contrast the religious beliefs and practices concerning diet, medications, and procedures for five of the religious groups discussed in this chapter.
4. Analyze the contributions of religious bodies to the United States (or Canadian) health care delivery system.
5. What effect do health care facilities that are owned and operated by religious groups have on the overall cost and quality of health care in the United States and Canada?

6. What religious rituals mark significant developmental milestones for children and adolescents? Identify the ritual or ceremony, the approximate age at which the child or adolescent participates in it, and the name of the religion(s) associated with it.

CRITICAL THINKING ACTIVITIES

1. Visit a church or worship center not of your own belief system and interview a member of the clergy or an official representative about the health-related beliefs of that religion. Discuss with him or her the implications of those beliefs for someone hospitalized for an acute illness or a chronic illness. Inquire about the ways in which nurses can be of most help to hospitalized members of this religion.

2. Interview members of various religions about their beliefs about health and illness. Compare these interviews with the published beliefs or official statements from these religions. Discuss the implications of the differences (if any) that you found.

3. Interview fellow students, classmates, or coworkers (if you are employed) about what they know of the health beliefs of various religions, especially those religions most often encountered among the patients with whom you work. Make a poster or prepare a presentation comparing the results of your interviews with the official beliefs of those religions. Share this information with your classmates.

4. Interview four or more members of the same religious group who are of various ages (i.e., children, teenagers, young adults, middle-aged adults, and elderly). Ask them about their religious beliefs and how they affect their health. Compare the results, commenting on similarities and differences.

5. Explore the meaning of various unique items of clothing worn by members of different religions. These may be in the form of items worn on the head or body. When are shoes removed? For which religious groups?

6. If you have thought about the previously stated exercises in terms of physical health, consider each of the questions from the perspective of mental health and spiritual health.

REFERENCES

Adams, G. R. (Project Coordinator). (1994). *Memory and mourning: American expressions of grief* [Multimedia exhibit]. Rochester, NY: Strong Museum.

Bunson, M. (2000). *Catholic Almanac.* Our Sunday Visitor, Inc; Huntington, IN.

Butler, S. M., Koenig. H. G., Puchalski, C., Cohen, C., & Sloan, R. (2003). *Is prayer good for your health? A critique of the scientific research.* Heritage Lecture #816. Accessed on March 18, 2007, at www.heritage.org/Research/Religion

Chapman, A. (1991). The Buddhist way of dying. *Nursing Praxis in New Zealand, 6*(2), 23–26.

Christian Science Publishing Society. (1978). *What is a Christian Science practitioner?* Boston: Christian Science Publishing Society.

Christian Science Publishing Society (1994). *Science and health.* Boston: Christian Science Publishing Society.

Donnermeyer, J. F. (1997). Amish society: An overview. *The Journal of Multicultural Nursing & Health, 3*(2), 6–12.

Duffy, S. (2006). Cultural concepts at the end of Life. *Nursing Older People, 18*(8), 10–14.

Dupre, M. E., Franzese, A. T., & Parrado, E. A. (2006). Religious attendance and mortality: Implications for the Black-White mortality crossover. *Demography, 43*(1), 141–164.

Ebersole, P., & Hess, P. (2003) *Toward healthy aging* (6th ed.). St. Louis, MO: C.V. Mosby.

Faulkner, J. E., & DeJong, C. F. (1966). Religiosity in 5 D: An empirical analysis. *Social Forces, 45,* 246–254.

Forsythe, E. (1991). Religious and cultural aspects of family planning. *Journal of the Royal Society of Medicine, 84*(3), 177–178.

Gordon, S. (2006). *Spirituality can soothe body and soul.* Accessed on March 18, 2007, at www.healthfinder.gov

Green, J. (1992a). Death with dignity: Christianity. *Nursing Times, 88*(3), 25–29.

Green, J. (1992b). Death with dignity: Jehovah's Witnesses. *Nursing Times, 88*(5), 36–37.

Greksa, L. P., & Korbin, J. E. (1997). Influence of changing occupational patterns on the use of commercial health insurance by the Old Order Amish. *The Journal of Multicultural Nursing & Health, 3*(2), 13–18.

Hickey, M. E., & Hall, T. R. (1993). Insulin therapy and weight change in Native American NIDDM patients. *Diabetes Care, 16*(1), 364–368.

Hinnell, J. R. (1984). *The Penguin dictionary of religions.* New York: Penguin Books.

Huttlinger, K., Krefting, L., Drevdahl, D., Tree, P., Bacca, E., & Benally, A. (1992). Doing battle: A metaphorical analysis of diabetes mellitus among Navajo people. *American Journal of Occupational Therapy, 46*(8), 706–712.

Johnson, T. M., Kurian, G. T., & Barett, D. B. (2001). World Christian Encyclopedia: A Comparative Survey of Churches and Religions in the Modern World. vol. 2. USA: Oxford University Press.

Kalish, R. A., & Reynolds, D. K. (1981). *Death and ethnicity: A psychocultural study.* New York: Baywood.

Kozak, D. (1991). *Devil sickness and devil songs.* Washington, DC: Smithsonian Institution Press.

Lyvers, M., Barling, N., & Harding-Cook, J. (2006). Effect of belief in "psychic healing" on self-reported pain in chronic pain sufferers. *Journal of Psychosomatic Research, 60*(1), 59–61.

Marty, M. M. (1990). *Health, medicine, and the faith traditions. Healthy people 2000: A role for America's religious communities.* Atlanta, GA: Emory University, The Carter Center, and the Park Ridge Center.

Moberg, D. (1971). *Spiritual well-being.* Washington, DC: White House Conference on Aging.

Moberg, D. (1981). Religion and the aging family. In P. Ebersole & P. Hess (Eds.), *Toward healthy aging* (pp. 349–351). St. Louis, MO: C.V. Mosby.

Musick, M. A., House, J., & Williams, D. (2004). Attendance at religious services and mortality in a national sample. *Journal of Health & Social Behavior, 45,* 198–213.

Nimer, M. (2002). *The North American Muslim resource guide to community life in the United States and Canada.* New York, NY: Routledge.

Pew Forum: Changing Faiths: Latinos and the transformation of American religion. http://pewforum.org/surveys/hispanic/. Accessed on May 24, 2007.

Roberts, L., Ahmed, I., & Hall, S. (2007). *Cochrane Database of Systematic Reviews, 1,* pp. 1–2. Accessed on March 18, 2007, at www.cochrane.org/clsysrev/articles/CD000368. html

Scherer, R. P. (1996). Hospital caregivers' own religion in relation to their perceptions of psychological inputs into health and healing. *Review of Religious Research, 37*(4), 302–324.

Smith, E. B. (1986). Surgery in Jehovah's Witnesses. *Journal of National Medical Association, 78*(7), 668–669.

Steiger, B. (1975). *Medicine talk.* New York: Doubleday.

Stolley, J. M., & Koenig, H. (1997). Religion/spirituality and health among elderly African Americans and Hispanics. *Journal of Psychosocial Nursing, 35*(11), 32–38.

Sugarman, J., Churchill, L. R., Moore, J. K., & Waugh, R. A. (1991). Medical, ethical, and legal issues regarding thrombolytic therapy in the Jehovah's Witnesses. *American Journal of Cardiology, 68*(15), 1525–1529.

University of Virginia Health System. (2006a). *Buddhist beliefs and practices affecting health care.* Retrieved March 18, 2007, from http://www.healthsystem.virginia.edu/internet/chaplaincy/buddhism.cfm

University of Virginia Health System. (2006b). *Hindu beliefs and practices affecting health care.* Retrieved March 18, 2007, from http://www.healthsystem.virginia.edu/internet/chaplaincy/hindu.cfm

University of Virginia Health System. (2006c). *Islamic beliefs and practices affecting health care.* Retrieved March 18, 2007, from http://www.healthsystem.virginia.edu/internet/chaplaincy/muslim.cfm

University of Virginia Health System. (2006d). *Jewish beliefs and practices affecting health care.* Retrieved March 18, 2007, from http://www.healthsystem.virginia.edu/internet/chaplaincy/jewish.cfm

University of Virginia Health System. (2006e). *Roman Catholic beliefs and practices affecting health care.* Retrieved March 18, 2007, from http://www.healthsystem.virginia.edu/internet/chaplaincy/romancatholic.cfm

U.S. Census Bureau. *2000 census of the population and housing data paper listing* (CPH-L-133). Washington, DC: U.S. Government Printing Office.

U.S. Conference of Catholic Bishops. (2007). Retrieved March 18, 2007, at www.usccb.org/coom/statisti.shtml

Vogel, V. J. (1970). *American Indian medicine.* Norman, OK: University of Oklahoma Press.

Weiss, D. W. (1988). Organ transplantation, medical ethics and Jewish law. *Transplantation Proceedings, 20*(1), 1071–1075.

Wenger, A. F. (1990). The culture care theory and the Old Order Amish. In M. M. Leininger (Ed.). *Culture care diversity and universality: A theory of nursing* (pp. 147–178). New York: National League for Nursing Press.

Wenger, A. F. (1991, April/May). Culture specific care and the Old Order Amish. *IMPRINT,* 80–85.

White, K. A. *Crisis of conscience: Reconciling religious health care providers' beliefs and patients' rights.* Accessed on March 14, 2007, at http:/www3.baylor.edu/-Charles_Kemp/Hispanic_health.htm

Woods, T. E., & Ironson, G. H. (1999). Religion and spirituality in the face of illness. *Journal of Health Psychology, 4*(3) 393–412.

World religious data: Current numbers of members and growth of various religions. (2007). http://www.religious tolerance.

Yearbook of American and Canadian churches, annual. (2006). New York: National Council of the Churches of Christ in the United States of America.

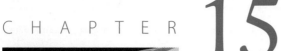

CHAPTER 15

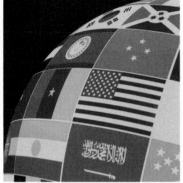

Cultural Competence
in Ethical Decision Making

Dula F. Pacquiao

KEY TERMS

Advance directives
American Nurses Association
   code of ethics
Autonomy
Beneficence
Categorical imperatives
Consequential theories of ethics
Cultural competence
Deontological theory of ethics

Emic
Ethic of care
Ethics
Etic
Fidelity
Health Insurance Portability
   and Accountability Act
Informed Consent
Justice

Nonmaleficence
Normative ethics
Patient Self-Determination
   Act
Patients' Bill of Rights
Principle-based ethics
Truth telling
Utilitarianism
Veracity

LEARNING OBJECTIVES

1. Compare moral beliefs and assumptions in Western and non-Western societies.
2. Describe how moral philosophies are socially and culturally constituted.
3. Define ethical concepts, principles, and theories.
4. Discuss cultural variability in ethical decision making.
5. Describe the culturally competent Model of Ethical Decision Making.
6. Use research findings relevant to ethical decision making.
7. Explain the significance of transcultural nursing in ethical care.

Contemporary society is marked by persistent and foundational moral disputes that are often unresolved by sound rational argument. Increasing population diversity brings a challenge to appreciate moral pluralism and understand disparate moral premises that individuals and groups bring into the situation (Englehardt, 2005). Health care practitioners are embedded in moral dilemmas because the work of health promotion, caring for and treating the sick, and comforting and protecting the suffering require judgments about resource allocation and decisions that are morally significant. Achieving a mutually satisfying resolution of conflicts in the context of cultural diversity is made more difficult by dwindling material and manpower resources. Cultural and humanistic factors are generally overlooked as health care increasingly becomes dominated by technological, economic, and social demands (Foley & Wurmser, 2004).

408

Increased cultural diversity in the workforce and client populations necessitates health care practitioners to evaluate the influence of their own moral assumptions, Western medical ethics, and organizational values on their work. Health care disparities demonstrate the unfair burden of suffering that can result from differential treatment of racial and ethnic minorities by practitioners (Institute of Medicine, 2002; Harrison & Falco, 2005). The federal mandate for **cultural competence** has a moral agenda for practitioners to remove barriers to access to care and eliminate health disparities. Ethical care requires proactive decisions so that health and social burden are not consistently borne by clients who are culturally different (Paasche-Orlow, 2004).

Ethical Concepts

A moral philosophy consists of beliefs and assumptions about what is right and wrong. This is the basis of ethics, which prescribes the proper action to take in a given situation. **Ethics** translates moral philosophies into action. **Normative ethics** defines actions that are morally right or wrong. The **American Nurses Association Code of Ethics** and the Canadian Nurses Association Code of Ethics are sets of principles or standards guiding professional nursing practice. They reflect the norms of valued beliefs and ideals in mainstream American and Canadian societies.

The **ethic of care** is drawn from psychological and feminist theories originated by Carol Gilligan. It emphasizes actions promoting positive relationships with and full understanding of the individual in his or her situational context. Under the ethic of care, practitioners need to develop empathy, compassion, and relationships that promote trust, growth, and well-being. This relationship is significant in caring for the frail and vulnerable individuals who are unable to advocate for themselves. Decisions about withdrawal of life support should take into consideration the individual's particular life context, (e.g.,

previous life, current situation, and relationships with significant others).

The **deontological theory of ethics** is derived from the work of Immanuel Kant, upholding reason as the basis for morality. Deontologists believe that human beings are duty bound to use reason. Reason yields universally applicable **categorical imperatives** that can be clearly, consistently, and practically used in all situations. Truth telling and respect for individual autonomy are considered intrinsically moral acts.

In contrast, **utilitarianism** is grounded in the belief that the utility or consequence of an action is the only relevant consideration in judging behaviors. Utilitarians believe in the idea of the greatest good for the greatest number. Proponents of utilitarianism such as Jeremy Bentham and John Stuart Mill argued that no action should be judged by itself but rather by its usefulness or end results (Bloch, & Green, 2006).

The contrasting perspective between deontology and utilitarianism is illustrated by the stem cell debate. Deontologists believe that preserving human life including that of an embryo is morally right. On the other hand, utilitarians believe that using human embryos to achieve cure for many illnesses, save lives, and improve the quality of life of many far outweigh the benefit of preserving the life of an embryo.

Principle-based ethics or principlism was introduced by Beauchamp & Childress (2001) in an attempt to reconcile the divergence between teleological and deontological models. It links moral decision making on scientific findings rather than universal rules. Principlism is based on the philosophical pragmatism of William James. The principles of **beneficence** and **nonmaleficence** require that care providers act in ways that benefit and cause no harm to consumers of their care. The decision to give larger doses of morphine to relieve the pain of a terminally ill patient with cancer is weighed carefully for its intended benefits against the possible harm it may cause, such as addiction, respiratory depression, and death. In most cases, promoting the patient's comfort and peaceful death is judged more beneficial over prolonging life and suffering. To do otherwise creates more harm than good.

The principle of **autonomy** is closely linked with respect for an individual's free will and includes the right to make choices about issues affecting one's being. Autonomous persons should be allowed to determine their own actions or delegate decision making to others when they become incapable of making such decisions. The **Patient Self-Determination Act** of 1991 is a legal protection of a person's autonomy or self-determination in these situations through advance directives. An individual's autonomy is ensured when a nurse provides appropriate information that could enhance the person's ability to make informed decisions about his or her care.

The principle of **justice** relates to the fair, equitable, and appropriate treatment or use of resources in light of what a person needs, weighed against the needs of others. The documents *Healthy People 2010* (U.S. Department of Health and Human Services, 2000) and *Achieving Health for All: A Framework for Health Promotion* (Health Canada, 2001) describe existing disparities in access to health care services and health outcomes among population groups in the United States and Canada. The allocation of resources to combat increasing infant mortality among Blacks, for example, applies the principle of distributive justice. The mandate for health care practitioners and organizations to provide a trained interpreter for patients who are less proficient in English, requiring allocation of resources for certain groups, is deemed fair and just (Office of Minority Health, 2001).

The principle of **fidelity** is the obligation to remain faithful to one's commitments. Nurses have an obligation to maintain standards of professional practice as a condition of continuing licensure. The principle of **veracity** upholds the virtues of being honest and telling the truth. **Truth telling** is recognized as a prerequisite to a trusting relationship. **Informed consent** requires veracity of information presented to clients and fidelity of practitioners to professional standards.

Contrasting Social Construction of Morality

Morals and philosophic beliefs are constituted within the social, historical, and cultural experiences of a society. These beliefs evolve as normative patterns of assumptions that serve as an implicit framework guiding the actions and thoughts of group members, which may or may not be shared by persons outside of the cultural group.

One of the most common sources of ethical conflicts in health care is rooted in the contrasting conceptualization of human beings in the Western and non-Western cultures. Lovejoy (1974) states that in Western cultures, there is a pervasive belief that human beings are endowed with the capacity for reason and action. Because reason is a universal capacity for all humans, it is through reason that humans can be expected to make valid and truthful judgments in any situations. The philosophic traditions of universalism and rationalism have shaped the Western concept of the person as the focus of moral reasoning. The person is the basic unit imbued with universal capacity for reason and action. Differences are attributed to deficits in cognitive skills, motivation, information, and/or linguistic tools (Shweder & Bourne, 1997). Approaches to ethical dilemmas, therefore, are based on the belief that by compensating for these deficits, a person can be expected to make a rational decision that is universally regarded as logical and morally acceptable.

However, not all human behaviors can be classified as simply rational or irrational. Culture can be arbitrary, and human beings create their own distinctive, symbolic realities. Many of our ideas and practices are beyond logic and experience (Shweder, 1997). In some groups, religious and spiritual dimensions highly influence behaviors. Among such ethnoreligious groups as devout Muslims, Hindus, and Jews, religion is embedded in everyday life. Decisions about euthanasia, for example, may not be acceptable to an Orthodox Jew whose beliefs uphold the sanctity of life. Jews generally consult their rabbi regarding matters

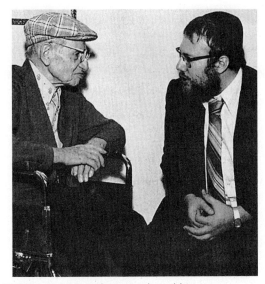

FIGURE 15-1. Consultation with a rabbi.

pertaining to life and death decisions (see Figure 15-1). Religion increases the awareness of the power and benevolence of God over humans; hence, earthly decisions are left to God, and the attitude is one of acceptance of fate rather than control over one's destiny. Members of Jehovah's Witnesses oppose blood transfusion as a life-saving measure, contradicting the logic of scientific reasoning. Similarly, Christian Scientists may prefer their own religious and spiritually based practices of healing to those of scientific medicine.

Cultural practices such as female circumcision, body piercing and tattooing, and taking home a newborn's afterbirth appear illogical and without any scientific basis (see Evidence-Based Practice 15-1). Yet these practices are supported by value–belief systems that are deeply entrenched in religious, philosophical, and social structure of certain groups. To professional practitioners, resistance to valid and scientifically proven measures belies common sense, but cultural traditions of some groups transcend rationality and logic. Indeed, common sense is not common after all; it is uniquely constructed within the social and cultural life contexts of human groups.

Another common source of moral conflict stems from contrasting views of a person between Western and non-Western cultures. In the West, individualism is the norm; the person is viewed as a self-contained entity, fully integrated and self-motivating, independent of social roles and relationships, and distinct from all others (Geertz, 1973). In contrast, among collectivistic cultures there is greater continuity and mutuality among group members. The Xhosa tribe in South Africa emphasizes collective decisions where tribal elders make major decisions about the distribution of human and material resources to provide care for their members (Figure 15-2).

Family and kinship patterns assign different roles, status, and power among group members. The social hierarchy governs decision making, interactions, roles, and obligations of members. Whereas Western health care providers value the individual's autonomy in decision making, filial piety and respect for the authority of one's elders are the guiding principles among traditional Asian cultures in making decisions about care. Influenced by the Confucian ethic, the Korean culture accepts inherent social inequality among family members as a condition for achieving collective harmony. By contrast, the Western value of instrumental individualism prizes the ability of individuals to make choices and rely upon themselves to achieve their purpose in life. While a traditional Chinese adult relies upon family members and the physician to make decisions, a typical American or Canadian adult expects to be given information so he or she can make a decision.

Respect for patient autonomy has become the focal context for health care decisions in the United States and Canada (Valente, 2004). Ethical principles are applied to ensure and maximize individual autonomy. The autonomy paradigm, which has been institutionalized in health care, underlines interactions with and expectations of patients and families by practitioners. The

Evidence-Based Practice 15–1:

Experiences of Circumcised Women with Swedish Health Care

Twenty-two African women from Eritrea, Somalia, and Sudan who were living in Sweden were interviewed regarding their experiences with the Swedish health care system. These women found themselves surrounded by doctors, midwives, and nurses who made them feel like objects of curiosity, staring at them without saying anything despite the presence of interpreters, and often speaking to each other without involving them. Pregnant women with more than two children met negative attitudes from midwives at health care centers who did not see them as capable of family-planning decisions. Many women stayed at home until late in pregnancy to avoid these negative encounters. Midwives were unaware of how to deliver infibulated women, failed to assess the women's unique needs, and often ignored their suggestions about how they should be delivered. Encounters with Swedish health care were viewed as a reenactment of their suffering, abandonment, and mutilation associated with circumcision.

Clinical Application

1. Identify the cultural and ethical conflicts in the previous situation.
2. Analyze implications of these conflicts on quality of care and patient safety.
3. Describe specific action modes to promote linkage between ethical and culturally competent practice for circumcised women outside of their sociocultural context.

Berggren, V., Bergstrom, S., & Edberg, A. K. (2006). Being different and vulnerable: Experiences of immigrant African women who have been circumcised and sought maternity care in Sweden. *Journal of Transcultural Nursing, 17* (1), 50–57.

Patient Self Determination Act of 1991 mandates health care practitioners to provide clients with information about advance directives. **Advance directives** are intended to assure patients' autonomy in situations when they can no longer make a decision. An individual's choices are presumably carried out on their behalf in the event that they cannot consciously and competently represent their own will. Although the intent of advance directives is laudable within the Western ethos of self-determination, other cultures subscribe to the belief that the fate of human beings is beyond their control.

The **Health Insurance Portability and Accountability Act** ensures confidentiality of an individual's health information. Health care practitioners are required to seek the patient's informed consent before any information is shared with others, including family members. This poses difficulty for collectivistic groups where family members decide which information is shared with the patient and other family members. The tension between managed care and individual rights to choose and seek redress for infractions of these rights created a long-drawn-out debate on the **Patients' Bill of Rights** in the U.S. Congress. It struck the core of individual rights versus limiting these rights to give cost-effective care to more people.

Ethics and Cultural Diversity

Ethical conflicts can arise from paternalistic attitudes of practitioners and their tendency to engage in cultural imposition. Contributing to

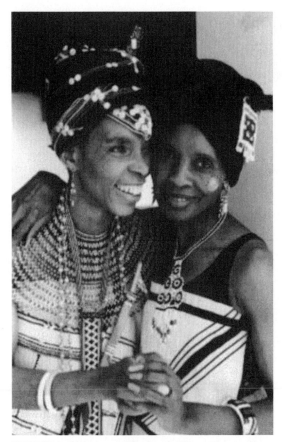

FIGURE 15-2. Women of the South African Xhosa tribe at a wedding of a family member. (Courtesy of Beatrice Mabutho)

this attitude is the belief that scientific, biomedical care is superior to other ways of caring and healing. Lack of knowledge of other cultures also breeds cultural imposition. Such is the case of a Mexican widow who is brought to the hospital by her adult daughter because of pain in her toes. On examination, the physician determined that her toes were gangrenous and needed immediate amputation. When presented the surgical consent, the patient and her daughter refused to sign. They insisted on speaking with the patient's oldest son who was residing in another state. When contacted, the patient's son refused to give consent until he consulted his uncle in Mexico. Unfortunately, the patient's brother said that he

should talk with the oldest brother living in rural Mexico who cannot be reached by phone. The surgeon was angered by the family's lack of understanding of the emergency nature of the surgery. The surgeon demanded that the patient's brothers and son meet with him. At this meeting, the family continued their refusal to sign the consent for surgery and took the patient home. After a month, the family took the patient back to the hospital and agreed to have her toes amputated because they witnessed how much she suffered (see Evidence-Based Practice 15–2).

The surgeon's anger and paternalistic attitude offended the family by denigrating their established age- and gender-based social hierarchy. The manner in which the surgeon responded to perceived disagreement and noncompliant behavior by the family created further mistrust of his morally good intentions that resulted in further suffering of the patient. A sense of cultural humility and openness to diverse pathways of decision making would no doubt have promoted positive interactions between the surgeon and the patient's brothers. This would have increased further understanding of each other's context of meanings and development of mutually respectful communication.

There are two perspectives in any given situation: the **emic** (insider's) view and the **etic** (outsider's) view. For example, the husband of a terminally ill patient (both are Filipino) was distressed by the nurse's suggestion that his wife should have a clear liquid diet until her nausea, vomiting, and diarrhea were relieved. From his emic perspective, providing food such as *arroz caldo* (rice and chicken soup) would promote health and signify caring. The nurse's etic interpretation of his behavior was that he lacked knowledge of appropriate care for the patient.

Cultural diversity requires us to switch our frames of understanding, recognizing the coequality of fundamentally different perspectives and the ability of each of several persistent yet incompatible frames to handle any and all new evidence (Shweder, 1997). Frame switching permits us to accept variances in common sense and to recognize that logic and science are lim-

Evidence-Based Practice 15–2:

Moral Conflicts in Medical-School Students

Researchers analyzed 688 cases of moral conflicts submitted by 327 third-year medical students in their bioethics course in one medical school over a period of 4 years. The most common ethical issues experienced were in surgery and obstetrics–gynecology. These included deliberate lies or deceptions by medical practitioners, refusal of recommended treatment by patients and/or patient surrogates, and insistence on futile treatment. Overt and subtle discrimination toward patients resulted in substandard or excessive treatment. Students were reluctant to speak up about moral conflict for fear of reprisal from superiors.

Clinical Application

1. Identify ethical theories or principles violated by the practitioners' behaviors.
2. Analyze the implications of power relationships that exist among participants.
3. Demonstrate application of Leininger's action modes to promote ethical care.

Caldicott, C. V., & Faber-Langendoen, K. (2005). Deception, discrimination and fear of reprisal: Lessons in ethics from third-year medical students. *Academic Medicine, 80*(9), 866–873.

ited in understanding differences. Belief in the universality of reason prevents us from considering other ways of life and appreciating other systems of meanings. Bracketing our own values and beliefs allows us to discover the emic ways of people from other cultures. The highest developmental phase of cultural competence is demonstrated when health practitioners lack strong cultural identification and have the ability to unconsciously adjust to a wide range of cultural beliefs (Crandall, George, Marion, & Davis, 2003).

Culturally Competent Model for Ethical Decision Making

Assumptions of Pacquiao's Model

The model is built on the following major premises (see Figure 15–3):

1. Access to cultural competent care is a basic human right.

2. Culturally congruent and competent care is by necessity ethical care.
3. The culture of health care organizations and professions reflects the dominant societal culture.
4. Cultural competence in ethical decision making requires awareness of personal, professional, and organizational cultural values and biases, as well as understanding their influence on interactions with others and with care decisions.
5. Cultural competence needs to occur at the practitioner, organizational, and societal or community levels.
6. Culturally competent ethical decisions use the modes of cultural preservation, accommodation, and repatterning separately or simultaneously.
7. Application of cultural action modes requires understanding of the values, beliefs, and lifeways of clients, families, and communities.

The three major components of the model are human rights, ethics, and cultural competence.

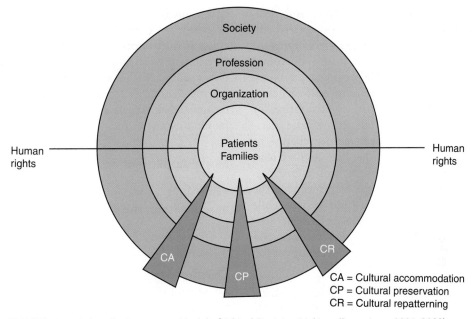

Human rights ————— Patients Families ————— Human rights

CA = Cultural accommodation
CP = Cultural preservation
CR = Cultural repatterning

FIGURE 15-3. Culturally Competent Model of Ethical Decision Making. (Pacquiano, 2001, 2003).

Figure 15–3 depicts the relationship of the components of the model. Access to culturally competent care is a basic human right. The model affirms the fundamental rights of individuals, families, groups, and populations to health care that is meaningful, supportive, and beneficial. Culturally competent care is achieved when ethical decisions preserve clients' fundamental right to meaningful and satisfying care that is grounded in their culturally constituted values and lifeways. This cultural context is paramount in achieving care that is judged moral and ethical by clients.

The Pacquiao model (Pacquiao, 2001) validates the rights of clients to become active participants in decisions about their care. Ethical care is culturally competent and demands that practitioners acknowledge the importance of culture, respect cultural differences, and minimize negative consequences of these differences. Culturally competent ethical decisions preserve human rights and dignity.

According to Leininger (Leininger & McFarland, 2006), caring is meaningful or beneficial

when a culture's care values, expressions, or patterns are known and used appropriately by care providers. Cultural conflicts arise from competing worldviews and moral assumptions, which lead to ethical dilemmas. Culturally congruent decisions are ethical because they respect and protect the inherent values and assumptions of people that have provided a context of meanings to their lives. Culturally congruent actions are the processes by which ethical principles are applied and human rights are preserved.

The action strategies suggested by Leininger are adopted in this model.

1. Cultural care preservation or maintenance—assistive, supportive, facilitative, or enabling professional actions and decisions that help people of a particular culture to retain and/or preserve relevant care values so that they can maintain their well-being, recover from illness, or face handicaps and/or death.

2. Cultural care accommodation or negotiation—assistive, supportive, facilitative, or

enabling professional actions and decisions that help people of a designated culture adapt to, or negotiate with, others for beneficial or satisfying health outcomes with professional care providers.

3. Cultural care repatterning or restructuring—assistive, supportive, facilitative, or enabling professional actions and decisions that help a client reorder, change, or greatly modify his or her lifeways for a new, different, and beneficial health care pattern, and maintenance of respect for the client's cultural values and beliefs while still providing a beneficial or healthier lifeway than before the changes were coestablished with the client (Leininger & McFarland, 2002, p. 84).

Figure 15-4 demonstrates the triad of ethical principles that are given priority in culturally competent ethical decision making. The concept of social justice and its correlates of fairness and distributive justice are the basis for decisions that are beneficent and nonmaleficent, particularly when clients have culturally different values, beliefs, and practices from the dominant norms of society and health care organizations and professions. While preserving individual autonomy through truth telling is paramount for mainstream Americans and Canadians, accommodating family requests to hold the truth from the client may be beneficial and cause less harm. Assuming a pluralistic framework instead of specific value-laden ethical perspectives allows the practitioner to reframe decisions that respect cultural differences and minimize the negative consequences of cultural imposition (Paasche-Orlow, 2004). Within this framework, an individualistic Westerner's value of self-autonomy is recognized equally as a non-Westerner's value of family solidarity.

Model Application

Table 15-1 provides a schema for using the model within the paradigm of the nursing process.

Assessment

The three component parts of assessment are (1) assessment of clients and families, (2) assessment of organizational culture, and (3) assessment of dominant professional and societal norms. Client and/or family assessment is focused on determining social and cultural variables influencing thoughts and behaviors. Data are collected to gain knowledge of cultural values, beliefs, and practices that can provide insight on behaviors relevant to care. Philosophic beliefs about life transitions such as birth, illness, and death can often be determined by assessing religious and spiritual traditions. Assessment includes ethnohistory, premigration and postmigration patterns, social organization and hierarchy, patterns of interaction, and family and community resources.

Assessment of staff and organizational cultures, organizational resources and allocation, and staff members' knowledge and skills in dealing with the client's culture will yield valuable information on the ability of the organization and care providers to handle situations. Most conflicts stem from inherent differences between the cultures of the clients and those of the organization and staff.

Dominant professional and societal norms are embedded in legal, ethical, and regulatory mandates. Awareness of these parameters will facilitate realistic collaboration between care

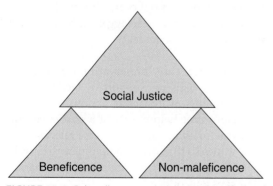

FIGURE 15-4. Culturally competent application of ethical principles.

TABLE 15-1. *Guide for Using the Culturally Competent Model*

Assessment

Client/families
Religion, spiritual, and philosophical beliefs and practices
Caring values, patterns, and expressions
Social organization and hierarchy
Roles and obligations of family members and kin
Differential acculturation of family/group members
Family and community resources
Cultural gatekeepers and brokers in the community
Communication norms and linguistic patterns
Experience with professional health care

Organizational culture
Personal culture and conflicting values among care providers
Professional cultural values, beliefs, and practices
Similarities and differences among clients, organizations, and professional cultures
Organizational policies and procedures
Organizational resources
Allocation of material resources
Support for culturally competent care
Interpretation and translation
Workforce cultural expertise
Staff development programs
Staffing

Dominant societal influences in organization
Legal mandates
Regulatory requirements
Professional code of ethics

Planning

Establish relationship with client(s)/families/communities
Define conflicting values, beliefs, and practices underlying problem
Define problems and priorities that reflect the emic perspectives of client(s)
Determine material and personnel resources needed
Determine aspects of action plans that need to be negotiated with participants

Intervention

Cultural care preservation or maintenance
Cultural care accommodation or negotiation
Cultural care repatterning or restructuring

Evaluation

Allow clients/families to identify outcomes and indices for achievement
Differentiate culturally meaningful outcomes from biomedical outcomes
Validate outcomes achievement with clients/families

providers and clients that protects the human rights of consumers, other patients, and staff. Assessing the societal and professional contexts promotes realistic decision making by addressing the needs of others external to the immediate situation.

Planning and Outcome Identification

Defining the problem and situation from the viewpoint of the client is the goal of the planning phase. Understanding the emic worldview of clients facilitates problem solving that preserves their human rights and cultural sets of meanings. Building relationships with clients, families, and groups is a prerequisite to forming respectful and trusting partnerships that enhance understanding of the problem from multiple perspectives.

Intervention

During the intervention phase, culturally congruent actions are implemented. All three strategies of preservation, negotiation, and repatterning may be used simultaneously. Using these nursing actions requires a relative perspective about the application of ethical principles of beneficence, nonmaleficence, and justice based on the life contexts of clients. These principles may be given different levels of priority across cultural groups. Understanding the cultural variables and the emic worldviews of clients is salient to the selection and implementation of actions. Culturally congruent actions are predicated on trusting relationships between consumers and practitioners and on interactions that integrate the cultural norms and language patterns of clients.

Outcomes Evaluation

Outcomes are achieved when the organization delivers on its commitment to culturally competent, ethical care. Policies should be in place such as allocation of resources for staff and management training and provision of interpreters for clients who are less proficient in English (see Evidence-Based Practice 15-3). Staff and management evaluation should reinforce and reward desired behaviors.

In evaluation, outcomes of care are not limited to the achievement of biomedical goals. Holistic indices inclusive of physical, psychological, social, cultural, and spiritual well-being are evaluated and monitored. The meanings and indices of outcomes of care may be different across cultural groups. Biomedical outcomes of care that define the effectiveness of professional health care may be secondary to other outcomes, such as observance of religious and spiritual beliefs. Clients' subjective, personal definition of, and affirmation of outcomes are paramount. Many meaningful outcomes may be variably expressed and may not be visible to outsiders to the culture. Receiving validation from clients and understanding their context of meanings will provide valuable information in identifying appropriate outcomes and indices of achievement.

Model Application in Case Studies

Defining Death

A teenager was rushed to the emergency room in critical condition after a motor vehicular accident. He was admitted to the critical care unit and placed on ventilatory assistance and fluid therapy. A diagnosis of massive and irreversible brain injury was made, and the physicians informed the family of imminent brain death. As soon as brain death was established, the parents were informed by the physician, who suggested discontinuing life support and encouraged them to consider organ donation. The parents reacted with anger, refused the physician's recommendations, and threatened to bring legal action if their son was transferred out of critical care. The ethical dilemma that ensued involved potential financial loss to the hospital for keeping a brain-dead patient in critical care; constant presence of large numbers of visitors who prayed at the patient's bedside, which created difficulty for other patients in the unit; and increased negative perceptions by staff of parental noncompliance with hospital policies and medical advice.

Defining the problem requires that practitioners should develop understanding of the family's values, beliefs, and practices as well as awareness of their own personal, professional, and organizational values and practices influencing their behaviors. Ethical dilemmas are characterized by diverse values, meanings, and decisions that parties bring into the situation. As born-

Evidence-Based Practice 15–3:

Physician Language Ability and Cultural Competence

This study explored how self-rated language ability and cultural competence of physicians affect health communication with Spanish-speaking, diabetic, low-income clients in two public hospital outpatient departments. Patients' interaction experiences were measured by using the Interpersonal Processes Instrument. Results revealed that patients were more likely to report better interpersonal processes of care when their primary care physician had higher self-rated language ability and cultural competence. Physicians who were fluent in Spanish elicited more of the patients' problems and concerns. In interpreter-mediated encounters, physicians made fewer facilitative remarks and were more likely to ignore patients' questions. Patients tended to express more concerns when speaking directly to their physicians.

Clinical Application

1. Identify ethical principles and theories that are violated when clients who are less proficient in English are not provided with appropriate interpretation.
2. Analyze the cultural values and moral premises of the Spanish culture that impact their interactions with healthcare professionals.
3. Describe ways by which practitioners can ensure greater understanding of patients' concerns when using interpreters.
4. Analyze the implications of power relationships that exist among participants.
5. Describe cultural accommodation of Spanish-speaking clients' valued communication patterns.

Fernandez, A., Schillinger, D., Grumbach, K., Rosenthal, A., Stewart, A. L., Wang, F., et al. (2004). Physician language ability and cultural competence: An exploratory study of communication with Spanish-speaking patients. *Journal of General Internal Medicine, 19,* 167–174.

again Christians, the parents believed in the sanctity of life over quality of life. Though accepting of the inevitability of their son's death, the parents viewed death holistically as the unity of body and soul. Brain death as a physical determinant was not acceptable as a marker of end of life. The family belonged to a close-knit congregation whose members believed that prayers are needed for the soul's redemption; the dying person is not left alone as the soul should leave the body in peace. The spiritual dimension superimposed the physical evidence of death.

Cultural repatterning of the hospital staff is needed to allow understanding of diverse beliefs and practices of the family and gain awareness of how their own values and beliefs negatively influenced their interactions with family members.

Cultural preservation of the family's valued beliefs and practices facilitates the communication of empathy and building of trust. Partnering with their religious leader and family decision maker accommodates their spiritual beliefs and practices while addressing organizational realities. Cultural negotiation becomes a necessity when preservation of cultural beliefs and practices is not fully possible. The religious leader is a trusted insider, who is knowledgeable about the family's beliefs and moral philosophies and an appropriate mediator between the family and staff. Continued respectful and trusting interactions between the family and staff can lead to mutual empathic understanding and respect (Kagawa-Singer & Kassim-Lakha, 2003). The staff needs to develop cultural humility

(Trevalon & Murray-Garcia, 1998)—a sense of openness and acceptance of differences in order to permit other frames of understanding of the situation to evolve. Ethical conflicts require that practitioners understand that they are not at the center stage of decisions, but instead they are partners in decision making through bridging by cultural experts and brokers. The staff should be comfortable with ambiguity and hone their skill in switching roles and frames of understanding.

Veracity and Autonomy

An elder Egyptian woman is admitted to the hospital, accompanied by her eldest son, with a diagnosis of metastatic breast cancer. The patient is a widow, and her son has assumed the role as decision maker after her husband's death. The son asked their Egyptian family physician to ask the hospital staff not to inform his mother that she has a terminal condition. He requested that the word *tumor* should be used instead of cancer when speaking to his mother. Before discharge, the attending physician wanted to refer the family to hospice. However, as the son refused to have his mother informed of her terminal condition to get an informed consent, the physician and nurses did not make the referral because they believed they were being coerced to lie to the patient. They upheld the principles of fidelity and truthfulness as legal mandates to ensure patient autonomy. The patient was subsequently discharged without hospice referral.

The problem stems from differential priorities between the staff and the client's son. As a devout Muslim, the son believes that one's fate is predestined, and humans are powerless in changing their fate. Prognostication is generally up to God and an inappropriate act for humans. As the major family decision maker, the client's son assumes responsibility for his mother's care. The ethical principle of beneficence and nonmaleficence guided his decision to prevent his mother from being burdened by the truth and its consequent hopelessness. In contrast, the staff's reactions demonstrate the dominant societal and organizational assumption that truth telling safeguards the client's right to know and ability

to reasonably make her own decision. Veracity is perceived as a precondition of autonomy.

Culturally competent ethical decision making by practitioners necessitates understanding the cultural, religious, and gender-based values, beliefs, and practices of the family. The staff needs to put aside their own personal and professional bias to gain a new understanding of the other's contextualized meanings. Cultural restructuring of the staff's own thinking allows them to create a new frame of understanding that permits cultural preservation and accommodation of the son's request. Partnering with the son and family physician can result in a mutually respectful and meaningful solution to the conflict.

Health care practitioners and organizations should develop partnerships with diverse communities to develop creative solutions and prevent future conflicts. The use of health care proxy designating family members to make decisions on behalf of clients has been found to be an acceptable alternative to informed consent and individual execution of advance directives in collectivistic cultures where status and authority are differentially assigned within an established social hierarchy. The model emphasizes development of cultural competence of diverse communities to enable them to effectively negotiate and use health care services. Hospitals should create advisory committees, representing the communities they serve to assist in policy development, that are meaningfully congruent with their values and priorities. Communities need to be culturally competent in making their needs and preferences known to health care practitioners and become actively involved in changing organizations towards cultural competence.

Summary

As health care becomes progressively multicultural, a different framework for decision making is needed—one built on an understanding of differences and similarities between populations and health care practitioners and organizations. Culturally competent and ethical care begins

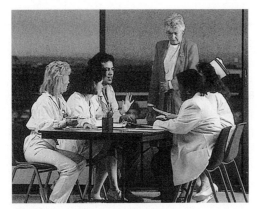

FIGURE 15-5. Assessment of the staff and organizational culture.

with an appreciation of the significant role of culture in health and caring. Cultural appreciation prompts practitioners to examine their own values and biases and engage in fully understanding the clients' context of meanings. Respecting and accommodating their unique life context allow for switching frames of understanding in order to work with cultural differences and design care that minimizes disadvantages associated with being different. Culturally competent ethical decisions promote empathic understanding, genuine respect, and greater appreciation of pluralistic perspectives about life and well-being. Culturally competent ethical decisions promote leveling of power differentials in health care and address the unequal burden of morbidity, mortality, and socioeconomic disadvantages across groups. Equity, fairness, and meaningfulness in caring are fully realized by cultural competent practitioners, organizations, and communities.

REVIEW QUESTIONS

1. Describe ethical dilemmas associated with the current state of health care and nursing.
2. Contrast the values that form the basis for moral philosophies of dominant and diverse groups in the United States and Canada.
3. Give examples of actions or decisions that demonstrate ethical theories and principles.
4. Explain why the application of the principles of veracity and autonomy may be problematic in some cultural groups.

CRITICAL THINKING ACTIVITIES

Identify an example of an ethical dilemma that you have encountered at work. Note that ethical dilemmas occur more frequently in clinical situations. For some of them, you may need some time to think before making a decision on your own, whereas other decisions are more complex and need referral to the ethics committee of the organization.

Identify the particulars of the situation:

1. What people are involved?
2. What is the setting?
3. How do different individuals or groups perceive the problem?
4. Identify conflicting values and beliefs at the individual, organizational, and societal levels that influence perceptions.
5. What assessment data about the situation are missing?
6. How can additional information be obtained?
7. Using the culturally competent Model of Ethical Decision Making, how would you redefine the problem?
8. What culturally congruent strategies do you recommend?

ETHICS RESOURCES

1. **Center for Bioethics**
   University of Pennsylvania
   3401 Market Street, Suite 320
   Philadelphia, PA 19104-3308
   Phone: (215) 898-7136
   Fax (215) 573-3036
   http://www.bioethics.upenn.edu/bioethics/?pageI
   d=10

2. **Alden March Bioethics Institute**
   47 New Scotland Avenue, MC 153
   Albany, NY 12208-3478
   Phone: (518) 262-6082
   Fax: (518) 262-6856
   http://www.bioethics.org

3. **Center for the Study of Bioethics**
   Medical College of Wisconsin
   8701 Watertown Plank Road
   Milwaukee, WI 53226
   Phone: (414) 456-8498
   bioethics@mcw.edu
   http://www.mcw.edu/bioethics/

4. **MacLean Center for Clinical Medical Ethics**
   University of Chicago
   5841 S. Maryland Avenue, MC 6098
   Chicago, IL 60637
   Phone: (773) 702-1453
   Fax: (773) 702-0090
   http://medicine.uchicago.edu/centers/ccme/

5. **Department of Bioethics**
   Case Western University
   School of Medicine, TA200
   10900 Euclid Ave.
   Cleveland, OH 44106-4976
   Phone: (216) 368-6196
   http://www.case.edu/med/bioethics/

6. **Center for Medical Ethics and Health Policy**
   Baylor College of Medicine
   One Baylor Plaza
   Houston, Texas 77030
   Phone: (713) 798-3500
   Fax: (713) 798-5678
   http://www.bcm.edu/ethics/

7. **Department of Bioethics/JJ60**
   Cleveland Clinic
   9500 Euclid Avenue
   Cleveland, OH 44195
   Phone: (216) 444-8720
   Fax: (216) 444-9275
   http://www.clevelandclinic.org/bioethics/

8. **Center for the Study of Society & Medicine**
   Columbia College of Physicians & Surgeons
   c/o 630 West 168th Street
   P&S Box 11
   New York, NY 10032
   Phone: (212) 305-4186
   Fax: (212) 305-6416
   http://www.societyandmedicine.columbia.edu/

9. **Center for Ethics, Emory University**
   1462 Clifton Road NE, Suite 302
   Atlanta, GA 30322
   Phone: (404) 727-4954
   http://ethics.emory.edu/index.html

10. **The Kennedy Institute of Ethics**
    Healy, 4th Floor
    Georgetown University
    Washington, DC 20057
    Phone: (202) 687-8099
    Fax: (202) 687-8089
    http://kennedyinstitute.georgetown.edu

11. **The National Catholic Bioethics Center**
    6399 Drexel Road
    Philadelphia, PA 19151
    Phone: (215) 877-2660
    Fax: (215) 877-2688
    http://www.ncbcenter.org/

12. **Center for Bioethics**
    University of Minnesota
    N504 Boynton Health Center
    410 Church Street SE
    Minneapolis, MN 55455
    Phone: (612) 624-9440
    Fax: (612) 624-9108
    http://www.bioethics.umn.edu/

13. **Center for Practical Bioethics**
    Harzfeld Building
    1111 Main Street, Suite 500
    Kansas City, MO 64105-2116
    Phone: (800) 344-3829
    Fax: (816) 221-1100, Fax: (816) 221-2002
    bioethic@practicalbioethics.org
    http://www.practicalbioethics.org

14. **National Center for Bioethics in Research & Health Care**
    Tuskegee University
    44-107
    Tuskegee, AL 36088
    Phone: (334) 724-4554
    Fax: (334) 727-7221
    http://www.tuskegee.edu

15. **The Bioethics Center**
    Brody School of Medicine at East Carolina
        University
    University Health Systems of East Carolina
    Greenville, North Carolina 27858-4354
    Phone: (252) 744-2361
    http://www.ecu.edu/bioethics/

16. **The Johns Hopkins Berman Institute of Bioethics**
    Johns Hopkins University
    100 North Charles Street, Suite 740
    Baltimore, MD 21201
    Phone: (410) 516-8500
    Fax: (410) 516-8504
    http://www.hopkinsmedicine.org/bioethics/
        contact.html

17. **The Hastings Center**
    21 Malcolm Gordon Road
    Garrison, NY 10524-4125
    Phone: (845) 424-4040
    Fax: (845) 424-4545
    www.thehastingscenter.org

REFERENCES

Beauchamp, T., & Childress, J. (2001). *Principles of biomedical ethics* (5th ed.). New York: Oxford University Press.

Berggren, V., Bergstrom, S., & Edberg, A. K. (2006). Being different and vulnerable: Experiences of immigrant African women who have been circumcised and sought maternity care in Sweden. *Journal of Transcultural Nursing, 17* (1), 50–57.

Bloch, S., & Green, S. A. (2006). An ethical framework for psychiatry. *British Journal of Psychiatry, 188*(1), 7–12.

Caldicott, C. V., & Faber-Langendoen, K. (2005). Deception, discrimination and fear of reprisal: Lessons in ethics from third-year medical students. *Academic Medicine, 80*(9), 866–873.

Crandall, S. J., George, G., Marion, G. S., & Davis, S. (2003). Applying theory to the design of cultural competency training for medical students: A case study. *Academic Medicine, 78,* 588–594.

Engelhardt, H. T. (2005). Critical care: Why there is no global bioethics. *Current Opinion in Critical Care, 11*(6), 605–609.

Fernandez, A., Schillinger, D., Grumbach, K., Rosenthal, A., Stewart, A. L., Wang, F., et al. (2004). Physician language ability and cultural competence: An exploratory study of communication with Spanish-speaking patients. *Journal of General Internal Medicine, 19,* 167–174.

Foley, R., & Wurmser, T. A. (2004). Culture diversity/A mobile workforce command creative leadership, new partnerships, and innovative approaches to integration. *Nursing Administration Quarterly, 28*(2), 122–128.

Geertz, C. (1973). *Interpretation of cultures.* New York: Basic Books.

Harrison, E., & Falco, S. (2005). Health disparity and the nurse advocate: Reaching out to alleviate suffering. *Advances in Nursing Science, 28*(3), 252–264.

Health Canada. (2001, October, 11). *Achieving health for all: A framework for health promotion.* Retrieved November 23, 2001, from http://www.hc-sc.gc.ca/hcs-sss/pubs/care-soins/2001-frame-plan-promotion/index_e.html

Institute of Medicine. (2002). *Unequal treatment: Confronting racial and ethnic disparities in health care.* Washington, DC: National Academy of Medicine.

Kagawa-Singer, M., & Kassim-Lakha, S. (2003). A strategy to reduce cross-cultural miscommunication and increase likelihood of improving health outcomes. *Academic Medicine, 78*(6), 577–587.

Leininger, M. M., & McFarland, M. R. (2002). *Transcultural nursing concepts, theories, research and practice.* NY: McGraw-Hill.

Leininger, M. M., & McFarland, M. R. (2006). *Culture care diversity and universality: A worldwide nursing theory* (2nd ed.). Boston, MA: Jones and Bartlett.

Lovejoy, A. O. (1974). *The great chain of being.* Cambridge, MA: Harvard University Press.

Office of Minority Health. (2001). *National Standards on Culturally and Linguistically Appropriate Services (CLAS) in Health Care (Final Report).* Washington, DC: Author. Retrieved from http://www.omhrc.gov/assets/pdf/checked/finalreport.pdf

Paasche-Orlow, M. (2004). The ethics of cultural competence. *Academic Medicine, 79*(4), 347–350.

Pacquiao, D. F. (2001). Addressing cultural incongruities of advance directives. *Bioethics Forum, 17*(1), 27–31.

Shweder, R. A. (1997). Anthropology's romantic rebellion against the enlightenment, or there's more to thinking than reason and evidence. In R. A. Shweder & R. A. LeVine (Eds.), *Culture theory: Essays on mind, self and emotion* (pp. 27–66). Cambridge, UK: Cambridge University Press.

Shweder, R. A., & Bourne, E. J. (1997). Does the concept of the person vary cross-culturally? In R. A. Shweder & R. A. LeVine (Eds.), *Culture theory: Essays on mind, self and emotion* (pp. 158–199). Cambridge, UK: Cambridge University Press.

Trevalon, M., & Murray-Garcia, J. (1998). Cultural humility versus cultural competence: A critical distinction in defining physician training outcomes in multicultural education. *Journal of Health Care for the Poor and Underserved, 9,* 117–126.

U.S. Department of Health and Human Services. (2000). *Healthy People 2010, Volume II.* Washington, DC: U.S. Government Printing Office.

Valente, S. M. (2004). End of life and ethnicity. *Journal of Nurses in Staff Development, 20*(6), 285–293.

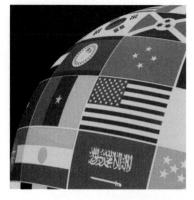

CHAPTER 16

Perspectives on International Nursing

Paula Herberg

LEARNING OBJECTIVES

1. Identify health issues from a global perspective (Millennium Development Goals).
2. Outline the services provided by international health/development aid organizations.
3. Discuss the role of international nursing and midwifery services.
4. Identify the parameters and challenges of international nursing as a career specialty.
5. Identify ways that nurses can prepare for international nursing.
6. Explore criteria for nurses to consider when choosing an international "sending" agency.
7. Identify selected health care agencies that send U.S. and Canadian nurses abroad.

Throughout this text, the emphasis has been largely on U.S. and Canadian cultures and subcultures. This chapter will provide a more global perspective and focus on the work that is done in the international arena to promote human development and health. The chapter will highlight the field of international nursing and the ways in which nurses from the United States and Canada can contribute to the global efforts to improve the health status of the world's peoples.

Health as a Global Concern

According to the International Council of Nurses (ICN, 2003), 30,000 children die each day from preventable diseases. The global toll from infectious diseases, malnutrition, and other effects of poverty and environmental pollutants is staggering. New forms of deadly viruses are discovered with seeming regularity, and health workers are not immune from contagion. (See Research

Application 16-1 for a study on African nurses who cared for Ebola victims.)

Health and illness statistics can only show a cross section of the real magnitude of the global disease burden. These statistics are readily available from reliable sources such as the United Nations (UN) (www.UN.org), the Centers for Disease Control and Prevention (CDC) (www.cdc.gov), the World Health Organization (WHO, 2007a) (www.who.org), and others. Using current WHO (2006a; 2006b) data, the following is a snapshot of global health concerns:

- Approximately 5 million people die from AIDS-related causes, including tuberculosis (TB), every year. By some estimates, 11 of every 1,000 adults age 15–49 worldwide is HIV infected. Globally, an estimated 13 million children under age 15 have lost one or both parents to AIDS.
- More than 150 million children under age 5 in the developing world are malnourished, including almost half the children in southern Asia.
- In 2002, there were 815 million hungry people in the developing world.
- More than 10 million children under age 5 die annually from six major causes: pneumonia, diarrhea, malaria, measles, neonatal pneumonia, preterm delivery, and asphyxia at birth.
- More than 500,000 women die each year from pregnancy-related causes. In 2002, 50% of the deaths were in Africa, 45% in Asia, 4% in Latin America, and less than 1% in more developed areas.
- Estimates of the number of cases of acute malaria are as high as 500 million. Young children living in sub-Saharan Africa account for 80% of malaria deaths (1–2 million annually).
- TB kills more than 1.7 million people a year. An estimated 8.8 million new cases were identified in 2003.
- In 2002, 1.1 billion people (one-sixth of the world's population) lacked access to safe drinking water. Sharp disparities are seen in access to sanitation between urban and rural areas.

Millennium Development Goals

In September 2000, world leaders met at the Millennium Summit and adopted the *UN Millennium Declaration*, endorsed by 189 countries (UN, 2006). The intent of the declaration was outlined in the identification of **Millennium Development Goals** (MDGs), to be reached by 2015. The MDGs represent commitments from governments to tackle and reduce poverty, hunger, ill health, and other inequalities.

The MDGs were set out as realistic, attainable goals aimed at relieving the worst of human suffering, including the overarching goal of cutting poverty in half. The MDGs served as a catalyst for change and began a process focused on improving living conditions for millions of people around the globe. The MDGs were based on the recognition that nations could assist each other through trade, **development aid**, debt relief, access to essential drugs, and technology transfer. Box 16-1 shows eight individual goals that were identified.

One important aspect of the MDGs is that they are not mutually exclusive. The MDGs emphasize that positive global development relies as much on health and education as on economic growth. Each of the MDGs has identified targets (16 in total) and indicators (48) that can be measured over time. As such, they serve as a blueprint for sustainable development and provide concrete measures of success and failure in each area. Of the MDGs, six focus specifically on health areas, and this includes nine targets and 17 indicators directly measuring health-related outcomes (see Table 16-1).

In 2002, the UN secretary-general commissioned the Millennium Project to develop an action plan to achieve the MDGs. This was headed by Professor Jeffrey Sachs and culminated in the 2005 report *Investing in Development: A Practical Plan to Achieve the Millennium Development Goals*. Work is now underway to provide

RESEARCH APPLICATION 16-1
Nursing During an Ebola Outbreak in Central Africa

Hewlett, B. L., & Hewlett, B. S. (2005). Providing care and facing death: Nursing during an Ebola outbreak in Central Africa. *Journal of Transcultural Nursing, 16*(4), 289-297.

Little research has been done to examine the experiences of nurses who work during outbreaks of deadly epidemics. In 1995, 2000, and again in 2003, outbreaks of Ebola hemorrhagic fever (EHF), one of the deadliest known viruses on Earth, occurred in Central Africa (Republic of the Congo and Uganda). Some of the earliest victims of Ebola were nurses. In the Democratic Republic of the Congo, approximately 20% of those who died were health care professionals. In Uganda, of the 224 victims, 14 were nurses.

This study used open-ended and semistructured interviews with individual nurses and small groups during the outbreaks in Uganda and the Republic of Congo in 2003. Three key themes emerged: (1) lack of protective gear, basic equipment, and other resources needed to provide care; (2) stigmatization by family, coworkers, and community; and (3) exceptional commitment to the nursing profession, even in the context of placing their own lives in jeopardy:

> My children were afraid of me, they were afraid to touch me. I wanted to quit, but I knew that if I quit all the others would want to quit. My husband was afraid and feared me.... We ate on separate plates and used separate silverware.

> —Ugandan Nurse (Hewlett & Hewlett, 2005, p. 289)

Clinical Application

The major themes identified by nurses in this study are present, to some degree, at all times when nurses work in areas where communicable diseases run rampant and unknown dangers in the environment exist, whether that is in rural villages or urban slums. Resources are generally always lacking. Stigmatization, discrimination, and folk beliefs and attitudes are prevalent, not only concerning Ebola, but also HIV and other infectious disease processes. During times of epidemics, health care workers, including nurses, often risk their own lives to provide care. This study provides insights into the experiences of nurses during such times. It highlights the need to understand the cultural models of illness: "Often health educators, and local, national, and international medical personnel were not aware or did not consider the possibility that existing traditional beliefs and practices actually contribute to EHF control efforts" (Hewlett & Hewlett, 2005, pp. 292-293).

This research demonstrates the potential benefit of indigenous cultural models and asks that international teams listen more closely to local nurses and communities. It points out the reality of permeable national and international borders with regards to newly emerging infectious diseases (Severe Acute Respiratory Syndrome [SARS] and bird flu, to name just two) and the globalization of diseases. What happens in a remote African village or Asian town cannot be ignored. The study provides some valuable lessons in how to deal more effectively with infection control.

needs assessments and identify baseline measures for each indicator in all countries, rich and poor. In 2004, Millennium Project personnel, in conjunction with the UN, selected "pilot countries" to help identify best practices for incorporating MDG targets and time lines into national strategies for poverty reduction. These pilot countries (Dominican Republic, Ethiopia,

Millennium Development Goals

Millennium Development Goals

MDG 1   Eradicate Extreme Poverty and Hunger
MDG 2   Achieve Universal Primary Education
MDG 3   Promote Gender Equity and Empower
        Women
MDG 4   Reduce Child Mortality
MDG 5   Improve Maternal Health
MDG 6   Combat HIV/AIDS, Malaria, and Other
        Diseases
MDG 7   Ensure Environmental Sustainability
MDG 8   Develop a Global Partnership for
        Development

Ghana, Kenya, Senegal, Tajikistan, and Yemen) will serve as models for other developing countries throughout the world (UN, 2006).

Five years after the identification of the MDGs, the World Economic Forum (2005) published a progress report on the success and failures of the world body to implement needed changes to reach MDG targets. This report card, based on a 10-point scale (10=target achieved), indicated the following:

Peace and Security	3/10
Poverty	5/10
Hunger	4/10
Education	4/10
Health	5/10

TABLE 16-1 Health in the Millennium Development Goals

MDG	Health Targets (by 2015)	Health Indicators
1. Eradicate poverty and hunger	1. Halve the proportion of people whose income is less than U.S. $1.00/day; 2. Halve the proportion of people who suffer from hunger	■ Prevalence of underweight children (< 5 y/o) ■ Proportion of population below minimum level of dietary energy consumption
4. Reduce child mortality	5. Reduce the under-5 mortality rate by two-thirds	■ Under-5 mortality rate ■ Infant mortality rate ■ Proportion of 1-year-olds immunized against measles
5. Improve maternal health	6. Reduce the maternal mortality ratio by three-quarters	■ Maternal mortality ratio ■ Proportion of births attended by skilled health personnel
6. Combat HIV/AIDS, malaria, and other diseases	7. Have halted and begun to reverse the spread of HIV/AIDS	■ HIV prevalence among young pregnant women (15–24 y/o) ■ Condom use rate of contraceptive prevalence rate ■ Ratio of school attendance by orphans vs. non-orphans aged 10–14 years
	8. Have halted and begun to reverse the incidence of malaria and other major diseases	■ Prevalence and death rates associated with malaria ■ Proportion of population using effective antimalaria prevention/treatment measures ■ TB prevalence and mortality rates ■ Proportion of TB cases detected and cured under DOTS (directly observed treatment short-course)

(Continued on following page)

TABLE 16-1 *Health in the Millennium Development Goals (continued)*		
MDG	**Health Targets (by 2015)**	**Health Indicators**
7. Ensure environmental sustainability	10. Halve the proportion of people without sustainable access to safe drinking water and sanitation	■ Proportion of population with sustainable access to improved water source, urban and rural
	11. By 2020, achieve a significant improvement in the lives of at least 100-million slum dwellers	■ Proportion of population with access to improved sanitation, urban and rural
8. Global partnership for development	17. In cooperation with pharmaceutical companies, provide access to affordable, essential drugs in developing countries	■ Proportion of population with sustainable access to affordable essential drugs

Modified from the World Health Organization. (2006). *Health in the Millennium Development Goals.* Retrieved January 2006 from http://www.who.int/mdg/goals/en/print.html

Environment	2/10
Human Rights	2/10

Reporting specifically on health, the report stated that "although the world did marginally better in 2005 than in 2004, moving from a score of 4 to 5, it remains far off the track on all its health goals" (p. 22).

Responding to Global Needs for Health, Development, and Humanitarian Assistance

Governments around the globe take the responsibility for meeting the needs of their citizens and responding to the best of their abilities. In some cases, however, outside assistance is beneficial to support or enhance the efforts of individual governments and to coordinate a global response to common concerns when needed. This has been the case in fields such as health, education, and humanitarian assistance.

In many instances, nurses participate in emergency relief work following natural disasters or volunteer their time for direct patient care services (operating room, clinics, etc.). These tend to be short term, isolated, or intermittent assignments, not taking the place of the nurses' usual employment. In other cases, nurses are involved in long-term "development" work at the systems level (sometimes referred to as *capacity building*), which often involves needs assessments, strategic planning, mentoring and education, policy discussions, financial analysis, and work with professional bodies inside the country to strengthen the ability of that sector (health care delivery, nursing education, regulatory bodies, for example) to perform. This is often a career choice that demands learning a new, development-oriented vocabulary and knowledge and/or skills.

There are several ways to categorize external assistance efforts. In this chapter, we will look at four categories. The first category, and one of the most widely used, is the *international* or *intergovernmental organizations* category. This is sometimes referred to as "multilateral aid." The second category contains the numerous *nongovernmental organizations(NGOs)* that work at international, national, and local levels around the globe. The third category represents *national government aid agencies* (also called "bilateral agencies") that provide humanitarian aid and assistance (such as the United States Agency for International Development [USAID]). The fourth category includes *professional organizations* that are international in scope. A list of major **development aid organizations** is shown in Box 16–2.

BOX 16-2

List of Development Aid Organizations

Major Government Aid/Donor Agencies

- Australia—Australian Agency for International Development (AusAID)
- Canada—Canadian International Development Agency (CIDA) and International Development Research Centre (IDRC)
- Denmark—Ministry of Foreign Affairs: Development Policy Section
- European Union—European Commission: Development Directorate-General
- France—Department for International Cooperation and French Development Agency (AfD)
- Germany—Deutsche Gesellschaft für Technische Zusammenarbeit (GTZ)
- Italy—Ministry of Foreign Affairs: Italian Development Cooperation Program
- Japan—Japan International Cooperation Agency (JICA)
- New Zealand—New Zealand Agency for International Development (NZAid)
- Norway—Ministry of Foreign Affairs: International Development Program and Norwegian Agency for Development Cooperation (NORAD)
- Spain—Spanish Agency for International Cooperation (AECI)
- Sweden—Sida
- Switzerland—Swiss Agency for Development Cooperation (SDC)
- United Kingdom—Department for International Development (DFID)
- United States—United States Agency for International Development (USAID) and the Peace Corps

Major Intergovernmental Organizations

- African Development Bank
- Asian Development Bank (ADB)
- European Bank for Reconstruction and Development
- Inter-American Development Bank
- International Bank for Reconstruction and Development (IBRD: The World Bank)

- International Fund for Agricultural Development (IFAD)
- International Monetary Fund (IMF)
- International Organization for Migration (IOM)
- Organization for Economic Cooperation and Development (OECD)
- United Nations (UN)
  - United Nations Children's Fund (UNICEF)
  - United Nations Development Program (UNDP)
  - United Nations Environment Programme (UNEP)
  - United Nations High Commissioner for Refugees (UNHCR)
  - World Food Program (WFP)
- World Health Organization (WHO)
  - Pan American Health Organization (PAHO)
- World Trade Organization (WTO)

Major Nongovernmental Organizations (NGOs)

- Amnesty, International
- CARE, Inc.
- Catholic Relief Services
- Council of World Churches
- Inter*Action*
- International Committee of the Red Cross (ICRC)
- International Rescue Committee (IRC)
- Joint Commission International
- Médécins Sans Frontières/Doctors Without Borders
- Mercy Corps
- Oxfam International
- Project HOPE (Health Opportunities for People Everywhere)
- Relief International
- Save the Children
- Voluntary Services Overseas
- World Vision

Professional Organizations

- International Council of Nurses
- Sigma Theta Tau International Honor Society of Nursing

Intergovernmental Organizations

Some organizations, which espouse common aims of international significance, are formed by member states (governments) through treaties or charters. Such treaties allow the organization to establish its own operating systems and governing mechanisms. Probably the best-known international organizations are the United Nations (UN) and the North Atlantic Treaty Organization (NATO).

The United Nations

In 1945, representatives of 50 countries met in San Francisco to develop a UN Charter. The UN was initiated on October 24, 1945, when the charter was ratified by a majority of countries, including China, France, the Soviet Union, the United Kingdom, and the United States. The purposes of the UN are to (1) maintain international peace and security, (2) develop friendly relations among nations, (3) cooperate in solving international economic, social, cultural, and humanitarian problems, 4) promote respect for human rights and fundamental freedoms, and 5) serve as a center for harmonizing the actions of nations in attaining these ends (UN, 2007a).

The UN is made up of six principal units: the General Assembly, Security Council, Economic and Social Council, Trusteeship Council, International Court of Justice, and Secretariat. The total UN institution, however, is much larger and contains 15 separate agencies and other individual programs or bodies. UN agencies offer several types of assistance.

Emergency Relief

The UN began relief operations in Europe following World War II (WWII) and continues to be a major provider of humanitarian relief operations worldwide. The UN has been recognized internationally as taking a lead role in responding to natural and man-made disasters by providing emergency relief and assistance where needed. In the last decade, civil wars have become a major cause of emergency situations. When natural disasters (floods, droughts, earthquakes) are added to the equation, emergencies affect millions of people and cause billions of dollars of damage. Unfortunately more than 90% (UN, 2006) of all disaster victims live in developing countries, where poverty and poorly developed infrastructures compound the problems.

Humanitarian Assistance

When needed, the UN is often among the first to offer humanitarian assistance. In one year alone, the UN raised more than $ 1.4 billion to assist 35 million people in 16 countries and regions (UN, 2006). The **UN High Commissioner for Refugees** (UNHCR) provides international assistance to more than 22 million refugees and displaced persons. The World Food Program delivers one-third of the world's emergency food assistance.

Prevention

The role of prevention in reducing the vulnerability of nations to disasters is another important activity of the UN. This includes developing early warning and detection systems and assisting disaster-prone countries to carry out contingency planning and preparedness measures. The **United Nations Development Program** (UNDP) is the primary agency for this activity. Headquartered in New York City, the UNDP is the UN's global development network. It publishes an annual Human Development Report available from the UNDP Web site (UNDP, 2006).

UN Volunteers

In 1970 the General Assembly created the UN Volunteers program to help implement development work requested by various member states. The UN Volunteers program reports to the UNDP through country offices worldwide. More than 30,000 UN volunteers have supported humanitarian peace, relief, and development operations in more than 166 countries since 1971 (UN, 2007b). If you are interested in more information about becoming a UN volunteer, check the Web site at http://www.unvolunteers.org/

The World Health Organization

The **World Health Organization (WHO)** is a part of the UN family and serves as the specialized agency for health. It was established in 1948 with the goal of promoting the attainment of the highest possible level of health by all peoples. In 1978, WHO changed the nature of the debate about "health" when it issued its now classic Alma-Ata declaration, defining health as "a state of complete physical, mental and social well-being and not merely the absence of disease or infirmity" (WHO, Regional Office for Europe, 2006). WHO is governed through the World Health Assembly (WHA), which convenes annually in Geneva, Switzerland, and contains 192 member states.

WHO has numerous branches and services. Its headquarters are in Geneva, Switzerland, and it convenes the WHA annually to discuss policy and other matters. Official delegations from around the world gather in Geneva for deliberations. Global nursing issues are often on the agenda. In fact, there is a dedicated WHO branch for Nursing and Midwifery Services (WHO, 2007b).

Nursing and Midwifery Services

The nursing and midwifery team at WHO headquarters is responsible for coordinating efforts across member countries. It links across WHO technical programs worldwide and coordinates common efforts with WHO regional and country offices, where WHO nurse advisors often reside. WHO has long focused its attention on the global status of nursing and midwifery. It has been a major agenda item throughout the 1990s and into the new millennium, as recently as 2003. WHO recognizes that nursing and midwifery services are vital to obtaining desired health outcomes and urges member states to give them priority attention. To this end, WHO has issued several resolutions on strengthening nursing and midwifery services to member states by (1) providing policy and technical advice, (2) facilitating capacity building and collaboration, and (3) supporting the enhancement of systems that generate evidence for decision making.

A recent WHO (2002) publication, *Nursing and Midwifery Services: Strategic Directions 2002–2008*, identifies five key areas for intervention: (1) human resource planning, (2) management of personnel, (3) evidence-based practice, (4) education, and (5) stewardship. The document addresses WHA Resolution 54.12, *Strengthening Nursing and Midwifery* (WHO, 2001) which promotes the achievement of WHO's health objectives as well as the UN MDGs.

The Pan American Health Organization

The **Pan American Health Organization (PAHO)** (2007) is a member of the UN system and serves as the Regional Office for the Americas of the WHO. PAHO has worked for more than 100 years as an international public health agency, improving the health and living standards of the countries of the Americas (includes the Caribbean, Central and South America, and the United States).

United Nations Children's Fund

The United Nations Children's Fund (UNICEF, 2007) works in more than 157 countries and employs more than 7,000 people. Its primary aim is to promote the rights of children and to overcome obstacles such as poverty, violence, disease, and discrimination (UNICEF, 2006). UNICEF focuses on (1) girls' education; (2) immunizations; (3) prevention and treatment of HIV/AIDS among young children and their families; (4) creation of protective environments for children to avoid abuse, violence, and exploitation; and (5) prevention of discrimination, against women and girls in particular.

Nongovernmental Organizations (NGOs)

Nongovernmental organizations (NGOs) are usually established by groups of individuals or associations as private enterprises. Nongovernmental organizations may be professional associations, foundations, multinational businesses, or simply groups with a common interest in humanitarian assistance activities (development and relief). They are not mandated by government agreements or charters. Many NGOs play an important role in the international health and development arena by virtue of the services they provide. However, they are not usually given any official governmental status. NGOs can be established at the local, regional, national, or international level. They can have secular or religious affiliations. The best-known NGO (actually an NGO hybrid) is probably the International Committee of the Red Cross (ICRC). Other well-known examples include Médécins Sans Frontières, Amnesty International, Save the Children, World Vision, and CARE, Inc. The following section contains a sampling of well-known NGOs.

International Committee of the Red Cross (ICRC) and International Federation of Red Cross and Red Crescent Societies

The International Committee of the Red Cross (ICRC) was established in 1863 as a humanitarian organization whose mission was to aid the victims of war and other internal violence. Today it is recognized as a major international relief organization. The ICRC includes the International Federation of Red Cross and Red Crescent Societies (2007), with 183 member states. The ICRC is a private association formed under the Swiss Civil Code but not mandated by governments. It is based on international law, specifically the Geneva Conventions and is recognized as having an "international legal status" (ICRC, 2007) unlike other NGOs. Therefore, it enjoys

certain privileges and immunities similar to those of UN agencies.

The federation's mission is *to improve the lives of vulnerable people* and focuses on four core areas: promoting humanitarian values, disaster relief, disaster preparedness, and community health. ICRC often deals with victims of natural disasters, poverty brought about by socioeconomic crises, and refugees.

Catholic Relief Services

Catholic Relief Services (CRS) was founded in 1943 by the Catholic bishops of the United States. They work in more than 90 countries to assist the poor and disadvantaged, alleviate suffering, and foster charity and justice as part of their faith-based mission. As the official international relief and development agency of the U.S. Catholic community, CRS is also committed to educating U.S. citizens to fulfill their moral responsibilities toward their global neighbors by helping the poor, working to remove the causes of poverty, and promoting social justice (Catholic Relief Services, 2006).

CARE, Inc.

CARE works with poor communities in more than 70 countries around the world to find lasting solutions to poverty. With a broad range of programs based on empowerment, equity, and sustainability, CARE seeks to facilitate change through (1) strengthening capacity for self-help, (2) providing economic opportunities, (3) delivering emergency relief, (4) influencing policy decisions at national and local levels, and (5) addressing discrimination in all its forms (CARE, 2007). CARE is one of the world's largest private international humanitarian organizations, which was founded in 1945 to provide relief to survivors of WWII. CARE programs are community based in areas such as education, health care, and economic development and use a combination of skills training, provision of resources, and knowledge building. Program areas include

- Agriculture and natural resources
- Education
- Emergency relief
- Health
- HIV/AIDS
- Nutrition
- Small economic activity development
- Water, sanitation, and environmental health

Project HOPE

The name Health Opportunities for People Everywhere (HOPE) is reflected in its mission: to achieve sustainable advances in health care around the world by implementing health education programs and providing humanitarian assistance in areas of need (Project HOPE, 2007). Initiated in 1958 as the S.S. HOPE, the world's first peacetime hospital ship, Project HOPE now conducts land-based training and health care education programs on five continents, including North America. More than 5,000 health care professionals and volunteer educators have worked for HOPE. It now provides approximately 100 million worth of resources to 20–30 countries each year. Project HOPE programs focus on

- Infectious disease: AIDS and TB
- Women's and children's health
- Health professional education (training of trainers)
- Health systems and facilities
- Humanitarian assistance

Oxfam International

Oxfam was founded in 1995 by a group of like-minded independent nongovernmental organizations that wanted to work together internationally to achieve greater impact in reducing poverty by their collective efforts (Oxfam, 2006). The name "Oxfam" comes from the Oxford Committee for Famine Relief, founded in Britain during WWII. Oxfam International is a confederation of 12 organizations based in Australia, Belgium, Canada, Germany, Great Britain, Hong Kong, Ireland, the Netherlands, New Zealand, Spain, and the United States who work together with over 3,000 partners in more than 100 countries to find lasting solutions to poverty, suffering, and injustice. Oxfam programs undertake

- Long term development
- Emergency work
- Research and lobbying
- Campaigning, alliance building, and media work

Save the Children

Save the Children was formed in 1932 by a group of concerned U.S. citizens reacting to the plight of Appalachia during the Depression. Today it is one of the leading international relief and development organizations (an alliance composed of 27 national Save the Children organizations) promoting the well-being of children and works in more than 100 countries. Save the Children works on the principle of self-sufficiency and helps families define and solve problems faced by children in their communities (Save the Children, 2007).

Doctors Without Borders/Médécins Sans Frontières (MSF)

MSF works in more than 70 countries to deliver emergency aid to those affected by armed conflict, disease, disasters, and other forms of exclusion from health care. It is an independent medical humanitarian organization founded in 1971. MSF consists of an international network with sections in 19 countries (MSF, 2007).

MSF is often one of the first to respond at the scene of an emergency (Lau, 2005). MSF volunteers (doctors, nurses, logisticians, water-and-sanitation experts, administrators, and other medical and nonmedical professionals) often work in very remote and/or dangerous parts of the world (Nestrell, 2004). They are available on short notice, usually dedicating 6 to 12 months to each assignment. MSF teams are composed of international volunteers and skilled local staff. Together, they work closely with national medical professionals, cooperate with other aid organizations, and carry out more than 3,800 aid missions annually.

Mercy Corps

Since 1979, Mercy Corps has provided more than $1 billion in assistance to people in 81 nations. Mercy Corps is a nonprofit organization with headquarters in Portland; Seattle; Cambridge; Washington, DC; and Edinburgh, Scotland. The agency's programs currently reach 7 million people in more than 35 countries (Mercy Corps, 2007). The organization was founded as Save the Refugees Fund, in response to the plight of Cambodian refugees fleeing the famine, war, and genocide of the "Killing Fields."

Mercy Corps pursues its mission through emergency relief services, sustainable economic development, and civil society initiatives. Mercy Corps has played an important role in responding to the massive tragedy of the Indian Ocean tsunami, war in Afghanistan, massive food shortages in North Korea, ethnic conflict in the Balkans, and economic transitions in Central Asia and the Caucasus.

World Vision

World Vision (2007) is a Christian relief and development organization dedicated to helping children and their communities worldwide by tackling the causes of poverty. The organization began in the 1950s working with orphaned children in the Korean War.

The program expanded into other Asian countries and eventually into Latin America, Africa, Eastern Europe, and the Middle East. In the 1960s, World Vision expanded its global relief efforts to people suffering from natural disasters.

By the 1970s, the organization had incorporated vocational and agricultural training for families into its efforts to promote self-sustainable change.

In 1990, World Vision began addressing the urgent needs of children orphaned by AIDS in Uganda and quickly expanded operations to other hard-hit African countries. By 2004, nearly 300,000 orphans and vulnerable children had been sponsored in AIDS-affected communities.

International Rescue Committee

Founded in 1933, the International Rescue Committee (IRC, 2007) is at work in 25 countries and is a global leader in emergency relief, rehabilitation, postconflict development, and resettlement services (IRC, 2006). The IRC delivers lifesaving aid in emergencies, helps those uprooted by war and fleeing from persecution, cares for war-traumatized children, and rehabilitates environmental and health care systems. IRC supports capacity building endeavors with local schools, organizations, and civil governments.

IRC is known for its work with refugees, providing emergency assistance: water, food, shelter, sanitation, and medical care in the immediate crisis, and then working with people to rebuild their lives by providing education, training, and economic assistance. IRC also helps thousands of refugees in the resettlement process in the United States.

Governmental Organizations

United States Agency for International Development (USAID)

In 1961, President John F. Kennedy signed into law the Foreign Assistance Act and thereby created the USAID. The United States has a long history of assisting others around the globe to overcome the effects of poverty, natural disasters, and oppression. USAID has its roots in the Marshall Plan reconstruction of Europe following

WWII and in President Harry Truman's Point Four Program. U.S. foreign assistance serves two purposes: furthering America's foreign policy and improving the lives of peoples in the developing world (USAID, 2007).

USAID is an independent agency of the federal government that receives guidance from the secretary of state. Spending less than one-half of 1% of the federal budget, USAID works around the world to achieve its goals in three areas: (1) economic growth, agriculture, and trade; (2) global health; and (3) democracy, conflict prevention, and humanitarian assistance. Assistance support is carried out in four global regions: sub-Saharan Africa, Asia and the Near East, Latin America and the Caribbean, and Europe and Eurasia.

USAID is located in Washington, DC, with field offices around the globe. The agency works in close partnerships with more than 300 U.S.-based private voluntary organizations, indigenous associations, colleges and universities, more than 3,500 American business companies, international NGOs, other governments, and other U.S. government bodies.

The Peace Corps

The Peace Corps was initiated in 1960, when then-Senator John F. Kennedy, in a speech to University of Michigan students, challenged them to spend 2 years serving their country in the cause of peace by living and working in developing countries. From that inspiration emerged the Peace Corps (Peace Corps, 2006). Since that time, more than 182,000 Peace Corps volunteers have worked in over 138 host countries on issues ranging from AIDS education, information technology, and environmental preservation.

The Peace Corps' mission is threefold: (1) helping interested countries meet their needs for trained personnel, (2) helping promote better understanding of Americans by others; and (3) helping to promote a better understanding of other peoples by all Americans. Today the Peace Corp continues to expand into new countries,

such as East Timor, and into new fields, such as information technology. In 2003, more than 1,000 new volunteers were included in President Bush's HIV/AIDS Act.

The Centers for Disease Control and Prevention (CDC)

The CDC started in 1946 as a malaria control agency. Today it is one of 13 major branches of the U.S. Department of Health and Human Services (CDC, 2007). The U.S. Department of Health and Human Services is the agency responsible for protecting the health and safety of all Americans and providing essential human services where needed. CDC is at the forefront of the nation's public health efforts. The CDC's work is often carried out in the field, involving national and international travel, collecting data, and developing strategic plans for intervention. It is recognized globally for its role in researching and investigating outbreaks of infectious disease and its action-oriented approach to control. The CDC also carries out educational campaigns on health and safety measures for the general public.

Canadian International Development Agency (CIDA)

The Canadian International Development Agency is a part of the Canadian government and administers foreign aid programs in developing countries (CIDA, 2007). It reports to the Canadian Parliament through the Minister for International Cooperation. CIDA's mission is to support sustainable development and reduce poverty in developing countries in order to promote a more equitable and prosperous world. CIDA works with other Canadian organizations, public and private, as well as other international organizations. Priorities identified focus on social development programs such as the treatment of sexually transmitted infections (STIs) in third-world countries; basic education and child protection, especially for girls; economic and environmental sustainability; programs that benefit women directly; and systems of good governance.

Professional Organizations

The International Council of Nurses

The **International Council of Nurses** (ICN) is an independent, nongovernmental federation of national nurses' associations representing more than 128 countries. Its headquarters are in Geneva, Switzerland. Founded in 1899, ICN is the oldest international professional organization in the health care field. The ICN works either through its own projects or in collaboration with other international organizations to promote health services. It encourages efforts by national nurses' associations to develop nursing standards and advance the economic position of nurses (ICN, 2007). ICN promotes its objectives through standard-setting programs, seminars, publications, and meetings. The official publication of the ICN is the *International Nursing Review*.

International organizations, notably WHO and UNICEF, work closely with the ICN on matters affecting health in all parts of the world. For example, ICN and WHO have issued a joint declaration on AIDS, dealing with the rights and responsibilities of nurses worldwide in caring for people infected with this disease. ICN also has worked with WHO to increase nurses' awareness and knowledge of the problems related to substance abuse and help nurses provide care for patients with addictions. The organization is active in such UN initiatives as Safe Motherhood and Occupational Health. ICN is involved with the UN Millennium Project and issued a comprehensive report, *Tackling the UN Millennium Development Goals* in 2003.

ICN advances the cause of nursing and nurses worldwide. It is particularly effective in the areas of professional practice, regulation, education, and socioeconomic welfare. ICN has pioneered an international classification of nursing practice—ICNP and the Leadership for Change Program. The ICN *Code for Nurses* has shaped the ethical practice of nursing in many countries throughout the world. ICN also provides a series of fact sheets for quick reference on a number of topics of interest to current health and social matters. Readers are encouraged to visit the ICN Web site at www.icn.ch

The World's Nurses

Although there is little global statistical information on nursing or midwifery personnel because of classification problems and lack of established information systems, it is widely accepted that there are insufficient nurses to care for the world's population. What is known is that the majority of nurses work in the developed world, and approximately one-quarter are in the United States. Although accepted benchmarks for nursing personnel (4–5 nurses per 1 physician) are reached in most Western countries, the ratio flattens in the developing world. In Pakistan, the nurse-to-physician ratio is reversed: 4–5 physicians for every nurse.

In addition to a lack of uniformity in classifying nursing and midwifery personnel, there are significant discrepancies in roles and functions, standards of performance, and quality of care by nurses in various parts of the world. The scope of practice for nurses varies widely from country to country. In parts of Africa and Asia, nurses may prescribe medications, perform some surgeries, suture wounds, and set fractured bones. In other places, they may not be allowed to take blood pressures or dress wounds. In yet other situations, nurses may consider bedside care (bathing and assisting with bedpans, for example) to be outside their realm of practice. In some cases apprenticeship training occurs, with on-the-job skill development and clinical instruction being supervised by staff nurses working on the unit.

Educational Preparation for Nurses

Each country has its own system of nursing education and career mobility. Curricula vary widely in content, length, standards, and evaluation criteria. General education required to enter the nursing program ranges from 6 to 13 years, and the length of the program varies from 1 to 4 years. There are general and specialty programs at the basic level of education. Specialization usually requires postbasic education. In some countries midwifery is a specialized field at the master's level; in others, it is the most basic level of preparation and is a stand-alone field, not connected to nursing.

Nurse Migration

Given the high demand for nursing services and the scarcity of nurses to meet that demand, it is not surprising that nurses are a mobile population. The important topic of foreign nurses migrating to the United States, United Kingdom, Australia, and Canada requires its own in-depth study and will not be covered in this chapter. The focus here is on U.S. and Canadian nurses who venture away from home.

Since the days of Florence Nightingale, highly trained nurses have traveled to all parts of the globe to practice their profession. Many young Englishwomen traveled to Germany for formal education as nurses. During the Crimean War, nurses traveled with Nightingale to Scutari to care for soldiers with battle wounds as well as infectious diseases such as cholera. Nightingale's hospital reforms reached from Europe to India (Nightingale, 1859). As early as 1867, graduates of the Saint Thomas Hospital Nursing School were found in Australia, Canada, Sweden, Germany, and most large hospitals in the United Kingdom and the United States.

North American Nurses Abroad

Early in the development of U.S. and Canadian nursing history, nurses prepared in the Nightingale tradition traveled abroad. In 1885 Linda Richards became the first U.S. nurse on record to engage in international nursing when she went to Japan under the auspices of the American Board of Missions to establish a school of nursing. Records from the Presbyterian Mission Board of Canada indicate that nurses were sent abroad more than 100 years ago, mainly to Taiwan, China, and India. The life of one exemplary missionary nurse, Ruth Harnar, is illustrated in Box 16–3.

Nurses in both the United States and Canada served in WWI and WWII. The MASH units of the Korean War are familiar to many through movies and television. With the creation of WHO in 1948 and the proliferation of technical assistance programs, nurses have become increasingly involved in international health. The ICRC has employed nurses as members of its relief teams for many years. In the 1960s with the establishment of USAID and CIDA, more funds became available for development, which expanded the number of health-related projects carried out. The demand for international nurses increased dramatically as agencies responded to the urgent health needs around the world. Today nurses have many opportunities to go abroad for the purposes of travel, research, education, consultation, and service in virtually all clinical practice specialty areas and administrative/management roles, as well as to assist in times of disaster relief. See Case Study 16–1 for a look at the realities of establishing and working in a refugee camp.

CASE STUDY 16-1 *Working in a Refugee Camp: A Personal Journey*

In early 1979 Cambodia's Khmer Rouge regime was overthrown, and amid the battles, hundreds of thousands of Cambodian citizens fled westwards toward the borders with Thailand and Laos. Before the end of the crisis, numerous camps and detention centers were established along these borders with the assistance of local governments, the UN High Commissioner for Refugees (UNHCR) and various international relief agencies.

By December, more than 150,000 refugees were being housed in Thailand. One of the first camps to open was Sa Kaeo, with an estimated population of about 30,000. These people arrived with only the clothes on their backs and handheld belongings. They were literally driven by truck from the border and dumped into the muddy fields of Sa Kaeo. The camp grew up around them. Many of these people were critically ill with malaria, diarrhea, kwashiorkor and other nutritional problems associated with months of starvation, respiratory diseases

BOX 16-3

Spotlight on Ruth May Harnar (1919–2004)

Dr. Ruth May Harnar[1], the daughter of missionaries, was born and reared in India. She knew at an early age she wanted to be a medical missionary and at age 12 began studying the Hindi language in earnest. She pursued her goal by completing her basic nursing education at Johns Hopkins University before returning to India in 1944, amid the chaos of WWII. She worked for the Division of Overseas Ministries of the Christian Church (Disciples of Christ). She returned to the United States to do her master's degree at the Frances Payne Bolton School of Nursing at Case Western Reserve University, graduating in 1952. In 1974 she completed her PhD in nursing education from Columbia University with a dissertation on the contributions made by church-based schools of nursing on nursing education in India.

Dr. Harnar devoted her life's work to helping educate Indian nurses and village health workers to serve community-based populations and in mission hospitals. She worked as nursing superintendent and acting director at Jackman Memorial Hospital in Bilaspur, India; as director of the graduate school for nurses at Indore, India; and in community health positions responsible for health assessments and immunization programs of approximately 1,200 school children annually. In 1947, Dr. Harnar and three Indian nurse colleagues served in the refugee camps that resulted from the partitioning of India and Pakistan when British rule ended.

Throughout her career, Dr. Harnar was known as a nurse educator. She developed a Hindi postgraduate syllabus approved by the India Nursing Council. She wrote curricula for nurses in training and administered final examinations throughout central India. She taught science and other subjects and helped organize a program of visual aids in the nursing schools and hospitals. In 1955 she made an extended trip to Nepal, where she worked in the medical and evangelistic programs of the United Church of Nepal. In the early 1970s, Dr. Harnar worked with the Voluntary Health Association of India in New Delhi, where she coauthored a curriculum for training village health workers and traveled throughout India to conduct

training sessions. This curriculum is still widely used throughout India and elsewhere in the region.

In the early 1980s, after retiring from the mission field, Dr. Harnar served as a visiting professor at the University of California, San Francisco (UCSF), School of Nursing, developing and teaching a new course in international nursing. In 1985 she moved to Geneva, Switzerland, to serve with the Christian Medical Commission of the World Council of Churches. In 1987, Dr. Harnar joined the faculty of the Aga Khan University in Karachi, Pakistan, to help develop a village health worker program and to assist in the startup of the Community Health Sciences (CHS) Department of the Medical College. She was responsible for the development and training of community health nurses and female health visitors for community-based health care programs in the poverty-stricken areas of Karachi in the rural Sindh province. Dr. Harnar's familiarity with South Asian culture and her fluency in Hindi/Urdu were of special importance in her work with staff, students, and community members. She also was a member of the initial planning team for the new RN to BSN program in the School of Nursing.

From 1992 until her death in November 2004, Dr. Harnar lived in a retirement community in Indianapolis, Indiana. She continued to be an active member of her church and shared her wealth of knowledge and experiences with the Nursing School at Indiana University. In 2002, the newly renovated nursing school building at Jackman Hospital in Bilaspur, India, was renamed the Jarvis and Harnar Nursing School.

In tribute to Dr. Harnar, John Bryant, former dean of the School of Public Health at Columbia University and a colleague at the Aga Khan University, said, "In the professional careers of those who work in the various corners of international health, one of the rich rewards is coming to know others who have dedicated their lives to enhancing the well-being of people who live in poverty and despair, to give them a chance for a life of health and dignity. Ruth Harnar was one of those precious persons who inspired us all and did so in joyful humility" (J. Bryant, personal communications, 2005).

[1]Thanks to the family and friends of Dr. Harnar for providing this information. Also, the Global Ministries *News* article on Dr. Harnar, retrieved August 4, 2005, from http://www.globalministries.org/news/harnar.htm

including TB and pneumonia, and infections caused by a variety of wounds. Pregnant women were numerous.

I arrived in Sa Kaeo at the beginning of November 1979 as part of a team of three nurses "loaned" by CARE, Inc., to the International Rescue Committee (IRC) to help establish the field hospital. I left by December 5th that same year. However, that 1 month at Sa Kaeo was one of the most grueling and rewarding experiences of my life.

The first night we were housed on the Thai border, and we slept on the floor of someone's house. We could hear the gun battles going on through the night. We made the 1-hour drive to the camp at sunrise the next morning and began what would become the customary process of checking in at the gate (as a military detention center, we all carried ID and had to cross a barbed-wire fence to enter the camp). Later we would find an apartment in Sa Kaeo. By now our IRC group had grown to three nurses and two physicians. Our team of five would be responsible for the care of all the patients in our charge—24/7. It rained just about every day; it was hot and humid, and the mosquitoes thrived. We were given Fansidar tablets to take (before it was known they were not a safe medication for malaria). We worked every day and occasionally round the clock. There were few breaks, no real times for meals, and very little food available, especially in the beginning. There were only primitive latrines.

Gradually the camp began to take shape. The hilly area became "residential"; tents and tarps were provided along with buckets and basins. The flat area became the "mess hall," and the field hospital grew beyond that, starting with a kind of "tent city."

Various aid agencies took on specific roles: The Israelis handled triage and ER/OR, the French and Germans handled maternity and pediatrics, the Thai Red Cross took on general medical patients, and the IRC was given the role of "ICU/acute med/surg." Each NGO had its own mandate. The UNHCR and CDC coordinated supplies and equipment, as well as rudimentary mortality and morbidity reports and other epidemiological studies. The engineers began to build water towers, outhouses, and more permanent wardlike structures (at least they had partial walls and a thatch roof). A quasi-permanent group of Thai food vendors took up residence just outside the barbed wire, providing the only "fast food" available to aid workers.

Around it all, we had to care for our patients. Our "ward" was designed with 120 cots—60 per side with a middle walkway. Most cots had more than one patient (especially if the patient were a mother or a child). The cots were about $2\frac{1}{2}$ feet from ground level, which made it hard on our backs. The ground was covered with small pebbles (certainly the engineers who designed it were not nurses!). All our patients were very ill. Many had cerebral malaria and were only semiconscious. Most were dehydrated and needed IVs. Many had diarrhea. There were wounds to be dressed. None of our patients spoke English, nor did our ward "helpers"—teenage girls who were well enough to work. We had no "systems" in place, but we knew they were needed.

So how did we cope? I like to think we did a great job because we were creative and we improvised, we were able to zero in on the basic essentials and not worry about much else, and we were willing to keep working even when exhausted:

- We divided the patients into two cohorts of 60 each (plus bedmates). Each patient was given an armband with a cot number and letter. We referred to our patients as "1A" or perhaps "3B," and we knew who we were talking about.
- We implemented a team task approach. Each half of the ward had a doctor–nurse team. We used 4x6 cards as charts. The doctor saw each patient and wrote orders on the cards (medications, IVs, dressings). Any other "comfort" measures were left to the ward helpers. They carried and emptied bedpans (mainly plastic buckets that required the patient to get out of the cot and use), changed sheets, gave sponge baths, provided drinks of water, and helped with running errands.
- We began each day at the "nurses' station," filling up syringes with set amounts of injectables, based on the ones we knew we needed: Imferon, penicillin, quinine, etc. We kept filled syringes in cups (we labeled the cups but not the syringes). We did the same with standard pills and tablets. This became our stock medication supply. The nurse took her set of cards, prepared her medication cart (a plastic laundry basket) with needed medications and supplies (by putting each item into small plastic cups), and carried a large water bottle. Each patient had his or her own cup at the bedside. In my month at Sa Kaeo, I learned three

Cambodian phrases: "where's your cup?," "swallow this," and "please or thank you."

- The two team nurses spent the day giving out meds and doing treatments to a minimum of 60 patients each.
- The third nurse was called the "IV nurse." She started and monitored all IVs in the ward (up to 100 of them on any given day). As we could not keep fluids going overnight because of lack of staff, each IV had to be started over again each morning.
- We worked very long days and carried flashlights to see in the dark. We did not take breaks except when absolutely necessary (luckily the new outhouses were close to our ward).
- On a rotation basis set up by UNHCR/CDC, each NGO took turns being the "night shift" for camp. This meant a doctor–nurse team worked a full 24 hours straight—the usual "day shift" plus being on call all night for the entire field hospital (about 1,000 patients). On those nights, we would be called out to deliver babies or see dying patients. We made two rounds of the entire field hospital, checking on especially sick patients. Otherwise we catnapped on the floor of the ward or in the supply tent. I remember the night the doctor and I each delivered a baby at the same time on two adjoining delivery tables! I had never delivered a baby before.

Over the course of a month, our patient population stabilized. We had many deaths in the first week, but it gradually tapered off. We were able to discharge patients. I saw sad, dirty, and hungry children begin to smile. We made sense of our workload and actually got to have breaks. IRC began hiring more permanent nurses to take our places. When we left in December, our ICU had been converted to the TB ward.

Some nurses work abroad because job prospects are better than in their home countries. Some do so as a means to an end: to allow them to travel and experience other cultures. Some want to compare nursing practices in other countries with their own. Military nurses are given foreign postings but care primarily for their own countrymen and women. Some nurses join overseas missionary groups in order to participate in faith-based activities, and others volunteer with emergency relief agencies because they "want to help" in times of disasters.

One image that comes to mind for many is that of traveling to an exotic locale, living in "primitive" conditions, having exciting and even dangerous encounters with locals, and working selflessly and tirelessly to aid the sick and injured. In fact, nurses have a broad range of options for working outside their home countries. These can be categorized as shown in Box 16–4.

Nurses can apply directly to public and private facilities (service and education) in host countries as long as they are able to work out visa and other requirements. Young graduates often seek employment in the United Kingdom or Europe as a means of paying for extended stays there. Nurses have also had a long tradition of working in the hospitals of the Middle East, especially Saudi Arabia, as employees of large U.S. or multinational oil companies. Other nurses take part in short-term health-related projects run by universities and/or church groups either as volunteers or paid staff. Many nurses volunteer to serve in times of disaster but do not intend to make long-term stays in the countries they serve. Embassies and consulates employ nurses abroad to care for their expatriate communities.

Although all these situations are legitimately international experiences, they do not define the field of international nursing in itself. The field

---

BOX 16-4

International Job Options for Nurses

Working for or in the host country directly
   Government or public facility
   Private facility
Working for an Intergovernmental Organization
Working for an International, National, or Local NGO
Working for a Bilateral Aid Agency and its Subcontractors
Working on a Grant-funded University or Research Project
Working for a Mission Group
Working for the Military

of international nursing, as discussed in the following section is a career option for nurses interested in more long-term commitments to an international health career. Some of the issues discussed, however, such as preparing to go abroad, are useful for all nurses who work outside their home country.

The Field of International Nursing

International nursing is a specialty because it consists of a unique body of knowledge with specific problems and domains of practice not shared by other recognized nursing specialties. International nursing is concerned with finding long-term sustainable solutions to problems of global importance to nursing. It is involved with development of individual nurses and capacity building of professional nursing systems at local

and state levels. It requires nurses to operate outside their own familiar comfort zones and to understand and function outside their own cultural base (language, interpersonal relationships, customs, and belief systems to name a few). The unique characteristics of international nursing are listed in Box 16-5.

There are many reasons for incorporating international nursing content into the curriculum and providing clinical learning opportunities whereby nurses and nursing students can experience other parts of the world. The globalization of nursing is a known fact. Political alignments and technology encourage mobility and an interchange of ideas so that national borders are less obvious and obscure. Nurses must increasingly see themselves as part of a global community in which problems, solutions, resources, and opportunities are shared.

BOX 16-5

Characteristics of International Nursing

1. Understanding the organizational structures, including communication and decision-making bodies, for health care policy and procedures at national, provincial or state, and local levels
2. Understanding the organizational structures, including communication and decision-making bodies, for nursing policy and procedures (regulations, practice standards, education, evaluation) at national, provincial or state, and local levels
3. Understanding and appreciating the status of nursing within the country and within specific health care systems (doctor–nurse relationships, decision making, authority, image, scope of practice)
4. Understanding and using concepts of development and capacity building
5. Assessing population health parameters in comparison with other countries
6. Experiencing challenges related to understanding and working within new or different systems of health care delivery and nurse practice regulations in other countries
7. Learning about the nursing role and clients' expectations of nurses

8. Working with counterparts who ultimately bear responsibility for nursing practice, education, and research in their nations
9. Functioning safely with unfamiliar equipment, supplies, and medications
10. Confronting ethical dilemmas having complex transnational components
11. Working with limited or unfamiliar health care resources
12. Collaborating with health care team members representing categories that may not exist in the United States or Canada
13. Learning about tropical illnesses and other health care problems unfamiliar in the nurse's home country (including cultural definitions of health, illness, and culture-bound syndromes)
14. Understanding and effectively working with political, social, economic, and cultural systems unlike those in the nurse's home country
15. Identifying and effectively using health care resources in the host country
16. Solving problems related to visas, immunizations, licenses, insurance, and other necessities of living in a foreign country

International nursing is not the same as transcultural nursing, although the two share many of the same tenets and philosophical underpinnings. However, the focus of international nursing extends beyond those areas of concern in transcultural nursing. The world is made up of many cultures, and the processes of learning how to deliver culturally sensitive high-quality nursing or health care to a diverse population is the realm of transcultural nursing. International nursing uses all the skills of transcultural nursing within a broader context of "development" or "capacity building."

International Nursing as a Career

The total number of persons whose primary professional focus is **international health** is unknown despite efforts to gather data. An estimated 9,000 U.S. health professionals are working in the international health field. Of these, 3,800 are considered long term or employed for 1 year or more; 1,700 are short term, usually consultants; and 3,200 are volunteers. Of the total, the largest category is nurses, followed by physicians and administrators. Of the long-term professionals, many work on 2- or 3-year contracts; however, a core of international health professionals (educators, administrators, consultants, and researchers) work their entire careers in the field.

As with other careers, international nursing has benefits and drawbacks. Travel is stimulating, but not all travel experiences are positive. Living abroad has many challenges. Interpersonal skills can be challenging when many health projects have multinational teams with nurses, physicians, and others from dozens of different countries. As shown in Research Application 16–2, the process of adjusting to nursing in another country is often stressful. Bolton (2004b) warns would-be international aid workers that this is not a traditional career path. It requires the ability to adapt to what he calls "intensely challenging" situations and to withstand periods of emotional strain. Case Study

16–2 highlights the emotional roller coaster of working in a health care environment in which the "norms" of behavior are not familiar.

CASE STUDY 16-2 *Two Afghan Girls: A Study in Contrasts*

Parween was admitted to the intensive care unit of a local hospital in Kabul, Afghanistan, during the morning hours of a cold winter day. She was 13 years old, dark haired, fair skinned, and pale. Her brown eyes were wide in both pain and fear. Pain due to her condition, which was vaginal bleeding of unknown origin. Fear because she had been admitted to a hospital—in and of itself a frightening experience but compounded by the fact that this hospital was known to have "foreigners" on the staff (a team of Canadian and U.S. nurses and doctors working for CARE, Inc.).

The ICU was referred to as the "model ward" in the hospital because it was intended to serve as a model of excellent patient care with up-to-date equipment. The unit was staffed by a female head nurse and four staff nurses (two men, two women) plus one "nana/bacha" team of housekeepers who functioned as nurse's aides. A female CARE nurse worked as counterpart to the head nurse. The model ward had four beds and very few high-tech features beyond the only defibrillator in the country at that time. There were basic supplies, linens, and medications.

Parween came to the model ward with her family, three older brothers. They had brought her from her village to the city for treatment. The bleeding had started at home and progressed to the point where the family realized some form of medical treatment was needed. However, she had not yet been examined by any physician, having been admitted from the ER directly to the unit. She was awake and alert but bleeding profusely. Her vital signs were taken, and a male lab technician drew blood to type and cross-match. Her three brothers stood guard around her bed. The head nurse started an IV. Blood was ordered and eventually started (by the CARE nurse).

Then the doctor entered the unit. The doctor was both male and foreign. The brothers would not let him near their sister. Following much discussion between the brothers and the head nurse, it was clear that the brothers were hesitant to let any-

RESEARCH APPLICATION **16-2**
Becoming a Foreign Nurse

Magnusdottir, H. (2005). Overcoming strangeness and communication barriers: A phenomenological study of becoming a foreign nurse. *International Nursing Review, 52,* 263–269.

Icelandic society has seen a shift in demographics in the last 10–15 years from a basically homogeneous population to an increasingly multicultural one because of the influx of foreign residents. In the health field, this has been largely caused by an increase in foreign nurses seeking employment. In 2003, foreign nurses at the largest hospital in Iceland accounted for 4.5% of the employed nurses and overall accounted for approximately 2.5% of all nurses working in Iceland.

This study used a phenomenological approach to explore the experience of foreign nurses working at three hospitals in Iceland. Based on the Vancouver school of phenomenological research, the participants were seen as co-researchers. Purposeful sampling was used to identify 11 registered nurses from seven countries who participated in unstructured interviews (dialogues) about the topic. The participants were asked to describe and reflect on their experiences of "...being a foreign nurse working at a hospital in Iceland." Thematic analysis was applied to the data.

The overriding theme emerging from the data was one of "growing through overcoming strangeness and communication barriers." Five key themes identified included (1) tackling the initial, multiple challenges; (2) becoming an outsider and the need to be included; (3) struggling with the language barrier; (4) adjusting to a different work culture; and (5) overcoming challenges to succeed. Working in a foreign country displaces people from their own culture and puts them in unfamiliar surroundings. This can result in powerful disorientation and feelings of conflict, frustration, and struggle. The author notes that one interesting finding was that experiences of nurses from neighboring countries that were linguistically and culturally close to Iceland (for example, like Canada and the United States) were initially as strenuous as the experiences of others from more distant lands.

Clinical Application
This study confirmed that the process of acculturation can be stressful and overwhelming, even painful and destabilizing, yet the end result is often positive. Being a "stranger" is a well-known phenomenon, and instances of racism and dislike of "the other" are realities to be addressed. Coworkers and supervisors may be more important than personal support systems when adjusting on the job. Language barriers are central to adjustment (as an instrument of communication and a vehicle of thought). Losing one's language was a major contributor to the nurses' loss of a sense of belonging. Nurses thinking about working overseas can use the insights in this study to help meet the challenges of a new working environment.

one examine their sister, given her age and the location of the bleeding. However, they agreed to let a female physician do the exam.

Unfortunately, most of the doctors in this hospital were male. As an adult medical/surgical facility, it was not seen as either a "women's or a maternity" hospital, where the majority of female physicians practiced. It took some time to find an appropriate physician. When she finally came, the brothers had a change of heart and would not let her examine their sister. They refused to consider any surgical procedures. Although they understood that without treatment their sister would most likely not survive, they choose comfort measures only over any form of "invasion of privacy" as they saw it. The brothers were not cold and unfeeling;

they wept and demonstrated the depth of their sadness over their sister's condition. They sat at her bedside constantly. They held her hand. They believed it was their duty to protect her honor. Parween died the next morning.

Gulalai was only 10 years old. She lived in northern Afghanistan, far from any real towns. One day she cut her foot while playing, and it became infected. As the infection spread, so did the pain. Her family knew she needed medical attention. There were no health posts or clinics anywhere near their home. They decided to bring her to the "big city," Kabul, for treatment. Her father and brother began the arduous trek, literally carrying Gulalai on their backs over the mountains to the nearest big town, where they hitched a ride in a truck to Kabul.

When they arrived at the CARE hospital days later, Gulalai had gangrene and was dangerously ill. After an examination, her family was told she needed immediate surgery if she was to have any chance to live. The doctors explained that they would need to amputate her left leg just above the knee. This was a major blow to the father and brother, not only because Gulalai was so near death, but because of the major implications of her losing a leg. The father worried about her ability to contribute to the family income if she could not work in the fields as she had before; he worried about how she would cope with the household chores that were part of her daily life, and how his wife would cope, caring for the other children, the chores, and a handicapped daughter. He wondered if she would be able to navigate the rough terrain on crutches. But most of all, the father and the brother worried about Gulalai's marriage prospects if she lost a leg. Would the families in their village shun her as a potential bride? Would she be destined to remain a spinster all her life? These were heavy concerns that needed to be weighed as they made the decision for Gulalai's treatment.

In the end, the father agreed to allow the surgery. He did not have all the answers, but he put his faith in Allah and said they would find a way to manage. Gulalai lost her leg and spent many months in the hospital recuperating. She became a familiar site walking the hallways with her crutches, her hair lightly covered with a shawl. She was shy but liked to smile. Her father and brother returned home but came back when she was discharged. They were so happy to see her healthy and mobile—they bought her a new pair of crutches, and then they all left the hospital.

In order to be successful in the international arena, the nurse needs a high degree of dedication, exceptional technical knowledge, and facility in informal diplomacy. Based on 16 years of personal experience, the author believes the following characteristics are critical for successful international nursing careers:

- High frustration tolerance and acceptance of ambiguity
- Resourcefulness
- Sense of adventure
- Open mind, flexible attitude
- Sense of humor
- Hardiness
- Cultural sensitivity and willingness to learn
- Enjoyment of diversity
- Language facility
- Ability to take criticism and intense scrutiny

When reflecting on their international experiences, most nurses who have spent substantial periods of time abroad indicate that they have learned from the exchange as well as contributed to improved health in the host country. Research on this subject reveals that nurses identify gaining increased knowledge in the following areas: cultural awareness, alternative health care delivery models, ways to include family members in nursing care, conservation of resources, nonbiomedical nursing interventions, and increased political awareness.

Preparation for International Nursing

Nurses often ask about academic qualifications and experience needed for international health work. There is in fact no identified standard set of educational or experiential requirements. All nurses who work overseas need to be clinically competent. Without earning the respect of the host country nurses, not much will happen. Local nurses expect you to be an expert in your field.

International nurses work with intelligent, skilled, and well-motivated professionals from all over the world. They are exposed to differing ideologies, methodologies, lifestyles, and languages. It is important that nurses have the skills, knowledge, and abilities needed to work with an international team. As Bolton (2004a) states, "Ideals cannot feed people." In addition to the obvious technical skills, nurses need good organizational management skills, people skills, oral presentation skills, teaching skills, research skills (most projects have built-in performance indicators that require quantitative and qualitative research methods), and writing abilities (projects require documentation and written reports; many require grant proposals and grant updates). Intergovernmental agencies and NGOs look for employees with a proven track record. Experience with a range of cultures and contexts is preferred. Employers want to gauge if you are likely to have an easy time learning a new language and adapting to new customs. In some cases, the first step is to gain experience by volunteering or serving as an intern on a project. The Peace Corps, Volunteer Services Overseas (VSO), and UN Volunteers are good places to start. Many universities offer courses in humanitarian assistance and international development, with or without internship experiences.

Academic Preparation

With increasing frequency U.S. and Canadian nurse educators are recognizing the importance of incorporating international nursing into the curriculum of baccalaureate, master's, and doctoral programs and in providing continuing-education courses with an international focus. Nurses and nursing students are expressing an increased interest in international nursing and are traveling, studying, and working abroad in greater numbers. Nursing students are seeking information about the appropriate ways in which to become prepared for the practice of nursing in other countries and are choosing programs that have internationalized their curriculum.

As nurses prepare for international work, they may ask, "How can I ever learn all I need to know about this culture so I won't appear foolish or alienate people?" First of all, recognize that it is impossible to learn all there is to know about another culture, regardless of how many years spent living in the country. By definition, the nurse will always be perceived as an outsider, stranger, or foreigner to some extent. See Case Study 16–3 for one nurse's experience preparing for an international position.

CASE STUDY 16-3 *Preparing for an International Nursing Assignment*

In 1974 Brenda Jones, age 27, had 2 years of pediatric nursing experience, a master's degree in pediatric nursing, and 2 years of experience teaching pediatrics in a large university school of nursing. She had always wanted to "do something" internationally, so she applied to several development aid agencies (NGOs) to see what was available. She was ready to commit to a multiyear assignment and was excited about the prospects of traveling and doing something useful in a developing country.

Two major NGOs interviewed Brenda. She was prepared to discuss her clinical skills and what she felt she had to offer but was surprised by how much of the interview was focused on (1) her health status, (2) her motivations for going abroad, and (3) her coping and adjusting skills in new environments, including her "hardiness tolerance" for things like lack of plumbing or toilet facilities, presence of scorpions and other insects, and living in a group or dormlike situation with other women. Both agencies wanted to know if she spoke a foreign language (even with 6 years of Spanish in school, she had to answer "no" to that question).

Brenda was faced with really examining her motivations for taking on this type of work. Bolton (2004a) reports that the ICRC sometimes asks applicants, "What are you running away from?" He points out that one needs strong motivations to leave one's home, family, and comfortable surroundings to go live and work in war zones or in impoverished environments. Citing Helen Fielding's novel *Cause Celeb*, he refers to a character wearing an "aide T-shirt questionnaire" that reads: a) Missionary? b) Mercenary? c) Misfit? d) Broken Heart? This tongue-in-cheek message points out the need to examine one's own motives carefully and to think about how they might impact performance.

Two weeks after the first interview, Brenda was offered a nursing position in Saigon, Vietnam, at a major NGO field hospital. Although excited at first, she was forced to decline the position after her parents' strong reaction to her serving in a war zone (a reaction she had not thought about sufficiently). In hindsight she realized preparing her family for the change was as important as preparing herself. She was later offered a position in an established NGO hospital in south Asia, in a country she knew next to nothing about; she accepted the position as a "nurse educator."

The human resources director at the NGO told Brenda she would be working in an adult, 100-bed medical/surgical hospital in the capital city. She would work with the nurses to ensure quality care in support of the NGO's physician internship training program. In addition, she would interface with the students who came to the hospital for clinical practice. She would be joining a team of U.S. and Canadian physicians, nurses, lab techs, and medical records personnel. She was told that none of the local nurses spoke English and that she would be expected to learn the local language.

Brenda had 1 month to prepare herself. The NGO stressed the importance of getting to know the country and sent her bulk documents to read containing information about the country: history, geography, politics, culture, ethnic groups, economy, and health care system. They included a large orientation manual for new employees with tips on how to pack (only two suitcases allowed), essential items to bring, what not to bring, and what to consider about dress in the country, norms of behavior, and dos and don'ts. The NGO sent bibliography lists with suggested readings, and Brenda scoured the library looking for titles. She checked the university library for government documents on the country. She read all the *National Geographic* magazine stories and even whatever novels she could find.

Finally, she thought about the language. Living in the Washington, D.C. area, she was able to connect with the Foreign Service Institute and ask for assistance. Although she was not eligible for training, they put her in contact with the language instructor. He was willing to give her private lessons. So, twice a week, after work, Brenda drove to Alexandria, Virginia, and met with her language instructor—for a total of eight lessons. He agreed to provide the lessons for free, stating, "If you are going to help my people, I am willing to help you." The encounter with a native speaker was invaluable. Beyond the basics of pronunciation, grammar, reading, and writing, Brenda learned firsthand about the land and its peoples, customs, and traditions. She even got to sample some local foods!

When Brenda arrived in country, she felt she had a start in getting to know the people. At least she could say "hello." She surprised the local driver, who took her from the airport to the city, with her ability to read road signs and bits of billboards in the local language. She was fortunate that her employer believed language training was crucial to success. On arrival, Brenda was told she would not start working at the hospital right away. Instead, she spent the first month in full-time language study (provided by the Peace Corps). The second month she had half-day lessons. Then she hired a private tutor (provided by the NGO) who continued her lessons during her entire 2-year stay in country.

Research on international health care indicates that most U.S. and Canadian nurses work with more than one culture, often rotating back and forth between an international assignment and a position in North America. Skills and attitudes that nurses can develop have been identified by the Peace Corps (2006) and include

1. Listening skills, including awareness of nonverbal cues
2. Careful observation
3. Patience, not always expecting "them" to take the lead in adjusting
4. Ability to take risks, try new things
5. Awareness of one's own values and cultural assumptions
6. Ability to identify culture resources in the community
7. Recognition that the reasons for one's feelings of frustration may be cultural in origin

Summarized in Box 16-6 are ways in which U.S. and Canadian nurses can prepare in advance and orient themselves to their host country, in addition to formal academic study.

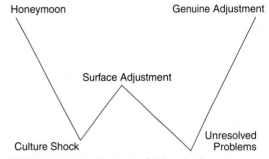

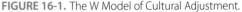

FIGURE 16-1. The W Model of Cultural Adjustment.

Patterns of Cultural Adjustment

Whenever people are immersed in another culture, they will go through a period of cultural adjustment. One of the more well-known patterns of cultural adjustment is the W model. Many variations on this theory exist, but the general pattern has been well documented in intercultural communications research. It is one of the few concepts agreed on by most professionals involved in cross-cultural education. Figure 16–1 illustrates the theory.

Cultural Adjustment

Five stages of cultural adaptation are illustrated as the points on W; this pattern may depend on the length of stay and the purpose of being in the other culture. The five stages are

1. Excitement, or the honeymoon period, which is characterized by enthusiasm resulting from the newness and sense of adventure.
2. Culture shock. The excitement is gone. Things are not "like back home"; social cues and relationships are difficult; there are feelings of alienation and homesickness and a temporary dislike of the host culture.
3. Surface adjustment. During this stage, the nurse is beginning to catch on; things are starting to make sense; rudimentary language (more accurate communication) skills are acquired, and the nurse is able to communicate some basic ideas and feelings, making some relationships in the local culture; the nurse begins to feel more comfortable.
4. Frustration and a deeper level of unresolved problems; the assignment period in the culture may seem very long, and the nurse may experience feelings of boredom, frustration, and isolation.
5. Genuine adjustment, which is characterized by acceptance of the new culture as just another way of living; the nurse may not always approve of cultural practices but understands the differences and begins to peel back some of the rich layers of the culture. The nurse has established genuine, real relationships with people in the host country.

All nurses experience the components identified in the cultural pattern when living in an unfamiliar culture. Some may decide that trying to adjust is too difficult and return home at the early "cultural shock" stage. Being aware that there is a pattern to feelings and reactions to the new culture is one step in making the nurse more effective in the international setting. Clients from other nations experience similar cultural patterns when they enter the United States or Canada. Shorter in duration, a phenomenon know as *reentry shock* can be expected when the nurse returns home. Reentry shock consists of feelings of general dissatisfaction, criticism for lifeways of his or her home country, and free-floating anxiety.

Going Abroad

In the next section, you will be given guidelines for making decisions about going abroad and choosing sending agencies that are congruent with your philosophical beliefs.

Motivation

Before choosing a sending agency, it is essential to examine one's motivation for going abroad. In studies of U.S. nurses engaging in international consultation, several reasons motivating nurses have been identified, including enjoyment of people from other cultures, interest in travel, moral convictions, religious beliefs, financial rewards, personal invitation by host country counterparts, cross-cultural exchange of ideas, professional commitment, and service to those in need. Identifying motivation and determining the goals and purposes for the international experience will facilitate selection of the appropriate type of position and sending agency.

Length of Time Abroad

Related to the motivation for going abroad is the length of time that you plan to spend overseas. Before contacting potential sending agencies, it is important to determine a time commitment, stated in terms of days, weeks, months, or years. Opportunities for short-term international experiences (less than 6 months) vary widely and are likely to require tradeoffs in benefits provided by the agency. Travel study programs usually assume that the applicant is willing to pay part or all of the expenses for the trip. Long-term international experiences offer a wide variety of opportunities, with contracts varying according to the agency's needs and resources.

Geographic Region

If a particular region is preferred, this must be matched with the sending agency's activities and projects. Some agencies specialize in a particular region, whereas others have programs on virtually every continent. The following reasons may motivate the nurse to choose a particular region or country: (1) political stability of the country, (2) personal or emotional reasons such as a significant other living in the area or familiarity with the language, and/or (3) matching host country needs with the expertise of the nurse.

Although global politics may shift rapidly, the Middle East, South Africa, and certain parts of Central and South America have a reputation for volatile politics including anti-American demonstrations. Personal safety is a concern, and careful research should be conducted before accepting an assignment in a politically unstable area. U.S. Department of State reports, information provided by the sending agency, informal discussions with recently returned visitors to the county, and current news sources may provide the necessary information to determine the safety of an area.

Reasonable Expectations of Sending Agencies

Although specific details will vary according to the sending agency, Box 16–7 is intended to provide guidelines for asking questions. Sending agencies expect questions and recognize that interviewing is a two-way process.

Negotiating a Contract

The preceding discussion has focused on some aspects that are reasonable to expect in a contractual agreement with a sending agency. Before

BOX 16-7

Guidelines for Choosing an International Sending Agency

Salary or Stipend

- What is the salary or stipend in U.S. or Canadian dollars?
- If any portion is paid in local currency, what is the exchange rate?
- What has been the history of fluctuation in the exchange rate during the past 2 years?
- What is the cost of living compared with the salary or stipend?
- What is the average cost for housing, food, transportation, and utilities in the host country? Will the sending agency cover any of these costs?
- Can local currency be exchanged for U.S. dollars? Can U.S. or Canadian dollars be used to purchase local currency?
- Can salary earned in the country be taken out of the country? If so, by what means? Bank transfer? Cashier's check? Cash and carry?
- What length of time is usually required for bank transactions? International transfers? Local banking needs?
- To which governments are taxes owed? What is the rate of taxation? How, when, and where should tax statements be processed or filed?

Travel to Host Country Assignment

- Is round-trip airfare paid by the agency? Are spouses and/or dependents sent or eligible for discounted fares?
- Is there a payback clause for early contract termination?
- Who makes travel arrangements? Is a confirmation by the ticket holder required?
- How frequently are return trips to the United States or Canada allowed and/or paid for by the agency?

Housing and Moving

- Does the agency provide housing? Is it in an expatriate community or in a local neighborhood?
- What is the type of housing provided? Are accommodations shared?
- Are there toilet and bathing facilities, central heating and/or air conditioning, running water, and window screens?
- What type of energy is used? What is the average monthly cost?
- Is there a reliable source of electricity available? If not, is there a generator?

- Is the housing furnished or unfurnished?
- What are the conditions of the move? By what means (air, land, sea)? Are travel and household insurance included? Amount of coverage provided? Who is responsible for packing?
- What household goods and commodities are reasonable to expect locally? At what cost?
- Does the agency have special arrangements for shipping items such as regular mail pouch service, agency deliveries, etc?
- If housing allowance is given, are family members included?
- Who is responsible for daily maintenance (housecleaning, cooking, gardening, upkeep)?
- What are the security arrangements?

Local Transportation

- Are vehicles available to staff for job-related travel? For personal use after hours and on weekends?
- What is the cost of gasoline? Maintenance of a vehicle? Does the agency employ a mechanic? Are reliable local mechanics available? Are replacement parts for vehicles available?
- Does the agency provide car loans? What are the terms? Is there a waiting list for vehicle purchases? If so, how long? What is the average price for a vehicle?
- What are the local regulations on drivers' licenses and automobile insurance?
- If vehicles are not available, what methods of local transportation are used by agency staff? Cost? Availability? Safety?
- Are employees expected to drive? Does the agency hire drivers? Are women permitted to drive vehicles? If not, when are drivers available? Costs?

Insurance Benefits

- What types of health, life, disability, and retirement insurance are available? Are family members included?
- In case of illness, what is the agency policy concerning treatment? What health care facilities may be accessed for personal and family health care?
- If local hospitals are used, what is the quality of care compared with the United States or Canada? What type of pediatric care is available locally for dependent children?

(Continued on following page)

BOX 16-7 (continued)

Guidelines for Choosing an International Sending Agency

- Is paid leave and/or airfare to the United States granted for health care emergencies? For compassionate leave?

Vacations and Holidays

- What U.S., Canadian, and/or local holidays does the agency recognize?
- What is the length and frequency of vacation or holiday absences? Are there limitations to travel during vacation?
- In politically volatile areas, are more frequent vacations or designated leaves (R&R) permitted and/or encouraged?
- Does the agency have an informal or formal network allowing for staff to vacation at a reduced cost?
- Do staff members offer hospitality to other agency members while traveling? Is it expected that all staff reciprocate by housing agency members during vacations and/or job-related travel?

Orientation Program

- What are the length, location, and nature of the agency orientation?
- Are language studies required? Where do language studies occur? Who pays for classes?
- Are local interpreters available? Are there any gender-related or age-related factors to consider when using an interpreter?

- Does the orientation include study of the political, economic, social, cultural, religious, and health-related aspects of the host country?
- Who is the U.S./Canadian ambassador to the host country? Where is the U.S./Canadian embassy/consulate located? Does the agency enjoy any special "privileges" (movies, commissary shopping, and access to information)?
- In case of natural disaster or political unrest, what is the emergency evacuation plan for expatriates? How are expatriates linked to their embassy/consulate emergency communication systems?

Other

- Are local and private schools available for children? In English? How hard are they to get into? Do they meet U.S./Canadian/international educational standards?
- Does the agency provide an educational stipend for dependent children? In country only?
- Does the agency provide employment opportunities for spouses? How easy is it to find work in the local economy? Are there special rules and regulations about spouses working in country?
- Does the agency provide advice about U.S./Canadian income tax laws and filing returns while overseas?

---

signing the contract, it is important to study the details carefully and to discuss any unclear matters with the agency representative. A written job description should accompany the contract along with a statement detailing the conditions surrounding contract termination by either the nurse or the sending agency.

Choosing an International Sending Agency

Because there are many agencies that send nurses abroad, it is impossible to provide an exhaustive list. The ones discussed in this chapter provide an overview of agencies that use nurses for health-related projects abroad. Not included were uni-

versities, foundations, private industries, study or travel groups, and the U.S. and Canadian military organizations. One Web site that can assist in the search for the right agency is InterAction (2006).

Nurses may affiliate themselves with a variety of sponsoring agencies. Sponsorship may be through a U.S. or Canadian organization or through the host country (ministry of health, university, hospital, school of nursing, public health agency, or private enterprise). Joint sponsorships, though relatively rare, also may occur. For example, some religious groups have both international and national organizations that may elect joint sponsorship.

Summary

With increasing frequency, U.S. and Canadian nurses are traveling, studying, researching, consulting, teaching, administering, and practicing nursing abroad. The decision to engage in an international interchange requires much thought and planning. Philosophical congruence with the sending agency or organization, selection of geographic area of interest, length of time available, and matching background with host-country needs are factors that interplay with the desire to go abroad.

Many U.S. and Canadian nurses are relatively naïve about negotiating a contract with a sending agency. An overview of reasonable questions to pursue with the agency has been provided, including discussions of salary or stipend, travel to the assignment site, housing and moving expenses, local transportation, insurance coverage, vacation and holiday leave, and orientation policies.

REFERENCES

Bolton, M. (2004a). *Aid agencies prefer professionals to inexperienced volunteers.* Retrieved April 1, 2007, from http://www.transitionsabroad.com/publications/magazine/0501/aid_agencies_prefer_professionals_to_volunteers.shtml

Bolton, M. (2004b). *Becoming an aid worker: An experienced professional explains how it's done.* Retrieved March 29, 2007, from http://www.transitionsabroad.com/publications/magazine/0409/becoming_an_international_aid_worker.shtml

Canadian International Development Agency. Homepage at http://www.acdi-cida.gc.ca/index-e.htm

CARE, Inc. (2007). Homepage at http://www.care.org/

Catholic Relief Services. (2006). Homepage at http://www.crs.org/

Centers for Disease Control and Prevention. (2007). Homepage at http://www.cdc.gov/

Global Ministries. (2004). *News: Ruth May Harnar.* Retrieved August 4, 2005, from http://www.globalministries.org/news/harnar.htm

Hewlett, B. L., & Hewlett, B. S. (2005). Providing care and facing death: Nursing during an Ebola outbreak in Central Africa. *Journal of Transcultural Nursing, 16*(4), 289–297.

InterAction. (2006). Homepage at www.interaction.org

International Committee of the Red Cross. (2007). Homepage in English at http://www.icrc.org/eng

International Council of Nurses. (2003). *Tackling the UN Millennium Development Goals. 2002–2003 Biennial Report.*

Geneva, Switzerland: Author. Retrieved April 1, 2007, from http://www.icn.ch/02-03BiennialReport.pdf

International Council of Nurses. (2007). Homepage at http://www.icn.ch/

International Federation of Red Cross and Red Crescent Societies. (2007). Homepage at http://www.ifrc.org/

International Rescue Committee. (2007). Homepage at http://www.theirc.org/

Lau, E., Médecins Sans Frontières. (2005). *Voices from the field: Aceh is completely smashed.* Retrieved December 2006 from www.doctorswithoutborders.org/news/voices/2005/01-2005_aceh.cfm/

Magnusdottir, H. (2005). Overcoming strangeness and communication barriers: A phenomenological study of becoming a foreign nurse. *International Nursing Review, 52,* 263–269.

Médecins Sans Frontières/Doctors Without Borders. (2007). Homepage at http://www.doctorswithoutborders.org/aboutus/index.cfm

Mercy Corps. (2007). Homepage at http://www.mercycorps.org/

Nestrell, J., Médecins Sans Frontières. (2004). *Voices from the field: Nurse Jessica Nestrell. Going upriver: MSF aid worker battles measles in Congo.* Retrieved December 2006 from www.doctorswithoutborders.org/news/voices/2004/10-2004_drc.cfm

Nightingale. (1859, 2007). Notes on nursing. Gloucestershire, UK: Tempus Publishing Group.

Oxfam. (2006). Homepage at http://www.oxfam.org.uk/

Pan American Health Organization. (2007). Homepage at http://www.paho.org/

Peace Corp. (2006). Homepage at http://www.peacecorps.gov/index.cfm

Project Hope. (2007). Homepage at http://www.projecthope.org/

Sachs, J. (2005). *Investing in development: A practical plan to achieve the Millennium Development Goals.* NY: UN Publications.

Save the Children. (2007). Homepage at http://www.savethechildren.org/

UNICEF. (2007). Homepage at http://www.unicef.org/

United Nations. (2006). *UN Millennium Project.* Accessed December 8, 2006, at www.unmillenniumproject.org

United Nations. (2007). Homepage in English at http://www.un.org/english/

United Nations. (2007). Volunteers' homepage at http://www.unv.org/

United Nations Development Program. (2006). *Human Development Report 2006: Beyond scarcity: Power, poverty and the global water crisis.* Retrieved from http://hdr.undp.org/hdr2006/pdfs/report/HDR06-complete.pdf

United States Agency for International Development. (2007). Homepage at http://www.usaid.gov/

World Economic Forum. (2005). *Global governance initiative. Annual Report 2006.* Washington, D.C.: Communications Development, Incorporated. Retrieved April 1, 2007 from http://www.weforum.org/pdf/Initiatives/GGI_Report06.pdf

World Health Organization. (2001). *Strengthening nursing and midwifery* (WHA 54.12). Geneva, Switzerland: Author.

World Health Organization. (2002). *Strategic directions for strengthening nursing and midwifery services.* Geneva, Switzerland: Author. Accessed June 2006 from http://whqlibdoc.who.int/publications/2002/924156217X.pdf

World Health Organization. (2006a). *Health and the Millennium Development Goals.* Retrieved January 1, 2006, from http://www.who.int/mdg/en/

World Health Organization. (2006b). *Health in the Millennium Development Goals.* Retrieved January 1, 2006, from http://www.who.int/mdg/goals/en

World Health Organization. (2006c). *The Nursing and Midwifery programme at WHO: What Nursing and Midwifery services mean to health.* Retrieved December 2006 from http://www.paho.org/English/DPM/SHD/HR/midwives-nurses-leafletWHA06-eng.pdf

World Health Organization. (2007a). Homepage at www.who.org

World Health Organization. (2007b). *Nursing and midwifery.* Retrieved from http://www.who.int/hrh/nursing_midwifery/en/

World Health Organization, Regional Office for Europe. (2006). *Declaration of Alma Ata.* Retrieved December 8, 2006, from http://www.euro.who.int/AboutWHO/Policy/20010827_1

World Vision. (2007). Homepage at http://www.worldvision.org

A

Andrews/Boyle Transcultural Nursing Assessment Guide for Individuals and Families

Joyceen S. Boyle and Margaret M. Andrews

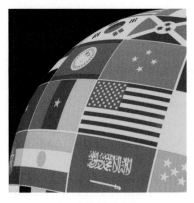

Biocultural Variations and Cultural Aspects of the Incidence of Disease

Does the client relate a health history associated with genetic or acquired conditions that are more prevalent for a specific cultural group (e.g., diabetes, hypertension, cardiovascular disease, sickle cell anemia, Tay-Sachs disease, G-6-PD deficiency, lactose intolerance)? Do his or her family members relate such a history?

Are there socioenvironmental conditions more prevalent among a specific cultural group that can be observed in a client or family members (e.g., lead poisoning, alcoholism, HIV/AIDS, drug abuse, ear infections, family violence, fetal alcohol syndrome, obesity, respiratory diseases)?

Are there diseases against which the client has an increased resistance (e.g., skin cancer in darkly pigmented individuals, malaria for those with sickle cell anemia)?

Does the client have distinctive features characteristic of a particular ethnic or cultural group (e.g., skin color, hair texture)? Do his or her family members have such features? Within the family group, are there variations in anatomy characteristics of a particular ethnic or cultural group (e.g., body structure, height, weight, facial shape and structure [nose, eye shape, facial contour], upper and lower extremities)?

How do anatomic, racial, and ethnic variations affect the physical and mental examination?

Communication

What language does the client speak at home with family members? In what language would the client prefer to communicate with you? What other languages does the client speak or read? What other languages do the client's family members speak or read?

What is the fluency level of the client in English—both written and spoken? What is the fluency level of the client's family members?

Does the client need an interpreter? Do his or her family members need an interpreter? Does the health care setting provide interpreters? Who would the client and his or her family members prefer to assist with interpretation? Is there anyone whom the client would prefer not to serve as an interpreter (e.g., member of the opposite sex, person younger or older than the client, member of a rival tribe, ethnic group, or nationality)?

What are the rules and style (formal or informal) of communication? How does the client prefer to be addressed? What do his or her family members prefer? What are the preferred terms for greeting?

How is it necessary to vary the technique and style of communication during the relationship with the client to accommodate his or her cultural background (e.g., tempo of conversation, eye contact, sensitivity to topical taboos, norms of confidentiality, and style of explanation)? How do these factors vary with family members, if at all?

What are the styles of individual and family members' nonverbal communication?

How does the client's nonverbal communication compare with that of individuals from other cultural groups? How does the client's style of nonverbal communication differ from the health care provider's style? How does it affect the client's relationships with you and with other members of the health care team? How does communication with the family influence the care environment?

How do the client and family members feel about health care providers who are not of the same cultural or religious background (e.g., Black, middle-class nurse; Hispanic of a different social class; Muslim or Jewish care provider)? Does the client prefer to receive care from a nurse of the same cultural background, gender, and/or age? How do family members react to care providers of different cultural backgrounds, age, and gender?

Cultural Affiliations

With what cultural group(s) does the client report affiliation (e.g., American, Hispanic, Irish, Black, Navajo, or combination)? It is becoming increasingly common for Americans to identify with two or more groups, such as Native American and African American. Tiger Woods, for example, has identified himself as being of Thai and African-American heritage. Equally important, to what degree does the client identify with the cultural group (e.g., "we" concept of solidarity or as a fringe member)?

How do the views of other family members coincide or differ from the client regarding cultural affiliations?

What is the preferred term that the cultural group chooses for itself?

Where was the client born? Where were his or her parents born? What are the generational similarities and differences in regards to cultural identification, language, customs, values, etc.?

Where has the client lived (country, city, or area within a country) and when (during what years of his or her life)? If the client has recently immigrated to the United States or other country, knowledge of prevalent diseases in his or her country of origin as well as sociopolitical history may be helpful. Current residence? Occupation? Occupation in home country?

Cultural Sanctions and Restrictions

How does the client's cultural group regard expression of emotion and feelings, spirituality, and religious beliefs? How are dying, death, and grieving expressed in a culturally appropriate manner?

How do men and women express modesty? Are there culturally defined expectations about male–female relationships, including the nurse–client relationship?

Does the client or family express any restrictions related to sexuality, exposure of various parts of the body, or certain types of surgery (e.g., vasectomy, hysterectomy, abortion)?

Are there restrictions against discussion of dead relatives or fears related to the unknown?

Developmental Considerations

Are there any distinct growth and development characteristics that vary with the cultural background of the client and family (e.g., bone density, psychomotor patterns of development, fat folds)?

What factors are significant in assessing children of various ages from the newborn period through adolescence (e.g., male and female circumcision, expected growth on standards grid, culturally acceptable age for toilet training, duration of breast-feeding, introduction of various types of foods, gender differences, discipline, and socialization to adult roles)?

What are the beliefs and practices associated with developmental life events such as pregnancy, birth, and death?

What is the cultural perception of aging (e.g., is youthfulness or the wisdom of old age more valued)?

How are elderly persons cared for within the cultural group (e.g., cared for in the home of adult children, placed in institutions for care)? What are culturally accepted roles for the elderly?

Economics

Who is the principal wage earner in the family and what is the income level? Is there more than one wage earner? Are there other sources of financial support? (*Note:* These may be potentially sensitive questions.)

What insurance coverage (health, dental, vision, pregnancy, cancer, or special conditions) does the client and his or her family have?

What impact does the economic status have on the client and his or her family's lifestyle and living conditions?

What has been the client and family's experience with the health care system in terms of reimbursement, costs, and insurance coverage?

Educational Background

What is the client's highest educational level obtained? What values do the family members express regarding educational achievements?

Does the client's educational level affect his or her knowledge level concerning his or her health literacy—how to obtain the needed care, teaching related to or learning about health care, and any written material that he or she is given in the health care setting (e.g., insurance forms, educational literature, information about diagnostic procedures and laboratory tests, admissions forms, etc.)? Does the client's educational level affect health behavior? As an example, cigarette smoking and obesity have been linked to economic levels.

Can the client read and write English, or is another language preferred? If English is the client's second language, are health-related materials available in the client's primary language? Are all family members fluent in English?

What learning style is most comfortable and familiar? Does the client prefer to learn through written materials, oral explanations, videos, and/or demonstrations?

Do the client and family members prefer intervention settings away from hospitals and clients, which may have negative connotations for them? Are community sites such as churches, schools, or adult day-care centers a good alternate choice for the client and his or her family, considering they are informal settings that may be more conducive for open discussion, demonstrations, and reinforcement of information and skills? Are the client and family more comfortable in their home setting?

Health-Related Beliefs and Practices

To what cause does the client attribute illness and disease or what factors influence the acquisition of illness and disease (e.g., divine wrath, imbalance in hot/cold, yin/yang, punishment for moral transgressions, a hex, soul loss, pathogenic organism, past behavior)? Is there congruence within the family on these beliefs?

What are the client's cultural beliefs about ideal body size and shape? What is the client's self-image in relation to the ideal?

How does the client describe his or her health-related condition? What names or terms are used? How does the client express pain?

What do the client and family members believe promotes health (e.g., eating certain foods, wearing amulets to bring good luck, sleeping, resting, getting good nutrition, reducing stress, exercising, praying or performing rituals to ancestors, saints, or other deities)?

What is the client's religious affiliation? How is the client actively involved in the practice of religion? Do other family members have the same religious beliefs and practices?

Does the client and his or her family rely on cultural healers (e.g., curandero, shaman, spiritualist, priest, minister)? Who determines when the client is sick and when he or she is healthy? Who influences the choice or type of healer and treatment that should be sought?

In what types of cultural healing or health promoting practices does the client engage (e.g., use of herbal remedies, potions, or massage; wearing of talismans, copper bracelets, or chains to discourage evil spirits; healing rituals; incantations; or prayers)? Do family members share these beliefs and practices?

How are biomedical or scientific health care providers perceived? How do the client and his or her family perceive nurses? What are the expectations of nurses and nursing care workers?

Who will care for the client at home? What accommodations will family members make to provide caregiving?

How does the client's family and cultural group view mental disorders? Are there differences in acceptable behaviors for physical versus psychological illnesses?

Kinship and Social Networks

Who makes up the client's social network (family, friends, peers, neighbors)? How do they influence the client's health or illness status? What is the composition of a "typical family" within the kinship network? What is the composition of the client's family?

How do members of the client's social support network define caring or caregiving? What is the role of various family members during health and illness episodes? Who makes decisions about health and health care?

How does the client's family participate in the promotion of health (e.g., lifestyle changes in diet, activity level, etc.) and nursing care (e.g., bathing, feeding, touching, being present) of the client?

Does the cultural family structure influence the client's response to health or illness (e.g., beliefs, strengths, weaknesses, and social class)?

What influence do ethnic, cultural, and/or religious organizations have on the lifestyle and

quality of life of the client (e.g., the National Association for the Advancement of Colored People [NAACP], churches [such as African-American Muslim, Jewish, Catholic, and others]) that may provide schools, classes, and/or community-based health care programs.

Are there special gender issues within this cultural group? Do the client and family members conform to traditional roles (e.g., women may be viewed as the caretakers of home and children, while men work outside the home and have primary decision-making responsibilities)?

Nutrition

What nutritional factors are influenced by the client's cultural background? What is the meaning of food and eating to the client and his or her family?

Does the client have any eating or nutritional disorders (e.g., anorexia, bulimia, obesity, lactose intolerance)? Do the client's family members have any similar disorders? How do the client and family view these conditions?

With whom does the client usually eat? What types of foods are eaten? What is the timing and sequencing of meals? What are the usual meal patterns?

What does the client define as food? What does the client believe constitutes a "healthy" versus an "unhealthy" diet? Are these beliefs congruent with what the client actually eats?

Who shops for and chooses food? Where are the foodstuffs purchased? Who prepares the actual meals? How are the family members involved in nutritional choices, values, and choices about food?

How are the foods prepared at home (type of food preparation, cook oil[s] used, length of time foods are cooked [especially vegetables], amount and type of seasoning added to various foods during preparation)? Who does the food preparation?

Has the client chosen a particular nutritional practice such as vegetarianism or abstinence from red meat or from alcoholic or fermented beverages? Do other family members adhere to these beliefs and practices?

Do religious beliefs and practices influence the client's or family's diet (e.g., amount, type, preparation, or delineation of acceptable food combinations, [e.g., kosher diets])? Does the client or client's family abstain from certain foods at regular intervals, on specific dates determined by the religious calendar, or at other times? Are there other food prohibitions or prescriptions?

If the client or client's family's religion mandates or encourages fasting, what does the term *fast* mean (e.g., refraining from certain types of foods, eating only during certain times of the day, skipping certain meals)? For what period of time are family members expected to fast? Are there exceptions to fasting (e.g., are pregnant women or children excluded from fasting)?

Are special utensils used (e.g., chopsticks, cookware, kosher restrictions)?

Does the client or client's family use home and folk remedies to treat illnesses (e.g., herbal remedies, acupuncture, cupping, or other healing rituals often involving eggs, lemons, candles)?

Religion and Spirituality

How does the client or family's religious affiliation affect health and illness (e.g., life events such as death, chronic illness, body image alteration, cause and effect of illness)?

What is the role of religious beliefs and practices during health and illness? Are there special rites or blessings for those with serious or terminal illnesses?

Are there healing rituals or practices that the client and family believe can promote well-being or hasten recovery from illness? If so, who performs these? What materials or arrangements are necessary for the nurse to have available for the practice of these rituals?

What is the role of significant religious representatives during health and illness? Are there recognized religious healers (e.g., Islamic imans, Christian Scientist practitioners or nurses, Catholic priests, Mormon elders, Buddhist monks)?

Values Orientation

What are the client's attitudes, values, and beliefs about his or her health and or illness status? Do family members have similar values and beliefs?

How do these influence behavior in terms of promotion of health and treatment of disease? What are the client's or family's attitudes, values, and beliefs about health care providers?

Does culture affect the manner in which the client relates to body image change resulting from illness or surgery (e.g., importance of appearance, beauty, strength, and roles in the cultural group)? Is there a cultural stigma associated with the client's illness (i.e., how is the illness or the manner in which it was contracted viewed by the family and larger culture)?

How do the client and his or her family view work, leisure, and education?

How does the client perceive and react to change?

How do the client and his or her family perceive changes in lifestyle related to current illness or surgery?

How do the client and his/her family view biomedical care or scientific health care (e.g., suspiciously, fearfully, acceptingly, unquestioningly, with awe)?

How does the client value privacy, courtesy, touch, and relationships with others?

How does the client relate to persons outside of his or her cultural group (e.g., withdrawal, suspicion, curiosity)?

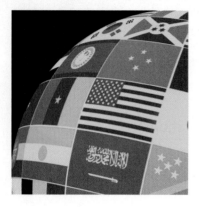

Components of a Cultural Assessment Applied: Native American (Navajo)

Family and Kinship Systems

- Navajos often have an extended family that consists of an older woman and her husband and unmarried children, together with married daughters and their husbands and unmarried children.
- The Navajo (or other Native Americans) have many unique categories of relatives.
- Descent is traced through the mother.
- Head of household is the husband, although the wife has a voice in decision making.
- Children are highly valued and are given responsibilities to make decisions about themselves.
- There is prestige with age as long as the elderly person can function independently.

Social Life

- The earth and nature are valued, and the individual should be in harmony with nature; this thought is interwoven with daily activities.
- Cooperation with others, rather than competition, is a cultural value.
- Life-cycle events are marked by special rituals; for example, the Blessing Way ceremony takes place shortly after the birth of a child.

- Like many other indigenous people, the Navajo have high rates of alcoholism, suicide, domestic violence, and homicide. Currently, abuse of drugs and HIV disease are becoming more common.
- Tribal and family ties are strong and contribute to a sense of belonging to a social group.
- Educational opportunities are often limited because of an inferior school system.
- Diet is often high in carbohydrates and fats; staple foods are corn, mutton, and fried bread.

Political Systems

- The system of tribal government was imposed by Whites.
- Poverty and high rates of unemployment are overriding concerns.
- The extended family has an economic as well as a social function.
- Control of resources (land, water) has been problematic, given the role of the U.S. government.
- Improving housing, sanitation, and work opportunities are major goals.
- A major problem is making deteriorated lands productive in an underpopulated region.

- Many Native American tribes have established large gambling casinos that have generated economic benefits for the tribes involved.

Language and Traditions

- Younger Navajos speak English. Reading, writing, and speaking English are taught in all the schools. Many elderly Navajo speak little or no English.
- The Navajo language contains many homonyms, words that have identical sounds but different meanings. The Navajo language is very specific.
- Periods of silence during communication show respect.
- Nonverbal communication is a high art form among the Navajo, and silence is highly respected. There may be little eye contact. Direct and prolonged eye contact is considered extremely rude and intrusive.
- Personal space is not an important need.
- The group has a history of oppression from the White dominant group.
- The "Long Walk" (a forced move of 300 miles to Fort Sumner in 1863) was a major calamity for the Navajo and remains a poignant chapter in cultural history that reinforces Native American culture and identity.

Worldview, Value Orientations, and Cultural Norms

- In all Native American cultures, interactions on all levels contain the fundamental element of respect. Respect is how a person presents himself or herself to the world and how a person acts, and it is tied to being Native American.
- The basic nature of human beings is neither good nor bad; both qualities exist in each person.
- Nature is more powerful than human beings.

- Individual success is not valued as highly as providing security to the extended family.
- Traditional Navajo views on the relationship of human beings with other human beings are both individualistic and collateral.
- The integrity of the individual must be respected. There is respect for the choice of an individual (even a child's decision is respected).
- There is also pressure for a Navajo to consider the extended family's welfare when making decisions.
- Time orientations are not strict; work and productivity are valued.

Religious Ideology

- Religion enters every phase of the traditional Navajo life, and an important emphasis is on curing illness.
- Many important Navajo ceremonies may be used with illness; theology and medicine are difficult to separate in traditional Navajo culture.
- Earth and nature are a part of the Navajo's cosmology, and health is viewed as harmony with the universe.
- Many Native Americans, including some Navajo, are members of the Native American Church.
- Peyote may be used in religious curing rituals to restore natural harmony. Peyote ceremonies may be conducted by special medicine men, known as *Roadmen*, who charge for their services.
- Certain individuals who are able to cause sickness in others may practice witchcraft.

Health Beliefs and Practices

- Health is a reflection of a correct relationship between human beings and the environment. Health is associated with good, blessing, and beauty, all of which are valued in life.

- All ailments, both physical and mental, are believed to have supernatural aspects. The Navajo frequently use both their traditional health care system, including traditional health care practitioners, and the modern health care system.
- There are two major types of traditional health care practitioners. The first is the diviner or diagnostician. Different methods, such as stargazing or hand trembling, are used to identify the cause of an illness. Then, once the cause of the illness has been determined, the individual seeks the second kind of practitioner, the singer, who provides the treatment that counters the cause of the disease and restores harmony.
- Different types of ceremonials as well as herbal medicines and traditional remedies may be used. Infants are placed in cradleboards, which have both traditional and religious significance.
- Cornmeal may be used in healing ceremonies.
- Women herbalists may prescribe herbs for specific and general reasons.

Health Concerns

- Unintentional injuries and violence reflect the combined effects of living conditions, environment, and behavior. All told, Native Americans have much higher death rates from alcoholism, tuberculosis, diabetes, accidents, suicide, pneumonia, influenza, and homicide (Strickland, Walsh & Cooper, 2006).
- Suicide is the third leading cause of death among Native American adolescents, age 15–24 years (Centers for Disease Control and Prevention [CDC], 2004). Suicide rates among Native American youth in the United States are two to three times the national average (Kirmayer, 1994).
- Fetal alcohol syndrome and domestic violence, both related to alcohol abuse, are common problems.
- The rate of fetal alcohol syndrome is six times that of other Americans. Alcohol-related mortality is four times that of the nation as a whole, and traumatic injury related to alcohol and substance abuse is a leading cause of death (U.S. Department of Health and Human Services, 1993).
- Heart disease and malignant neoplasms are leading causes of death for Native Americans (Spector, 2003).
- Obesity, hypertension, and diabetes are also health concerns in Native American groups.
- Mortality in adults from infectious diseases is twice that of the general population, and tuberculosis remains a pressing health problem (U.S. Department of Health and Human Services, 2000). In fact, tuberculosis was 475% greater in Native Americans than in the U.S. population (CDC, 2000).
- Reservations remain poor and often are geographically isolated. Geographic access to health care is a concern.

Adapted from Spector, 2003; Huff & Kline, 1999.

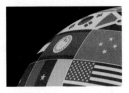

INDEX

Key to page references: *b* refers to material located in a box; *c* refers to a case study; *e* refers to evidence-based practice; *f* refers to a figure; *r* refers to a research application; *t* refers to a table